Translational and Clinical Research in Autism Spectrum Disorders

Translational and Clinical Research in Autism Spectrum Disorders

Editor: Paul Spencer

AMERICAN
MEDICAL PUBLISHERS
www.americanmedicalpublishers.com

AMERICAN
MEDICAL PUBLISHERS
www.americanmedicalpublishers.com

Cataloging-in-Publication Data

Translational and clinical research in autism spectrum disorders / edited by Paul Spencer.
p. cm.
Includes bibliographical references and index.
ISBN 978-1-63927-902-9
1. Autism spectrum disorders. 2. Autism spectrum disorders--Research. 3. Developmental disabilities.
4. Autism spectrum disorders--Diagnosis. 5. Autism spectrum disorders--Treatment. I. Spencer, Paul.
RC553.A88 T73 2023
616.858 82--dc23

American Medical Publishers,
41 Flatbush Avenue,
1st Floor, New York,
NY 11217, USA

ISBN 978-1-63927-902-9 (Hardback)

Contents

Preface

The main aim of this book is to educate learners and enhance their research focus by presenting diverse topics covering this vast field. This is an advanced book which compiles significant studies by distinguished experts in the area of analysis. This book addresses successive solutions to the challenges arising in the area of application, along with it; the book provides scope for future developments.

Autism spectrum disorder (ASD) is a neurodevelopmental disorder that affects how a person perceives and interacts with others, leading to problems in social interaction and communication. Limited and repetitive patterns of conduct are also part of the disorder. While autism is a lifelong disease, the extent to which these challenges limit a person's capacity to function varies from person to person. The term 'spectrum disorders' signifies the wide variety of symptoms and severity associated with autism. Genetic factors are primarily the reason for the disorder's occurrence. ASD appears early in childhood and is related to social, scholastic, and occupational challenges. Autism signs appear as early as the first year of life. Some of the complications linked with the disease include difficulties in school and successful learning, work issues, inability to live independently, social isolation, and family stress. This book is a collection of translational and clinical researches on autism. The readers would gain knowledge that would broaden their perspective about autism spectrum disorders.

It was a great honour to edit this book, though there were challenges, as it involved a lot of communication and networking between me and the editorial team. However, the end result was this all-inclusive book covering diverse themes in the field.

Finally, it is important to acknowledge the efforts of the contributors for their excellent chapters, through which a wide variety of issues have been addressed. I would also like to thank my colleagues for their valuable feedback during the making of this book.

Editor

1

Emerging role of the KCNT1 Slack channel in intellectual disability

Grace E. Kim and Leonard K. Kaczmarek*

Departments of Pharmacology and Cellular & Molecular Physiology, Yale University School of Medicine, New Haven, CT, USA

Correspondence:
Leonard K. Kaczmarek, Departments of Pharmacology and Cellular & Molecular Physiology, Yale University School of Medicine, New Haven, CT 06520, USA
e-mail: leonard.kaczmarek@yale.edu

The sodium-activated potassium K_{Na} channels Slack and Slick are encoded by *KCNT1* and *KCNT2*, respectively. These channels are found in neurons throughout the brain, and are responsible for a delayed outward current termed I_{KNa}. These currents integrate into shaping neuronal excitability, as well as adaptation in response to maintained stimulation. Abnormal Slack channel activity may play a role in Fragile X syndrome, the most common cause for intellectual disability and inherited autism. Slack channels interact directly with the fragile X mental retardation protein (FMRP) and I_{KNa} is reduced in animal models of Fragile X syndrome that lack FMRP. Human Slack mutations that alter channel activity can also lead to intellectual disability, as has been found for several childhood epileptic disorders. Ongoing research is elucidating the relationship between mutant Slack channel activity, development of early onset epilepsies and intellectual impairment. This review describes the emerging role of Slack channels in intellectual disability, coupled with an overview of the physiological role of neuronal I_{KNa} currents.

Keywords: Slack, KCNT1, intellectual disability, Fragile X syndrome, epilepsy

INTRODUCTION

An influx of sodium ions through sodium channels or neurotransmitter receptors triggers a sodium-sensitive potassium current (I_{KNa}), which is found in a diverse range of neuronal cell types. In many cases, I_{KNa} is mediated by the phylogenetically related K_{Na} channel subunits Slack and Slick (Bhattacharjee and Kaczmarek, 2005). Where Slack or Slick is expressed, I_{KNa} contributes to a late afterhyperpolarization that follows repetitive firing. I_{KNa} also regulates neuronal excitability and the rate of adaptation in response to repeated stimulation at high frequencies. Alterations in I_{KNa} have pathophysiological consequences, as suggested by reports of human mutations found in the Slack-encoding gene *KCNT1* (Barcia et al., 2012; Heron et al., 2012; Martin et al., 2014). Slack channels are hence associated with several early onset epileptic encephalopathies. Epilepsies associated with each one of the Slack mutations are in turn associated with a severe delay in cognitive development. Importantly, these new findings strengthened an earlier connection between Slack channels and Fragile X syndrome (FXS); Slack channels interact with FMRP (Fragile X Mental Retardation protein; Brown et al., 2010), which is absent in FXS patients. FXS as a condition is also associated with an increased incidence of childhood seizures, and is the most commonly inherited form of intellectual disability and autism. These observations suggest that Slack channels are developmentally important modulators of cell plasticity underlying normal cognitive development.

This review summarizes studies that have focused on the physiological and pathophysiological role of I_{KNa}, with a particular focus on Slack channels, and also discusses implications for future research. The review is divided into the following parts. First, we describe the properties of Slack channels and physiological functions of the I_{KNa} current, drawing from both historical and more recent studies. Next, we compare and contrast some of the features of FXS and three epileptic encephalopathies (malignant migrating partial seizures of infancy, MMPSI; autosomal dominant nocturnal frontal lobe epilepsy, ADNFLE; and Ohtahara syndrome, OS; Barcia et al., 2012; Heron et al., 2012; Martin et al., 2014) that can result from mutations in Slack channels. In the last section, we cover the mechanisms by which Slack channel activity is altered in these conditions. In particular, we focus on the extent to which the development of intellectual disability can be attributed to the occurrence of the seizures themselves vs. alterations in cellular signaling pathways likely to be disrupted by Slack mutations.

PROPERTIES OF KCNT1 SLACK CHANNELS

The *KCNT1* gene encodes the sodium-activated potassium channel called Slack (named for Sequence like a calcium-activated K^+ channel). Slack channels resemble the well-known voltage-gated Kv channels in their topography and assembly. Like the Kv channels, Slack subunits have six hydrophobic, transmembrane segments (S1–S6) along with a pore-lining loop that is found between S5 and S6 (**Figure 1**). These subunits assemble as tetramers to form a functional channel that is voltage-dependent (Joiner et al., 1998). However, unlike the Kv family of channels, which use a set of positively charged residues along the S4 segment to sense changes in transmembrane voltage (Aggarwal and MacKinnon, 1996; Seoh et al., 1996), Slack channels have no charged residues in S4, and the corresponding mechanism for voltage-sensing in Slack channels is not yet understood. Another distinguishing feature of Slack channels is their very large cytoplasmic C-terminal domain, which is over 900 amino acids in length (Joiner et al., 1998), making Slack channels the

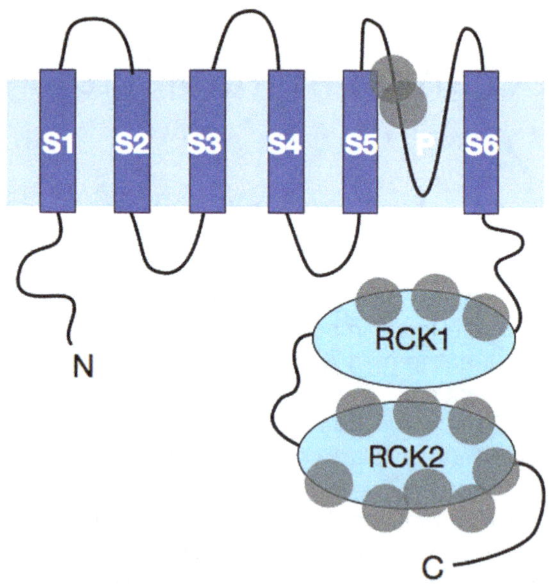

FIGURE 1 | A schematic diagram of Slack subunit topography. Slack subunits have six transmembrane domains. These hydrophobic transmembrane segments are labeled as S1–S6, with the pore region between S5 and S6 indicated with the letter P. Four of these subunits assemble into a functional channel. Both the N- and C-terminal ends are cytosolic in Slack, with C-terminus being one of the longest found among all potassium channels. The C-terminus contains two RCK (regulators of K^+ conductance) domains that stack on top of each other and form a gating ring underneath the channel opening pore. Gray circles represent the general locations where human mutations have been found. A total of thirteen distinct mutations have been found to date, and these mutations are discussed further in the text.

largest know potassium channel subunits. In comparison, the C-terminal domain of one of the longest Kv family *eag* channels is only ~650 amino acids in length (Warmke and Ganetzky, 1994).

The unitary conductance of the Slack channels expressed in heterologous systems ranges from 88 to 180 pS in symmetrical potassium solutions (Yuan et al., 2003; Chen et al., 2009; Zhang et al., 2012), while single channel conductances measured for Na^+-activated K^+ channels in native neurons range from 122 to 198 pS (Yang et al., 2007; Tamsett et al., 2009). At least three observations can explain the wide range and difference in the two expression systems. One confounding factor in measuring channel conductance is that both native I_{KNa} channels and Slack channels in expression systems are known to have multiple subconductance states, which in patch clamp experiments appear as brief, flickering short steps alternating with time spent in the fully open or the closed state (Yuan et al., 2003; Brown et al., 2008). We will revisit this particular property of Slack channels in our discussion of the pathophysiological consequences of aberrant changes in Slack channel activity. Secondly, diversity in the properties of native I_{KNa} can stem from the existence of multiple splice isoforms of Slack channels (Brown et al., 2008), and the fact that some Slack isoforms can form heteromers with related channel subunits such as Slick subunits (Joiner et al., 1998; Yang et al., 2007; Chen et al., 2009). Encoded by *KCNT2*, Slick subunits are distinct in their channel kinetic behavior and unitary conductances (Bhattacharjee et al., 2003). Heteromeric Slack/Slick channels also have properties that are yet different from those of either subunits expressed alone, and their response to modulation by protein kinases also differs from that of the homomeric channels (Chen et al., 2009). Evidence that Slack and Slick channels are co-expressed has been provided in auditory brainstem neurons, olfactory bulb and a number of other neurons (Bhattacharjee et al., 2005; Chen et al., 2009). Finally, in addition to the Slack and Slick channels, which are phylogenetically related (Salkoff et al., 2006), the evolutionarily more distant $K_{ir}3$ inward rectifier potassium channels are also sensitive to cytoplasmic sodium ions, further increasing the diversity of native I_{KNa} channels. (Petit-Jacques et al., 1999).

SLACK ENTERS INTO PROTEIN–PROTEIN INTERACTIONS WITH OTHER MEMBRANE PROTEINS AND CYTOPLASMIC SIGNALING PROTEINS

The Slack channel subunit interacts directly with the mRNA-binding protein FMRP, which regulates the probability of Slack channel opening (Brown et al., 2010; Zhang et al., 2012). Evidence for direct Slack channel-FMRP binding was first found in a yeast-two-hybrid assay, and confirmed by co-immunoprecipitation from synaptosomal lysates isolated from mouse brainstem and olfactory bulbs (Brown et al., 2010). This interaction appeared to be evolutionarily conserved, as the same finding was demonstrated in large bag cell neurons of the marine mollusk *Aplysia californica* (Zhang et al., 2012). Moreover, messenger RNA targets of FMRP can be co-immunoprecipitated with Slack from wild type mice but not from the $fmr^{-/y}$ mice lacking FMRP (Brown et al., 2010). Addition of an N-terminal fragment of FMRP (FMRP 1–298) that retains the majority of the known FMRP protein–protein interaction domains, but lacks the major mRNA binding sites to Slack channels in excised inside-out patches substantially increased channel mean open time (Brown et al., 2010). In part, this increase in Slack channel activity occurs by eliminating subconductance states and favoring openings to the fully open state.

Slack channel subunits also interact directly with TMEM16C (ANO3), a transmembrane protein found in non-peptidergic nociceptive neurons (Huang et al., 2013). Though closely related to the Ca^{2+}-activated Cl^- channels TMEM16A and B, TMEM16C itself alone does not appear to function as an ion channel. Slack and TMEM16C can exist together in a protein complex and are colocalized in nociceptive neurons. Similar to FMRP, the presence of TMEM16C substantially increases the activity of Slack channels. Further discussion of the biological role of this interaction in nociceptive neurons is provided later in this review, but for now we turn to discuss neuronal cell types that express K_{Na} channels.

LOCALIZATION OF SLACK AND SLICK SUBUNITS

Cloning of the K_{Na} Slack and Slick genes, *KCNT1* and *KCNT2*, and the development of specific antibodies have enabled a detailed study of their expression in the brain (Bhattacharjee et al., 2003, 2005; Yuan et al., 2003). These studies have confirmed that highest levels of Slack and Slick channels are found in the brain, with detection of lower levels in the heart and the kidney (Joiner et al., 1998; Yuan et al., 2003; Bhattacharjee et al., 2005; Brown et al., 2008).

In situ hybridization and immunohistochemistry were systematically performed in the adult rat brain, and demonstrated that Slack transcripts and protein are abundantly expressed in neurons throughout all regions of the brain, including the brainstem, cerebellum, frontal cortex and the hippocampus (Bhattacharjee et al., 2002; Santi et al., 2006; Brown et al., 2008). Similar results are also reported in the mouse brain, where abundant mRNA expression has been found in the brainstem and the olfactory bulb (Brown et al., 2008).

PHYSIOLOGICAL FUNCTIONS OF THE SLACK CHANNEL

I_{KNa} IS A MAJOR COMPONENT OF THE DELAYED OUTWARD CURRENT IN NEURONS

The term I_{KNa} was first coined by Bader et al. (1985), who described in avian neurons an outward K^+ current with dependence on $[Na^+]_i$ (**Table 1**). An independent study concurrently described similar currents in neurons isolated from the Crayfish (Hartung, 1985). In both studies, researchers observed changes in the outward K^+ current in the presence and absence of the Na^+ channel inhibitor tetrodotoxin (TTX), and concluded that a component of the neuronal outward current was sensitive to Na^+ influx. Similar reports soon followed in a number of neuronal cell types, which led to the recognition of a previously unrecognized outward current that was sensitive to Na^+ influx (Haimann et al., 1990; Dryer, 1991; Bischoff et al., 1998). A partial list of such cell types includes medial nucleus of the trapezoid body (MNTB), trigeminal, mitral, vestibular, and dorsal root ganglion (DRG) nociceptive neurons. Importantly, this list demonstrates that Slack channels are involved in the olfactory, auditory, vestibular and pain-sensing systems, all of which are critical to normal development and learning. For a more comprehensive review of Slack channel expression patterns, the reader is advised to Refs. (Bhattacharjee and Kaczmarek, 2005; Kaczmarek, 2013).

SLACK CHANNEL SUBUNITS ARE REQUIRED FOR I_{KNa}

That Slack channel subunits contribute to I_{KNa} currents was demonstrated in later studies, using neonatal neurons isolated from the rat olfactory bulb, as well as in corpus striatum (Budelli et al., 2009; Lu et al., 2010). A component of the outward current similar to the I_{KNa} reported in the earlier studies was suppressed upon knocking-down Slack expression using the siRNA technique (Budelli et al., 2009). These studies contributed the surprising discovery that I_{KNa} represents a very major fraction of the total outward current of these neurons.

Levels of I_{KNa} channels are particularly high in mitral cells of the olfactory bulb (Egan et al., 1992; Bhattacharjee et al., 2002), in which the other major component of K^+ current is carried by the voltage-dependent potassium channel subunit Kv1.3 (Kues and Wunder, 1992). The activity of Kv1.3 channels helps determine the firing patterns of mitral cells in response to odorant stimulation and/or glucose presence (Tucker et al., 2013). A very interesting phenotype results when Kv1.3 channels are deleted by homologous recombination in mice (Fadool et al., 2004). Levels of both I_{KNa} current and of Slack channel protein expression are substantially increased in Kv1.$3^{-/-}$ mice (Lu et al., 2010). This I_{KNa} could be directly attributed to the Slack subunits by again knocking down Slack subunits with the siRNA technique, which suppressed the I_{KNa} currents (Lu et al., 2010). Loss of Kv1.3 channels, together with the upregulation of I_{KNa} currents, altered the kinetics of inactivation of K^+ currents in the mitral cells, resulting in a decrease in action potential height and an increased adaptation of action potential firing in response to maintained stimulation (Fadool

Table 1 | Physiological role of Slack-mediated I_{KNa} in specific neuronal cell types (selected references).

Neuronal type	Animal/Age	I_{KNa} contribution	Reference
Ciliary and trigeminal ganglia	E7–8, chick or quail embryos	Sodium-dependent outward current	Bader et al. (1985)
Layer V neurons of sensorimotor cortex	Cats	sAHP, cellular excitability	Schwindt et al. (1989)
Spinal cord neurons	Lamprey (*Lampetra fluviatilis*)	sAHP, neuronal frequency regulation	Wallen et al. (2007)
MNTB principal neurons	P11, 129SV/EMS mice	Accuracy of timing of APs to high-frequency stimulation	Yang et al. (2007)
Olfactory bulb tufted/mitral cells, corpus striatum medium spiny neuron (MSN)	P2, rat pups	Delayed outward current	Budelli et al. (2009)
Olfactory bulb mitral cells	<1 m, C57BL/6 Kv1.$3^{-/-}$ mice	Compensatory increase in Slack expression in Kv1.$3^{-/-}$ mitral cells, leading to increased delayed outward current	Lu et al. (2010)
Peptidergic nociceptors in dorsal root ganglion (DRG)	E15, Sprague-Dawley rat embryos	APD, firing accommodation to stimulus, cellular excitability	Nuwer et al. (2010)
Non-peptidergic nociceptors in DRG	<1 m, F344 rats	APD, firing threshold, cellular excitability	Huang et al. (2013)
Vestibular afferent neurons (VAN)	<1 m, Sprague-Dawley rats	APD, rate of repolarization, amplitude of AHP, phase locking of APs	Cervantes et al. (2013)

MNTB, medial nucleus of the tripezoid body; DRG, dorsal root ganglion; E, embryonic; P, post-natal; m, month; sAHP, slow afterhyperpolarization; AP, action potential; APD, action potential duration.

et al., 2004). Remarkably, these changes were associated with the development of increased numbers of olfactory glomeruli in the olfactory bulb and a 10,000-fold increase in the sensitivity of the $Kv1.3^{-/-}$ mice to odorant stimuli.

CONTRIBUTION OF I_{KNa} TO NEURONAL FIRING PATTERNS: REGULATION OF ADAPTATION TO MAINTAINED STIMULATION

In many neurons, I_{KNa} currents contribute to a long-lasting slow afterhyperpolarization (sAHP), which results from a slowly developing outward current evoked during sustained stimulation (Vergara et al., 1998). The period of reduced excitability afforded by sAHP is thought to protect the cell from repetitive, tetanic activity, and has been studied in layer V neurons of the sensorimotor cortex of the cat (Schwindt et al., 1988a,b). It has been shown that whereas the early part of the sAHP is dependent on Ca^{2+} influx during stimulation, the late part is Na^{+}-sensitive. Furthermore, this late component of the sAHP is sufficient to reduce cellular excitability in the cat sensorimotor cortex layer V neurons (Schwindt et al., 1989). Performing slice recordings in the absence of Ca^{2+}, Schwindt et al. (1989) showed that neuronal firing rate is attenuated for many tens of seconds following stimulation, matching the duration of Na^{+}-dependent sAHP.

Similar Na^{+}-dependent sAHPs have also been observed in a number of other neurons, including hippocampal pyramidal cells (Gustafsson and Wigstrom, 1983) and spinal cord neurons (Wallen et al., 2007). In motor neurons from the lamprey spinal cord, stimulation of action potentials at increasingly higher rates (from 2 to 8 Hz) progressively prolongs the time it takes for the membrane potential to return to baseline, an effect that can be attributed to the duration of the evoked sAHP. At lower firing rates, the Ca^{2+}-sensitive early phase of the sAHP dominates the rate of recovery to the resting state. However, the contribution of the late I_{KNa}-dependent phase of the sAHP to this effect becomes more significant with increasing firing frequencies. It appears then that the I_{KNa}-mediated sAHP is likely to be a physiological modulator of neuronal excitability during rapid firing (Wallen et al., 2007).

ROLE OF SLACK CHANNELS IN NOCICEPTION

Two studies focusing on the pain-sensing DRG nociceptors have shed further light on the role of I_{KNa} in neuronal excitability (Nuwer et al., 2010; Huang et al., 2013). In one study, siRNA-mediated technology was utilized to knock down Slack channels in the embryonic rat peptidergic nociceptors, demonstrating that these Slack-knockdown neurons were hyperexcitable compared to control neurons (Nuwer et al., 2010). The second study showed that the voltage threshold for action potential generation is significantly reduced in nociceptive neurons isolated from a $TMEM16C^{-/-}$ rat (Gadotti and Zamponi, 2013; Huang et al., 2013). As was described earlier in this review, TMEM16C is a transmembrane protein found in non-peptidergic nociceptive neurons that binds Slack channel subunits and increases their channel activity. Consistent with this, the neurons from $TMEM16C^{-/-}$ rats had reduced I_{KNa} currents. The $TMEM16C^{-/-}$ rats also had increased thermal and mechanical sensitivity, as revealed in behavioral studies. That this increased sensitivity could be directly attributed to the change in Slack I_{KNa} current was confirmed by an *in vivo* Slack knockdown experiment in animals, which induced the same pattern of heightened sensitivities (Huang et al., 2013).

ROLE OF SLACK CHANNELS IN TEMPORAL ACCURACY OF ACTION POTENTIAL FIRING

Slack/Slick channels are also expressed in high abundance in neurons of the MNTB within the auditory brainstem (Bhattacharjee et al., 2002; Yang et al., 2007). These neurons are capable of firing at rates up to ~800 Hz with high temporal accuracy, a feature that is required for accurate determination of the location of sounds in space. Current clamp and voltage clamp experiments have demonstrated that activation of I_{KNa} currents increases temporal accuracy in these neurons at high rates of stimulation, in large part by increasing the membrane conductance close to the threshold for action potential generation (Yang et al., 2007). This reduces the time constant of the membrane and allows the timing of action potentials to be closely matched to the pattern of incoming stimuli. Pharmacological activation of Slack channels in these neurons has been shown to further increase timing accuracy in these cells, a finding that is consistent with numerical simulations of the firing patterns of these cells with and without I_{KNa} currents (Yang et al., 2007).

I_{KNa} currents also shape the neuronal firing in the vestibular system, which consists of four vestibular nuclei that receive input from the vestibular afferent neurons (Fitzpatrick and Day, 2004). The afferent neurons transmit information about head movements to help the organism stabilize gaze and maintain proper balance. Vestibular afferent neurons have characteristic resting discharge rates that adapt upon detecting angular and linear accelerations, thereby relaying vestibular information (Grillner et al., 1995). Cervantes et al. (2013) characterized I_{KNa} currents in rat vestibular ganglion neurons, and found that I_{KNa} currents regulate the phase-locking of action potential firing to a stimulus, as well as the firing regularity and discharge patterns of these neurons.

The summarized studies have demonstrated that I_{KNa} currents are a major physiological component of the outward current in neurons, where these currents help regulate intrinsic electrical excitability, as well as the manner in which neurons respond to patterns of incoming stimulation. These studies have led Budelli et al. (2009) to conclude "*in clinical and pharmacological studies, this previously unseen current system that is active during normal physiology represents a new and promising pharmacological target for drugs dealing with seizure and psychotropic disorders,*" an early prediction that would be realized by the finding of human mutations in Slack channels.

SLACK CHANNELS IN COGNITIVE DISORDERS

Given that Slack channels appear as modulators of neuronal excitability and of neuronal adaptation to stimulation in a wide range of species, it is not surprising that alterations in Slack channel activity may have significant pathophysiological consequences. Furthermore, what is known about these pathologies strongly suggests that Slack channel activity is a critical component that ensures normal cognitive development. The finding that Slack channel activity is increased by direct complex formation with FMRP, the RNA-binding protein that is deleted in FXS, implicates Slack channel function in this syndrome (Brown et al., 2010). More specifically, there may be a clinically significant relationship between Slack channel activity and development of intellectual disability in FXS. Increasing evidence supports this hypothesis: epilepsy patients who have profound intellectual disability carry mutations in the Slack-encoding *KCNT1*. More than a dozen different *KCNT1* mutations have now been reported in the literature, in connection with three different types of seizures that occur in infancy or childhood, MMPSI, ADNFLE, and OS (Barcia et al., 2012; Heron et al., 2012; Martin et al., 2014). These findings strongly indicate a pathophysiological role for Slack channels in the abnormal development of intellectual function.

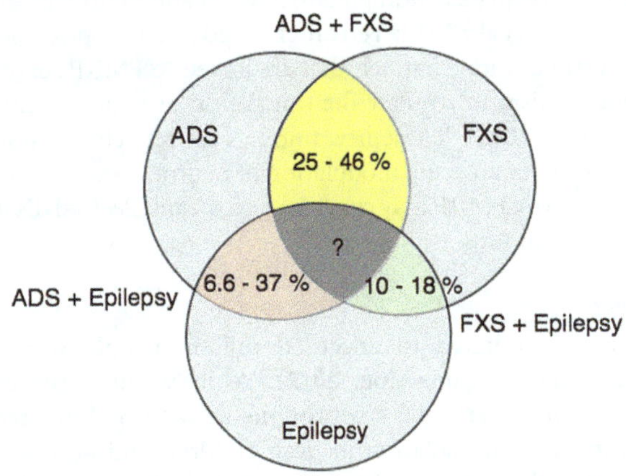

FIGURE 2 | Co-diagnosis rates among FXS, ASD and epilepsy patients. This diagram shows the prevalence of co-diagnosis in fragile x syndrome (FXS), autism spectrum disorder (ASD) and epilepsy patients, as reported in Refs. (Musumeci et al., 1999; Muhle et al., 2004; Abrahams and Geschwind, 2008; Amiet et al., 2008; Bailey et al., 2008; Hernandez et al., 2009; Yasuhara, 2010; Jokiranta et al., 2014).

INTELLECTUAL DISABILITIES

Seizures can have variations in onset and frequency, and may occur during childhood with little or no intellectual impairment [Engel and International League Against Epilepsy (ILAE), 2001]. A case in point is ADNFLE, epilepsy that can be caused by mutations either in the α-4, α-2 or β-2 subunits of the neuronal nicotinic acetylcholine receptor, encoded by the *CHRNA4, CHRNA2,* or *CHRNB2* genes respectively, or by mutations in the Slack channel. Severe intellectual disability, however, only occurs in those patients who carry Slack mutations (Heron et al., 2012). This implies that the seizure episodes themselves are unlikely to be the prime determinant of intellectual function. Intellectual disability is a salient feature in all patients diagnosed with FXS, and in some patients with epilepsy and/or autism spectrum disorder (ASD). Below, we explore the overlap in clinical manifestation among these three types of patient groups.

Fragile X syndrome, childhood epilepsies and ASD are notable for their heterogeneity of clinical manifestations in the behavioral and cognitive domains. Different combinations of these three disorders have also occurred together in patients. Numerous studies have reported a range of percentages for the prevalence of such overlapping patient groups, and are shown in **Figure 2**. The co-diagnosis rate of an ASD disorder in male Fragile X patients ranges from 25 to 46% (Muhle et al., 2004; Abrahams and Geschwind, 2008; Bailey et al., 2008; Hernandez et al., 2009). The corresponding rate for epilepsy in male Fragile X patients is lower, ranging from 10 to 18% (Musumeci et al., 1999; Muhle et al., 2004; Bailey et al., 2008), whereas the occurrence of epilepsy in ASD patients varies more widely from 6.6 to 37% (Amiet et al., 2008; Yasuhara, 2010; Jokiranta et al., 2014). Such a wide variation likely reflects methodological differences, as well as heterogeneity in sample population and etiology of the diseases. Even so, these studies are helpful in demonstrating the overlap among FXS, childhood epilepsy and ASD at the clinical diagnostic level. More pertinent to our discussion in this review, these findings raise the possibility that there could be a molecular link that controls intellectual disability development in each of the three clinical diseases.

FRAGILE X SYNDROME

Fragile X syndrome is caused by functional absence of the FMRP, which usually arises due to hypermethylation and subsequent silencing of its gene *fmr1*, found on the X chromosome (Pieretti et al., 1991). FMRP is highly expressed throughout the brain in neurons, where it is found in both pre- and post-synaptic processes (Christie et al., 2009). One well-characterized function of this RNA-binding protein is to suppress the translation of these target mRNAs. Through mechanisms that are not fully understood, neuronal activity can release the suppression of some mRNAs (Khandjian et al., 2004; Stefani et al., 2004), leading to an activity-dependent increase in protein synthesis in synaptosomal regions (Bassell and Warren, 2008). FMRP binds to polyribosomes and specific mRNAs in neuronal dendrites, leading to the concept that it regulates local translation at these sites. FMRP is required for a number of forms of synaptic plasticity including mGluR1-mediated long-term depression (LTD; Li et al., 2002).

As described earlier, FMRP can also form complexes with Slack channel protein (Brown et al., 2010; Zhang et al., 2012), and in this manner directly regulate Slack channel activity. I_{KNa} currents were compared in MNTB neurons recorded in brain slices from the FMRP-deficient $Fmr1^{-/y}$ mice vs. those from wild-type mice. As expected, outward I_{KNa} currents were smaller in $Fmr1^{-/y}$ MNTB neurons, even though Slack subunit levels are not decreased (Brown et al., 2010). Conversely, increases in levels of FMRP can enhance I_{KNa} currents. This was demonstrated by the finding that introduction of the FMRP N-terminal 1–298 fragment into bag cell neurons of *Aplysia* increases I_{KNa} currents and hyperpolarizes the resting membrane potential (Zhang et al., 2012). These findings suggest a more versatile role for FMRP in both the presynaptic and postsynaptic elements of neurons, in addition to its function in the suppression of translation.

Slack is not the only ion channel that can interact with FMRP. Both the large-conductance calcium-activated BK potassium channel and $Ca_V2.2$ voltage-dependent calcium channel have recently been shown to interact directly with FMRP, and these interactions regulate action potential width and neurotransmitter release (Deng et al., 2013; Ferron et al., 2014). It is possible that the activation of ion channels that are linked to FMRP serves as a local mechanism to regulate the translation of neuronal mRNAs (Zhang et al., 2012). These new findings collectively suggest that dysregulation of an acute modulation of neuronal excitability and transmission by FMRP may contribute to the intellectual disability associated with FXS.

EPILEPSY

Epilepsy is estimated to affect 50 million people worldwide (World Health Organization, 2012). While seizures, presenting as abnormal patterns of synchronous activity in EEG recordings, can occur in isolation in both children and adults, these are distinguished from epilepsy, in which such abnormal activity is recurrent, and which may have an enduring clinical impact. The impact can manifest as neurobiological, cognitive, psychological, and/or social changes (Fisher et al., 2005). Although over 30 different kinds of epileptic seizures, or syndromes, are recognized as of 2013, each syndrome has considerable variation in etiology and health outcome [Engel and International League Against Epilepsy (ILAE), 2001; Berg et al., 2010].

Some epilepsies are channelopathies, and human mutations in a number of genes encoding ligand-gated receptors or ion channels have been found in epilepsy patients (Steinlein et al., 1995; Scheffer and Berkovic, 1997; Charlier et al., 1998; Zuberi et al., 1999; Escayg et al., 2000; Brenner et al., 2005). The advancement and wider use of sequencing technologies such as whole exome sequencing, which can identify *de novo* mutations in single probands, are reshaping the genomics approach to understanding epileptogenesis, and rapidly expanding the list of proteins mutated in epilepsy patients. In this next section, we consider in particular the three types of seizures associated with mutations in the Slack-encoding *KCNT1* gene, accompanied by a summary table of selected clinical reports from the literature.

Table 2 | Summary of clinical reports on MMPSI patients.

No. of patients reviewed	96
No. of Refs. Reviewed	16
Males	42.5%
Age at onset	
Average	7.6 week
Range	1 day – 7 month
Prognosis	
Developmental delay	71%
Normal development	1%
Hypotonia	56%
Deceased	21%
Causes – brain abnormalities	
Normal	16
Atrophy	24
Delayed myelination	12
Encephalopathy	57
Thin corpus callosum	3
Other lesions	4
Other findings	7
Not considered	5
Causes – genetic alterations (out of those sequenced)	
SCN1A	2/32
KCNT1	10/30
TBC1D24	2/15
Not considered	47

MALIGNANT MIGRATING PARTIAL SEIZURES IN INFANCY

Malignant migrating partial seizures in infancy was first described by Coppola et al. (1995), as a new distinct early onset (<6 months) seizure type with a characteristic random pattern of electrical discharges recorded on the brain electrical encephalogram (EEG). Since then, numerous other groups have also identified patients who fit these original criteria, selected references of which are reviewed and summarized in **Table 2** (Coppola et al., 1995, 2006, 2007; Okuda et al., 2000; Veneselli et al., 2001; Gross-Tsur et al., 2004; Marsh et al., 2005; Hmaimess et al., 2006; Caraballo et al., 2008; Carranza Rojo et al., 2011; Sharma et al., 2011; Barcia et al., 2012; Lee et al., 2012; Ishii et al., 2013; McTague et al., 2013; Milh et al., 2013). Ongoing analyses of these patients using EEGs, brain imaging and DNA sequence analysis continue to shape the field's understanding of this focal seizure in infancy.

Patients diagnosed with MMPSI are unlikely to achieve intellectual growth, learning, and other developmental milestones. Following an early onset, MMPSI seizures increase in frequency to the point of halting normal development; patients also lose any developmental progress they had previously accomplished (Coppola et al., 1995). Even when the seizures diminish in frequency, very few patients resume neurodevelopmental growth. The end results are severe delays in development and profound intellectual disability. Not surprisingly, absence of language and hypotonia are also commonly noted in these patients. In capturing the bleak prognosis for MMPSI patients, a study of 14 patients concluded, "the highest developmental level maintained beyond 1 year of age in all patients was partial head control, rolling and visual fixation" (McTague et al., 2013). Out of the 96 patients considered in **Table 2**, 20 were reported as deceased.

Possible cause(s) for seizure development in MMPSI patients has remained elusive until recently. Neurometabolic, blood gas and serum tests are typically normal, and brain lesions are rarely observed in affected patients (Nabbout and Dulac, 2008). Besides microcephaly, or abnormally small heads, that progressively appeared in 57 out of 91 examined patients reported in the literature (**Table 2**), the brain appears to be without any other structural lesions at presentation.

Genetic etiologies for MMPSI were first made in 2011, with the discovery of *SCN1A* (Nav1.1) mutations (Carranza Rojo et al.,

Table 3 | Summary of clinical reports on ADNFLE patients.

No. of patients reviewed	114
No. of Refs. reviewed	6
Males	48%
Age at onset	
Average	10.9 year
Range	1–30 year
Deceased	N/A

2011), followed by *TBC1D24* (protein name the same; Milh et al., 2013) and *KCNT1* (Slack) mutations (Barcia et al., 2012; Epi et al., 2013; Ishii et al., 2013; McTague et al., 2013; Vanderver et al., 2014). Of special note, Slack channel mutations have been found in 50% of patients examined (Barcia et al., 2012). Detailed characterizations of these Slack mutations are presented at the end of this section.

AUTOSOMAL DOMINANT NOCTURNAL FRONTAL LOBE EPILEPSY

Autosomal dominant nocturnal frontal lobe epilepsy is a focal seizure that occurs predominantly during sleep with a typical onset in late childhood. The mean age among more than 110 patients reported in six different case reports was 10.9 years (**Table 3**; Scheffer et al., 1995; Oldani et al., 1998; Phillips et al., 1998; Nakken et al., 1999; Derry et al., 2008; Heron et al., 2012). ADNFLE patients are sometimes misdiagnosed as having sleep disorders rather than suffering a seizure attack, because the seizure attacks often disrupt sound sleep (Oldani et al., 1998).

That a genetic mutation can result in ADNFLE in an affected family was first suggested by chromosome linkage and confirmed later by sequencing of the gene for the nicotinic α4 acetylcholine receptor subunit (*CHRNA4*; Steinlein et al., 1995). For this reason, ADNFLE is most commonly associated with mutations in acetylcholine receptor subunits (Steinlein et al., 1995; De Fusco et al., 2000; Aridon et al., 2006). Statistically, however, only 20% of ADNFLE patients with a family history of seizures, and 5% of those without, have a mutation in one of these genes (Kurahashi and Hirose, 2002).

More recently, mutations in *KCNT1* (Slack) have been identified as a novel genetic etiology for ADNFLE, but these too seem to be a cause in a minority of affected families (Heron et al., 2012). Nevertheless, it is interesting that several observations distinguish the families harboring a *KCNT1* mutation from those with a different mutation. As a notable example, the occurrence of intellectual disability and other psychiatric illnesses appear to be greatly increased in those families with a *KCNT1* mutation (Heron et al., 2012). This is in contrast to ADNFLE patients without mutations in Slack, in whom intelligence and other neurologic functions are largely unimpaired (Phillips et al., 1998). Penetrance of the mutation is also increased to 100% in the families with Slack mutations, when that of acetylcholine receptor mutations has been estimated to be only 70% (Heron et al., 2012). These results further implicate Slack channels in intellectual development.

OHTAHARA SYNDROME

Originally described as an early infantile epileptic encephalopathy with suppression-bursts (Ohtahara et al., 1976), OS is one of the earliest seizures in its presentation (Clarke et al., 1987). Among 82 patients reported in 27 different publications (Robain and Dulac, 1992; Miller et al., 1998; Ohno et al., 2000; Ohtsuka et al., 2000; Krasemann et al., 2001; Quan et al., 2001; Trinka et al., 2001; Krsek et al., 2002; Yamatogi and Ohtahara, 2002; Hmaimess et al., 2005; Kato et al., 2007, 2010, 2013; Saitsu et al., 2008, 2010, 2012a,b; Absoud et al., 2010; Cazorla et al., 2010; Fullston et al., 2010; Giordano et al., 2010; Seo et al., 2010; Choi et al., 2011; Eksioglu et al., 2011; Milh et al., 2011; Nakamura et al., 2013; Touma et al., 2013), the first seizure was seen within 3 weeks of life (**Table 4**). Common prognosis and known etiologies of OS are summarized below.

A majority of OS patients show severe developmental delay, including intellectual disability. Greater than 80% of OS patients reported in the literature have a developmental delay, while only 10% are described as showing normal development (**Table 4**). OS patients also appear to have increased vulnerability to other ailments such as pneumonia and virus infections (Krasemann

Table 4 | Summary of clinical reports on OS patients.

No. of patients reviewed	82
No. of Refs. reviewed	27
Males	60%
Age at onset	
Average	2.56 week
Range	1 day – 4 month
Prognosis	
Evolution to WS	43%
Developmental delay	83%
Normal development	10%
Hypotonia	52%
Deceased	22%
Causes – brain abnormalities (out of those considered)	
Normal	17/67
Atrophy	28/67
Delayed myelination	13/67
Encephalopathy	8/67
Thin corpus callosum	9/67
Other lesions	9/67
Other findings	13/67
Not considered	15
Causes – genetic alterations (out of those sequenced)	
SCN2A	12/25
KCNT1	3/25
KCNQ2	13/25
STXBP1	20/45
Other genes	8/45
Not considered	37

et al., 2001; Quan et al., 2001), and these complications have been a cause of death in more than 20% of patients. It remains a challenge to reverse or overcome these prognoses, since these seizures have pronounced pharmacological resistance (Beal et al., 2012). Nevertheless, surgical intervention may hold some promise for patients in whom brain abnormalities can be identified as the basis of the seizures (Malik et al., 2013). Macroscopic and microscopic brain abnormalities are the predominant causes of seizure development in OS patients, and common defects are enumerated in **Table 4** (Robain and Dulac, 1992; Trinka et al., 2001; Low et al., 2007; Saitsu et al., 2008; Nakamura et al., 2013). In more than one-fifth of the patients, however, no brain abnormalities can be detected.

Genetic etiologies have also been identified in a subset of OS patients. To date, alterations in five different genes have been found in patients: ion channels *KCNQ2* (Kv7.2; Saitsu et al., 2012a; Kato et al., 2013), *SCN2A* (Nav1.2; Nakamura et al., 2013; Touma et al., 2013), and *KCNT1* (Slack; Martin et al., 2014); the transcription factor ARX (Kato et al., 2007; Absoud et al., 2010; Giordano et al., 2010; Fullston et al., 2010; Eksioglu et al., 2011); and the synaptic binding protein *STXBP1* (Saitsu et al., 2008, 2010, 2011; Mignot et al., 2011; Milh et al., 2011). Interestingly, mutations in *SCN2A* and *KCNT1* have also been found in patients diagnosed with MMPSI.

Many earlier studies (prior to 2011) were selective in their approach, sequencing only one or a few selected genes of interest. A growing number of researchers are now utilizing whole exomic or genomic sequencing for such patients (Majewski et al., 2011), however, and it is foreseeable that a more comprehensive estimate of the prevalence of these epileptogenic alleles will emerge within the next decade.

MECHANISMS UNDERLYING CHANGES IN HUMAN SLACK MUTANTS

Slack mutants have been tested for change in channel activity in *Xenopus laevis* oocytes and HEK 293 cells using two-electrode voltage clamping. These studies have shown that, surprisingly, currents generated by the Slack mutants are greatly increased over those in wild type channels. Peak current amplitudes of mutant Slack currents are increased by 3- to 12-fold, with no change in levels of Slack protein (Barcia et al., 2012; Martin et al., 2014; Milligan et al., 2014).

One alteration in the biophysical properties of the mutant Slack channels is that the occurrence of subconductance states is greatly reduced compared to that in wild type channels. As we described earlier, subconductances appear as brief, flickering short steps alternating with time spent in the fully open or the closed state in single channel patch clamp experiments. The wild type channel spends most of its time transitioning between the closed or subconductance states (Joiner et al., 1998). However, mutant channels are more likely to open immediately to a fully open state rather than to a subconductance state, resulting in an overall increase in current during depolarization of the membrane (Barcia et al., 2012). A similar reduction in occurrence of subconductance states was also seen in FMRP-mediated positive regulation of Slack channel activity (Brown et al., 2010).

A second mechanism for increased current in at least two of the mutant channels is that they render the channels in a state that mimics constitutive channel phosphorylation by protein kinase C (Barcia et al., 2012). Wild type Slack channels undergo phosphorylation by this enzyme at a site (Serine 407) in their large C-terminal cytoplasmic domain, leading to an ~3-fold increase in peak current amplitude. Protein kinase C was pharmacologically activated in *Xenopus* oocytes expressing Slack channels, and the peak current amplitude compared in the mutants and wild type channels using two-electrode voltage clamping. The results showed that unlike in the wild type channel, which showed an increase in channel activity, it remained unchanged in mutant channels (Barcia et al., 2012). Thus in these channels the mutations both mimicked and occluded the effects of activation by protein kinase C.

Other mechanisms for the enhanced currents in the Slack mutants are under investigation. These channels are sensitive to cytoplasmic levels of Na^+. In patch clamp experiments it has been found, however, that the Na^+-sensitivity of the mutant channels is not different from that of the wild type channels. Nevertheless, other potential mechanisms, such as shifts in voltage-dependence, may also contribute to the enhanced currents in mutant channels.

The unexpected finding that a gain-of-function change in a K^+ channel can induce a hyperexcitable state of the brain has a precedence in the BK channel, a mutation of which can lead to generalized epilepsy and paroxysmal dyskinesia (GEPD; Yang et al., 2010). BK channels are activated by $[Ca^{2+}]_i$, and can contribute to the rapid hyperpolarizations that follow action potentials, thereby regulating cellular excitability. An electrophysiological study of the mutant BK channel in *Xenopus* oocytes showed that the mutant channel has increased Ca^{2+} sensitivity, resulting in an overall increase in BK channel activity (Yang et al., 2010).

Several possible changes at the cellular/neuronal network level could account for how aberrant electrical activities of the brain may arise from increased K^+ channel activity, some of which have been suggested by others (Du et al., 2005). First, an increase in K^+ current could cause more rapid neuronal repolarization, shortening the duration of action potentials. A more rapid repolarization can indirectly increase cell excitability by increasing the rate at which voltage-dependent Na^+ channels recover from inactivation. Next, more pronounced hyperpolarizations resulting from BK or Slack channel hyperactivity may also potentiate hyperpolarization-activated cation channel (I_h) currents, aberrantly triggering network excitability. It is also possible that the enhancement of K^+ current may occur selectively in inhibitory neurons. This could lead to a selective suppression of the activity of inhibitory interneurons, thereby producing an imbalance of excitation to inhibition (Du et al., 2005). Finally, increases in K^+ current early in development could alter the formation of normal patterns of synaptic connections, predisposing the nervous system to develop circuits that generate epileptiform discharges. After close to a decade, however, these hypotheses have yet to be tested experimentally, perhaps due in part because of a lack of a specific knock-in mouse or other animal models.

Malignant migrating partial seizures of infancy, OS, and ADNFLE have traditionally been regarded as distinct seizures with considerable heterogeneity in etiology and prognosis. OS and MMPSI are two of the first epilepsies known to affect newborns, and both produce devastating changes in neurodevelopment. ADNFLE, on the other hand, is typically less disruptive of normal development and life, and seizures are often successfully controlled with antiepileptic drugs. The recent discoveries that Slack mutants have been uncovered in patients diagnosed with one of these three seizures, and that they all share in common severe intellectual disability and other developmental delays together give rise to an emerging role for Slack channels in intellectual disability. The evidence suggests that a key physiological role of Slack may be its control over cellular or network excitability in regions of the brain involved in intellectual development.

CONCLUSION

Slack channels are physiologically important regulators of neuronal excitability and adaptability to changing patterns of sensory stimulation. In this review, we have considered how alterations in Slack channel activity can have pathophysiological ramifications, in conditions such as FXS and early onset epileptic encephalopathies. In addition to FXS, which has a well-established genetic link to the development of intellectual disability, the three seizures related to Slack mutants – OS, MMPSI and ADNFLE – also notably share a common manifestation of intellectual disability in their patients. These new findings make a strong argument that Slack channels may be a common link that can describe the occurrence of intellectual disability in these patients, suggesting that Slack channels could be critical modulators of cognitive development.

REFERENCES

Abrahams, B. S., and Geschwind, D. H. (2008). Advances in autism genetics: on the threshold of a new neurobiology. *Nat. Rev. Genet.* 9, 341–355. doi: 10.1038/nrg2346

Absoud, M., Parr, J. R., Halliday, D., Pretorius, P., Zaiwalla, Z., and Jayawant, S. (2010). A novel ARX phenotype: rapid neurodegeneration with Ohtahara syndrome and a dyskinetic movement disorder. *Dev. Med. Child Neurol.* 52, 305–307. doi: 10.1111/j.1469-8749.2009.03470.x

Aggarwal, S. K., and MacKinnon, R. (1996). Contribution of the S4 segment to gating charge in the Shaker K+ channel. *Neuron* 16, 1169–1177. doi: 10.1016/S0896-6273(00)80143-9

Amiet, C., Gourfinkel-An, I., Bouzamondo, A., Tordjman, S., Baulac, M., Lechat, P., et al. (2008). Epilepsy in autism is associated with intellectual disability and gender: evidence from a meta-analysis. *Biol. Psychiatry* 64, 577–582. doi: 10.1016/j.biopsych.2008.04.030

Aridon, P., Marini, C., Di Resta, C., Brilli, E., De Fusco, M., Politi, F., et al. (2006). Increased sensitivity of the neuronal nicotinic receptor alpha 2 subunit causes familial epilepsy with nocturnal wandering and ictal fear. *Am. J. Hum. Genet.* 79, 342–350. doi: 10.1086/506459

Bader, C. R., Bernheim, L., and Bertrand, D. (1985). Sodium-activated potassium current in cultured avian neurones. *Nature* 317, 540–542. doi: 10.1038/317540a0

Bailey, D. B. Jr., Raspa, M., Olmsted, M., and Holiday, D. B. (2008). Co-occurring conditions associated with FMR1 gene variations: findings from a national parent survey. *Am. J. Med. Genet. A* 146A, 2060–2069. doi: 10.1002/ajmg.a.32439

Barcia, G., Fleming, M. R., Deligniere, A., Gazula, V. R., Brown, M. R., Langouet, M., et al. (2012). *De novo* gain-of-function KCNT1 channel mutations cause malignant migrating partial seizures of infancy. *Nat. Genet.* 44, 1255–1259. doi: 10.1038/ng.2441

Bassell, G. J., and Warren, S. T. (2008). Fragile X syndrome: loss of local mRNA regulation alters synaptic development and function. *Neuron* 60, 201–214. doi: 10.1016/j.neuron.2008.10.004

Beal, J. C., Cherian, K., and Moshe, S. L. (2012). Early-onset epileptic encephalopathies: ohtahara syndrome and early myoclonic encephalopathy. *Pediatr. Neurol.* 47, 317–323. doi: 10.1016/j.pediatrneurol.2012.06.002

Berg, A. T., Berkovic, S. F., Brodie, M. J., Buchhalter, J., Cross, J. H., van Emde Boas, W., et al. (2010). Revised terminology and concepts for organization of seizures and epilepsies: report of the ILAE Commission on Classification and Terminology, 2005–2009. *Epilepsia* 51, 676–685. doi: 10.1111/j.1528-1167.2010.02522.x

Bhattacharjee, A., Gan, L., and Kaczmarek, L. K. (2002). Localization of the Slack potassium channel in the rat central nervous system. *J. Comp. Neurol.* 454, 241–254. doi: 10.1002/cne.10439

Bhattacharjee, A., Joiner, W., Wu, M., Yang, Y., Sigworth, F., and Kaczmarek, L. (2003). Slick (Slo2.1), a rapidly-gating sodium-activated potassium channel inhibited by ATP. *J. Neurosci.* 23, 11681–11691.

Bhattacharjee, A., and Kaczmarek, L. (2005). For K+ channels, Na+ is the new Ca2+. *Trends Neurosci.* 28, 422–428. doi: 10.1016/j.tins.2005.06.003

Bhattacharjee, A., von Hehn, C., Mei, X., and Kaczmarek, L. (2005). Localization of the Na+-activated K+ channel Slick in the rat central nervous system. *J. Comp. Neurol.* 484, 80–92. doi: 10.1002/cne.20462

Bischoff, U., Vogel, W., and Safronov, B. V. (1998). Na+-activated K+ channels in small dorsal root ganglion neurones of rat. *J. Physiol.* 510(Pt 3), 743–754. doi: 10.1111/j.1469-7793.1998.743bj.x

Brenner, R., Chen, Q. H., Vilaythong, A., Toney, G. M., Noebels, J. L., and Aldrich, R. W. (2005). BK channel beta4 subunit reduces dentate gyrus excitability and protects against temporal lobe seizures. *Nat. Neurosci.* 8, 1752–1759. doi: 10.1038/nn1573

Brown, M., Kronengold, J., Gazula, V., Chen, Y., Strumbos, J., Sigworth, F., et al. (2010). Fragile X mental retardation protein controls gating of the sodium-activated potassium channel Slack. *Nat. Neurosci.* 13, 819–821. doi: 10.1038/nn.2563

Brown, M., Kronengold, J., Gazula, V., Spilianakis, C., Flavell, R., von Hehn, C., et al. (2008). Amino-termini isoforms of the Slack K+ channel, regulated by alternative promoters, differentially modulate rhythmic firing and adaptation. *J. Physiol.* 586, 5161–5179. doi: 10.1113/jphysiol.2008.160861

Budelli, G., Hage, T. A., Wei, A., Rojas, P., Jong, Y. J., O'Malley, K., et al. (2009). Na+-activated K+ channels express a large delayed outward current in neurons during normal physiology. *Nat. Neurosci.* 12, 745–750. doi: 10.1038/nn.2313

Caraballo, R. H., Fontana, E., Darra, F., Cassar, L., Negrini, F., Fiorini, E., et al. (2008). Migrating focal seizures in infancy: analysis of the electroclinical patterns in 17 patients. *J. Child Neurol.* 23, 497–506. doi: 10.1177/0883073807309771

Carranza Rojo, D., Hamiwka, L., McMahon, J. M., Dibbens, L. M., Arsov, T., Suls, A., et al. (2011). *De novo* SCN1A mutations in migrating partial seizures of infancy. *Neurology* 77, 380–383. doi: 10.1212/WNL.0b013e318227046d

Cazorla, M. R., Verdu, A., Montes, C., and Ayuga, F. (2010). Early infantile epileptic encephalopathy with unusual favourable outcome. *Brain Dev.* 32, 673–676. doi: 10.1016/j.braindev.2009.08.007

Cervantes, B., Vega, R., Limon, A., and Soto, E. (2013). Identity, expression and functional role of the sodium-activated potassium current in vestibular ganglion afferent neurons. *Neuroscience* 240, 163–175. doi: 10.1016/j.neuroscience.2013.02.052

Charlier, C., Singh, N. A., Ryan, S. G., Lewis, T. B., Reus, B. E., Leach, R. J., et al. (1998). A pore mutation in a novel KQT-like potassium channel gene in an idiopathic epilepsy family. *Nat. Genet.* 18, 53–55. doi: 10.1038/ng0198-53

Chen, H., Kronengold, J., Yan, Y., Gazula, V., Brown, M., Ma, L., et al. (2009). The N-terminal domain of Slack determines the formation and trafficking of Slick/Slack heteromeric sodium-activated potassium channels. *J. Neurosci.* 29, 5654–5665. doi: 10.1523/JNEUROSCI.5978-08.2009

Choi, E. M., Min, K. T., Cho, J. S., and Choi, S. H. (2011). Anesthetic experience of a patient with Ohtahara syndrome – a case report. *Korean J. Anesthesiol.* 60, 124–127. doi: 10.4097/kjae.2011.60.2.124

Christie, S. B., Akins, M. R., Schwob, J. E., and Fallon, J. R. (2009). The FXG: a presynaptic fragile X granule expressed in a subset of developing brain circuits. *J. Neurosci.* 29, 1514–1524. doi: 10.1523/JNEUROSCI.3937-08.2009

Clarke, M., Gill, J., Noronha, M., and McKinlay, I. (1987). Early infantile epileptic encephalopathy with suppression burst: ohtahara syndrome. *Dev. Med. Child Neurol.* 29, 520–528. doi: 10.1111/j.1469-8749.1987.tb02512.x

Coppola, G., Operto, F. F., Auricchio, G., D'Amico, A., Fortunato, D., and Pascotto, A. (2007). Temporal lobe dual pathology in malignant migrating partial seizures in infancy. *Epileptic Disord.* 9, 145–148.

Coppola, G., Plouin, P., Chiron, C., Robain, O., and Dulac, O. (1995). Migrating partial seizures in infancy: a malignant disorder with developmental arrest. *Epilepsia* 36, 1017–1024. doi: 10.1111/j.1528-1157.1995.tb00961.x

Coppola, G., Veggiotti, P., Del Giudice, E. M., Bellini, G., Longaretti, F., Taglialatela, M., et al. (2006). Mutational scanning of potassium, sodium and chloride ion channels in malignant migrating partial seizures in infancy. *Brain Dev.* 28, 76–79. doi: 10.1016/j.braindev.2005.05.002

De Fusco, M., Becchetti, A., Patrignani, A., Annesi, G., Gambardella, A., Quattrone, A., et al. (2000). The nicotinic receptor beta 2 subunit is mutant in nocturnal frontal lobe epilepsy. *Nat. Genet.* 26, 275–276. doi: 10.1038/81566

Deng, P. Y., Rotman, Z., Blundon, J. A., Cho, Y., Cui, J., Cavalli, V., et al. (2013). FMRP regulates neurotransmitter release and synaptic information transmission by modulating action potential duration via BK channels. *Neuron* 77, 696–711. doi: 10.1016/j.neuron.2012.12.018

Derry, C. P., Heron, S. E., Phillips, F., Howell, S., MacMahon, J., Phillips, H. A., et al. (2008). Severe autosomal dominant nocturnal frontal lobe epilepsy associated with psychiatric disorders and intellectual disability. *Epilepsia* 49, 2125–2129. doi: 10.1111/j.1528-1167.2008.01652.x

Dryer, S. E. (1991). Na^+-activated K^+ channels and voltage-evoked ionic currents in brain stem and parasympathetic neurones of the chick. *J. Physiol.* 435, 513–532.

Du, W., Bautista, J. F., Yang, H., Diez-Sampedro, A., You, S. A., Wang, L., et al. (2005). Calcium-sensitive potassium channelopathy in human epilepsy and paroxysmal movement disorder. *Nat. Genet.* 37, 733–738. doi: 10.1038/ng1585

Egan, T. M., Dagan, D., Kupper, J., and Levitan, I. B. (1992). Properties and rundown of sodium-activated potassium channels in rat olfactory bulb neurons. *J. Neurosci.* 12, 1964–1976.

Eksioglu, Y. Z., Pong, A. W., and Takeoka, M. (2011). A novel mutation in the aristaless domain of the ARX gene leads to Ohtahara syndrome, global developmental delay, and ambiguous genitalia in males and neuropsychiatric disorders in females. *Epilepsia* 52, 984–992. doi: 10.1111/j.1528-1167.2011.02980.x

Engel, J., and International League Against Epilepsy (ILAE). (2001). A proposed diagnostic scheme for people with epileptic seizures and with epilepsy: report of the ILAE Task Force on Classification and Terminology. *Epilepsia* 42, 796–803. doi: 10.1046/j.1528-1157.2001.10401.x

Epi, K. C., Epilepsy Phenome/Genome, P., Allen, A. S., Berkovic, S. F., Cossette, P., Delanty, N., et al. (2013). *De novo* mutations in epileptic encephalopathies. *Nature* 501, 217–221. doi: 10.1038/nature12439

Escayg, A., MacDonald, B. T., Meisler, M. H., Baulac, S., Huberfeld, G., An-Gourfinkel, I., et al. (2000). Mutations of SCN1A, encoding a neuronal sodium channel, in two families with GEFS+2. *Nat. Genet.* 24, 343–345. doi: 10.1038/74159

Fadool, D. A., Tucker, K., Perkins, R., Fasciani, G., Thompson, R. N., Parsons, A. D., et al. (2004). Kv1.3 channel gene-targeted deletion produces "Super-Smeller Mice" with altered glomeruli, interacting scaffolding proteins, and biophysics. *Neuron* 41, 389–404. doi: 10.1016/S0896-6273(03)00844-4

Ferron, L., Nieto-Rostro, M., Cassidy, J. S., and Dolphin, A. C. (2014). Fragile X mental retardation protein controls synaptic vesicle exocytosis by modulating N-type calcium channel density. *Nat. Commun.* 5, 3628. doi: 10.1038/ncomms4628

Fisher, R. S., van Emde Boas, W., Blume, W., Elger, C., Genton, P., Lee, P., et al. (2005). Epileptic seizures and epilepsy: definitions proposed by the International League Against Epilepsy (ILAE) and the International Bureau for Epilepsy (IBE). *Epilepsia* 46, 470–472. doi: 10.1111/j.0013-9580.2005.66104.x

Fitzpatrick, R. C., and Day, B. L. (2004). Probing the human vestibular system with galvanic stimulation. *J. Appl. Physiol.* 96, 2301–2316. doi: 10.1152/japplphysiol.00008.2004

Fullston, T., Brueton, L., Willis, T., Philip, S., MacPherson, L., Finnis, M., et al. (2010). Ohtahara syndrome in a family with an ARX protein truncation mutation (c.81C > G/p.Y27X). *Eur. J. Hum. Genet.* 18, 157–162. doi: 10.1038/ejhg.2009.139

Gadotti, V. M., and Zamponi, G. W. (2013). TMEM16C cuts pain no SLACK. *Nat. Neurosci.* 16, 1165–1166. doi: 10.1038/nn.3497

Giordano, L., Sartori, S., Russo, S., Accorsi, P., Galli, J., Tiberti, A., et al. (2010). Familial Ohtahara syndrome due to a novel ARX gene mutation. *Am. J. Med. Genet. A* 152a, 3133–3137. doi: 10.1002/ajmg.a.33701

Grillner, S., Deliagina, T., Ekeberg, O., el Manira, A., Hill, R. H., Lansner, A., et al. (1995). Neural networks that co-ordinate locomotion and body orientation in lamprey. *Trends Neurosci.* 18, 270–279. doi: 10.1016/0166-2236(95)93914-J

Gross-Tsur, V., Ben-Zeev, B., and Shalev, R. S. (2004). Malignant migrating partial seizures in infancy. *Pediatr. Neurol.* 31, 287–290. doi: 10.1016/j.pediatrneurol.2004.05.001

Gustafsson, B., and Wigstrom, H. (1983). Hyperpolarization following long-lasting tetanic activation of hippocampal pyramidal cells. *Brain Res.* 275, 159–163. doi: 10.1016/0006-8993(83)90429-8

Haimann, C., Bernheim, L., Bertrand, D., and Bader, C. R. (1990). Potassium current activated by intracellular sodium in quail trigeminal ganglion neurons. *J. Gen. Physiol.* 95, 961–979. doi: 10.1085/jgp.95.5.961

Hartung, K. (1985). Potentiation of a transient outward current by Na+ influx in crayfish neurons. *Pflugers Arch.* 404, 41–44. doi: 10.1007/BF00581488

Hernandez, R. N., Feinberg, R. L., Vaurio, R., Passanante, N. M., Thompson, R. E., and Kaufmann, W. E. (2009). Autism spectrum disorder in fragile X syndrome: a longitudinal evaluation. *Am. J. Med. Genet. A* 149A, 1125–1137. doi: 10.1002/ajmg.a.32848

Heron, S. E., Smith, K. R., Bahlo, M., Nobili, L., Kahana, E., Licchetta, L., et al. (2012). Missense mutations in the sodium-gated potassium channel gene KCNT1 cause severe autosomal dominant nocturnal frontal lobe epilepsy. *Nat. Genet.* 44, 1188–1190. doi: 10.1038/ng.2440

Hmaimess, G., Kadhim, H., Nassogne, M. C., Bonnier, C., and van Rijckevorsel, K. (2006). Levetiracetam in a neonate with malignant migrating partial seizures. *Pediatr. Neurol.* 34, 55–59. doi: 10.1016/j.pediatrneurol.2005.06.011

Hmaimess, G., Raftopoulos, C., Kadhim, H., Nassogne, M. C., Ghariani, S., de Tourtchaninoff, M., et al. (2005). Impact of early hemispherotomy in a case of Ohtahara syndrome with left parieto-occipital megalencephaly. *Seizure* 14, 439–442. doi: 10.1016/j.seizure.2005.05.004

Huang, F., Wang, X., Ostertag, E. M., Nuwal, T., Huang, B., Jan, Y. N., et al. (2013). TMEM16C facilitates Na^+-activated K^+ currents in rat sensory neurons and regulates pain processing. *Nat. Neurosci.* 16, 1284–1290. doi: 10.1038/nn.3468

Ishii, A., Shioda, M., Okumura, A., Kidokoro, H., Sakauchi, M., Shimada, S., et al. (2013). A recurrent KCNT1 mutation in two sporadic cases with malignant migrating partial seizures in infancy. *Gene* 531, 467–471. doi: 10.1016/j.gene.2013.08.096

Joiner, W. J., Tang, M. D., Wang, L. Y., Dworetzky, S. I., Boissard, C. G., Gan, L., et al. (1998). Formation of intermediate-conductance calcium-activated potassium channels by interaction of Slack and Slo subunits. *Nat. Neurosci.* 1, 462–469. doi: 10.1038/2176

Jokiranta, E., Sourander, A., Suominen, A., Timonen-Soivio, L., Brown, A. S., and Sillanpaa, M. (2014). Epilepsy among children and adolescents with autism spectrum disorders: a population-based study. *J. Autism Dev. Disord.* doi: 10.1007/s10803-014-2126-6 [Epub ahead of print].

Kaczmarek, L. K. (2013). Slack, slick and sodium-activated potassium channels. *ISRN Neurosci.* 2013. doi: 10.1155/2013/354262

Kato, M., Koyama, N., Ohta, M., Miura, K., and Hayasaka, K. (2010). Frameshift mutations of the ARX gene in familial Ohtahara syndrome. *Epilepsia* 51, 1679–1684. doi: 10.1111/j.1528-1167.2010.02559.x

Kato, M., Saitoh, S., Kamei, A., Shiraishi, H., Ueda, Y., Akasaka, M., et al. (2007). A longer polyalanine expansion mutation in the ARX gene causes early infantile epileptic encephalopathy with suppression-burst pattern (Ohtahara syndrome). *Am. J. Hum. Genet.* 81, 361–366. doi: 10.1086/518903

Kato, M., Yamagata, T., Kubota, M., Arai, H., Yamashita, S., Nakagawa, T., et al. (2013). Clinical spectrum of early onset epileptic encephalopathies caused by KCNQ2 mutation. *Epilepsia* 54, 1282–1287. doi: 10.1111/epi.12200

Khandjian, E. W., Huot, M. E., Tremblay, S., Davidovic, L., Mazroui, R., and Bardoni, B. (2004). Biochemical evidence for the association of fragile X mental retardation protein with brain polyribosomal ribonucleoparticles. *Proc. Natl. Acad. Sci. U.S.A.* 101, 13357–13362. doi: 10.1073/pnas.0405398101

Krasemann, T., Hoovey, S., Uekoetter, J., Bosse, H., Kurlemann, G., and Debus, O. M. (2001). Early infantile epileptic encephalopathy (Ohtahara syndrome) after maternal electric injury during pregnancy: etiological considerations. *Brain Dev.* 23, 359–362. doi: 10.1016/S0387-7604(01)00238-8

Krsek, P., Sebronova, V., Prochazka, T., Maulisova, A., and Komarek, V. (2002). Successful treatment of Ohtahara syndrome with chloral hydrate. *Pediatr. Neurol.* 27, 388–391. doi: 10.1016/S0887-8994(02)00464-2

Kues, W. A., and Wunder, F. (1992). Heterogeneous expression patterns of mammalian potassium channel genes in developing and adult rat brain. *Eur. J. Neurosci.* 4, 1296–1308. doi: 10.1111/j.1460-9568.1992.tb00155.x

Kurahashi, H., and Hirose, S. (2002). "Autosomal dominant nocturnal frontal lobe epilepsy," in *GeneReviews*, eds R. Pagon, M. Adam, and T. Bird (Seattle, WA: University of Washington).

Lee, E. H., Yum, M. S., Jeong, M. H., Lee, K. Y., and Ko, T. S. (2012). A case of malignant migrating partial seizures in infancy as a continuum of infantile epileptic encephalopathy. *Brain Dev.* 34, 768–772. doi: 10.1016/j.braindev.2011.11.011

Li, J., Pelletier, M. R., Perez Velazquez, J. L., and Carlen, P. L. (2002). Reduced cortical synaptic plasticity and GluR1 expression associated with fragile X mental retardation protein deficiency. *Mol. Cell. Neurosci.* 19, 138–151. doi: 10.1006/mcne.2001.1085

Low, C., Garzon, E., Carrete, H., Vilanova, L. C., Yacubian, E. M., and Sakamoto, A. C. (2007). Early destructive lesions in the developing brain: clinical and electrographic correlates. *Arq. Neuropsiquiatr.* 65, 416–422. doi: 10.1590/S0004-282X2007000300010

Lu, S., Das, P., Fadool, D., and Kaczmarek, L. (2010). The slack sodium-activated potassium channel provides a major outward current in olfactory neurons of Kv1.3-/- super-smeller mice. *J. Neurophysiol.* 103, 3311–3319. doi: 10.1152/jn.00607.2009

Majewski, J., Schwartzentruber, J., Lalonde, E., Montpetit, A., and Jabado, N. (2011). What can exome sequencing do for you? *J. Med. Genet.* 48, 580–589. doi: 10.1136/jmedgenet-2011-100223

Malik, S. I., Galliani, C. A., Hernandez, A. W., and Donahue, D. J. (2013). Epilepsy surgery for early infantile epileptic encephalopathy (ohtahara syndrome). *J. Child Neurol.* 28, 1607–1617. doi: 10.1177/0883073812464395

Marsh, E., Melamed, S. E., Barron, T., and Clancy, R. R. (2005). Migrating partial seizures in infancy: expanding the phenotype of a rare seizure syndrome. *Epilepsia* 46, 568–572. doi: 10.1111/j.0013-9580.2005.34104.x

Martin, H. C., Kim, G. E., Pagnamenta, A. T., Murakami, Y., Carvill, G., Meyer, E., et al. (2014). Clinical whole-genome sequencing in severe early-onset epilepsy reveals new genes and improves molecular diagnosis. *Hum. Mol. Genet.* 23, 3200–3211. doi: 10.1093/hmg/ddu030

McTague, A., Appleton, R., Avula, S., Cross, J. H., King, M. D., Jacques, T. S., et al. (2013). Migrating partial seizures of infancy: expansion of the electroclinical, radiological and pathological disease spectrum. *Brain* 136, 1578–1591. doi: 10.1093/brain/awt073

Mignot, C., Moutard, M. L., Trouillard, O., Gourfinkel-An, I., Jacquette, A., Arveiler, B., et al. (2011). STXBP1-related encephalopathy presenting as infantile spasms and generalized tremor in three patients. *Epilepsia* 52, 1820–1827. doi: 10.1111/j.1528-1167.2011.03163.x

Milh, M., Falace, A., Villeneuve, N., Vanni, N., Cacciagli, P., Assereto, S., et al. (2013). Novel compound heterozygous mutations in TBC1D24 cause familial malignant migrating partial seizures of infancy. *Hum. Mutat.* 34, 869–872. doi: 10.1002/humu.22318

Milh, M., Villeneuve, N., Chouchane, M., Kaminska, A., Laroche, C., Barthez, M. A., et al. (2011). Epileptic and nonepileptic features in patients with early onset epileptic encephalopathy and STXBP1 mutations. *Epilepsia* 52, 1828–1834. doi: 10.1111/j.1528-1167.2011.03181.x

Miller, S. P., Dilenge, M. E., Meagher-Villemure, K., O'Gorman, A. M., and Shevell, M. I. (1998). Infantile epileptic encephalopathy (Ohtahara syndrome) and migrational disorder. *Pediatr. Neurol.* 19, 50–54. doi: 10.1016/S0887-8994(98)00009-5

Milligan, C. J., Li, M., Gazina, E. V., Heron, S. E., Nair, U., Trager, C., et al. (2014). KCNT1 gain of function in 2 epilepsy phenotypes is reversed by quinidine. *Ann. Neurol.* 75, 581–590. doi: 10.1002/ana.24128

Muhle, R., Trentacoste, S. V., and Rapin, I. (2004). The genetics of autism. *Pediatrics* 113, e472–e486. doi: 10.1542/peds.113.5.e472

Musumeci, S. A., Hagerman, R. J., Ferri, R., Bosco, P., Dalla Bernardina, B., Tassinari, C. A., et al. (1999). Epilepsy and EEG findings in males with fragile X syndrome. *Epilepsia* 40, 1092–1099. doi: 10.1111/j.1528-1157.1999.tb00824.x

Nabbout, R., and Dulac, O. (2008). Epileptic syndromes in infancy and childhood. *Curr. Opin. Neurol.* 21, 161–166. doi: 10.1097/WCO.0b013e3282f7007e

Nakamura, K., Kato, M., Osaka, H., Yamashita, S., Nakagawa, E., Haginoya, K., et al. (2013). Clinical spectrum of SCN2A mutations expanding to Ohtahara syndrome. *Neurology* 81, 992–998. doi: 10.1212/WNL.0b013e3182a43e57

Nakken, K. O., Magnusson, A., and Steinlein, O. K. (1999). Autosomal dominant nocturnal frontal lobe epilepsy: an electroclinical study of a Norwegian family with ten affected members. *Epilepsia* 40, 88–92. doi: 10.1111/j.1528-1157.1999.tb01993.x

Nuwer, M. O., Picchione, K. E., and Bhattacharjee, A. (2010). PKA-induced internalization of slack KNa channels produces dorsal root ganglion neuron hyperexcitability. *J. Neurosci.* 30, 14165–14172. doi: 10.1523/JNEUROSCI.3150-10.2010

Ohno, M., Shimotsuji, Y., Abe, J., Shimada, M., and Tamiya, H. (2000). Zonisamide treatment of early infantile epileptic encephalopathy. *Pediatr. Neurol.* 23, 341–344. doi: 10.1016/S0887-8994(00)00197-1

Ohtahara, S., Ishida, T., Oka, E., Yamatogi, Y., and Inoue, H. (1976). On the specific age dependent epileptic syndrome: the early-infantile epileptic encephalopathy with suppression-burst (in Japanese). *No To Hottatsu (Tokyo)* 8, 270–280.

Ohtsuka, Y., Sato, M., Sanada, S., Yoshinaga, H., and Oka, E. (2000). Suppression-burst patterns in intractable epilepsy with focal cortical dysplasia. *Brain Dev.* 22, 135–138. doi: 10.1016/S0387-7604(00)00090-5

Okuda, K., Yasuhara, A., Kamei, A., Araki, A., Kitamura, N., and Kobayashi, Y. (2000). Successful control with bromide of two patients with malignant migrating partial seizures in infancy. *Brain Dev.* 22, 56–59. doi: 10.1016/S0387-7604(99)00108-4

Oldani, A., Zucconi, M., Asselta, R., Modugno, M., Bonati, M. T., Dalpra, L., et al. (1998). Autosomal dominant nocturnal frontal lobe epilepsy. A video-polysomnographic and genetic appraisal of 40 patients and delineation of the epileptic syndrome. *Brain* 121(Pt 2), 205–223. doi: 10.1093/brain/121.2.205

Petit-Jacques, J., Sui, J. L., and Logothetis, D. E. (1999). Synergistic activation of G protein-gated inwardly rectifying potassium channels by the betagamma subunits of G proteins and Na^+ and Mg^{2+} ions. *J. Gen. Physiol.* 114, 673–684. doi: 10.1085/jgp.114.5.673

Phillips, H. A., Scheffer, I. E., Crossland, K. M., Bhatia, K. P., Fish, D. R., Marsden, C. D., et al. (1998). Autosomal dominant nocturnal frontal-lobe epilepsy: genetic heterogeneity and evidence for a second locus at 15q24. *Am. J. Hum. Genet.* 63, 1108–1116. doi: 10.1086/302047

Pieretti, M., Zhang, F. P., Fu, Y. H., Warren, S. T., Oostra, B. A., Caskey, C. T., et al. (1991). Absence of expression of the FMR-1 gene in fragile X syndrome. *Cell* 66, 817–822. doi: 10.1016/0092-8674(91)90125-I

Quan, L., Zhu, B. L., Ishida, K., Taniguchi, M., Li, D. R., Kamikodai, Y., et al. (2001). Sudden death of an infant with 'an early epileptic encephalopathy'. *Forensic Sci. Int.* 124, 62–67. doi: 10.1016/S0379-0738(01)00568-0

Robain, O., and Dulac, O. (1992). Early epileptic encephalopathy with suppression bursts and olivary-dentate dysplasia. *Neuropediatrics* 23, 162–164. doi: 10.1055/s-2008-1071334

Saitsu, H., Hoshino, H., Kato, M., Nishiyama, K., Okada, I., Yoneda, Y., et al. (2011). Paternal mosaicism of an STXBP1 mutation in OS. *Clin. Genet.* 80, 484–488. doi: 10.1111/j.1399-0004.2010.01575.x

Saitsu, H., Kato, M., Koide, A., Goto, T., Fujita, T., Nishiyama, K., et al. (2012a). Whole exome sequencing identifies KCNQ2 mutations in Ohtahara syndrome. *Ann. Neurol.* 72, 298–300. doi: 10.1002/ana.23620

Saitsu, H., Kato, M., Shimono, M., Senju, A., Tanabe, S., Kimura, T., et al. (2012b). Association of genomic deletions in the STXBP1 gene with Ohtahara syndrome. *Clin. Genet.* 81, 399–402. doi: 10.1111/j.1399-0004.2011.01733.x

Saitsu, H., Kato, M., Mizuguchi, T., Hamada, K., Osaka, H., Tohyama, J., et al. (2008). *De novo* mutations in the gene encoding STXBP1 (MUNC18-1) cause early infantile epileptic encephalopathy. *Nat. Genet.* 40, 782–788. doi: 10.1038/ng.150

Saitsu, H., Kato, M., Okada, I., Orii, K. E., Higuchi, T., Hoshino, H., et al. (2010). STXBP1 mutations in early infantile epileptic encephalopathy with suppression-burst pattern. *Epilepsia* 51, 2397–2405. doi: 10.1111/j.1528-1167.2010.02728.x

Salkoff, L., Butler, A., Ferreira, G., Santi, C., and Wei, A. (2006). High-conductance potassium channels of the SLO family. *Nat. Rev. Neurosci.* 7, 921–931. doi: 10.1038/nrn1992

Santi, C., Ferreira, G., Yang, B., Gazula, V., Butler, A., Wei, A., et al. (2006). Opposite regulation of Slick and Slack K+ channels by neuromodulators. *J. Neurosci.* 26, 5059–5068. doi: 10.1523/JNEUROSCI.3372-05.2006

Scheffer, I. E., and Berkovic, S. F. (1997). Generalized epilepsy with febrile seizures plus. A genetic disorder with heterogeneous clinical phenotypes. *Brain* 120(Pt 3), 479–490. doi: 10.1093/brain/120.3.479

Scheffer, I. E., Bhatia, K. P., Lopes-Cendes, I., Fish, D. R., Marsden, C. D., Andermann, E., et al. (1995). Autosomal dominant nocturnal frontal lobe epilepsy. A distinctive clinical disorder. *Brain* 118(Pt 1), 61–73. doi: 10.1093/brain/118.1.61

Schwindt, P. C., Spain, W. J., and Crill, W. E. (1989). Long-lasting reduction of excitability by a sodium-dependent potassium current in cat neocortical neurons. *J. Neurophysiol.* 61, 233–244.

Schwindt, P. C., Spain, W. J., Foehring, R. C., Chubb, M. C., and Crill, W. E. (1988a). Slow conductances in neurons from cat sensorimotor cortex *in vitro* and their role in slow excitability changes. *J. Neurophysiol.* 59, 450–467.

Schwindt, P. C., Spain, W. J., Foehring, R. C., Stafstrom, C. E., Chubb, M. C., and Crill, W. E. (1988b). Multiple potassium conductances and their functions in neurons from cat sensorimotor cortex *in vitro*. *J. Neurophysiol.* 59, 424–449.

Seo, J. H., Lee, Y. M., Lee, J. S., Kim, S. H., and Kim, H. D. (2010). A case of Ohtahara syndrome with mitochondrial respiratory chain complex I deficiency. *Brain Dev.* 32, 253–257. doi: 10.1016/j.braindev.2008.12.020

Seoh, S. A., Sigg, D., Papazian, D. M., and Bezanilla, F. (1996). Voltage-sensing residues in the S2 and S4 segments of the Shaker K+ channel. *Neuron* 16, 1159–1167. doi: 10.1016/S0896-6273(00)80142-7

Sharma, S., Sankhyan, N., Ramesh, K., and Gulati, S. (2011). Child neurology: epilepsy of infancy with migrating focal seizures. *Neurology* 77, e21–e24. doi: 10.1212/WNL.0b013e3182267b4f

Stefani, G., Fraser, C. E., Darnell, J. C., and Darnell, R. B. (2004). Fragile X mental retardation protein is associated with translating polyribosomes in neuronal cells. *J. Neurosci.* 24, 7272–7276. doi: 10.1523/JNEUROSCI.2306-04.2004

Steinlein, O. K., Mulley, J. C., Propping, P., Wallace, R. H., Phillips, H. A., Sutherland, G. R., et al. (1995). A missense mutation in the neuronal nicotinic acetylcholine receptor alpha 4 subunit is associated with autosomal dominant nocturnal frontal lobe epilepsy. *Nat. Genet.* 11, 201–203. doi: 10.1038/ng1095-201

Tamsett, T. J., Picchione, K. E., and Bhattacharjee, A. (2009). NAD+ activates KNa channels in dorsal root ganglion neurons. *J. Neurosci.* 29, 5127–5134. doi: 10.1523/JNEUROSCI.0859-09.2009

Touma, M., Joshi, M., Connolly, M. C., Grant, P. E., Hansen, A. R., Khwaja, O., et al. (2013). Whole genome sequencing identifies SCN2A mutation in monozygotic twins with Ohtahara syndrome and unique neuropathologic findings. *Epilepsia* 54, e81–e85. doi: 10.1111/epi.12137

Trinka, E., Rauscher, C., Nagler, M., Moroder, T., Ladurner, G., Irnberger, E., et al. (2001). A case of Ohtahara syndrome with olivary-dentate dysplasia and agenesis of mamillary bodies. *Epilepsia* 42, 950–953. doi: 10.1046/j.1528-1157.2001.042007950.x

Tucker, K., Cho, S., Thiebaud, N., Henderson, M. X., and Fadool, D. A. (2013). Glucose sensitivity of mouse olfactory bulb neurons is conveyed by a voltage-gated potassium channel. *J. Physiol.* 591, 2541–2561. doi: 10.1113/jphysiol.2013.254086

Vanderver, A., Simons, C., Schmidt, J. L., Pearl, P. L., Bloom, M., Lavenstein, B., et al. (2014). Identification of a novel *de novo* p.Phe932Ile KCNT1 mutation in a patient with leukoencephalopathy and severe epilepsy. *Pediatr. Neurol.* 50, 112–114. doi: 10.1016/j.pediatrneurol.2013.06.024

Veneselli, E., Perrone, M. V., Di Rocco, M., Gaggero, R., and Biancheri, R. (2001). Malignant migrating partial seizures in infancy. *Epilepsy Res.* 46, 27–32. doi: 10.1016/S0920-1211(01)00197-8

Vergara, C., Latorre, R., Marrion, N. V., and Adelman, J. P. (1998). Calcium-activated potassium channels. *Curr. Opin. Neurobiol.* 8, 321–329. doi: 10.1016/S0959-4388(98)80056-1

Wallen, P., Robertson, B., Cangiano, L., Low, P., Bhattacharjee, A., Kaczmarek, L. K., et al. (2007). Sodium-dependent potassium channels of a Slack-like subtype contribute to the slow afterhyperpolarization in lamprey spinal neurons. *J. Physiol.* 585, 75–90. doi: 10.1113/jphysiol.2007.138156

Warmke, J. W., and Ganetzky, B. (1994). A family of potassium channel genes related to eag in Drosophila and mammals. *Proc. Natl. Acad. Sci. U.S.A.* 91, 3438–3442. doi: 10.1073/pnas.91.8.3438

Yamatogi, Y., and Ohtahara, S. (2002). Early-infantile epileptic encephalopathy with suppression-bursts, Ohtahara syndrome; its overview referring to our 16 cases. *Brain Dev.* 24, 13–23. doi: 10.1016/S0387-7604(01)00392-8

Yang, B., Desai, R., and Kaczmarek, L. (2007). Slack and Slick K_{Na} channels regulate the accuracy of timing of auditory neurons. *J. Neurosci.* 27, 2617–2627. doi: 10.1523/JNEUROSCI.5308-06.2007

Yang, J., Krishnamoorthy, G., Saxena, A., Zhang, G., Shi, J., Yang, H., et al. (2010). An epilepsy/dyskinesia-associated mutation enhances BK channel activation by potentiating Ca2+ sensing. *Neuron* 66, 871–883. doi: 10.1016/j.neuron.2010.05.009

Yasuhara, A. (2010). Correlation between EEG abnormalities and symptoms of autism spectrum disorder (ASD). *Brain Dev.* 32, 791–798. doi: 10.1016/j.braindev.2010.08.010

Yuan, A., Santi, C., Wei, A., Wang, Z., Pollak, K., Nonet, M., et al. (2003). The sodium-activated potassium channel is encoded by a member of the Slo gene family. *Neuron* 37, 765–773. doi: 10.1016/S0896-6273(03)00096-5

Zhang, Y., Brown, M. R., Hyland, C., Chen, Y., Kronengold, J., Fleming, M. R., et al. (2012). Regulation of neuronal excitability by interaction of fragile x mental retardation protein with slack potassium channels. *J. Neurosci.* 32, 15318–15327. doi: 10.1523/JNEUROSCI.2162-12.2012

Zuberi, S. M., Eunson, L. H., Spauschus, A., De Silva, R., Tolmie, J., Wood, N. W., et al. (1999). A novel mutation in the human voltage-gated potassium channel gene (Kv1.1) associates with episodic ataxia type 1 and sometimes with partial epilepsy. *Brain* 122(Pt 5), 817–825. doi: 10.1093/brain/122.5.817

2

Impaired activity-dependent neural circuit assembly and refinement in autism spectrum disorder genetic models

Caleb A. Doll[1] and Kendal Broadie[1,2] *

[1] *Department of Biological Sciences, Vanderbilt University, Nashville, TN, USA*
[2] *Kennedy Center for Research on Human Development, Vanderbilt University, Nashville, TN, USA*

Correspondence:
Kendal Broadie, Department of Biological Sciences, Vanderbilt University, 6270A MRBIII, Nashville, TN 37232-8548, USA
e-mail: kendal.broadie@vanderbilt.edu

Early-use activity during circuit-specific critical periods refines brain circuitry by the coupled processes of eliminating inappropriate synapses and strengthening maintained synapses. We theorize these activity-dependent (A-D) developmental processes are specifically impaired in autism spectrum disorders (ASDs). ASD genetic models in both mouse and *Drosophila* have pioneered our insights into normal A-D neural circuit assembly and consolidation, and how these developmental mechanisms go awry in specific genetic conditions. The monogenic fragile X syndrome (FXS), a common cause of heritable ASD and intellectual disability, has been particularly well linked to defects in A-D critical period processes. The fragile X mental retardation protein (FMRP) is positively activity-regulated in expression and function, in turn regulates excitability and activity in a negative feedback loop, and appears to be required for the A-D remodeling of synaptic connectivity during early-use critical periods. The *Drosophila* FXS model has been shown to functionally conserve the roles of human FMRP in synaptogenesis, and has been centrally important in generating our current mechanistic understanding of the FXS disease state. Recent advances in *Drosophila* optogenetics, transgenic calcium reporters, highly-targeted transgenic drivers for individually-identified neurons, and a vastly improved connectome of the brain are now being combined to provide unparalleled opportunities to both manipulate and monitor A-D processes during critical period brain development in defined neural circuits. The field is now poised to exploit this new *Drosophila* transgenic toolbox for the systematic dissection of A-D mechanisms in normal versus ASD brain development, particularly utilizing the well-established *Drosophila* FXS disease model.

Keywords: fragile X syndrome, synaptogenesis, synapse elimination, E/I ratio, optogenetics, *Drosophila*

INTRODUCTION

The recent passing of David Hubel (September 22, 2013) occurs in the midst of a rich era of research into the activity-dependent (A-D) formation and refinement of neural circuitry during normal brain development and in neurodevelopmental disease states. Hubel and Wiesel's pioneering studies on monocular deprivation and activity manipulations in the cat visual system (Hubel and Wiesel, 1959, 1962, 1970; Wiesel and Hubel, 1963) laid the foundation for our understanding of the A-D assembly and pruning of synaptic connections. All synapses formed through the reciprocal, highly orchestrated crosstalk between axons and dendrites face the bottleneck decision of elimination versus long-term maintenance and strengthening to form a stable partnership (dendrite stabilization review, Koleske, 2013; intrinsic dendrite development, Puram and Bonni, 2013). Although early synaptogenesis proceeds via largely activity-independent mechanisms, the refinement of synapses is a progressive, A-D process most active during the early-use critical periods of postnatal development, when synaptic arrays are most amenable to pruning and *de nova* additions (Hensch, 2004). Following this refinement period, A-D modulation is greatly reduced in the mature brain, except for maintenance of the synaptic plasticity underlying behavioral adaptation (Rice and Barone, 2000; rodent visual cortex, Nataraj and Turrigiano, 2011). Recent advances in biotechnology provide high-fidelity readouts of neural activity, as well as precise, non-invasive methods for the bidirectional manipulation of neural activity (Chen et al., 2013; Lin et al., 2013b), generating the means to study A-D developmental processes at a previously inconceivable level.

Autism spectrum disorders (ASDs) are defined by social interaction impairments (Abrahams and Geschwind, 2008), frequently accompanied by sensory hypersensitivity, cognitive deficits, and A-D seizures (Kim and Lord, 2012; Kim et al., 2013b). The improper development of neural circuitry likely lies at the heart of ASDs, particularly the A-D processes of solidifying appropriate synaptic connections and concomitantly pruning superfluous or incorrect connections (Zoghbi and Bear, 2012). The apparently diverse genetic bases of the wide spectrum of autism-related disorders makes genetic modeling a challenge (Sanders et al., 2012), but recent hypotheses suggest that the variety of genetic variants associated with ASDs may converge on a more manageable set of core molecular pathways (Murdoch and State, 2013). With this in mind, targeted mouse and *Drosophila* animal model systems harboring deficiencies in ASD-linked human genes often show comparable phenotypic and behavioral defects to human patients (Hagerman et al., 2009; van Alphen et al., 2013). Among the strongest primary research contributions have come from models of fragile X syndrome (FXS), a monogenic disorder that is the leading heritable contributor to the autism spectrum (Harris et al., 2008; McBride et al., 2012). In both mouse and *Drosophila* FXS models, there is clear and consistent evidence that the causal fragile X mental retardation protein (FMRP) is directly activity-regulated and in turn regulates A-D processes of neural circuit assembly and refinement (Wang et al., 2010a,b; Wondolowski and Dickman, 2013). Preclinical studies with these animal models have already advanced to a number of human clinical trials [e.g., metabotropic glutamate receptor (mGluR) therapeutics], and groundbreaking tools to assess and manipulate A-D synapse and circuit development show great promise toward major breakthroughs in ASD therapeutic intervention strategies (Akerboom et al., 2013; Paz et al., 2013; Sukhotinsky et al., 2013).

In this review article, we seek to highlight recent advances in our understanding of A-D synaptic development in the normal and ASD brain, particularly focused on recent work from mouse and *Drosophila* genetic models. We will only mention is passing electrophysiological investigations of synaptic plasticity at maturity, which is the focus of many excellent reviews (Malenka and Bear, 2004; Nelson and Turrigiano, 2008; Castillo et al., 2011). Likewise, the broad genetic and molecular details of A-D neural circuit assembly have recently been presented elsewhere (Flavell and Greenberg, 2008; West and Greenberg, 2011; Ebert and Greenberg, 2013). Our main focus will be on the A-D basis of ASDs, and particularly on FXS, as the leading heritable contributor to this neurodevelopmental disease condition (Hagerman and Hagerman, 2002). Starting with a brief review of normal experience-dependent synaptic changes (Part 1), we will then focus on correlates between the ASD disease state and A-D circuit formation (Part 2), and finally finish with a detailed review of the recent technological advances for the manipulation and monitoring of A-D processes (Part 3) during neural circuit development.

PART 1: NORMAL ACTIVITY-DEPENDENT NEURODEVELOPMENT

Hebb (1949) theorized that neural activity would code neural circuit connectivity through a mechanism of coincident synapse elimination and consolidation. This theory was first tested in the cat visual cortex, with the first visual response recordings made in the 1950s (Bishop and Clare, 1951, 1952, 1955; Clare and Bishop, 1954; Jung, 1958), coincident with the pioneering work of Kuffler (1953) defining ganglion cell specificity/organization and producing some of the first primary evidence of higher order processing. Kuffler's students went on to establish the principles of A-D mechanisms (**Figure 1A**), including Horace Barlow's characterization of selectivity and lateral inhibition in the frog retina (Barlow, 1953a,b), and David Hubel and Torsten Wiesel's work on the basis of A-D (and later experience-dependent) synaptic development in the cat retinal system. Hubel and Wiesel first demonstrated that individual striatal cortical neurons (primary visual cortex) respond preferentially to slits of light (Hubel and Wiesel, 1959), providing a mechanism by which cortex organization enables higher order perception (Hubel and Wiesel, 1962). Their subsequent studies using monocular deprivation revealed profound changes in cortex development, with active-pathway axons from the lateral geniculate nucleus (LGN) dramatically out-competing inactive axons for cortex innervation of striatal cortical neurons (Wiesel and Hubel, 1963). The LGN innervated by the monocularly deprived retinal axons was also thinner, demonstrating a sensory experience-dependent restructuring of the developing neural circuit (Wiesel and Hubel, 1963).

Hubel and Wiesel went on to perform an extended series of A-D developmental studies, establishing a critical period for visual cortical development in kittens, and demonstrating that adult cats show no comparable experience-dependent morphological or electrophysiological changes (Wiesel and Hubel, 1963, 1965a,b; Hubel and Wiesel, 1970; Wiesel, 1982; Cohen and Greenberg, 2008). Following these pioneering studies, A-D morphological changes were similarly revealed in other areas of the sensory cortex. As one example, upon trimming whiskers in specific rows, axonal projections in the rat somatosensory cortex were reduced from non-deprived columns into deprived columns (axons from column A generally innervate column B; if the B column is deprived of input, the A axon receives no postsynaptic response and collapses), and increased horizontal axonal projections between non-deprived columns (Broser et al., 2008). Whisker trimming on the rat's snout from birth leads to a smaller contralateral motor area that evokes abnormal motor activity, a phenomenon not seen in adult rats (Huntley, 1997), again indicating a transient developmental window. Neuromuscular junction (NMJ) innervation is another classic system for studying A-D remodeling (Schuster, 2006). Motor axons compete to target individual muscle fibers during the early-use neonatal period (Sanes and Lichtman, 1999), and NMJ development in the first couple of neonatal weeks displays a progression of A-D synapse elimination, functional reinforcement, and eventual structural consolidation (Lichtman and Colman, 2000; Walsh and Lichtman, 2003). Consistently, impeding neural activity results in slowed synaptic refinement in the mouse neuromusculature, and enhancing activity increases the rate of development (Thompson, 1985).

Humans show similar mechanisms of A-D neural circuit development (**Figure 1B**). For example, the auditory cortex displays an early age critical window of experience-dependent maturation, with professional musicians developing asymmetric brain features when exposed to music before the age of 7. Specifically, development of absolute pitch correlates with a larger left planum temporale (Schlaug et al., 1995), and enlarged cortical representation of the left hand in dexterous string players (Elbert et al., 1995; Schlaug et al., 1995). Auditory cortical development may actually represent a more extensive (or indefinite) critical period, as compared to other sensory modalities (Kilgard and Merzenich, 1998; Chang and Merzenich, 2003). This relative extension may result from a late peak of parvalbumin-expressing (PV+) interneurons, as described in ferret brain development (Gao et al., 2000). The emergence of these inhibitory interneurons is progressive (Honig et al., 1996) and vital for the proper formation of cortical circuits (**Figure 1C**; Powell et al., 2012). The auditory critical period is not open ended, however, as childhood ear infections leading to long-term deficits in auditory perceptual acuity can occur if not treated before the age of 7 (Popescu and Polley, 2010). These select

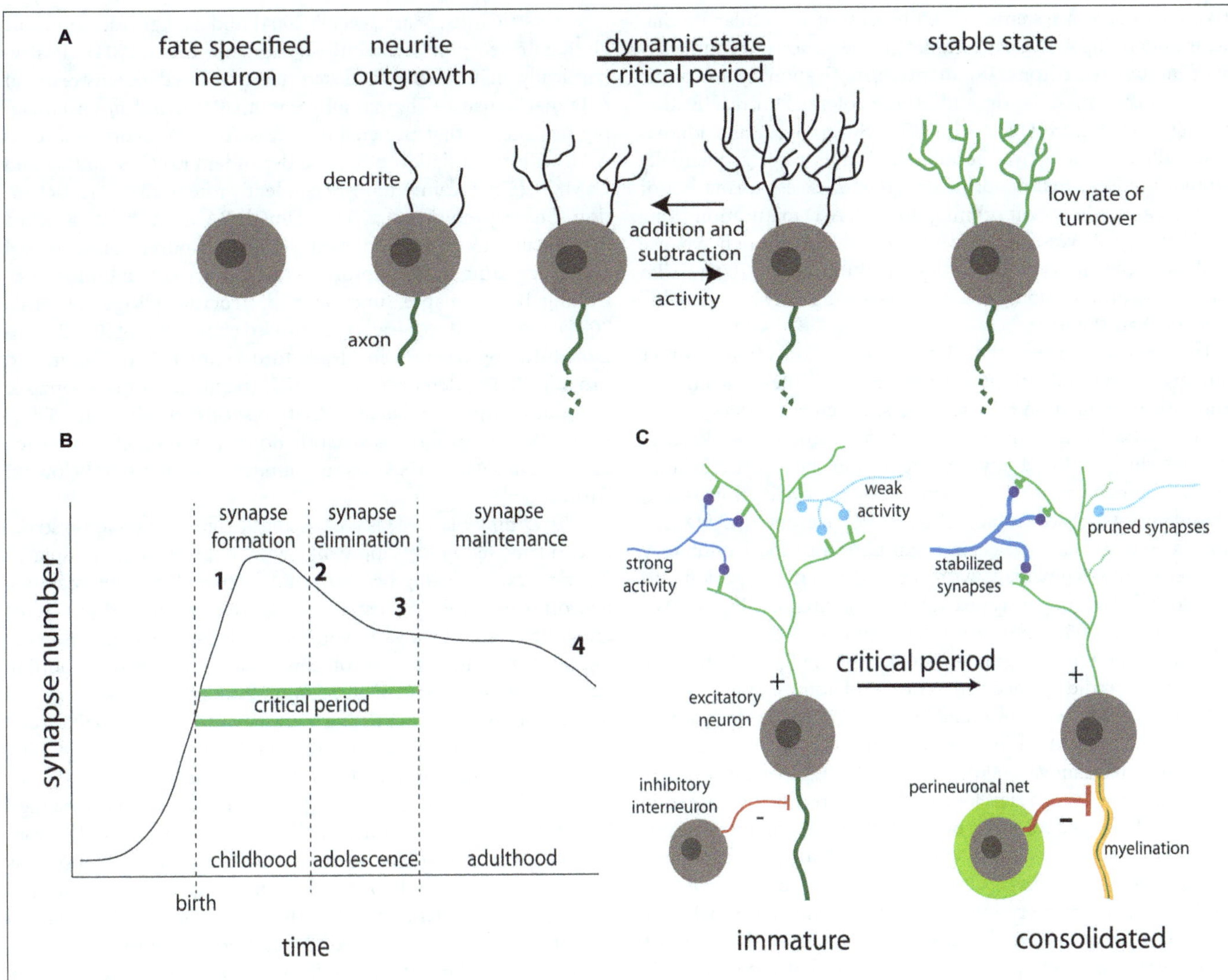

FIGURE 1 | Activity-dependent synaptic remodeling during critical periods. (A) Progression of dendrite development. Highly dynamic dendrites occur in the A-D critical period prior to consolidation of relatively stable mature connections (Kreutz and Sala, 2012). **(B)** Synapse number changes as a function of age. Defects in synaptogenesis (formation, pruning, and stabilization) correlate with onset of specific neurological disorder classes, including intellectual disability (1), ASDs (2), schizophrenia (3), and Alzheimer's disease (4) (for example, Penzes et al., 2011). **(C)** Activity-dependent synapse changes occur during the critical period, in which synaptic partnerships are solidified or dissolved prior to consolidation, coinciding with inhibitory interneuron innervation, progressive myelination and the formation of extracellular perineuronal nets (Hensch, 2003).

examples illustrate normal A-D development within single sensory modalities. ASD symptoms may manifest through faulty A-D development in a number of sensory systems, with impairments of higher-order cognition circuitry developing after formation of primary sensory circuitry (Belmonte et al., 2004; Geschwind and Levitt, 2007). Although ASD diagnoses focuses on higher order cognitive tasks such as social communication, language and cognitive development, and repetitive behaviors (Zwaigenbaum et al., 2013), precursor deficits in primary sensory processing are characteristic (Marco et al., 2011). A more detailed discussion of ASD phenotypes is presented in Part 2.

CRITICAL PERIODS OF NEURAL CIRCUIT DEVELOPMENT

The highly dynamic nature of synaptic connectivity is largely a transient feature of neurodevelopment: long-term imaging of dendritic spines in adult mice reveals that most mature synapses are relatively stable (Grutzendler et al., 2002). The critical window (or critical period) theory has emerged to explain the decline in synaptic dynamics as the brain develops, and as a mechanistic foundation toward understanding ASD disease states (**Figure 1**; Hensch, 2004). A critical period defines a temporary developmental window of heightened sensitivity to sensory stimuli, which drive connectivity changes (Holtmaat and Svoboda, 2009), with A-D modulation reduced after the window passes, as reflected by the decrease in spine turnover as the brain matures (Trachtenberg et al., 2002; Holtmaat et al., 2005; Zuo et al., 2005). The key critical period hallmarks include (1) competition between circuit elements, (2) neural activity regulation, (3) structural solidification of maintained connections, (4) sharply-defined experience-dependent window, (5) variable/hierarchical timing and duration of windows across systems, (6) a diversity of molecular mechanisms underlying A-D modulation, (7) emergence and connectivity of inhibitory neurons, (8) attention/motivation by aminergic and cholinergic modulation, and (9) the potential for reactivation in adulthood (**Figure 1**; Hensch, 2004). Synaptogenesis underlies these hallmarks in critical periods, and takes place sequentially through initial axonal/dendritic outgrowth, excess formation of synapses, and subsequent pruning through A-D maturation (Katz and Shatz, 1996; West and Greenberg, 2011). Although synapse regulation continues throughout life (Holtmaat et al., 2005; Grillo et al., 2013), peak synaptogenesis occurs during early postnatal life (Pan and Gan, 2008).

The terminal periods of critical windows coincide with other hallmarks of neurodevelopment (**Figure 1C**). These include the progressive myelination of nerve fibers, which is a process essential for cortical function; mice caged in isolation 2 weeks after weaning show reduced myelin and diminished cortical function (Makinodan et al., 2012). Importantly, myelination is also delayed in FXS (Pacey et al., 2013). Also relevant to ASD disease states is the emergence and maturation of local inhibitory (I) interneurons coincident with the end of critical periods, to provide balance to young excitatory (E) circuits (**Figure 1C**; Hensch, 2004, 2005). The correct development of E/I ratio is critical to neural circuit output, and defects in the E/I ratio balance is a leading candidate mechanism for explaining the emergence of ASD disease states (Gatto and Broadie, 2010). Both hyperexcitation and hypoinhibition are recurring themes in numerous ASD models (Casanova, 2006). More generally, genetic disruption of cortical interneuron development causes regional GABAergic deficits, epilepsy and ASD-like behavioral changes in mice (Powell et al., 2003). As one example, mice deficient for the axon guidance receptor *neuropilin 2* display reduced cortical interneuron numbers and are more prone to seizure following neuronal excitation (Gant et al., 2009). Thus, the critical period theory must include the temporally phased regulation of first excitatory and then inhibitory synapses, such that A-D synapse selection generates the appropriate E/I synapse ratio balance. There are other hallmarks of critical period cessation, including the A-D establishment of the perineuronal network, a matrix of chondroitin sulfate proteoglycans (**Figure 1C**; Ye and Miao, 2013). Roles of glycan modifications in ASD models will be further discussed below in Part 2.

ACTIVITY-DEPENDENT SYNAPSE MECHANISMS IN *Drosophila*

Synaptic ultrastructure and function is remarkably conserved across species, for example, comparing mammalian brain glutamatergic synapses to *Drosophila* NMJ glutamatergic synapses (Schuster, 2006). Moreover, the underlying molecular elements of synapses are similarly extremely well conserved, allowing mutually complementary studies in animals ranging from rodents to flies (Featherstone and Broadie, 2000; Koles and Budnik, 2012). Most A-D work in *Drosophila* has focused on axonal (presynaptic) development (Rohrbough et al., 2003), whereas most comparable work in mouse has focused on dendritic (postsynaptic) spines. However, the *Drosophila* NMJ postsynaptic domain is well described and clearly subject to extensive A-D remodeling. It contains two functional classes of ionotropic glutamate receptors (iGluRs; Marrus et al., 2004) and a single metabotropic glutamate receptor (DmGluRA; Bogdanik et al., 2004). Postsynaptically, iGluRs are trafficked and stabilized downstream of A-D mechanisms (Thomas and Sigrist, 2012), and *in vivo* imaging has shown that presynaptic release of dense core vesicles is A-D, with potentiation of release dependent on Ca^{2+} influx and CaMKII (Ca^{2+}/calmodulin-dependent protein kinase II) activation (Shakiryanova et al., 2007). DmGluRA nulls show increased A-D facilitation and decreased synaptic boutons of increased size, suggesting the receptor acts as an activity monitor controlling both synapse function and structure (Bogdanik et al., 2004). DmGluRA loss leads to increased expression of iGluRs, and DmGluRA over-expression leads to decreased iGluRs (Pan and Broadie, 2007), demonstrating a tight regulation of postsynaptic receptor composition as an activity response mechanism. These A-D processes in the postsynaptic domain are directly impacted in the *Drosophila* FXS disease model as discussed below in Part 2.

The *Drosophila* NMJ is a particularly dynamic synaptic structure during early development, with A-D growth modulated during larval crawling behavior and mediated via glutamatergic neurotransmission (Schuster, 2006). Live imaging shows NMJ growth proceeds by a variety of mechanisms: stretching of existing boutons and insertion of new boutons in between, adding new boutons to the end of an existing strand, *de novo* addition and branch formation from existing boutons (Zito et al., 1999). A crude method to increase NMJ transmission is through chronic rearing at 29–30°C, which results in accelerated synapse growth (Sigrist et al., 2003; Zhong and Wu, 2004). Spaced depolarization via high K^+ saline application leads to the rapid extension and retraction of short filopodia, and the formation of synaptic boutons (Ataman et al., 2006). Reduced membrane excitability via inward current mutants (*paralytic* Na^+ channel) or other Na^+ channel loss-of-function (*tipE* or $mle^{nap-ts1}$) leads to improper synaptic refinement (Jarecki and Keshishian, 1995; White et al., 2001), with significantly smaller synaptic boutons (Lnenicka et al., 2003). Acute depolarization of the NMJ leads to the formation of "ghost boutons," that initially lack presynaptic active zones and postsynaptic iGluRs, which appear on a timescale of hours (Ataman et al., 2006, 2008). Generation of genetically targetable channels, such as the voltage-dependent UAS-EKO and UAS-Kir2.1 (Baines et al., 2001; Paradis et al., 2001), and the constitutively open UAS-dORK potassium channel shunt (White et al., 2001) allow a more precise dissection of the effects of activity regulating NMJ synaptic morphology. Recent advances in bioengineering have taken advantage of channel variants for genetically targeted hyperexcitation in *Drosophila*, including the *transient receptor potential* (TrpA1; Hamada et al., 2008) and TrpM8 thermogenic channels (Peabody et al., 2009), the constitutively active NaChBac channel (Nitabach et al., 2006), the expanding family of channelrhodopsin (ChR2) variants (Schroll et al., 2006; Ataman et al., 2008), and the hyperpolarizing eNpHR3.0 channel (Inada et al., 2011). These new methods will be more fully described below in Part 3.

Beyond neurotransmission *per se*, proper formation of the *Drosophila* NMJ entails other A-D *trans*-synaptic signaling mechanisms. Wnt signaling via wingless (Wg; Packard et al., 2002;

Korkut and Budnik, 2009) functions downstream of activity (high K^+ depolarization, ChR stimulation) to regulate both structural and functional development (Ataman et al., 2008; Korkut et al., 2009). Similarly in mammals, activity regulates *Wnt2* transcription, which stimulates dendritic arborization in hippocampal cultures (Wayman et al., 2006). Bone morphogenetic protein (BMP) signaling via glass bottom boat (Gbb; McCabe et al., 2003; Keshishian and Kim, 2004) leads to NMJ stabilization through LIM kinase 1 activity, preventing retraction and synapse loss (Eaton and Davis, 2005). Recent use of *Shaker* K^+ channel mutants (or raising temperature to 30°C) to increase excitability, shows that retrograde BMP signaling is required for A-D NMJ growth and maturation (Berke et al., 2013). Heparan sulfate proteoglycan (HSPG) co-receptors of such signaling ligands (Ren et al., 2009), including Dally-like protein (Dlp) and Syndecan (Sdc), play important roles in NMJ synaptogenesis (Johnson et al., 2006; Dani et al., 2012). Importantly, HSPGs interact closely with FMRP to modulate *trans*-synaptic signaling in the *Drosophila* FXS disease model (Friedman et al., 2013), suggesting a link to A-D processes. Laminin A (LanA) is another extracellular synaptic protein of interest that is downregulated in response to activity to regulate synaptic architecture: LanA expression is inversely correlated with NMJ size, and is regulated by larval crawling activity, synapse excitation, postsynaptic response, and Wnt signaling (Tsai et al., 2012). These A-D processes in the presynaptic domain are directly impacted in the *Drosophila* FXS disease model as discussed below in Part 2.

Although A-D development has been explored at length at the *Drosophila* NMJ, more limited studies have examined A-D mechanisms in the brain, mainly focusing on the mushroom body (MB) learning and memory center (Zars et al., 2000; Margulies et al., 2005). These studies have been enhanced by recent generation of more targeted Gal4 drivers and new optogenetic tools allowing cell-autonomous, single-cell resolution dissection of A-D mechanisms in normal and disease states (Chiang et al., 2011). Using the mosaic analysis with a repressible cell marker (MARCM) clonal technique (Lee and Luo, 2001), characterization of MB axons shows critical period development at the level of individual cells: synaptic branches display significant A-D pruning during the early-use period following eclosion, but become relatively static at maturity (Tessier and Broadie, 2008). Importantly, sensory deprivation (SD) elevated synaptic branch number during this critical period, whereas activity depolarization of single-cell MARCM clones by ChR2 optical stimulation significant decreased synaptic branching during this same critical period (Tessier and Broadie, 2008). Similarly, recent work silencing olfactory sensory neurons (via UAS-Kir2.1; Limb3b-Gal4 or UAS-DorK; Limb3b) lead to immature axonal morphology, including broad axon terminals and multiple filopodia (Prieto-Godino et al., 2012). Silencing of a limited subset of projection neurons innervating the MB (UAS-dORK1.deltaC; Mz19-Gal4) leads to increased size, number, and active zone density of axon terminals within the microglumeruli of the MB calyx (Kremer et al., 2010). These A-D processes in the brain MB learning/memory center are directly impacted in the *Drosophila* FXS disease model, as discussed below in Part 2.

Information on A-D mechanisms regulating dendrites in the *Drosophila* genetic model is more limited, but this research focus is rapidly expanding. For example, motor neuron dendrite structural development has been shown to be regulated downstream of high K^+ depolarization (Hartwig et al., 2008; Zwart et al., 2013). Moreover, a role for synaptic activity in dendritic remodeling has been shown via targeted transgenic tetanus toxin expression (UAS-TNT; Sweeney et al., 1995) blocking neurotransmitter release from cholinergic interneurons (Cha-Gal4; UAS-TNT) leads to increased dendritic structural complexity (Tripodi et al., 2008). Dendritic refinement in serotonergic neuron pupal development is also modulated by activity: hyperpolarization via UAS-Kir2.1 caused increased dendritic length, which was proposed to be due to A-D Wnt/Wg signaling with a pro-retraction role in sensory-input dendritic refinement (Singh et al., 2010). Similarly, the silencing of olfactory sensory neurons (via UAS-Kir2.1; Orco-Gal4) led to enhanced dendritic occupancy of the antennal lobe by projection neurons (Prieto-Godino et al., 2012). However, it is also clear that A-D differences may be found across different neuronal types or developmental stages. For example, increased firing of RP2 motor neurons caused by dominant negative *Shaker* and *eag* K^+ channel mutations resulted in increased dendritic complexity, whereas Kir2.1 silencing resulted in decreased dendritic structure (Timmermans et al., 2013). Moreover, constitutively active CaMKII also led to increased dendrite length and branching (Timmermans et al., 2013). Use of the temperature-gated TrpA1 channel to activate neuron firing demonstrated that MN5 flight motor neuron dendrites respond to activity differently over time: increased activity before pupal day 6 caused decreased dendritic branching (Vonhoff et al., 2013), whereas increased activity later in development caused increased branching (Duch et al., 2008), again suggesting differential A-D critical periods.

Mammalian models of dendritogenesis display similar A-D mechanisms to those characterized above in *Drosophila.* For example, increased neural activity and glutamatergic signaling led to dendritic spine outgrowth (Jontes and Smith, 2000; Antar et al., 2006), and spine turnover rates in young mice were shown to be sensory experience-dependent (Trachtenberg et al., 2002). Long-term SD through whisker trimming led to dendritic spine pruning that was more prominent in young mice (Zuo et al., 2005), and spine synapse densities changed upon rearing or training in enriched environments (Greenough et al., 1985; Beaulieu and Colonnier, 1987; Moser et al., 1995). Spaced depolarization of hippocampal neurons in culture led to extension of new spines, a process correlated with A-D MAPK activation (Wu et al., 2001). Recent advances in live imaging have elegantly provided *in vivo* evidence of A-D dendritic spine dynamics (Alvarez and Sabatini, 2007; Holtmaat and Svoboda, 2009). As one example, the immediate early gene Arc/Arg3.1 functions to eliminate surplus climbing fibers (CF) onto Purkinje cell synapses in the cerebellum, a process that is accelerated with ChR2 depolarizing stimulation for 2 days and suppressed by targeted CF knockdown of voltage-gated Ca^{2+} channels (Mikuni et al., 2013). Limited regions of the adult brain remain amenable to similar changes, for example, hippocampal spine density increased in adult rats following spatial learning (Moser et al., 1995), and multiphoton imaging of dendritic spines during mGluR-induced long-term depression (LTD) showed spine shrinkage and spine elimination that persisted for up to 24 h (Ramiro-Cortes and Israely, 2013), but in general these synaptic dynamics are confined to critical periods of synaptogenesis during defined developmental windows.

ACTIVITY-DEPENDENT TRANSCRIPTIONAL AND TRANSLATIONAL REGULATION OF SYNAPTOGENESIS

Activity-dependent gene transcription clearly leads to developmental changes in synaptic connectivity. Mouse studies of the transcriptional regulator methyl CpG binding protein 2 (MeCP2) are one elegant example, with knock-in mouse lacking the *neuronal activity-induced phosphorylation* (NAIP) sequence showing increased excitatory synaptogenesis (Li et al., 2011). MeCP2 is phosphorylated in response to activity and subsequent Ca^{2+} influx (CaMKII-dependent), leading to regulation of dendritic branching, spine morphogenesis, and A-D induction of brain-derived neurotrophic factor (BDNF) transcription (Zhou et al., 2006). Importantly, MeCP2-deficient mice exhibit delayed maturation of cortical synaptogenesis and neuronal architecture defects (Fukuda et al., 2005), and human MeCP2 mutations are causally associated with the ASD Rett syndrome (Amir et al., 1999). Indeed, many ASD candidate genes are expressed synaptically to modulate synapse function/morphology, and are directly regulated by synaptic activity (Zoghbi and Bear, 2012). Calcium influx has a profound impact on gene transcription (Greer and Greenberg, 2008). As one example, A-D Ca^{2+} influx leads to dephosphorylation of myocyte enhancing factor 2 (MEF2) by calcineurin, causing dissociation with histone deacetylases, CBP recruitment and ultimately, transcription-dependent synapse elimination (Flavell et al., 2006; Barbosa et al., 2008; Pulipparacharuvil et al., 2008). MEF2 activation also leads to suppression of excitatory synapse number via Arc (Flavell et al., 2006; Flavell and Greenberg, 2008), perhaps through Arc-mediated AMPA receptor internalization (Niere et al., 2012). This MEF2-regulated synapse elimination has been correlated with the acquisition of learning and memory abilities (Barbosa et al., 2008), such as those impacted in ASD disease states. Activity similarly regulates cAMP response element-binding protein (CREB), serum response factor (SRF), FBJ murine osteosarcoma viral oncogene (Fos; Greenberg et al., 1986), and neuronal PAS domain protein 4 (NPAS4; Lin et al., 2008), leading to the A-D transcriptional regulation of synaptic proteins, including ASD-associated BDNF, Arc, and ubiquitin-protein ligase E3A (Ube3A; Cohen and Greenberg, 2008; Greer and Greenberg, 2008). CREB and NPAS4 transcriptional activity, via BDNF A-D activation, also leads to a reduced number of inhibitory synapses on excitatory neurons (Hong et al., 2008; Lin et al., 2008), suggesting roles in the developmental regulation of E/I ratio.

Activity-dependent localized synaptic translation permits a rapid and synapse-specific response, which is particularly important in governing the multitude of differentially active synapses occurring at a distance from the cell body. RNA-binding proteins and translational regulation have been demonstrated in both axonal growth cones and mature axons (Hornberg and Holt, 2013), ostensibly permitting local protein production in presynaptic boutons. Highly motile RNA granules containing inactive ribosomes (Krichevsky and Kosik, 2001; Elvira et al., 2006), suggest neurons have evolved mechanisms to bypass translation initiation locally at the synapse (Costa-Mattioli et al., 2009; Batish et al., 2012). Assays of local translation using ribopuromycylation to visualize ribosomes associated with nascent peptide chains (David et al., 2012) demonstrate that mRNAs are transported alongside paused polyribosomes at hippocampal synapse, thereby bypassing the rate-limiting step of translation initiation (Graber et al., 2013). Importantly, these polyribosomes co-localize with RNA-binding FMRP and Staufen 2 (Antar et al., 2005; Elvira et al., 2006; Napoli et al., 2008; Darnell et al., 2011; Lebeau et al., 2011), and defects in A-D translational control can lead to ASD states, with unregulated translation causing synaptic impairment driving behavioral dysfunction (Santini et al., 2013). This topic will be explored at length in Part 2.

The strongest link between translation control and A-D synaptogenesis is the RNA-binding FMRP, which regulates translational initiation (Napoli et al., 2008), mRNA transport (Bassell and Warren, 2008), and translational elongation of mRNAs encoding synaptic proteins (Darnell et al., 2011). FMRP is strongly upregulated during critical periods of neural circuit refinement, where it associates with mobile RNA granules in dendrites, spines, filopodia, and growth cones that translocate in response to the level of neuronal activity (Antar et al., 2005; Cook et al., 2011). Importantly, FMRP is positivity upregulated by neuronal activity (Antar et al., 2004; Gabel et al., 2004; Tessier and Broadie, 2008; Wang et al., 2008b), and regulates multiple A-D processes including synapse elimination (Pfeiffer et al., 2010). Studies at the *Drosophila* NMJ first demonstrated that FMRP negatively regulates cytoskeletal targets, including the MAP1B/Futsch (Zhang et al., 2001) mediator of microtubule-associated synaptic growth (Roos et al., 2000). Interestingly, A-D transcriptional and translational control are linked through FMRP, as the activity of MEF2 in synapse elimination is wholly dependent on FMRP function, and occurs cell autonomously in the postsynaptic neuron (Pfeiffer et al., 2010). In *Fmr1* knockout (KO) hippocampal culture, acute expression of FMRP (via timed transfection) at an early postnatal period leads to synapse growth, but FMRP during the second postnatal week led to suppression of synapse formation (Zang et al., 2013). Interestingly, MEF2 activity is progressively increased upon depolarization (via high K^+ treatment) over the same developmental period (Zang et al., 2013). These recent studies highlight both the impact of FMRP on synaptic growth and the importance of developmental timing within critical periods of development. In the following section (Part 2) we will elaborate the molecular details of FXS and other ASDs, highlighting A-D changes in the development of synaptic connectivity.

PART 2: ACTIVITY-DEPENDENT MECHANISMS IN ASD DISEASE STATES

For ASD diagnosis, children must display three core symptoms before 3 years of age: (1) atypical social behavior, (2) disrupted verbal/non-verbal communication, and (3) unusual patterns of restricted interests or repetitive behaviors (Geschwind and Levitt, 2007). It has been proposed that a "disconnect" between brain regions involved in higher-order associations lies at the root of these ASD behaviors (Frith, 2004; Courchesne and Pierce, 2005; for historical context, Geschwind, 1965a,b). For example, this disconnect may occur between a pair of higher-order association cortices (or several such centers), which represent input from multiple sensory modalities in cortical space (Geschwind and Levitt, 2007). More evidence for this disconnect theory comes from prefrontal cortex and anterior cingulate disconnection for joint attention (foundation of language and social behavior; Mundy, 2003), and demonstrated disconnect in functional magnetic resources imaging (fMRI) studies (Koshino et al., 2005). The root of this hypothesis is based on the hierarchical development of cortical circuitry (LeBlanc and Fagiolini, 2011; i.e., disrupted development of the initial architecture, e.g., via shifts in critical periods) results in faulty substrates for subsequent A-D mechanisms that are crucial for reorganization, pruning, and solidification of synapses within circuits. Primary sensory cortices develop progressively, with critical periods that are variable in time and often non-overlapping (Kroon et al., 2013). Furthermore, individual modalities develop progressively, as the critical periods of rodent somatosensory cortex begin at the subcortical level and then progress to cortical levels (Feldmeyer et al., 2013). The "missed window" theory of ASDs may help explain the root of auditory, visual, and somatosensory dysfunction in information processing, which drives the socialization and communication deficits defining ASDs (LeBlanc and Fagiolini, 2011). In terms of basic brain architecture, ASDs may emerge through faulty subcortical development, which precedes thalamic as well as subsequent cortical development (Kroon et al., 2013). Evidence for this theory includes early incidence of motor developmental delay, social impairment, and epileptic seizures (Zoghbi and Bear, 2012).

The hierarchical model of ASD brain development is built upon evidence that alterations in primary sensory modalities underlie higher order cognition defects. Broadly speaking, these primary sensory alterations appear to lessen in severity with age, although the severity of primary sensory impairments clearly correlates with the degree of social interaction impairment (Ben-Sasson et al., 2009; Simmons et al., 2009). Neuronal activity is essential for circuit development (Lendvai et al., 2000; Spitzer, 2006), and this activity is both intrinsically generated (Golshani et al., 2009; Rochefort et al., 2009) and sensory derived, as shown in primary visual cortex (Siegel et al., 2012). However, this A-D component of circuit development is obviously built upon genetic foundations, and several hundred genes are associated with ASDs (State and Sestan, 2012). Clinical characterizations of ASDs are highly suggestive of A-D synaptic defects (Toro et al., 2010; Ebert and Greenberg, 2013). For example, FXS patients display hypersensitivity to numerous sensory stimuli (Miller et al., 1999), as well as abnormal sensory gating in prepulse inhibition trials (Hessl et al., 2009). In addition, attention deficit/hyperactivity disorder (Murray, 2010) and developmentally transient epilepsy are also associated with FXS (Musumeci et al., 1999; Berry-Kravis, 2002) strongly indicating a core A-D impairment.

Although it is understandably difficult to model ASD behaviors in animals, several recent studies demonstrate inventive ways to address this essential issue. For example, *Fmr1* KO mice display many behavioral disruptions similar to human FXS patients, including susceptibility to audiogenic seizure, hyperactivity, learning and memory deficits, and social interaction abnormalities (Kooy, 2003; Bear et al., 2004; Hagerman et al., 2009). Some studies report that *Fmr1* KO mice show increased anxiety-related activity during social interaction (Mines et al., 2010), whereas other studies show *decreased* anxiety in open field studies (Michalon et al., 2014). It is quite clear that behavioral phenotypic effects are heavily dependent on genetic background (Spencer et al., 2011). However, *Fmr1* KO mice in the C57 background show consistent impairments in social interaction behaviors (Baker et al., 2010). Research in mice has also focused on single sensory modalities, showing that *Fmr1* KO mice display altered auditory processing (Rotschafer and Razak, 2013). Although higher cognition is difficult to test in mice, recent research using a touchscreen operant conditioning paradigm (which facilitates a conflict between sensory-driven and task-dependent signals, thereby increasing cognitive load) demonstrates that *Fmr1* KO mice display defects in learning under heavy cognitive demand (Dickson et al., 2013). The *Drosophila* FXS model similarly shows disruptions closely resembling human FXS patients, including hyperactivity, learning/memory deficits, and social interaction abnormalities (Bolduc et al., 2008, 2010a,b; Coffee et al., 2010, 2012; Tessier and Broadie, 2012).

CRITICAL PERIOD DEVELOPMENT OF E/I RATIOS IN ASDs

Autism spectrum disorders have been ascribed to altered E/I synaptic balance, which likely reflects defects in A-D synapse elimination/addition specific to different classes of synapse (Rubenstein and Merzenich, 2003; Hensch, 2005; Ramocki and Zoghbi, 2008; Gatto and Broadie, 2010). Neural circuits must carefully balance excitatory and inhibitory connections during critical period development, and theories of synaptic homeostasis posit that compensatory alterations prevent runaway signaling (Turrigiano and Nelson, 2004; Maffei and Fontanini, 2009). The appearance of altered E/I ratio is linked with critical periods of brain development, as runaway hyperexcitable circuits fail to mature properly without inhibitory input (Rubenstein and Merzenich, 2003; Rippon et al., 2007). In support of this idea, postmortem neocortex tissue from ASD patients shows reduced vertical arrays of glutamatergic and GABAergic mini-columns and disordered peripheral neuropil space (Casanova, 2006). Moreover, ASD postmortem studies reveal a reduction in glutamic acid decarboxylase (GAD), the rate-limiting enzyme in GABA synthesis (Fatemi et al., 2002). On the postsynaptic membrane, samples from ASD patient brains also contain reduced GABA-A receptor expression (Fatemi et al., 2009a,b). Crucially, excitatory circuits must be balanced by GABAergic inhibitory interneurons that form connections progressively during late-stage critical period development (Bacci et al., 2005). Competing theories of both hypoinhibition (GABAergic deficits) and hyperexcitation (excitatory excess) underlying autistic disease states are well known (Gatto and Broadie, 2010). However, many results support hypoinhibition models that complement hyperexcitation models; these models are not necessarily mutually exclusive and may represent two counterbalancing underpinnings of ASD disease states.

Fragile X syndrome is among the best-characterized ASD disease states. FMRP is found at the synapse, positivity upregulated by

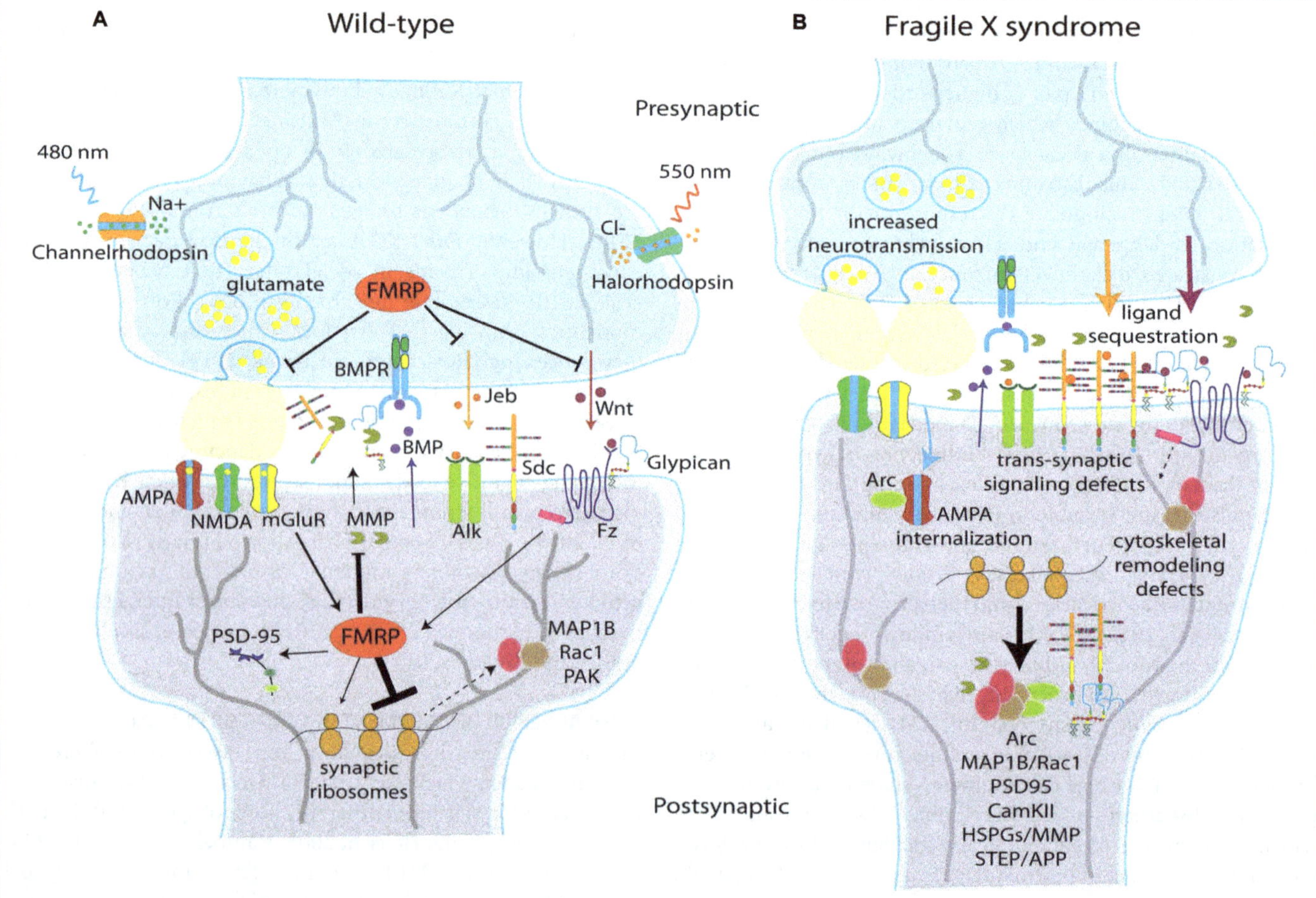

FIGURE 2 | Synaptic changes in the Fragile X syndrome disease state. Schematic depictions of glutamatergic synapses in wild type **(A)** and FXS **(B)** conditions showing molecular changes in the response to activity. Data reflect human FXS patient studies, as well as mouse and *Drosophila* FXS animal models. **(A)** In wild-type, FMRP regulates glutamate release and anterograde *trans*-synaptic signaling (e.g., Jeb and Wnt), but does not demonstrably affect retrograde signaling (e.g., BMP; Friedman et al., 2013). FMRP acts as a translational repressor limiting synthesis of cytoskeletal regulators (e.g., MAP1B, Rac1, PAK; Zhang et al., 2001; Bongmba et al., 2011; Dolan et al., 2013), AMPA-R regulators (e.g., Arc; Costa et al., 2012; Niere et al., 2012), MMPs (Bilousova et al., 2009), and heparan sulfate proteoglycans (HSPGs: Dlp and Syd; Dani et al., 2012). FMRP is activity regulated downstream of mGluR signaling, but likely responds to other activity signals as well. **(B)** In the FXS state, lack of FMRP leads to increased neurotransmission, increased HSPG production (which in turn sequester anterograde *trans*-synaptic signaling molecules), increased MMP synthesis/activity, cytoskeletal remodeling defects, and changes in postsynaptic AMPA glutamate receptor cycling. Two engineered rhodopsin variants allow non-invasive modulation of neural activity: channelrhodopsin responds to 480 nm blue light to gate Na^+ influx (depolarization), and halorhodopsin responds to 550 nm amber light to gate Cl^- influx (hyperpolarization; Fenno et al., 2011).

neuronal activity and regulates A-D processes including synapse elimination (**Figure 2**; Antar et al., 2004; Gabel et al., 2004; Tessier and Broadie, 2008; Wang et al., 2008a; Pfeiffer et al., 2010). FXS may be characterized by a failure to remove immature synaptic connections and properly balance E/I synapse ratio during critical period development (Comery et al., 1997; Irwin et al., 2000, 2001; Galvez et al., 2005; McKinney et al., 2005). For example, *Fmr1* KO mice display brain-region specific increases and decreases in GAD expression (D'Hulst et al., 2006; Adusei et al., 2010); increased in cortex, brainstem, and diencephalon (El Idrissi et al., 2005), and decreased in amygdala (Olmos-Serrano et al., 2010). FMRP also regulates GABA-A receptor expression (Liu et al., 2013), as *Fmr1* KOs show reduced GABA-R subunit mRNA (D'Hulst et al., 2006; Gantois et al., 2006) and protein (El Idrissi et al., 2005; Curia et al., 2009; Adusei et al., 2010). Recent work suggests that the timing rather than the absolute expression levels of $GABA_A$Rs α1, α2, and gephyrin are altered in *Fmr1* KO mice (Kratovac and Corbin, 2013), once again supporting the theory of critical period dysfunction. It is now clear that GABAergic changes are regionally specific, as *Fmr1* KO mice display reduced inhibitory synapses within the basolateral amygdala (Olmos-Serrano et al., 2010), yet increased inhibitory synapses are noted in CA1 region of hippocampus (Dahlhaus and El-Husseini, 2010), providing direct evidence of E/I imbalance. *Fmr1*-deficient mice exhibit defects in GABAergic neocortical circuits (Selby et al., 2007), with differences in the neocortical E/I balance (Gibson et al., 2008). There is some conflicting data from functional GABAergic studies, with decreased tonic inhibition in recordings from subicular neurons (Curia et al., 2009), decreased tonic and phasic inhibition in the amygdala (Olmos-Serrano et al., 2010), and increased inhibitory transmission in striatal spiny neurons (Centonze et al., 2008) all reported in the mouse FXS model. A recent study reports a cell-specific presynaptic role for FMRP in excitatory neurotransmission onto inhibitory interneurons in layer 4 of mouse cortex (Patel et al., 2013), with mice mosaic for *Fmr1* displaying decreased glutamate release probability. This defect was not observed in neurotransmission between excitatory neurons, showing a cell-specific role for FMRP and a potential mechanistic basis for E/I imbalance in the FXS disease state.

The opposing side of the E/I ratio – excitatory signaling – is even better explored in ASD models, especially in the FXS disease state (Rubenstein and Merzenich, 2003). Excitatory neurons are intrinsically more excitable in *Fmr1* KO mice (Gibson et al., 2008), with elevated Ca^{2+} signaling (Goncalves et al., 2013) and excitatory networks that are structurally hyperconnected (although individual excitatory connections are slower; Testa-Silva et al., 2012). Excessive mGluR signaling, as a reporter of glutamatergic synapse activity state, is widely reported (Bear et al., 2004; Bear, 2005). The mGluR theory of FXS suggests that disease symptoms are due to exaggerated downstream consequences of aberrant mGluR1/5 signaling. Crucially, FMRP is locally synthesized in response to mGluR activation (Weiler et al., 1997), and mGluR-mediated hippocampal LTD is exaggerated in *Fmr1* KO mice (Huber et al., 2002; Nosyreva and Huber, 2006). FMRP is dephosphorylated (by PP2A) upon stimulation of group I mGluRs, which leads to a rapid increase in translation (Narayanan et al., 2007). In line with these studies, mGluR5 heterozygosity rescues many of *Fmr1* KO mice phenotypes (Dolen et al., 2007). Also, group 1 mGluR antagonists [e.g., MPEP (2-methyl-6-(phenylethynyl)-pyridine)] ameliorate several behavioral phenotypes in *Fmr1* KO mice (Yan et al., 2005; Choi et al., 2010b). Recent mechanistic studies show that mGluRA activation starts a cascade of events leading to FMRP phosphorylation and subsequent synthesis of Arc, and ultimately mGluR-associated LTD (Niere et al., 2012). In addition, activation of serotonin 7 receptors (5-HT7) can reverse mGluR-induced AMPA internalization in FXS model mice, effectively correcting mGluR-LTD (Costa et al., 2012). Although initial formation of auditory cortex is normal in *Fmr1* KO mice, mutants fail to undergo experience-dependent reorganization, suggesting an altered auditory critical period that is mGluR-dependent, as MPEP suppressed the sound-induced reorganization phenotype (Kim et al., 2013a). Sensory-dependent reorganization of auditory cortex has been explored at length, with A-D changes in hippocampus including neurogenesis, learning and memory, and neural connectivity (Chaudhury et al., 2013).

There are some caveats with the mouse FXS model. One issue is the timing of the FMRP loss, as in mouse models the *Fmr1* gene is deleted and therefore not expressed (Mientjes et al., 2006), whereas the human gene is silenced via methylation during embryonic development, but is expressed at early stages (Willemsen et al., 2002). Furthermore, human patients may display *Fmr1* mosaicism across cell types, due to methylation specificity or variable presence of a premutation (Stoger et al., 2011). Finally, mouse *Fmr1* phenotypic effects are often surprisingly mild, transient, and heavily dependent on genetic background (Spencer et al., 2011). Although the *Drosophila* FXS model does not address the first two issues, *dfmr1* null phenotypes are generally both more robust and more penetrant (Tessier and Broadie, 2012). Excitatory synaptic signaling (glutamatergic and cholinergic) pathways have both been extensively studied in the *Drosophila* FXS model (**Figure 2**). Electrophysiological studies indicate increased excitability, A-D synaptic vesicle cycling and neurotransmission in *dfmr1* null glutamatergic synapses (Zhang et al., 2001; Gatto and Broadie, 2008). *Drosophila* FMRP and sole mGluR (DmGluRA) display mutual feedback regulation, as FMRP expression increases with the loss of *dmGluRA*, and DmGluRA expression increases with loss of *dfmr1* (Pan et al., 2008). Crucially, many FXS phenotypes are ameliorated by feeding of mGluR antagonists (e.g., MPEP; McBride et al., 2005; Choi et al., 2011), and MPEP phenocopies the genetic loss of *dmGluRA* (Pan and Broadie, 2007; Pan et al., 2008). Importantly, *dfmr1*; *dmGluRA* double null mutants partially rescue excitatory defects witnessed under high frequency stimulation paradigms (Repicky and Broadie, 2009), providing a partial genetic basis for a hyperexcitable state in FXS. In the absence of FMRP, increased mGluR function leads to decreased cyclic AMP, which is further correlated with deficits in olfactory learning and memory (Kanellopoulos et al., 2012). Intriguingly, cAMP positively regulates transcription of *dfmr1*, via PKA and CREB (Kanellopoulos et al., 2012), thereby linking glutamatergic signaling and FMRP at the nucleus. In addition, recent work in our laboratory has identified alterations in the inhibitory circuitry of *dfmr1* null flies. *dfmr1* mutants are characterized by reduced GAD expression in the adult brain, developmental stage-specific dysmorphia in GABAergic axons innervating the MB calyx, and altered GABAergic Ca^{2+} dynamics (Gatto et al., 2014). This data importantly implicates altered inhibitory neurotransmission in the *Drosophila* model of FXS, and further validates the conservation of FMRP function in the fruit fly brain.

DYSMORPHIC SYNAPSES IN ASD DISEASE STATES

Most ASD human studies on synaptic dysmorphia focus on the dendritic domain. For example, ASD patients display increased dendritic spine densities on cortical projection neurons (Hutsler and Zhang, 2010). FXS patients also display elevated spine density, with processes displaying elongated, "tortuous" structures (Irwin et al., 2001), perhaps suggestive of defects in synapse elimination. Similar dendritic dysmorphia are common in many other neurological disease states (Marin-Padilla, 1972; Purpura, 1974; Kaufmann and Moser, 2000), which may reflect developmental arrest or an attempted compensation for the lack of functionally mature spines (Fiala et al., 1998). In particular, it should be noted that these dendritic phenotypes are not restricted to the autism spectrum (sociolinguist deficits), as individuals with schizophrenia (perception deficits) and Alzheimer's disease (memory dysfunction) also display abnormal dendritic spine architectures (Penzes et al., 2011). These three forms of neurological dysfunction are distinct in symptomology, yet this specificity may be rooted in the timing and onset of synaptic dysfunction (**Figure 1B**).

Protrusion dynamics are just as important for synaptogenesis in genetic model systems (Ziv and Smith, 1996; Luikart et al., 2008). In the mouse FXS model, for example, there is delayed functional spine formation in the hippocampus (Braun and Segal, 2000), and ultimately fewer spines with mature, bulbous morphology (Irwin et al., 2000). SD leads to changes in spine protrusion dynamics in neonatal mice (Lendvai et al., 2000), demonstrating A-D regulation. Specifically, *Fmr1* KO mice deficits may result from deficits in experience-dependent plasticity during critical periods of synaptic refinement (Dolen et al., 2007; Bureau et al., 2008). During *in vivo* time lapse imaging through cranial windows in neonatal mice, layer 2/3 neurons show a dramatic decrease in dendritic spine dynamics during the first 2 weeks as mushroom-shaped spines replace filopodia and protospines, whereas *Fmr1* KO mice show developmental delays in the downregulation of spine turnover and the transition to mature spines (Cruz-Martin et al., 2010). Importantly, mGluR blockage accentuated these phenotypes in *Fmr1* KO mice (Cruz-Martin et al., 2010), providing a different link to A-D synaptic remodeling in the FXS disease state.

The dynamic nature of dendrites enhances their ability to sample the extracellular space for suitable presynaptic terminals (Ziv and Smith, 1996; Bonhoeffer and Yuste, 2002). Immature synapses from as adhesions between dendritic filopodia and axons (Fiala et al., 1998). Perturbations in these dynamics lead to altered synaptogenesis, for example, as demonstrated in Ephrin B-deficient (Kayser et al., 2008) and neurotrophin-deficient (Luikart et al., 2008) conditions. Following initial contact, spine dynamics are necessary for A-D remodeling (Lendvai et al., 2000; Yuste and Bonhoeffer, 2001, Yuste and Bonhoeffer, 2004; Holtmaat et al., 2006), and then strongly downregulated at the end of the critical period of synapse selection (Ziv and Smith, 1996). In FXS animal models, the failure to stabilize dendritic spines in developmental critical periods suggests *Fmr1* null protrusions have problems maintaining proper balance between stability and dynamism (Antar et al., 2006; Pfeiffer and Huber, 2007), resulting in fewer mature synaptic connections (Cruz-Martin et al., 2010). FMRP presumably modulates synaptic stability through regulation of mRNAs coding for dendritic spine regulators (Bagni and Greenough, 2005; Bassell and Warren, 2008), such as the key postsynaptic scaffold PSD-95 (postsynaptic density protein 95) as one example (**Figure 2**; Zalfa et al., 2007). Recent reviews outline the spine dysmorphia in the mouse FXS model in more detail (He and Portera-Cailliau, 2013).

Differences in axonal development in the mouse FXS model have not been as extensively studied. However, FMRP is localized at axon growth cones, which are far less dynamic in *Fmr1* KO mice (Antar et al., 2006). More thorough studies in the *Drosophila* FXS model demonstrate progressive differences in axonal projection and synaptic process pruning in the central brain MB of *dfmr1* null mutants (Tessier and Broadie, 2012). The *Drosophila* model demonstrates defects in the development of neuronal architecture (Zhang et al., 2001) and inappropriate A-D pruning (Tessier and Broadie, 2009) throughout the brain. For example, the synapses of small ventrolateral neurons (sLNvS) in the circadian regulation circuitry are overelaborated in *dfmr1* nulls (Dockendorff et al., 2002; Gatto and Broadie, 2009), a developmental phenotype that can be rescued only during the late pupal/early adult critical period, but not in early pupal stages or in mature adult stages (Gatto and Broadie, 2009), demonstrating a transient critical period requirement for FMRP. In the MB circuit, FMRP is required to limit outgrowth during an early phase and to subsequently prune synaptic branches in a later phase, and both phases are dependent on activity input (Tessier and Broadie, 2008). Furthermore, MB neurons in *dfmr1* nulls demonstrate age-dependent increases in calcium signaling dynamics, as well as deficient expression of several calcium-binding proteins (Tessier and Broadie, 2011), suggesting activity is driving a calcium signaling cascade coupling structural and functional developmental changes in the FXS disease state. Collectively, these defects all map to the early-use, A-D critical period of synaptic remodeling.

A-D TRANSLATION MISREGULATION IN THE ASD FRAGILE X SYNDROME

Autism spectrum disorders have been linked to hundreds of genes (Abrahams and Geschwind, 2008; Toro et al., 2010; Devlin and Scherer, 2012), and the number keeps jumping higher, with candidates in pathways affecting many distinct neuronal functions (Delorme et al., 2013). Importantly, however, many of these genes are modulated by neural activity, either directly or indirectly (Morrow et al., 2008; Chahrour et al., 2012; Ebert and Greenberg, 2013), and a number are known to be involved in A-D neural circuit modification (Toro et al., 2010). Rare *de novo* mutations have implicated a large network of genes directly involved in synaptogenesis and synaptic function (Gilman et al., 2011). Nevertheless, ASD modeling is made difficult by the underlying genetic diversity, and this difficulty is compounded by the array of symptoms described in human conditions and debates about appropriate genetic models (Crawley, 2007). The genetic bases of autism can be divided into a number of molecular groups: (1) chromatin remodeling, (2) cytoskeletal dynamics, (3) synaptic scaffolds, (4) neurotransmitter receptors and transporters, (5) second messengers, (6) cell adhesion molecules, and (7) secreted proteins (Persico and Bourgeron, 2006). Clearly the genetic basis of ASDs is massive area, and we focus here only on the FXS disease state, which may be an A-D translation control point for a number of these protein classes.

The monogenic FXS disease state (Verkerk et al., 1991) is typically caused by an unstable 5′ trinucleotide expansion in the promoter region of the *Fmr1* gene leading to hypermethylation and transcriptional silencing (Leehey et al., 2008). FXS patients exhibit delayed developmental trajectories, working memory deficits, circadian defects, hypersensitivity to sensory input, seizures, increased anxiety and hyperactivity (Harris et al., 2008), and a 30% comorbidity with autism (Zingerevich et al., 2009). Furthermore, FMRP may be associated with other neurological disease states, as schizophrenic patients have reduced FMRP in the periphery (Kovacs et al., 2013) and cerebellum (Fatemi et al., 2010), correlating with poor performance on perceptual integration tasks (Kelemen et al., 2013). The expanding web of FMRP associations (Bourgeois et al., 2009; Hagerman et al., 2010; Fatemi and Folsom, 2011) underlines the importance of this mRNA-binding translational regulator, with hundreds of candidate mRNA targets (Miyashiro et al., 2003; Darnell et al., 2011; Bagni et al., 2012). FMRP forms large cytosolic ribonuclear particles (RNPs), which are associated with mRNA transport, stability, and translation control (Bagni et al., 2012). RNP transport dynamics are altered in *Fmr1* KO mice, with reduced kinesin-associated mRNAs (Dictenberg et al., 2008). However, FMRP does not appear to be necessary for steady-state maintenance or constitutive localization of the majority of its target mRNAs (Steward et al., 1998; Dictenberg et al., 2008), although direct measurement of protein synthesis in hippocampal slices (Dolen et al., 2007), hippocampal culture (Osterweil et al., 2010), and synaptosomes (Muddashetty et al., 2007) shows global elevations in the *Fmr1* KO mouse.

Fragile X mental retardation protein is such an important focus because it is poised to directly and quickly respond to activity changes at the synapse. FMRP transports mRNA within the neuron and specifically at synapses in an A-D manner via association with microtubule-associated motor proteins (Kanai et al., 2004; Antar et al., 2005; Ferrari et al., 2007; Dictenberg et al., 2008; Charalambous et al., 2013). Targets of FMRP (Billuart and Chelly, 2003) include the small GTPase *Rac1* and its effector p-21 activated kinase (*PAK*), functioning as actin regulators (Bokoch, 2003). Rac1 is necessary for dendritic spine development, loss of FMRP leads to over-activation of Rac1 (**Figure 2B**), and Rac1 pharmacological inhibition leads to suppression of LTD in *Fmr1* KO mice (Bongmba et al., 2011). In addition, A-D stimulation of hippocampal synapses leads to increased phosphorylated PAK in wild-type, but not *Fmr1* KO mice, and mutants were unable to maintain actin cytoskeletal A-D changes (Chen et al., 2010). Moreover, small molecule inhibition of PAK suppresses *Fmr1* null phenotypes including dendritic spine morphology, seizures, hyperactivity, and repetitive movements (Dolan et al., 2013). Another target, PSD-95 is an adaptor protein associated with glutamatergic receptors (Sheng and Kim, 2002); mice deficient in PSD-95 show dendritic spine dysmorphia in striatum and hippocampus (Vickers et al., 2006). FMRP may regulate PSD-95 partially through stabilization of PSD-95 mRNA, a process that is enhanced with mGluR activation (**Figure 2A**; Zalfa et al., 2007). FMRP also associates with *futsch/MAP1B* mRNA, a microtubule regulator of synaptic growth (Roos et al., 2000), that can be localized at the growth cone of developing axons (Antar et al., 2006), and is localized within FMRP–RNP granules in cultured hippocampal neurons (Antar et al., 2005). FMRP and *futsch* associate in co-immunoprecipitation assays, and its expression is inversely correlated with FMRP expression (Zhang et al., 2001). Importantly, *futsch* loss of function corrects the synaptic overgrowth phenotype in *dfmr1* nulls (**Figure 2B**; Zhang et al., 2001). Application of the axon guidance molecule Semaphorin-3A (Sema3A) to hippocampal culture leads to MAP1B protein synthesis, but this response is attenuated in *Fmr1* null neurons (Li et al., 2009), thereby linking the activity of an axon guidance molecule with local FMRP-dependent translation. More recent work has shown that FMRP regulation of *futsch* is downstream of BMP and Spartin signaling (Nahm et al., 2013), thereby linking a key *trans*-synaptic signaling pathway with cytoskeletal changes in presynaptic neurons.

Several recent studies have provided new mechanistic insights about FMRP function at the synapse. Two recently identified FMRP targets are striatal-enriched protein tyrosine phosphatase (STEP) and amyloid precursor protein (APP), which appear to underlie at least a portion of mouse *Fmr1* phenotypes, as genetic reduction of either can suppress audiogenic seizure, anxiety, and social deficits in the disease model condition (Westmark et al., 2011; Goebel-Goody et al., 2012; **Figure 2**). Another target of FMRP is *Arc* mRNA (Zalfa et al., 2003), an A-D immediate early gene (Link et al., 1995) strongly linked to synaptic function (Park et al., 2008). Importantly, Arc protein functions to stimulate endocytosis of AMPA glutamate receptors (Chowdhury et al., 2006), an action correlated with the A-D induction of LTD (Park et al., 2008). FMRP plays an important modulatory role in this A-D process, acting as a translational repressor of *Arc* synthesis during mGluR-LTD (Niere et al., 2012). FMRP also regulates several potassium ion channels. For example, FMRP interacts with Kv3.1b mRNA in brainstem synaptosomes, and the A-D increase in Kv3.1b channel expression in wild type mice is abolished in *Fmr1* null mice (Strumbos et al., 2010). Moreover, FMRP can directly interact with potassium channel proteins to regulate channel kinetics, including Slack channels (Brown et al., 2010) and the β4 subunit of BK channels (Deng et al., 2013). Therefore, FMRP can no longer be described as solely a translational regulator, with protein–protein interactions regulating excitability demonstrating an additional vital role for FMRP function.

The final area of focus for FMRP regulation lies in the extracellular space. Both mouse and *Drosophila* FXS models have recently been documented to show large increase in the levels of synaptic matrix metalloproteases (MMPs), a family of extracellular proteases involved in synaptic development, function, and plasticity (**Figures 2A,B**; Rivera et al., 2010). MMPs cleave secreted as well as membrane-anchored proteins during synaptogenesis and A-D synaptic remodeling (Ethell and Ethell, 2007). Specifically, MMP-9 expression and activity are increased in *Fmr1* KO mice (Bilousova et al., 2009), with MMP-9 locally translated at synaptodendritic domains in an A-D manner (Dziembowska et al., 2012). MMP-9 mRNA is transported and regulated by FMRP, and increased MMP-9 expression is found in *Fmr1* null synaptosomes from mouse hippocampus (Janusz et al., 2013). Crucially, a drug inhibitor of MMPs, minocycline, effectively restores synaptic architecture and behavioral defects in the mouse FXS model (**Figure 2**; Bilousova et al., 2009). The mechanistic link between MMPs and ASDs may lie with MMP substrates, especially the HSPGs, which are well-established proteolytic targets of MMPs (Choi et al., 2012). HSPGs bind a variety of molecules, including growth factors, morphogens, and cell surface receptors, effectively modulating a hosts of biological functions (Bishop et al., 2007). In BTBR autism mouse models (Scattoni et al., 2011), hippocampal sclerosis (HS) immunoreactivity is reduced (Meyza et al., 2012). Conditional inactivation (neuronal specific) of *Ext1*, an essential enzyme for HS synthesis, leads to defective glutamatergic neurotransmission and behavioral abnormalities similar to autistic phenotypes (Irie et al., 2012). Disruption of HSPGs in *Drosophila* leads to *trans*-synaptic signaling defects at the NMJ (Dani et al., 2012), causing impairments of synaptic structural and functional development. Moreover, in the *Drosophila* FXS model, both MMP mutation and the minocycline MMP inhibitor (MMPIs) treatment effectively suppresses synaptic architecture defects in motor neurons, clock neurons, and neurons of the central brain MB learning/memory center (Siller and Broadie, 2011). Perhaps linking these two mechanisms, the *Drosophila* FXS model displays dramatic upregulation of synaptic HSPGs (**Figure 2**), including a GPI-anchored Glypican and transmembrane Syndecan (Sdc; Friedman et al., 2013). These elevated co-receptors in turn inappropriately sequester Jelly Belly (Jeb) and Wnt Wg *trans*-synaptic signaling ligands to alter intercellular communication between pre- and postsynaptic cells during synaptogenesis (**Figures 2A,B**). Genetic correction of the synaptic HSPG upregulation in *dfmr1* null mutants corrects both structural overelaboration and elevated neurotransmission (Friedman et al., 2013), demonstrating this signaling mechanism to be causative to A-D synaptogenic defects in this FXS disease state model. Based on these extensive studies in mice and flies, MMPIs are currently in development for FXS therapeutics as discussed below.

ASD THERAPEUTIC AVENUES

The A-D model of ASDs, especially as it applies to the regulation of critical period development of appropriate E/I synaptic ratios, suggests a number of therapeutic strategies. For example, the overabundant mGluR signaling theory underlying FXS dysfunction is supported by numerous mGluR mutant studies in mouse and *Drosophila* animal models (Bear et al., 2004, 2008; Bear, 2005; McBride et al., 2005; Dolen et al., 2007, 2010; Pan and Broadie, 2007; Dolen and Bear, 2008; Pan et al., 2008; Repicky and Broadie, 2009). Importantly, mGluR antagonists (such as MPEP) effectively rescue many of the mouse and *Drosophila* FXS model cellular and behavioral defects associated with FXS (McBride et al., 2005; Pan and Broadie, 2007; Bolduc et al., 2008; Dolen and Bear, 2008; Choi et al., 2010a; Dolen et al., 2010). MPEP is not available for human use due to toxicity, but new generation mGluR antagonists are in development (Levenga et al., 2010; Wang et al., 2010b; Pop et al., 2013). For example, chronic application of the mGluR antagonist CTEP suppresses learning and memory deficits and leads to regional improvements in brain function in *Fmr1* KO mice, as determined by perfusion imaging as an indirect measure of neural activity (Michalon et al., 2014), although it is important to note that CTEP also affected wild-type learning and memory. This first use of functional imaging in a mouse ASD model is an important step forward. Current FXS patient clinical trials include other mGluR antagonists (e.g., mavoglurant; Gantois et al., 2013) as well as GABA-B receptor agonists (e.g., arbaclofen; Henderson et al., 2012). Fenobam, a selective mGluR antagonist, improved prepulse inhibition in 6 of 12 FXS patients (Berry-Kravis et al., 2009). mGluR reverse agonists in phase II and III clinical trials were recently extended to younger children (Levenga et al., 2010), recognizing the early developmental focus likely necessary for effective intervention. For illustration, the rescue of spine morphology in cultured neurons from *Fmr1* KO mice by mGluR blockage is effective in young neurons but less so in older neurons (Su et al., 2011). Thus, it is important for interventions to target A-D critical periods.

On this opposing side of the E/I balance lies the therapeutic potential to increase GABA levels or potentiate GABA receptors, with the goal to alleviating FXS symptoms of hypoinhibition (Paluszkiewicz et al., 2011; Coghlan et al., 2012). Altered GABAergic inhibition is a common thread in many neurodevelopmental disorders and represent an important focus for therapeutics. Pharmacological approaches to GABAergic modulation address several components of inhibitory neurotransmission, including the GABA reuptake blockers Riluzole (Mantz et al., 1994; Jahn et al., 2008; Erickson et al., 2011b) and Tiagabine (Nielsen et al., 1991), $GABA_AR$ activators Ganaxolone (Biagini et al., 2010; Reddy and Rogawski, 2010) and Gaboxadol (Deacon et al., 2007; Lundahl et al., 2007; Olmos-Serrano et al., 2010), $GABA_BR$ activator Arbaclofen (Pacey et al., 2009), and Vigabatrin, an inhibitor of GABA catabolism (French et al., 1996; Coppola et al., 1997). Acamprosate is also interesting, as a drug that both antagonizes mGluR5 (Blednov and Harris, 2008) and agonizes $GABA_ARs$ (Mann et al., 2008). A small uncontrolled trial with three adult FXS patients showed improvement in social behavior and communication after 16–28 weeks on acamprosate (Erickson et al., 2010), and similar gains in social communication were found in a small uncontrolled sample of autistic children (Erickson et al., 2011a).

Alternative pharmaceutical approaches to FXS focus on MMP and perhaps HSPG function in the synaptomatrix (Siller and Broadie, 2011; Dani and Broadie, 2012; Dani et al., 2012; Friedman et al., 2013). One obvious approach is the use of MMPIs, of which a large collection has been developed for human clinical trials on inflammatory and vascular diseases (Hu et al., 2007). For example, the tetracycline-derivative minocycline acting as an MMPI spurs maturation of hippocampal dendritic spines and represses anxiety and memory defects in the FXS mouse model (Bilousova et al., 2009), and similarly suppresses synaptic architecture defects in motor neurons, clock neurons, and MB learning/memory center neurons in the *Drosophila* FXS model (Siller and Broadie, 2011). The drug therefore offers a directed approach toward deficits in A-D mechanisms at the synapse as it aims to correct overactive MMP in the absence of FMRP. Minocycline has previously been successful in treating a variety of neurological disorders, including multiple sclerosis, Huntington's disease, Parkinson's disease, and Alzheimer's disease (Wang et al., 2003; Choi et al., 2007; Kim and Suh, 2009). Minocycline treatments led to a long-term reduction in hyperactivity and audiogenic seizures in young, but not old mice (Dansie et al., 2013). In human trials, minocycline led to improved language, behavior, and attention in FXS patients in an uncontrolled study (Utari et al., 2010), and a recent 3-month double-blind, placebo-controlled trial with young FXS patients showed improvements in anxiety, mood, and clinical global impression (CGI) of FXS individuals given minocycline (Leigh et al., 2013). The mechanistic link between minocycline and MMPs in human patients has also been explored, as reduced MMP-9 activity correlates with CGI improvements in FXS patients (Dziembowska et al., 2013). Finally, the PAK-associated cytoskeletal changes in FXS models have been pharmaceutically targeted, with significant suppression of FXS phenotypes in the *Fmr1* null mouse (Dolan et al., 2013). There may be a clinical path forward targeting PAK and/or downstream cytoskeletal perturbations.

A quite different avenue for ASD treatment targets A-D critical period development via environmental enrichment and training intervention following early diagnosis (Dawson et al., 2010; Woo and Leon, 2013). To illustrate the impact of environmental input on cognitive development, Romanian orphans who received limited sensory stimulation can have profound social and cognitive defects, and many develop post-institutional autistic syndrome (Hoksbergen et al., 2005), suggesting that an ASD-like state can be achieved through purely environmental impoverishment. Thankfully many of these children make significant cognitive and social gains upon adoption and placement into enriched environments (Nelson et al., 2007). Importantly, enriched environments increase sensory input activity and have profound effects on A-D synaptic dynamics (Greenough et al., 1985; Beaulieu and Colonnier, 1987; Moser et al., 1995). In animal models, FXS mutant mice display a host of striking improvements when reared in enriched environments, including greater spine hippocampal spine density (Lauterborn et al., 2013) and improved spike timing long-term potentiation (LTP; Meredith et al., 2007). As a group of syndromes with strong links to A-D synaptic developmental defects, enrichment approaches are popular in ASD treatments (Reichow and Volkmar, 2010; Warren et al., 2011). For example, a peer-mediated theater-based intervention strategy for ASD children showed significant gains in core social deficits (Corbett et al., 2013). Similarly, a recent 6-month controlled trial showed significant gains in autistic children who underwent sensorimotor enrichment through olfactory and tactile stimulation and exercises for other cross-sensory stimulation (Woo and Leon, 2013). These behavioral intervention strategies are, crucially, focusing on multisensory domains and may enable great improvements in both social and cognitive abilities of ASD children.

PART 3: *IN VIVO* MANIPULATION/READOUT OF ACTIVITY-DEPENDENT CHANGES

The recent emergence of tools to non-invasively drive and monitor neural activity represents a pioneering step forward for A-D neurodevelopmental studies. Compared to the relatively narrow and invasive strategies of traditional electrophysiology (Biran et al., 2005; Bjornsson et al., 2006), new optogenetic techniques provide simultaneous access to groups of neurons, which can be selectively targeted with a range of transgenic drivers (Kim and Jun, 2013). On the one hand, new optogenetic techniques using engineered rhodopsin variants have enormously advanced our ability to control activity with pulsed application of specific wavelengths of light in defined populations of neurons (Fenno et al., 2011). On the other hand, optical recording techniques, such as calcium sensors and voltage-sensitive fluorescent reporters, provide individual and massed readouts of neural activity throughout the imaged circuitry, albeit at a cost in sensitivity and temporal resolution compared to electrophysiological recordings (Grienberger and Konnerth, 2012; Mutoh et al., 2012). Thus, these new transgenic techniques provide unprecedented abilities to both drive and record *in vivo* neural activity, and therefore show great promise for the systematic dissection of A-D critical period mechanisms at the heart of ASD disease states.

Techniques for detecting neural calcium flux have been progressing for decades (Shimomura et al., 1962; Tsien et al., 1985), taking advantage of Ca^{2+} dynamics as a readout of neural activity (Berridge et al., 2003). Resting Ca^{2+} concentrations in neurons are typically <100 nM and rise 10- to 100-fold following a single action potential (Berridge et al., 2000), providing the ability to monitor spike number, timing, frequency, and levels of synaptic input (Yasuda et al., 2004). Genetically encoded calcium indicators (GECIs), such as the frGECIs and GCamps (Kotlikoff, 2007), have revolutionized *in vivo* Ca^{2+} imaging. The latest generations of GCamp sensors are especially exciting, as they display ultra-sensitive kinetics and stably provide readout of neural activity over extensive periods of time (Akerboom et al., 2012; Chen et al., 2013). For instance, GCamp6 effectively records neural activity from large groups of neurons to small synaptic compartments, in animals ranging from *Drosophila* to mice (Chen et al., 2013). The recent development of red-shifted GECIs reduces tissue scattering, phototoxicity, and background fluorescence, and allows the simultaneous use of other tools, such as ChR2, which is activated with 480 nm light and would therefore overlap and interfere with traditional green fluorescent protein (GFP)-based calcium sensors (Akerboom et al., 2013). The tandem development of multiphoton imaging and GECIs now provide exquisite access for activity monitoring.

Although Ca^{2+} imaging serves as readout for diverse forms of A-D changes (e.g., depolarization, influx, store release, second messenger cascades), the direct detection of changes in membrane voltage would represent a more specific, direct readout of electrical activity. Small fluorescent hydrophobic dyes have long been able to detect changes in membrane potential, and can also be used to characterize propagation of electrical signals through a given circuit (Salzberg et al., 1973). However, these dyes have low penetrance to deep areas of the brain, and are not genetically targetable. Early generations of genetically encoded voltage indicator proteins (GEVIs) overcame some of these limitations (Siegel and Isacoff, 1997; Barnett et al., 2012), but failed to reliably demonstrate robust signals in intact animals. In contrast, the recently developed ArcLight system is a voltage sensor probes (VSP)-based fluorescent voltage sensor with greatly increased signal-to-noise ratio (Jin et al., 2012). In intact *Drosophila* brains, the ArcLight system effectively reports both action potentials and subthreshold events, demonstrating beautiful sensitivity (Cao et al., 2013). The *in vivo* applications for this new tool are exciting. For example, ArcLight has provided the ability to record rhythmic activity in *Drosophila* clock neurons, which have so far been inaccessible to electrophysiology approaches (Cao et al., 2013). Thus, GEVIs and GECIs are exciting new tools that grant non-invasive and increasingly penetrant representations of *in vivo* neural activity.

OPTOGENETIC CONTROL OF NEURONAL ACTIVITY

Optogenetic techniques have revolutionized the ability to direct and dissect A-D processes during critical period development (Williams and Deisseroth, 2013). Delivery of engineered rhodopsin variants into targeted neurons provides a non-invasive means to control neuronal firing rates via pulses of specific wavelengths of light. ChR2 facilitate depolarization of the membrane by gating influx of Na^{+} ions when illuminated by blue light (see **Figure 2A**; Fenno et al., 2011). Conversely, halorhodopsins (eNpHR) respond to amber light by mediating Cl^{-} ion influx, thereby hyperpolarizing the membrane and inhibiting firing (**Figure 2A**; Zhang et al., 2007; Gradinaru et al., 2008). To date, most optogenetic studies have been either electrophysiological or behavioral work in mature animals including, for example, an alternative to deep brain stimulation in Parkinson's disease model mice (Gradinaru et al., 2009), reduction of anxiety (Tye et al., 2011), serotonergic modulation of behavior (Warden et al., 2012), dopaminergic depression alleviation (Tye et al., 2013), and memory extinction (Van den Oever et al., 2013). However, developmental applications of optogenetic A-D modulation are beginning to appear. For example, ChR2-expressing *Drosophila* MB neurons respond to short blue light illumination (6 h) during critical period development with significant decreases in synaptic process branching, but this A-D synaptic pruning is completely abolished in FXS model animals (Tessier and Broadie, 2008, 2012). In mouse, ChR2 optogenetic stimulation causes a lasting increase in postsynaptic spine density and increased concentration of CaMKII, when paired with glutamate uncaging (Zhang et al., 2008). Furthermore, optogenetics is now capable of producing cortical maps, and can be coupled with Ca^{2+} imaging for readouts of activity alterations (Patterson et al., 2013). In addition, the coupling of optogenetic stimulation and immediate early active gene *NPAS4* mRNA facilitates identification of transfected neurons in mice (Bepari et al., 2012). The capacity to manipulate A-D neuronal structure and function *in vivo* in a developmental context is simply remarkable, and recent studies highlight the promise of these rapidly evolving techniques.

In the past year, optogenetics techniques have particularly begun to blossom. For example, delivery of ChR2 to thalamic neurons was recently shown to effectively silence cortical seizures in mice (Paz et al., 2013). Conversely, expression of eNpHR in hippocampal neurons also provided protection against seizures (Sukhotinsky et al., 2013). Halorhodopsin channels can also provide *in vivo* inhibition of motor activity (Liske et al., 2013). The emergence of red-shifted GECIs and optogenetic channels now facilitates dual transgenic manipulation and functional readout in the same animal (Akerboom et al., 2013). Combinatorial dye labeling can also facilitate the simultaneous detection of structural and functional changes without the use of genetics (Siegel and Lohmann, 2013). The development of optochemical G protein-coupled receptors (GPCRs), including light-agonized mGluRs, have been shown to be fast, bistable means to effectively suppress excitability and inhibit neurotransmitter release both in brain slices and *in vivo* (Levitz et al., 2013). The InSynC (inhibition of synapses with chromophore-assisted light inactivation) technique has been developed to directly inhibit neurotransmitter release, via a genetically encoded singlet oxygen generator (miniSOG) fused to two synaptic proteins, vesicle-associated membrane protein 2 (VAMP2) and synaptophysin (Lin et al., 2013b). Multiphoton uncaging of glutamate and GABA analogs has been demonstrated on individual dendritic spines in hippocampal slices (Hayama et al., 2013). Red-shifted excitatory optogenes (ReaChR) have improved membrane trafficking, higher photocurrents and faster kinetics, scatter less in passing through the tissue, and have been capable of driving action potentials in awake mice with illumination through the intact skull (Lin et al., 2013a).

Despite the justifiable excitement, it is important to note also important caveats to optogenetic applications, particularly for the use in A-D developmental studies. First, it was recently reported that long-term expression of ChR2 can alter axonal morphology in mice (Miyashita et al., 2013). In addition, high-level, long-term expression of fluorescent probes can lead to structural artifacts and phototoxicity (Packer et al., 2013). Second, optogenetics are generally delivered through viral means in mammalian models, and it has recently been reported that adeno-associated viruses (AAVs) can form tissue deposits after injection, which can lead to continued infection over time and alterations in the expression of the optogene (Packer et al., 2013). This problem may be avoided with single cell electroporation (Judkewitz et al., 2009), but this limits the applications. Third, extreme stimulation can lead to an exhaustion of synaptic transmission (Kittelmann et al., 2013). Therefore, it is important to modulate the expression and long-term, high frequency use of optogenes, and to use appropriate controls to detect any artifacts. Alternative approaches to optogenetics include the use of genetically targeted TrpA1 channels, which are a class of temperature-gated excitatory cation channels for depolarizing neurons (Viswanath et al., 2003; Dhaka et al., 2006; Hamada et al., 2008). Work in *Drosophila* illustrates the power of TrpA1 manipulations, specifically in comparison to ChR2 optogenetics, as neurons expressing TrpA1 can show stronger and longer lasting electrophysiological effects (Pulver et al., 2009).

Drosophila METHODS FOR STUDYING A-D DEVELOPMENTAL MECHANISMS

The "relative" simplicity of the *Drosophila* brain (hundreds of thousands of neurons) provides a high level of understanding about clonal lineages and connectivity among small, defined populations of neurons, even down to the individually identified single neuron level (Chou et al., 2010; Chiang et al., 2011; Lovick et al., 2013; Takemura et al., 2013; Wong et al., 2013). Importantly, *Drosophila* genetics allows precise delivery of transgenic tools to these targeted neuronal populations using the GAL4/UAS bipartite system (Jones, 2009), and with the MARCM technique for clonal analysis down to the individually identified single neuron level (Lee and Luo, 2001; Ostrovsky et al., 2013). Our lab has utilized these techniques particularly to analyze individually identified neurons in the FXS disease model (Pan and Broadie, 2007; Tessier and Broadie, 2008; Gatto and Broadie, 2009; Siller and Broadie, 2011), as our best-defined *Drosophila* ASD model. More recently, *Drosophila* has gained an expansive catalog of highly selective neuronal GAL4 drivers, which utilize limited regulatory sequences for exquisitely limited expression (Jenett et al., 2012; Manning et al., 2012). These new tools are providing the capacity to target defined neuronal circuits within the *Drosophila* brain at a never-before achieved level of resolution. The use of selective drivers for high-resolution morphological readouts of individual neurons, in combination with non-invasive methods of activity modulation, will greatly enhance our understanding of A-D mechanisms of synapse remodeling. We predict that the utilization of these new classes of neural drivers (in MB, projection neuron, fan body, ellipsoid body, retina, etc.), in combination with both optogenetic and alternative activity modulation techniques, will provide much better dissection of neuron class-specific A-D developmental mechanisms within the next few years. These studies will lead to a deeper understanding of ASD model disease states within precise maps of brain circuits, such as the MB (Parnas et al., 2013;

Perisse et al., 2013) and antennal lobes (Tanaka et al., 2012), which will provide a foundation for deciphering the molecular genetic bases of these disease states and engineering effecting treatment strategies.

What are the current limitations on this use of the *Drosophila* system? For optogenetics, *Drosophila* requires an essential co-factor, all-trans retinal (ATR), for ChR2 activation (Schroll et al., 2006; Ataman et al., 2008), although this feature does provide a useful control. Moreover, fluorescent tags on optogenetic channels label targeted neurons to grant cell-autonomous morphological readouts of A-D modifications, but fail to illuminate their synaptic partners, although clever mapping techniques are being developed [e.g., Genetic Reconstitution Across Synaptic Partners (GRASP); Feinberg et al., 2008]. For example, the GRASP technique was recently used to synaptically link MB Kenyon cells with modulatory aminergic neurons (Pech et al., 2013). In a similar fashion, the CaLexA (calcium-dependent nuclear import of Lexa) neural tracing method may be useful for mapping synaptic partners (Masuyama et al., 2012). Alternatively, synaptic mapping studies may be more suited for larger subsets of neurons (broader GAL4 drivers), which are coupled to known targets and could then be assayed through standard immunohistochemistry. Further downstream, the use of immediate early neural genes, may help illuminate downstream effects of activity modulation (e.g., *Dhr38*; Fujita et al., 2013). Importantly, use of the multiple methods now available for A-D manipulations during neurodevelopmental studies (e.g., ChR2, eNpHR, TrpA1, NaChBac) in the *Drosophila* FXS model can be used to directly test whether targeted brain circuitry is capable of responding appropriately to activity during defined developmental critical periods. Moreover, the capacity to genetically target subsets of neurons may allow suppression of downstream ASD-related phenotypes. For example, in the *Drosophila* FXS model, hypoinhibition (e.g., reduced GABAergic input) might be suppressed by increased depolarization of inhibitory interneurons using a GAD:Gal4 driver crossed to ChR2, and hyperexcitation (e.g., elevated mGluR activity) could similarly be suppressed by selectively hyperpolarizing specific groups of glutamatergic neurons with halorhodopsin. Such studies in the particularly well-characterized *Drosophila* FXS model could ultimately lead to new intervention strategies in FXS patients and, by extension, the treatment of other patient groups suffering ASDs.

ACKNOWLEDGMENTS

We thank Dr. Cheryl Gatto for critical input on this manuscript. This work is supported by NIH grant R01 MH096832 to Kendal Broadie.

REFERENCES

Abrahams, B. S., and Geschwind, D. H. (2008). Advances in autism genetics: on the threshold of a new neurobiology. *Nat. Rev. Genet.* 9, 341–355. doi: 10.1038/nrg2346

Adusei, D. C., Pacey, L. K., Chen, D., and Hampson, D. R. (2010). Early developmental alterations in GABAergic protein expression in fragile X knockout mice. *Neuropharmacology* 59, 167–171. doi: 10.1016/j.neuropharm.2010.05.002

Akerboom, J., Carreras Calderon, N., Tian, L., Wabnig, S., Prigge, M., Tolo, J., et al. (2013). Genetically encoded calcium indicators for multi-color neural activity imaging and combination with optogenetics. *Front. Mol. Neurosci.* 6:2. doi: 10.3389/fnmol.2013.00002

Akerboom, J., Chen, T. W., Wardill, T. J., Tian, L., Marvin, J. S., Mutlu, S., et al. (2012). Optimization of a GCaMP calcium indicator for neural activity imaging. *J. Neurosci.* 32, 13819–13840. doi: 10.1523/JNEUROSCI.2601-12.2012

Alvarez, V. A., and Sabatini, B. L. (2007). Anatomical and physiological plasticity of dendritic spines. *Annu. Rev. Neurosci.* 30, 79–97. doi: 10.1146/annurev.neuro.30.051606.094222

Amir, R. E., Van Den Veyver, I. B., Wan, M., Tran, C. Q., Francke, U., and Zoghbi, H. Y. (1999). Rett syndrome is caused by mutations in X-linked MECP2, encoding methyl-CpG-binding protein 2. *Nat. Genet.* 23, 185–188. doi: 10.1038/13810

Antar, L. N., Afroz, R., Dictenberg, J. B., Carroll, R. C., and Bassell, G. J. (2004). Metabotropic glutamate receptor activation regulates fragile X mental retardation protein and FMR1 mRNA localization differentially in dendrites and at synapses. *J. Neurosci.* 24, 2648–2655. doi: 10.1523/JNEUROSCI.0099-04.2004

Antar, L. N., Dictenberg, J. B., Plociniak, M., Afroz, R., and Bassell, G. J. (2005). Localization of FMRP-associated mRNA granules and requirement of microtubules for activity-dependent trafficking in hippocampal neurons. *Genes Brain Behav.* 4, 350–359. doi: 10.1111/j.1601-183X.2005.00128.x

Antar, L. N., Li, C., Zhang, H., Carroll, R. C., and Bassell, G. J. (2006). Local functions for FMRP in axon growth cone motility and activity-dependent regulation of filopodia and spine synapses. *Mol. Cell. Neurosci.* 32, 37–48. doi: 10.1016/j.mcn.2006.02.001

Ataman, B., Ashley, J., Gorczyca, D., Gorczyca, M., Mathew, D., Wichmann, C., et al. (2006). Nuclear trafficking of *Drosophila* Frizzled-2 during synapse development requires the PDZ protein dGRIP. *Proc. Natl. Acad. Sci. U.S.A.* 103, 7841–7846. doi: 10.1073/pnas.0600387103

Ataman, B., Ashley, J., Gorczyca, M., Ramachandran, P., Fouquet, W., Sigrist, S. J., et al. (2008). Rapid activity-dependent modifications in synaptic structure and function require bidirectional Wnt signaling. *Neuron* 57, 705–718. doi: 10.1016/j.neuron.2008.01.026

Bacci, A., Huguenard, J. R., and Prince, D. A. (2005). Modulation of neocortical interneurons: extrinsic influences and exercises in self-control. *Trends Neurosci.* 28, 602–610. doi: 10.1016/j.tins.2005.08.007

Bagni, C., and Greenough, W. T. (2005). From mRNP trafficking to spine dysmorphogenesis: the roots of fragile X syndrome. *Nat. Rev. Neurosci.* 6, 376–387. doi: 10.1038/nrn1667

Bagni, C., Tassone, F., Neri, G., and Hagerman, R. (2012). Fragile X syndrome: causes, diagnosis, mechanisms, and therapeutics. *J. Clin. Invest.* 122, 4314–4322. doi: 10.1172/JCI63141

Baines, R. A., Uhler, J. P., Thompson, A., Sweeney, S. T., and Bate, M. (2001). Altered electrical properties in *Drosophila* neurons developing without synaptic transmission. *J. Neurosci.* 21, 1523–1531

Baker, K. B., Wray, S. P., Ritter, R., Mason, S., Lanthorn, T. H., and Savelieva, K. V. (2010). Male and female Fmr1 knockout mice on C57 albino background exhibit spatial learning and memory impairments. *Genes Brain Behav.* 9, 562–574. doi: 10.1111/j.1601-183X.2010.00585.x

Barbosa, A. C., Kim, M. S., Ertunc, M., Adachi, M., Nelson, E. D., Mcanally, J., et al. (2008). MEF2C, a transcription factor that facilitates learning and memory by negative regulation of synapse numbers and function. *Proc. Natl. Acad. Sci. U.S.A.* 105, 9391–9396. doi: 10.1073/pnas.0802679105

Barlow, H. B. (1953a). Action potentials from the frog's retina. *J. Physiol.* 119, 58–68.

Barlow, H. B. (1953b). Summation and inhibition in the frog's retina. *J. Physiol.* 119, 69–88.

Barnett, L., Platisa, J., Popovic, M., Pieribone, V. A., and Hughes, T. (2012). A fluorescent, genetically-encoded voltage probe capable of resolving action potentials. *PLoS ONE* 7:e43454. doi: 10.1371/journal.pone.0043454

Bassell, G. J., and Warren, S. T. (2008). Fragile X syndrome: loss of local mRNA regulation alters synaptic development and function. *Neuron* 60, 201–214. doi: 10.1016/j.neuron.2008.10.004

Batish, M., Van Den Bogaard, P., Kramer, F. R., and Tyagi, S. (2012). Neuronal mRNAs travel singly into dendrites. *Proc. Natl. Acad. Sci. U.S.A.* 109, 4645–4650. doi: 10.1073/pnas.1111226109

Bear, M. F. (2005). Therapeutic implications of the mGluR theory of fragile X mental retardation. *Genes Brain Behav.* 4, 393–398. doi: 10.1111/j.1601-183X.2005.00135.x

Bear, M. F., Dolen, G., Osterweil, E., and Nagarajan, N. (2008). Fragile X: translation in action. *Neuropsychopharmacology* 33, 84–87. doi: 10.1038/sj.npp.1301610

Bear, M. F., Huber, K. M., and Warren, S. T. (2004). The mGluR theory of fragile X mental retardation. *Trends Neurosci.* 27, 370–377. doi: 10.1016/j.tins.2004.04.009

Beaulieu, C., and Colonnier, M. (1987). Effect of the richness of the environment on the cat visual cortex. *J. Comp. Neurol.* 266, 478–494. doi: 10.1002/cne.9026 60404

Belmonte, M. K., Cook, E. H. Jr., Anderson, G. M., Rubenstein, J. L., Greenough, W. T., Beckel-Mitchener, A., et al. (2004). Autism as a disorder of neural information processing: directions for research and targets for therapy. *Mol. Psychiatry* 9, 646–663. doi: 10.1038/sj.mp.4001499

Ben-Sasson, A., Hen, L., Fluss, R., Cermak, S. A., Engel-Yeger, B., and Gal, E. (2009). A meta-analysis of sensory modulation symptoms in individuals with autism spectrum disorders. *J. Autism Dev. Disord.* 39, 1–11. doi: 10.1007/s10803-008-0593-3

Bepari, A. K., Sano, H., Tamamaki, N., Nambu, A., Tanaka, K. F., and Takebayashi, H. (2012). Identification of optogenetically activated striatal medium spiny neurons by Npas4 expression. *PLoS ONE* 7:e52783. doi: 10.1371/journal.pone.00 52783

Berke, B., Wittnam, J., Mcneill, E., Van Vactor, D. L., and Keshishian, H. (2013). Retrograde BMP signaling at the synapse: a permissive signal for synapse maturation and activity-dependent plasticity. *J. Neurosci.* 33, 17937–17950. doi: 10.1523/JNEUROSCI.6075-11.2013

Berridge, M. J., Bootman, M. D., and Roderick, H. L. (2003). Calcium signalling: dynamics, homeostasis and remodelling. *Nat. Rev. Mol. Cell Biol.* 4, 517–529. doi: 10.1038/nrm1155

Berridge, M. J., Lipp, P., and Bootman, M. D. (2000). Signal transduction. The calcium entry pas de deux. *Science* 287, 1604–1605. doi: 10.1126/science.287.5458.1604

Berry-Kravis, E. (2002). Epilepsy in fragile X syndrome. *Dev. Med. Child Neurol.* 44, 724–728. doi: 10.1111/j.1469-8749.2002.tb00277.x

Berry-Kravis, E., Hessl, D., Coffey, S., Hervey, C., Schneider, A., Yuhas, J., et al. (2009). A pilot open label, single dose trial of fenobam in adults with fragile X syndrome. *J. Med. Genet.* 46, 266–271. doi: 10.1136/jmg.2008.063701

Biagini, G., Panuccio, G., and Avoli, M. (2010). Neurosteroids and epilepsy. *Curr. Opin. Neurol.* 23, 170–176. doi: 10.1097/WCO.0b013e32833735cf

Billuart, P., and Chelly, J. (2003). From fragile X mental retardation protein to Rac1 GTPase: new insights from Fly CYFIP. *Neuron* 38, 843–845. doi: 10.1016/S0896-6273(03)00362-3

Bilousova, T. V., Dansie, L., Ngo, M., Aye, J., Charles, J. R., Ethell, D. W., et al. (2009). Minocycline promotes dendritic spine maturation and improves behavioural performance in the fragile X mouse model. *J. Med. Genet.* 46, 94–102. doi: 10.1136/jmg.2008.061796

Biran, R., Martin, D. C., and Tresco, P. A. (2005). Neuronal cell loss accompanies the brain tissue response to chronically implanted silicon microelectrode arrays. *Exp. Neurol.* 195, 115–126. doi: 10.1016/j.expneurol.2005.04.020

Bishop, G. H., and Clare, M. (1951). Radiation path from geniculate to optic cortex in cat. *J. Neurophysiol.* 14, 496–505.

Bishop, G. H., and Clare, M. H. (1952). Sites of origin of electric potentials in striate cortex. *J. Neurophysiol.* 15, 201–220.

Bishop, G. H., and Clare, M. H. (1955). Organization and distribution of fibers in the optic tract of the cat. *J. Comp. Neurol.* 103, 269–304. doi: 10.1002/cne.901030204

Bishop, J. R., Schuksz, M., and Esko, J. D. (2007). Heparan sulphate proteoglycans fine-tune mammalian physiology. *Nature* 446, 1030–1037. doi: 10.1038/nature05817

Bjornsson, C. S., Oh, S. J., Al-Kofahi, Y. A., Lim, Y. J., Smith, K. L., Turner, J. N., et al. (2006). Effects of insertion conditions on tissue strain and vascular damage during neuroprosthetic device insertion. *J. Neural Eng.* 3, 196–207. doi: 10.1088/1741-2560/3/3/002

Blednov, Y. A., and Harris, R. A. (2008). Metabotropic glutamate receptor 5 (mGluR5) regulation of ethanol sedation, dependence and consumption: relationship to acamprosate actions. *Int. J. Neuropsychopharmacol.* 11, 775–793. doi: 10.1017/S1461145708008584

Bogdanik, L., Mohrmann, R., Ramaekers, A., Bockaert, J., Grau, Y., Broadie, K., et al. (2004). The *Drosophila* metabotropic glutamate receptor DmGluRA regulates activity-dependent synaptic facilitation and fine synaptic morphology. *J. Neurosci.* 24, 9105–9116. doi: 10.1523/JNEUROSCI.2724-04.2004

Bokoch, G. M. (2003). Biology of the p21-activated kinases. *Annu. Rev. Biochem.* 72, 743–781. doi: 10.1146/annurev.biochem.72.121801.161742

Bolduc, F. V., Bell, K., Cox, H., Broadie, K. S., and Tully, T. (2008). Excess protein synthesis in *Drosophila* fragile X mutants impairs long-term memory. *Nat. Neurosci.* 11, 1143–1145. doi: 10.1038/nn.2175

Bolduc, F. V., Bell, K., Rosenfelt, C., Cox, H., and Tully, T. (2010a). Fragile X mental retardation 1 and filamin a interact genetically in *Drosophila* long-term memory. *Front. Neural Circuits* 3:22. doi: 10.3389/neuro.04.022.2009

Bolduc, F. V., Valente, D., Nguyen, A. T., Mitra, P. P., and Tully, T. (2010b). An assay for social interaction in *Drosophila* fragile X mutants. *Fly (Austin)* 4, 216–225. doi: 10.4161/fly.4.3.12280

Bongmba, O. Y., Martinez, L. A., Elhardt, M. E., Butler, K., and Tejada-Simon, M. V. (2011). Modulation of dendritic spines and synaptic function by Rac1: a possible link to fragile X syndrome pathology. *Brain Res.* 1399, 79–95. doi: 10.1016/j.brainres.2011.05.020

Bonhoeffer, T., and Yuste, R. (2002). Spine motility. Phenomenology, mechanisms, and function. *Neuron* 35, 1019–1027. doi: 10.1016/S0896-6273(02)00906-6

Bourgeois, J. A., Coffey, S. M., Rivera, S. M., Hessl, D., Gane, L. W., Tassone, F., et al. (2009). A review of fragile X premutation disorders: expanding the psychiatric perspective. *J. Clin. Psychiatry* 70, 852–862. doi: 10.4088/JCP.08m04476

Braun, K., and Segal, M. (2000). FMRP involvement in formation of synapses among cultured hippocampal neurons. *Cereb. Cortex* 10, 1045–1052. doi: 10.1093/cercor/10.10.1045

Broser, P., Grinevich, V., Osten, P., Sakmann, B., and Wallace, D. J. (2008). Critical period plasticity of axonal arbors of layer 2/3 pyramidal neurons in rat somatosensory cortex: layer-specific reduction of projections into deprived cortical columns. *Cereb. Cortex* 18, 1588–1603. doi: 10.1093/cercor/bhm189

Brown, M. R., Kronengold, J., Gazula, V. R., Chen, Y., Strumbos, J. G., Sigworth, F. J., et al. (2010). Fragile X mental retardation protein controls gating of the sodium-activated potassium channel Slack. *Nat. Neurosci.* 13, 819–821. doi: 10.1038/nn.2563

Bureau, I., Shepherd, G. M., and Svoboda, K. (2008). Circuit and plasticity defects in the developing somatosensory cortex of FMR1 knock-out mice. *J. Neurosci.* 28, 5178–5188. doi: 10.1523/JNEUROSCI.1076-08.2008

Cao, G., Platisa, J., Pieribone, V. A., Raccuglia, D., Kunst, M., and Nitabach, M. N. (2013). Genetically targeted optical electrophysiology in intact neural circuits. *Cell* 154, 904–913. doi: 10.1016/j.cell.2013.07.027

Casanova, M. F. (2006). Neuropathological and genetic findings in autism: the significance of a putative minicolumnopathy. *Neuroscientist* 12, 435–441. doi: 10.1177/1073858406290375

Castillo, P. E., Chiu, C. Q., and Carroll, R. C. (2011). Long-term plasticity at inhibitory synapses. *Curr. Opin. Neurobiol.* 21, 328–338. doi: 10.1016/j.conb.2011.01.006

Centonze, D., Rossi, S., Mercaldo, V., Napoli, I., Ciotti, M. T., De Chiara, V., et al. (2008). Abnormal striatal GABA transmission in the mouse model for the fragile X syndrome. *Biol. Psychiatry* 63, 963–973. doi: 10.1016/j.biopsych.2007.09.008

Chahrour, M. H., Yu, T. W., Lim, E. T., Ataman, B., Coulter, M. E., Hill, R. S., et al. (2012). Whole-exome sequencing and homozygosity analysis implicate depolarization-regulated neuronal genes in autism. *PLoS Genet.* 8:e1002635. doi: 10.1371/journal.pgen.1002635

Chang, E. F., and Merzenich, M. M. (2003). Environmental noise retards auditory cortical development. *Science* 300, 498–502. doi: 10.1126/science.1082163

Charalambous, D. C., Pasciuto, E., Mercaldo, V., Pilo Boyl, P., Munck, S., Bagni, C., et al. (2013). KIF1Bbeta transports dendritically localized mRNPs in neurons and is recruited to synapses in an activity-dependent manner. *Cell. Mol. Life Sci.* 70, 335–356. doi: 10.1007/s00018-012-1108-0

Chaudhury, S., Nag, T. C., Jain, S., and Wadhwa, S. (2013). Role of sound stimulation in reprogramming brain connectivity. *J. Biosci.* 38, 605–614. doi: 10.1007/s12038-013-9341-8

Chen, L. Y., Rex, C. S., Babayan, A. H., Kramar, E. A., Lynch, G., Gall, C. M., et al. (2010). Physiological activation of synaptic Rac > PAK (p-21 activated kinase) signaling is defective in a mouse model of fragile X syndrome. *J. Neurosci.* 30, 10977–10984. doi: 10.1523/JNEUROSCI.1077-10.2010

Chen, T. W., Wardill, T. J., Sun, Y., Pulver, S. R., Renninger, S. L., Baohan, A., et al. (2013). Ultrasensitive fluorescent proteins for imaging neuronal activity. *Nature* 499, 295–300. doi: 10.1038/nature12354

Chiang, A. S., Lin, C. Y., Chuang, C. C., Chang, H. M., Hsieh, C. H., Yeh, C. W., et al. (2011). Three-dimensional reconstruction of brain-wide wiring networks in *Drosophila* at single-cell resolution. *Curr. Biol.* 21, 1–11. doi: 10.1016/j.cub.2010.11.056

Choi, C. H., Mcbride, S. M., Schoenfeld, B. P., Liebelt, D. A., Ferreiro, D., Ferrick, N. J., et al. (2010a). Age-dependent cognitive impairment in a *Drosophila* fragile X model and its pharmacological rescue. *Biogerontology* 11, 347–362. doi: 10.1007/s10522-009-9259-6

Choi, H. C., Kim, Y. I., Song, H. K., Kim, J. E., Kim, D. S., and Kang, T. C. (2010b). Effects of selective serotonin reuptake inhibitors on GABAergic inhibition in the hippocampus of normal and pilocarpine induced epileptic rats. *Brain Res.* 1357, 131–141. doi: 10.1016/j.brainres.2010.08.010

Choi, C. H., Schoenfeld, B. P., Bell, A. J., Hinchey, P., Kollaros, M., Gertner, M. J., et al. (2011). Pharmacological reversal of synaptic plasticity deficits in the mouse model of fragile X syndrome by group II mGluR antagonist or lithium treatment. *Brain Res.* 1380, 106–119. doi: 10.1016/j.brainres.2010.11.032

Choi, S., Kim, J. Y., Park, J. H., Lee, S. T., Han, I. O., and Oh, E. S. (2012). The matrix metalloproteinase-7 regulates the extracellular shedding of syndecan-2 from colon cancer cells. *Biochem. Biophys. Res. Commun.* 417, 1260–1264. doi: 10.1016/j.bbrc.2011.12.120

Choi, Y., Kim, H. S., Shin, K. Y., Kim, E. M., Kim, M., Kim, H. S., et al. (2007). Minocycline attenuates neuronal cell death and improves cognitive impairment in Alzheimer's disease models. *Neuropsychopharmacology* 32, 2393–2404. doi: 10.1038/sj.npp.1301377

Chou, Y. H., Spletter, M. L., Yaksi, E., Leong, J. C., Wilson, R. I., and Luo, L. (2010). Diversity and wiring variability of olfactory local interneurons in the *Drosophila* antennal lobe. *Nat. Neurosci.* 13, 439–449. doi: 10.1038/nn.2489

Chowdhury, S., Shepherd, J. D., Okuno, H., Lyford, G., Petralia, R. S., Plath, N., et al. (2006). Arc/Arg3.1 interacts with the endocytic machinery to regulate AMPA receptor trafficking. *Neuron* 52, 445–459. doi: 10.1016/j.neuron.2006.08.033

Clare, M. H., and Bishop, G. H. (1954). Responses from an association area secondarily activated from optic cortex. *J. Neurophysiol.* 17, 271–277.

Coffee, R. L. Jr., Tessier, C. R., Woodruff, E. A. III, and Broadie, K. (2010). Fragile X mental retardation protein has a unique, evolutionarily conserved neuronal function not shared with FXR1P or FXR2P. *Dis. Model. Mech.* 3, 471–485. doi: 10.1242/dmm.004598

Coffee, R. L. Jr., Williamson, A. J., Adkins, C. M., Gray, M. C., Page, T. L., and Broadie, K. (2012). In vivo neuronal function of the fragile X mental retardation protein is regulated by phosphorylation. *Hum. Mol. Genet.* 21, 900–915. doi: 10.1093/hmg/ddr527

Coghlan, S., Horder, J., Inkster, B., Mendez, M. A., Murphy, D. G., and Nutt, D. J. (2012). GABA system dysfunction in autism and related disorders: from synapse to symptoms. *Neurosci. Biobehav. Rev.* 36, 2044–2055. doi: 10.1016/j.neubiorev.2012.07.005

Cohen, S., and Greenberg, M. E. (2008). Communication between the synapse and the nucleus in neuronal development, plasticity, and disease. *Annu. Rev. Cell Dev. Biol.* 24, 183–209. doi: 10.1146/annurev.cellbio.24.110707.175235

Comery, T. A., Harris, J. B., Willems, P. J., Oostra, B. A., Irwin, S. A., Weiler, I. J., et al. (1997). Abnormal dendritic spines in fragile X knockout mice: maturation and pruning deficits. *Proc. Natl. Acad. Sci. U.S.A.* 94, 5401–5404. doi: 10.1073/pnas.94.10.5401

Cook, D., Sanchez-Carbente Mdel, R., Lachance, C., Radzioch, D., Tremblay, S., Khandjian, E. W., et al. (2011). Fragile X related protein 1 clusters with ribosomes and messenger RNAs at a subset of dendritic spines in the mouse hippocampus. *PLoS ONE* 6:e26120. doi: 10.1371/journal.pone.0026120

Coppola, G., Terraciano, A. M., and Pascotto, A. (1997). Vigabatrin as add-on therapy in children and adolescents with refractory epilepsy: an open trial. *Brain Dev.* 19, 459–463. doi: 10.1016/S0387-7604(97)00063-6

Corbett, B. A., Swain, D. M., Coke, C., Simon, D., Newsom, C., Houchins-Juarez, N., et al. (2013). Improvement in social deficits in autism spectrum disorders using a theatre-based, peer-mediated intervention. *Autism Res.* doi: 10.1002/aur.1341 [Epub ahead of print].

Costa, L., Spatuzza, M., D'Antoni, S., Bonaccorso, C. M., Trovato, C., Musumeci, S. A., et al. (2012). Activation of 5-HT7 serotonin receptors reverses metabotropic glutamate receptor-mediated synaptic plasticity in wild-type and Fmr1 knockout mice, a model of fragile X syndrome. *Biol. Psychiatry* 72, 924–933. doi: 10.1016/j.biopsych.2012.06.008

Costa-Mattioli, M., Sossin, W. S., Klann, E., and Sonenberg, N. (2009). Translational control of long-lasting synaptic plasticity and memory. *Neuron* 61, 10–26. doi: 10.1016/j.neuron.2008.10.055

Courchesne, E., and Pierce, K. (2005). Why the frontal cortex in autism might be talking only to itself: local over-connectivity but long-distance disconnection. *Curr. Opin. Neurobiol.* 15, 225–230. doi: 10.1016/j.conb.2005.03.001

Crawley, J. N. (2007). Mouse behavioral assays relevant to the symptoms of autism. *Brain Pathol.* 17, 448–459. doi: 10.1111/j.1750-3639.2007.00096.x

Cruz-Martin, A., Crespo, M., and Portera-Cailliau, C. (2010). Delayed stabilization of dendritic spines in fragile X mice. *J. Neurosci.* 30, 7793–7803. doi: 10.1523/JNEUROSCI.0577-10.2010

Curia, G., Papouin, T., Seguela, P., and Avoli, M. (2009). Downregulation of tonic GABAergic inhibition in a mouse model of fragile X syndrome. *Cereb. Cortex* 19, 1515–1520. doi: 10.1093/cercor/bhn159

Dahlhaus, R., and El-Husseini, A. (2010). Altered neuroligin expression is involved in social deficits in a mouse model of the fragile X syndrome. *Behav. Brain Res.* 208, 96–105. doi: 10.1016/j.bbr.2009.11.019

Dani, N., and Broadie, K. (2012). Glycosylated synaptomatrix regulation of trans-synaptic signaling. *Dev. Neurobiol.* 72, 2–21. doi: 10.1002/dneu.20891

Dani, N., Nahm, M., Lee, S., and Broadie, K. (2012). A targeted glycan-related gene screen reveals heparan sulfate proteoglycan sulfation regulates WNT and BMP trans-synaptic signaling. *PLoS Genet.* 8:e1003031. doi: 10.1371/journal.pgen.1003031

Dansie, L. E., Phommahaxay, K., Okusanya, A. G., Uwadia, J., Huang, M., Rotschafer, S. E., et al. (2013). Long-lasting effects of minocycline on behavior in young but not adult fragile X mice. *Neuroscience* 246, 186–198. doi: 10.1016/j.neuroscience.2013.04.058

Darnell, J. C., Van Driesche, S. J., Zhang, C., Hung, K. Y., Mele, A., Fraser, C. E., et al. (2011). FMRP stalls ribosomal translocation on mRNAs linked to synaptic function and autism. *Cell* 146, 247–261. doi: 10.1016/j.cell.2011.06.013

David, A., Dolan, B. P., Hickman, H. D., Knowlton, J. J., Clavarino, G., Pierre, P., et al. (2012). Nuclear translation visualized by ribosome-bound nascent chain puromycylation. *J. Cell Biol.* 197, 45–57. doi: 10.1083/jcb.201112145

Dawson, G., Rogers, S., Munson, J., Smith, M., Winter, J., Greenson, J., et al. (2010). Randomized, controlled trial of an intervention for toddlers with autism: the Early Start Denver Model. *Pediatrics* 125, e17–e23. doi: 10.1542/peds.2009-0958

Deacon, S., Staner, L., Staner, C., Legters, A., Loft, H., and Lundahl, J. (2007). Effect of short-term treatment with gaboxadol on sleep maintenance and initiation in patients with primary insomnia. *Sleep* 30, 281–287.

Delorme, R., Ey, E., Toro, R., Leboyer, M., Gillberg, C., and Bourgeron, T. (2013). Progress toward treatments for synaptic defects in autism. *Nat. Med.* 19, 685–694. doi: 10.1038/nm.3193

Deng, P. Y., Rotman, Z., Blundon, J. A., Cho, Y., Cui, J., Cavalli, V., et al. (2013). FMRP regulates neurotransmitter release and synaptic information transmission by modulating action potential duration via BK channels. *Neuron* 77, 696–711. doi: 10.1016/j.neuron.2012.12.018

Devlin, B., and Scherer, S. W. (2012). Genetic architecture in autism spectrum disorder. *Curr. Opin. Genet. Dev.* 22, 229–237. doi: 10.1016/j.gde.2012.03.002

Dhaka, A., Viswanath, V., and Patapoutian, A. (2006). Trp ion channels and temperature sensation. *Annu. Rev. Neurosci.* 29, 135–161. doi: 10.1146/annurev.neuro.29.051605.112958

D'Hulst, C., De Geest, N., Reeve, S. P., Van Dam, D., De Deyn, P. P., Hassan, B. A., et al. (2006). Decreased expression of the GABAA receptor in fragile X syndrome. *Brain Res.* 1121, 238–245. doi: 10.1016/j.brainres.2006.08.115

Dickson, P. E., Corkill, B., Mckimm, E., Miller, M. M., Calton, M. A., Goldowitz, D., et al. (2013). Effects of stimulus salience on touchscreen serial reversal learning in a mouse model of fragile X syndrome. *Behav. Brain Res.* 252, 126–135. doi: 10.1016/j.bbr.2013.05.060

Dictenberg, J. B., Swanger, S. A., Antar, L. N., Singer, R. H., and Bassell, G. J. (2008). A direct role for FMRP in activity-dependent dendritic mRNA transport links filopodial-spine morphogenesis to fragile X syndrome. *Dev. Cell* 14, 926–939. doi: 10.1016/j.devcel.2008.04.003

Dockendorff, T. C., Su, H. S., Mcbride, S. M., Yang, Z., Choi, C. H., Siwicki, K. K., et al. (2002). *Drosophila* lacking dfmr1 activity show defects in circadian output and fail to maintain courtship interest. *Neuron* 34, 973–984. doi: 10.1016/S0896-6273(02)00724-9

Dolan, B. M., Duron, S. G., Campbell, D. A., Vollrath, B., Shankaranarayana Rao, B. S., Ko, H. Y., et al. (2013). Rescue of fragile X syndrome phenotypes in Fmr1 KO mice by the small-molecule PAK inhibitor FRAX486. *Proc. Natl. Acad. Sci. U.S.A.* 110, 5671–5676. doi: 10.1073/pnas.1219383110

Dolen, G., and Bear, M. F. (2008). Role for metabotropic glutamate receptor 5 (mGluR5) in the pathogenesis of fragile X syndrome. *J. Physiol.* 586, 1503–1508. doi: 10.1113/jphysiol.2008.150722

Dolen, G., Carpenter, R. L., Ocain, T. D., and Bear, M. F. (2010). Mechanism-based approaches to treating fragile X. *Pharmacol. Ther.* 127, 78–93. doi: 10.1016/j.pharmthera.2010.02.008

Dolen, G., Osterweil, E., Rao, B. S., Smith, G. B., Auerbach, B. D., Chattarji, S., et al. (2007). Correction of fragile X syndrome in mice. *Neuron* 56, 955–962. doi: 10.1016/j.neuron.2007.12.001

Duch, C., Vonhoff, F., and Ryglewski, S. (2008). Dendrite elongation and dendritic branching are affected separately by different forms of intrinsic motoneuron excitability. *J. Neurophysiol.* 100, 2525–2536. doi: 10.1152/jn.90758.2008

Dziembowska, M., Milek, J., Janusz, A., Rejmak, E., Romanowska, E., Gorkiewicz, T., et al. (2012). Activity-dependent local translation of matrix metalloproteinase-9. *J. Neurosci.* 32, 14538–14547. doi: 10.1523/JNEUROSCI.6028-11.2012

Dziembowska, M., Pretto, D. I., Janusz, A., Kaczmarek, L., Leigh, M. J., Gabriel, N., et al. (2013). High MMP-9 activity levels in fragile X syndrome are lowered by minocycline. *Am. J. Med. Genet. A* 161A, 1897–1903. doi: 10.1002/ajmg.a.36023

Eaton, B. A., and Davis, G. W. (2005). LIM kinasel controls synaptic stability downstream of the type II BMP receptor. *Neuron* 47, 695–708. doi: 10.1016/j.neuron.2005.08.010

Ebert, D. H., and Greenberg, M. E. (2013). Activity-dependent neuronal signalling and autism spectrum disorder. *Nature* 493, 327–337. doi: 10.1038/nature11860

Elbert, T., Pantev, C., Wienbruch, C., Rockstroh, B., and Taub, E. (1995). Increased cortical representation of the fingers of the left hand in string players. *Science* 270, 305–307. doi: 10.1126/science.270.5234.305

El Idrissi, A., Ding, X. H., Scalia, J., Trenkner, E., Brown, W. T., and Dobkin, C. (2005). Decreased GABA(A) receptor expression in the seizure-prone fragile X mouse. *Neurosci. Lett.* 377, 141–146. doi: 10.1016/j.neulet.2004.11.087

Elvira, G., Wasiak, S., Blandford, V., Tong, X. K., Serrano, A., Fan, X., et al. (2006). Characterization of an RNA granule from developing brain. *Mol. Cell. Proteomics* 5, 635–651. doi: 10.1074/mcp.M500255-MCP200

Erickson, C. A., Early, M., Stigler, K. A., Wink, L. K., Mullett, J. E., and Mcdougle, C. J. (2011a). An open-label naturalistic pilot study of acamprosate in youth with autistic disorder. *J. Child Adolesc. Psychopharmacol.* 21, 565–569. doi: 10.1089/cap.2011.0034

Erickson, C. A., Weng, N., Weiler, I. J., Greenough, W. T., Stigler, K. A., Wink, L. K., et al. (2011b). Open-label riluzole in fragile X syndrome. *Brain Res.* 1380, 264–270. doi: 10.1016/j.brainres.2010.10.108

Erickson, C. A., Mullett, J. E., and Mcdougle, C. J. (2010). Brief report: acamprosate in fragile X syndrome. *J. Autism Dev. Disord.* 40, 1412–1416. doi: 10.1007/s10803-010-0988-9

Ethell, I. M., and Ethell, D. W. (2007). Matrix metalloproteinases in brain development and remodeling: synaptic functions and targets. *J. Neurosci. Res.* 85, 2813–2823. doi: 10.1002/jnr.21273

Fatemi, S. H., and Folsom, T. D. (2011). The role of fragile X mental retardation protein in major mental disorders. *Neuropharmacology* 60, 1221–1226. doi: 10.1016/j.neuropharm.2010.11.011

Fatemi, S. H., Folsom, T. D., Reutiman, T. J., and Thuras, P. D. (2009a). Expression of GABA(B) receptors is altered in brains of subjects with autism. *Cerebellum* 8, 64–69. doi: 10.1007/s12311-008-0075-3

Fatemi, S. H., Reutiman, T. J., Folsom, T. D., and Thuras, P. D. (2009b). GABA(A) receptor downregulation in brains of subjects with autism. *J. Autism Dev. Disord.* 39, 223–230. doi: 10.1007/s10803-008-0646-7.

Fatemi, S. H., Halt, A. R., Stary, J. M., Kanodia, R., Schulz, S. C., and Realmuto, G. R. (2002). Glutamic acid decarboxylase 65 and 67 kDa proteins are reduced in autistic parietal and cerebellar cortices. *Biol. Psychiatry* 52, 805–810. doi: 10.1016/S0006-3223(02)01430-0

Fatemi, S. H., Kneeland, R. E., Liesch, S. B., and Folsom, T. D. (2010). Fragile X mental retardation protein levels are decreased in major psychiatric disorders. *Schizophr. Res.* 124, 246–247. doi: 10.1016/j.schres.2010.07.017

Featherstone, D. E., and Broadie, K. (2000). Surprises from *Drosophila*: genetic mechanisms of synaptic development and plasticity. *Brain Res. Bull.* 53, 501–511. doi: 10.1016/S0361-9230(00)00383-X

Feinberg, E. H., Vanhoven, M. K., Bendesky, A., Wang, G., Fetter, R. D., Shen, K., et al. (2008). GFP Reconstitution Across Synaptic Partners (GRASP) defines cell contacts and synapses in living nervous systems. *Neuron* 57, 353–363. doi: 10.1016/j.neuron.2007.11.030

Feldmeyer, D., Brecht, M., Helmchen, F., Petersen, C. C., Poulet, J. F., Staiger, J. F., et al. (2013). Barrel cortex function. *Prog. Neurobiol.* 103, 3–27. doi: 10.1016/j.pneurobio.2012.11.002

Fenno, L., Yizhar, O., and Deisseroth, K. (2011). The development and application of optogenetics. *Annu. Rev. Neurosci.* 34, 389–412. doi: 10.1146/annurev-neuro-061010-113817

Ferrari, F., Mercaldo, V., Piccoli, G., Sala, C., Cannata, S., Achsel, T., et al. (2007). The fragile X mental retardation protein-RNP granules show an mGluR-dependent localization in the post-synaptic spines. *Mol. Cell. Neurosci.* 34, 343–354. doi: 10.1016/j.mcn.2006.11.015

Fiala, J. C., Feinberg, M., Popov, V., and Harris, K. M. (1998). Synaptogenesis via dendritic filopodia in developing hippocampal area CA1. *J. Neurosci.* 18, 8900–8911.

Flavell, S. W., Cowan, C. W., Kim, T. K., Greer, P. L., Lin, Y., Paradis, S., et al. (2006). Activity-dependent regulation of MEF2 transcription factors suppresses excitatory synapse number. *Science* 311, 1008–1012. doi: 10.1126/science.1122511

Flavell, S. W., and Greenberg, M. E. (2008). Signaling mechanisms linking neuronal activity to gene expression and plasticity of the nervous system. *Annu. Rev. Neurosci.* 31, 563–590. doi: 10.1146/annurev.neuro.31.060407.125631

French, J. A., Mosier, M., Walker, S., Sommerville, K., and Sussman, N. (1996). A double-blind, placebo-controlled study of vigabatrin three g/day in patients with uncontrolled complex partial seizures. Vigabatrin Protocol 024 Investigative Cohort. *Neurology* 46, 54–61. doi: 10.1212/WNL.46.1.54

Friedman, S. H., Dani, N., Rushton, E., and Broadie, K. (2013). Fragile X mental retardation protein regulates trans-synaptic signaling in *Drosophila. Dis. Model. Mech.* 6, 1400–1413. doi: 10.1242/dmm.012229

Frith, C. (2004). Is autism a disconnection disorder? *Lancet Neurol.* 3, 577. doi: 10.1016/S1474-4422(04)00875-0

Fujita, N., Nagata, Y., Nishiuchi, T., Sato, M., Iwami, M., and Kiya, T. (2013). Visualization of neural activity in insect brains using a conserved immediate early gene, Hr38. *Curr. Biol.* 23, 2063–2070. doi: 10.1016/j.cub.2013.08.051

Fukuda, T., Itoh, M., Ichikawa, T., Washiyama, K., and Goto, Y. (2005). Delayed maturation of neuronal architecture and synaptogenesis in cerebral cortex of Mecp2-deficient mice. *J. Neuropathol. Exp. Neurol.* 64, 537–544.

Gabel, L. A., Won, S., Kawai, H., Mckinney, M., Tartakoff, A. M., and Fallon, J. R. (2004). Visual experience regulates transient expression and dendritic localization of fragile X mental retardation protein. *J. Neurosci.* 24, 10579–10583. doi: 10.1523/JNEUROSCI.2185-04.2004

Galvez, R., Smith, R. L., and Greenough, W. T. (2005). Olfactory bulb mitral cell dendritic pruning abnormalities in a mouse model of the Fragile-X mental retardation syndrome: further support for FMRP's involvement in dendritic development. *Brain Res. Dev. Brain Res.* 157, 214–216. doi: 10.1016/j.devbrainres.2005.03.010

Gant, J. C., Thibault, O., Blalock, E. M., Yang, J., Bachstetter, A., Kotick, J., et al. (2009). Decreased number of interneurons and increased seizures in neuropilin 2 deficient mice: implications for autism and epilepsy. *Epilepsia* 50, 629–645. doi: 10.1111/j.1528-1167.2008.01725.x

Gantois, I., Pop, A. S., De Esch, C. E., Buijsen, R. A., Pooters, T., Gomez-Mancilla, B., et al. (2013). Chronic administration of AFQ056/Mavoglurant restores social behaviour in Fmr1 knockout mice. *Behav. Brain Res.* 239, 72–79. doi: 10.1016/j.bbr.2012.10.059

Gantois, I., Vandesompele, J., Speleman, F., Reyniers, E., D'Hooge, R., Severijnen, L. A., et al. (2006). Expression profiling suggests underexpression of the GABA(A) receptor subunit delta in the fragile X knockout mouse model. *Neurobiol. Dis.* 21, 346–357. doi: 10.1016/j.nbd.2005.07.017

Gao, W. J., Wormington, A. B., Newman, D. E., and Pallas, S. L. (2000). Development of inhibitory circuitry in visual and auditory cortex of postnatal ferrets: immunocytochemical localization of calbindin- and parvalbumin-containing neurons. *J. Comp. Neurol.* 422, 140–157. doi: 10.1002/(SICI)1096-9861(20000619)422:1<140::AID-CNE9>3.0.CO;2-0

Gatto, C. L., and Broadie, K. (2008). Temporal requirements of the fragile X mental retardation protein in the regulation of synaptic structure. *Development* 135, 2637–2648. doi: 10.1242/dev.022244

Gatto, C. L., and Broadie, K. (2009). Temporal requirements of the fragile X mental retardation protein in modulating circadian clock circuit synaptic architecture. *Front. Neural Circuits* 3:8. doi: 10.3389/neuro.04.008.2009

Gatto, C. L., and Broadie, K. (2010). Genetic controls balancing excitatory and inhibitory synaptogenesis in neurodevelopmental disorder models. *Front. Synaptic Neurosci.* 2:4. doi: 10.3389/fnsyn.2010.00004

Gatto, C. L., Pereira, D., and Broadie, K. (2014). GABAergic circuit dysfunction in the *Drosophila* Fragile X syndrome model. *Neurobiol. Dis.* doi: 10.1016/j.nbd.2014.01.008 [Epub ahead of print].

Geschwind, D. H., and Levitt, P. (2007). Autism spectrum disorders: developmental disconnection syndromes. *Curr. Opin. Neurobiol.* 17, 103–111. doi: 10.1016/j.conb.2007.01.009

Geschwind, N. (1965a). Disconnexion syndromes in animals and man. I. *Brain* 88, 237–294. doi: 10.1093/brain/88.2.237

Geschwind, N. (1965b). Disconnexion syndromes in animals and man. II. *Brain* 88, 585–644. doi: 10.1093/brain/88.3.585

Gibson, J. R., Bartley, A. F., Hays, S. A., and Huber, K. M. (2008). Imbalance of neocortical excitation and inhibition and altered UP states reflect network hyperexcitability in the mouse model of fragile X syndrome. *J. Neurophysiol.* 100, 2615–2626. doi: 10.1152/jn.90752.2008

Gilman, S. R., Iossifov, I., Levy, D., Ronemus, M., Wigler, M., and Vitkup, D. (2011). Rare de novo variants associated with autism implicate a large functional network of genes involved in formation and function of synapses. *Neuron* 70, 898–907. doi: 10.1016/j.neuron.2011.05.021

Goebel-Goody, S. M., Wilson-Wallis, E. D., Royston, S., Tagliatela, S. M., Naegele, J. R., and Lombroso, P. J. (2012). Genetic manipulation of STEP reverses behavioral abnormalities in a fragile X syndrome mouse model. *Genes Brain Behav.* 11, 586–600. doi: 10.1111/j.1601-183X.2012.00781.x

Golshani, P., Goncalves, J. T., Khoshkhoo, S., Mostany, R., Smirnakis, S., and Portera-Cailliau, C. (2009). Internally mediated developmental desynchronization of neocortical network activity. *J. Neurosci.* 29, 10890–10899. doi: 10.1523/JNEUROSCI.2012-09.2009

Goncalves, J. T., Anstey, J. E., Golshani, P., and Portera-Cailliau, C. (2013). Circuit level defects in the developing neocortex of fragile X mice. *Nat. Neurosci.* 16, 903–909. doi: 10.1038/nn.3415

Graber, T. E., Hebert-Seropian, S., Khoutorsky, A., David, A., Yewdell, J. W., Lacaille, J. C., et al. (2013). Reactivation of stalled polyribosomes in synaptic plasticity. *Proc. Natl. Acad. Sci. U.S.A.* 110, 16205–16210. doi: 10.1073/pnas.1307747110

Gradinaru, V., Mogri, M., Thompson, K. R., Henderson, J. M., and Deisseroth, K. (2009). Optical deconstruction of parkinsonian neural circuitry. *Science* 324, 354–359. doi: 10.1126/science.1167093

Gradinaru, V., Thompson, K. R., and Deisseroth, K. (2008). eNpHR: a natronomonas halorhodopsin enhanced for optogenetic applications. *Brain Cell Biol.* 36, 129–139. doi: 10.1007/s11068-008-9027-6

Greenberg, M. E., Ziff, E. B., and Greene, L. A. (1986). Stimulation of neuronal acetylcholine receptors induces rapid gene transcription. *Science* 234, 80–83. doi: 10.1126/science.3749894

Greenough, W. T., Hwang, H. M., and Gorman, C. (1985). Evidence for active synapse formation or altered postsynaptic metabolism in visual cortex of rats reared in complex environments. *Proc. Natl. Acad. Sci. U.S.A.* 82, 4549–4552. doi: 10.1073/pnas.82.13.4549

Greer, P. L., and Greenberg, M. E. (2008). From synapse to nucleus: calcium-dependent gene transcription in the control of synapse development and function. *Neuron* 59, 846–860. doi: 10.1016/j.neuron.2008.09.002

Grienberger, C., and Konnerth, A. (2012). Imaging calcium in neurons. *Neuron* 73, 862–885. doi: 10.1016/j.neuron.2012.02.011

Grillo, F. W., Song, S., Teles-Grilo Ruivo, L. M., Huang, L., Gao, G., Knott, G. W., et al. (2013). Increased axonal bouton dynamics in the aging mouse cortex. *Proc. Natl. Acad. Sci. U.S.A.* 110, E1514–E1523. doi: 10.1073/pnas.1218731110

Grutzendler, J., Kasthuri, N., and Gan, W. B. (2002). Long-term dendritic spine stability in the adult cortex. *Nature* 420, 812–816. doi: 10.1038/nature01276

Hagerman, R., Hoem, G., and Hagerman, P. (2010). Fragile X and autism: intertwined at the molecular level leading to targeted treatments. *Mol. Autism* 1, 12. doi: 10.1186/2040-2392-1-12

Hagerman, R. J., Berry-Kravis, E., Kaufmann, W. E., Ono, M. Y., Tartaglia, N., Lachiewicz, A., et al. (2009). Advances in the treatment of fragile X syndrome. *Pediatrics* 123, 378–390. doi: 10.1542/peds.2008-0317

Hagerman, R. J., and Hagerman, P. J. (2002). The fragile X premutation: into the phenotypic fold. *Curr. Opin. Genet. Dev.* 12, 278–283. doi: 10.1016/S0959-437X(02)00299-X

Hamada, F. N., Rosenzweig, M., Kang, K., Pulver, S. R., Ghezzi, A., Jegla, T. J., et al. (2008). An internal thermal sensor controlling temperature preference in *Drosophila. Nature* 454, 217–220. doi: 10.1038/nature07001

Harris, S. W., Hessl, D., Goodlin-Jones, B., Ferranti, J., Bacalman, S., Barbato, I., et al. (2008). Autism profiles of males with fragile X syndrome. *Am. J. Ment. Retard.* 113, 427–438. doi: 10.1352/2008.113:427-438.

Hartwig, C. L., Worrell, J., Levine, R. B., Ramaswami, M., and Sanyal, S. (2008). Normal dendrite growth in *Drosophila* motor neurons requires the AP-1 transcription factor. *Dev. Neurobiol.* 68, 1225–1242. doi: 10.1002/dneu.20655

Hayama, T., Noguchi, J., Watanabe, S., Takahashi, N., Hayashi-Takagi, A., Ellis-Davies, G. C., et al. (2013). GABA promotes the competitive selection of dendritic spines by controlling local Ca^{2+} signaling. *Nat. Neurosci.* 16, 1409–1416. doi: 10.1038/nn.3496

He, C. X., and Portera-Cailliau, C. (2013). The trouble with spines in fragile X syndrome: density, maturity and plasticity. *Neuroscience* 251, 120–128. doi: 10.1016/j.neuroscience.2012.03.049

Hebb, D. O. (1949). *The Organization of Behavior: A Neuropsychological Theory.* New York: Wiley.

Henderson, C., Wijetunge, L., Kinoshita, M. N., Shumway, M., Hammond, R. S., Postma, F. R., et al. (2012). Reversal of disease-related pathologies in the fragile X mouse model by selective activation of GABAB receptors with arbaclofen. *Sci. Transl. Med.* 4, 152ra128. doi: 10.1126/scitranslmed.3004218.

Hensch, T. K. (2003). Controlling the critical period. *Neurosci. Res.* 47, 17–22. doi: 10.1016/S0168-0102(03)00164-0

Hensch, T. K. (2004). Critical period regulation. *Annu. Rev. Neurosci.* 27, 549–579. doi: 10.1146/annurev.neuro.27.070203.144327

Hensch, T. K. (2005). Critical period plasticity in local cortical circuits. *Nat. Rev. Neurosci.* 6, 877–888. doi: 10.1038/nrn1787

Hessl, D., Berry-Kravis, E., Cordeiro, L., Yuhas, J., Ornitz, E. M., Campbell, A., et al. (2009). Prepulse inhibition in fragile X syndrome: feasibility, reliability, and implications for treatment. *Am. J. Med. Genet. B Neuropsychiatr. Genet.* 150B, 545–553. doi: 10.1002/ajmg.b.30858

Hoksbergen, R., Ter Laak, J., Rijk, K., Van Dijkum, C., and Stoutjesdijk, F. (2005). Post-institutional autistic syndrome in Romanian adoptees. *J. Autism Dev. Disord.* 35, 615–623. doi: 10.1007/s10803-005-0005-x

Holtmaat, A., and Svoboda, K. (2009). Experience-dependent structural synaptic plasticity in the mammalian brain. *Nat. Rev. Neurosci.* 10, 647–658. doi: 10.1038/nrn2699

Holtmaat, A., Wilbrecht, L., Knott, G. W., Welker, E., and Svoboda, K. (2006). Experience-dependent and cell-type-specific spine growth in the neocortex. *Nature* 441, 979–983. doi: 10.1038/nature04783

Holtmaat, A. J., Trachtenberg, J. T., Wilbrecht, L., Shepherd, G. M., Zhang, X., Knott, G. W., et al. (2005). Transient and persistent dendritic spines in the neocortex in vivo. *Neuron* 45, 279–291. doi: 10.1016/j.neuron.2005.01.003

Hong, E. J., Mccord, A. E., and Greenberg, M. E. (2008). A biological function for the neuronal activity-dependent component of Bdnf transcription in the development of cortical inhibition. *Neuron* 60, 610–624. doi: 10.1016/j.neuron.2008.09.024

Honig, L. S., Herrmann, K., and Shatz, C. J. (1996). Developmental changes revealed by immunohistochemical markers in human cerebral cortex. *Cereb. Cortex* 6, 794–806. doi: 10.1093/cercor/6.6.794

Hornberg, H., and Holt, C. (2013). RNA-binding proteins and translational regulation in axons and growth cones. *Front. Neurosci.* 7:81. doi: 10.3389/fnins.2013.00081

Hu, J., Van Den Steen, P. E., Sang, Q. X., and Opdenakker, G. (2007). Matrix metalloproteinase inhibitors as therapy for inflammatory and vascular diseases. *Nat. Rev. Drug Discov.* 6, 480–498. doi: 10.1038/nrd2308

Hubel, D. H., and Wiesel, T. N. (1959). Receptive fields of single neurones in the cat's striate cortex. *J. Physiol.* 148, 574–591.

Hubel, D. H., and Wiesel, T. N. (1962). Receptive fields, binocular interaction and functional architecture in the cat's visual cortex. *J. Physiol.* 160, 106–154.

Hubel, D. H., and Wiesel, T. N. (1970). The period of susceptibility to the physiological effects of unilateral eye closure in kittens. *J. Physiol.* 206, 419–436.

Huber, K. M., Gallagher, S. M., Warren, S. T., and Bear, M. F. (2002). Altered synaptic plasticity in a mouse model of fragile X mental retardation. *Proc. Natl. Acad. Sci. U.S.A.* 99, 7746–7750. doi: 10.1073/pnas.122205699

Huntley, G. W. (1997). Differential effects of abnormal tactile experience on shaping representation patterns in developing and adult motor cortex. *J. Neurosci.* 17, 9220–9232.

Hutsler, J. J., and Zhang, H. (2010). Increased dendritic spine densities on cortical projection neurons in autism spectrum disorders. *Brain Res.* 1309, 83–94. doi: 10.1016/j.brainres.2009.09.120

Inada, K., Kohsaka, H., Takasu, E., Matsunaga, T., and Nose, A. (2011). Optical dissection of neural circuits responsible for *Drosophila* larval locomotion with halorhodopsin. *PLoS ONE* 6:e29019. doi: 10.1371/journal.pone.0029019

Irie, F., Badie-Mahdavi, H., and Yamaguchi, Y. (2012). Autism-like socio-communicative deficits and stereotypies in mice lacking heparan sulfate. *Proc. Natl. Acad. Sci. U.S.A.* 109, 5052–5056. doi: 10.1073/pnas.1117881109

Irwin, S. A., Galvez, R., and Greenough, W. T. (2000). Dendritic spine structural anomalies in fragile-X mental retardation syndrome. *Cereb. Cortex* 10, 1038–1044. doi: 10.1093/cercor/10.10.1038

Irwin, S. A., Patel, B., Idupulapati, M., Harris, J. B., Crisostomo, R. A., Larsen, B. P., et al. (2001). Abnormal dendritic spine characteristics in the temporal and visual cortices of patients with fragile-X syndrome: a quantitative examination. *Am. J. Med. Genet.* 98, 161–167. doi: 10.1002/1096-8628(20010115)98:2<161::AID-AJMG1025>3.0.CO;2-B

Jahn, K., Schlesinger, F., Jin, L. J., Dengler, R., Bufler, J., and Krampfl, K. (2008). Molecular mechanisms of interaction between the neuroprotective substance riluzole and GABA(A)-receptors. *Naunyn Schmiedebergs Arch. Pharmacol.* 378, 53–63. doi: 10.1007/s00210-008-0290-y

Janusz, A., Milek, J., Perycz, M., Pacini, L., Bagni, C., Kaczmarek, L., et al. (2013). The fragile X mental retardation protein regulates matrix metalloproteinase 9 mRNA at synapses. *J. Neurosci.* 33, 18234–18241. doi: 10.1523/JNEUROSCI.2207-13.2013

Jarecki, J., and Keshishian, H. (1995). Role of neural activity during synaptogenesis in *Drosophila. J. Neurosci.* 15, 8177–8190.

Jenett, A., Rubin, G. M., Ngo, T. T., Shepherd, D., Murphy, C., Dionne, H., et al. (2012). A GAL4-driver line resource for *Drosophila* neurobiology. *Cell Rep.* 2, 991–1001. doi: 10.1016/j.celrep.2012.09.011

Jin, L., Han, Z., Platisa, J., Wooltorton, J. R., Cohen, L. B., and Pieribone, V. A. (2012). Single action potentials and subthreshold electrical events imaged in neurons with a fluorescent protein voltage probe. *Neuron* 75, 779–785. doi: 10.1016/j.neuron.2012.06.040

Johnson, K. G., Tenney, A. P., Ghose, A., Duckworth, A. M., Higashi, M. E., Parfitt, K., et al. (2006). The HSPGs Syndecan and Dallylike bind the receptor phosphatase LAR and exert distinct effects on synaptic development. *Neuron* 49, 517–531. doi: 10.1016/j.neuron.2006.01.026

Jones, W. D. (2009). The expanding reach of the GAL4/UAS system into the behavioral neurobiology of *Drosophila. BMB Rep.* 42, 705–712. doi: 10.5483/BMBRep.2009.42.11.705

Jontes, J. D., and Smith, S. J. (2000). Filopodia, spines, and the generation of synaptic diversity. *Neuron* 27, 11–14. doi: 10.1016/S0896-6273(00)00003-9

Judkewitz, B., Rizzi, M., Kitamura, K., and Hausser, M. (2009). Targeted single-cell electroporation of mammalian neurons in vivo. *Nat. Protoc.* 4, 862–869. doi: 10.1038/nprot.2009.56

Jung, R. (1958). Excitation, inhibition and coordination of cortical neurones. *Exp. Cell Res.* 14, 262–271.

Kanai, Y., Dohmae, N., and Hirokawa, N. (2004). Kinesin transports RNA: isolation and characterization of an RNA-transporting granule. *Neuron* 43, 513–525. doi: 10.1016/j.neuron.2004.07.022

Kanellopoulos, A. K., Semelidou, O., Kotini, A. G., Anezaki, M., and Skoulakis, E. M. (2012). Learning and memory deficits consequent to reduction of the fragile X mental retardation protein result from metabotropic glutamate receptor-mediated inhibition of cAMP signaling in *Drosophila. J. Neurosci.* 32, 13111–13124. doi: 10.1523/JNEUROSCI.1347-12.2012

Katz, L. C., and Shatz, C. J. (1996). Synaptic activity and the construction of cortical circuits. *Science* 274, 1133–1138. doi: 10.1126/science.274.5290.1133

Kaufmann, W. E., and Moser, H. W. (2000). Dendritic anomalies in disorders associated with mental retardation. *Cereb. Cortex* 10, 981–991. doi: 10.1093/cercor/10.10.981

Kayser, M. S., Nolt, M. J., and Dalva, M. B. (2008). EphB receptors couple dendritic filopodia motility to synapse formation. *Neuron* 59, 56–69. doi: 10.1016/j.neuron.2008.05.007

Kelemen, O., Kovacs, T., and Keri, S. (2013). Contrast, motion, perceptual integration, and neurocognition in schizophrenia: the role of fragile-X related mechanisms. *Prog. Neuropsychopharmacol. Biol. Psychiatry* 46, 92–97. doi: 10.1016/j.pnpbp.2013.06.017.

Keshishian, H., and Kim, Y. S. (2004). Orchestrating development and function: retrograde BMP signaling in the *Drosophila* nervous system. *Trends Neurosci.* 27, 143–147. doi: 10.1016/j.tins.2004.01.004

Kilgard, M. P., and Merzenich, M. M. (1998). Cortical map reorganization enabled by nucleus basalis activity. *Science* 279, 1714–1718. doi: 10.1126/science.279.5357.1714

Kim, H., Gibboni, R., Kirkhart, C., and Bao, S. (2013a). Impaired critical period plasticity in primary auditory cortex of fragile X model mice. *J. Neurosci.* 33, 15686–15692. doi: 10.1523/JNEUROSCI.3246-12.2013

Kim, S. H., Thurm, A., Shumway, S., and Lord, C. (2013b). Multisite study of new autism diagnostic interview-revised (ADI-R) algorithms for toddlers and young preschoolers. *J. Autism Dev. Disord.* 43, 1527–1538. doi: 10.1007/s10803-012-1696-4

Kim, H. S., and Suh, Y. H. (2009). Minocycline and neurodegenerative diseases. *Behav. Brain Res.* 196, 168–179. doi: 10.1016/j.bbr.2008.09.040

Kim, S. A., and Jun, S. B. (2013). Optical measurement of neural activity in the brain. *Exp. Neurobiol.* 22, 158–166. doi: 10.5607/en.2013.22.3.158

Kim, S. H., and Lord, C. (2012). Combining information from multiple sources for the diagnosis of autism spectrum disorders for toddlers and young preschoolers from 12 to 47 months of age. *J. Child Psychol. Psychiatry* 53, 143–151. doi: 10.1111/j.1469-7610.2011.02458.x

Kittelmann, M., Liewald, J. F., Hegermann, J., Schultheis, C., Brauner, M., Steuer Costa, W., et al. (2013). In vivo synaptic recovery following optogenetic hyperstimulation. *Proc. Natl. Acad. Sci. U.S.A.* 110, E3007–E3016. doi: 10.1073/pnas.1305679110

Koles, K., and Budnik, V. (2012). Wnt signaling in neuromuscular junction development. *Cold Spring Harb. Perspect. Biol.* 4. doi: 10.1101/cshperspect.a008045

Koleske, A. J. (2013). Molecular mechanisms of dendrite stability. *Nat. Rev. Neurosci.* 14, 536–550. doi: 10.1038/nrn3486

Kooy, R. F. (2003). Of mice and the fragile X syndrome. *Trends Genet.* 19, 148–154. doi: 10.1016/S0168-9525(03)00017-9

Korkut, C., Ataman, B., Ramachandran, P., Ashley, J., Barria, R., Gherbesi, N., et al. (2009). Trans-synaptic transmission of vesicular Wnt signals through Evi/Wntless. *Cell* 139, 393–404. doi: 10.1016/j.cell.2009.07.051

Korkut, C., and Budnik, V. (2009). WNTs tune up the neuromuscular junction. *Nat. Rev. Neurosci.* 10, 627–634. doi: 10.1038/nrn2681

Koshino, H., Carpenter, P. A., Minshew, N. J., Cherkassky, V. L., Keller, T. A., and Just, M. A. (2005). Functional connectivity in an fMRI working memory task in high-functioning autism. *Neuroimage* 24, 810–821. doi: 10.1016/j.neuroimage.2004.09.028

Kotlikoff, M. I. (2007). Genetically encoded Ca^{2+} indicators: using genetics and molecular design to understand complex physiology. *J. Physiol.* 578, 55–67. doi: 10.1113/jphysiol.2006.120212

Kovacs, T., Kelemen, O., and Keri, S. (2013). Decreased fragile X mental retardation protein (FMRP) is associated with lower IQ and earlier illness onset in patients with schizophrenia. *Psychiatry Res.* 210, 690–693. doi: 10.1016/j.psychres.2012.12.022

Kratovac, S., and Corbin, J. G. (2013). Developmental changes in expression of inhibitory neuronal proteins in the fragile X Syndrome mouse basolateral amygdala. *Brain Res.* 1537, 69–78. doi: 10.1016/j.brainres.2013.08.052

Kremer, M. C., Christiansen, F., Leiss, F., Paehler, M., Knapek, S., Andlauer, T. F., et al. (2010). Structural long-term changes at mushroom body input synapses. *Curr. Biol.* 20, 1938–1944. doi: 10.1016/j.cub.2010.09.060

Kreutz, M. R., and Sala, C. (2012). *Synaptic Plasticity: Dynamics, Development and Disease.* New York: Springer. doi: 10.1007/978-3-7091-0932-8

Krichevsky, A. M., and Kosik, K. S. (2001). Neuronal RNA granules: a link between RNA localization and stimulation-dependent translation. *Neuron* 32, 683–696. doi: 10.1016/S0896-6273(01)00508-6

Kroon, T., Sierksma, M. C., and Meredith, R. M. (2013). Investigating mechanisms underlying neurodevelopmental phenotypes of autistic and intellectual disability disorders: a perspective. *Front. Syst. Neurosci.* 7:75. doi: 10.3389/fnsys.2013.00075

Kuffler, S. W. (1953). Discharge patterns and functional organization of mammalian retina. *J. Neurophysiol.* 16, 37–68.

Lauterborn, J. C., Jafari, M., Babayan, A. H., and Gall, C. M. (2013). Environmental enrichment reveals effects of genotype on hippocampal spine morphologies in the mouse model of fragile X syndrome. *Cereb. Cortex* doi: 10.1093/cercor/bht249 [Epub ahead of print].

Lebeau, G., Miller, L. C., Tartas, M., Mcadam, R., Laplante, I., Badeaux, F., et al. (2011). Staufen 2 regulates mGluR long-term depression and Map1b mRNA distribution in hippocampal neurons. *Learn. Mem.* 18, 314–326. doi: 10.1101/lm.2100611

LeBlanc, J. J., and Fagiolini, M. (2011). Autism: a "critical period" disorder? *Neural Plast.* 2011, 921680. doi: 10.1155/2011/921680

Lee, T., and Luo, L. (2001). Mosaic analysis with a repressible cell marker (MARCM) for *Drosophila* neural development. *Trends Neurosci.* 24, 251–254. doi: 10.1016/S0166-2236(00)01791-4

Leehey, M. A., Berry-Kravis, E., Goetz, C. G., Zhang, L., Hall, D. A., Li, L., et al. (2008). FMR1 CGG repeat length predicts motor dysfunction in premutation carriers. *Neurology* 70, 1397–1402. doi: 10.1212/01.wnl.0000281692.98200.f5

Leigh, M. J., Nguyen, D. V., Mu, Y., Winarni, T. I., Schneider, A., Chechi, T., et al. (2013). A randomized double-blind, placebo-controlled trial of minocycline in children and adolescents with fragile X syndrome. *J. Dev. Behav. Pediatr.* 34, 147–155. doi: 10.1097/DBP.0b013e318287cd17

Lendvai, B., Stern, E. A., Chen, B., and Svoboda, K. (2000). Experience-dependent plasticity of dendritic spines in the developing rat barrel cortex in vivo. *Nature* 404, 876–881. doi: 10.1038/35009107

Levenga, J., De Vrij, F. M., Oostra, B.A., and Willemsen, R. (2010). Potential therapeutic interventions for fragile X syndrome. *Trends Mol. Med.* 16, 516–527. doi: 10.1016/j.molmed.2010.08.005

Levitz, J., Pantoja, C., Gaub, B., Janovjak, H., Reiner, A., Hoagland, A., et al. (2013). Optical control of metabotropic glutamate receptors. *Nat. Neurosci.* 16, 507–516. doi: 10.1038/nn.3346

Li, C., Bassell, G. J., and Sasaki, Y. (2009). Fragile X mental retardation protein is involved in protein synthesis-dependent collapse of growth cones induced by semaphorin-3A. *Front. Neural Circuits* 3:11. doi: 10.3389/neuro.04.011.2009

Li, H., Zhong, X., Chau, K. F., Williams, E. C., and Chang, Q. (2011). Loss of activity-induced phosphorylation of MeCP2 enhances synaptogenesis, LTP and spatial memory. *Nat. Neurosci.* 14, 1001–1008. doi: 10.1038/nn.2866

Lichtman, J. W., and Colman, H. (2000). Synapse elimination and indelible memory. *Neuron* 25, 269–278. doi: 10.1016/S0896-6273(00)80893-4

Lin, J. Y., Knutsen, P. M., Muller, A., Kleinfeld, D., and Tsien, R. Y. (2013a). ReaChR: a red-shifted variant of channelrhodopsin enables deep transcranial optogenetic excitation. *Nat. Neurosci.* 16, 1499–1508. doi: 10.1038/nn.3502

Lin, J. Y., Sann, S. B., Zhou, K., Nabavi, S., Proulx, C. D., Malinow, R., et al. (2013b). Optogenetic inhibition of synaptic release with chromophore-assisted light inactivation (CALI). *Neuron* 79, 241–253. doi: 10.1016/j.neuron.2013.05.022

Lin, Y., Bloodgood, B. L., Hauser, J. L., Lapan, A. D., Koon, A. C., Kim, T. K., et al. (2008). Activity-dependent regulation of inhibitory synapse development by Npas4. *Nature* 455, 1198–1204. doi: 10.1038/nature07319

Link, W., Konietzko, U., Kauselmann, G., Krug, M., Schwanke, B., Frey, U., et al. (1995). Somatodendritic expression of an immediate early gene is regulated by synaptic activity. *Proc. Natl. Acad. Sci. U.S.A.* 92, 5734–5738 doi: 10.1073/pnas.92.12.5734

Liske, H., Towne, C., Anikeeva, P., Zhao, S., Feng, G., Deisseroth, K., et al. (2013). Optical inhibition of motor nerve and muscle activity in vivo. *Muscle Nerve* 47, 916–921. doi: 10.1002/mus.23696

Liu, B., Li, L., Chen, J., Wang, Z., Li, Z., and Wan, Q. (2013). Regulation of GABAA receptors by fragile X mental retardation protein. *Int. J. Physiol. Pathophysiol. Pharmacol.* 5, 169–176.

Lnenicka, G. A., Spencer, G. M., and Keshishian, H. (2003). Effect of reduced impulse activity on the development of identified motor terminals in *Drosophila* larvae. *J. Neurobiol.* 54, 337–345. doi: 10.1002/neu.10133

Lovick, J. K., Ngo, K. T., Omoto, J. J., Wong, D. C., Nguyen, J. D., and Hartenstein, V. (2013). Postembryonic lineages of the *Drosophila* brain: I. Development of the lineage-associated fiber tracts. *Dev. Biol.* 384, 228–257. doi: 10.1016/j.ydbio.2013.07.008

Luikart, B. W., Zhang, W., Wayman, G. A., Kwon, C. H., Westbrook, G. L., and Parada, L. F. (2008). Neurotrophin-dependent dendritic filopodial motility: a convergence on PI3K signaling. *J. Neurosci.* 28, 7006–7012. doi: 10.1523/JNEUROSCI.0195-08.2008

Lundahl, J., Staner, L., Staner, C., Loft, H., and Deacon, S. (2007). Short-term treatment with gaboxadol improves sleep maintenance and enhances slow wave sleep in adult patients with primary insomnia. *Psychopharmacology (Berl.)* 195, 139–146. doi: 10.1007/s00213-007-0866-0

Maffei, A., and Fontanini, A. (2009). Network homeostasis: a matter of coordination. *Curr. Opin. Neurobiol.* 19, 168–173. doi: 10.1016/j.conb.2009.05.012

Makinodan, M., Rosen, K. M., Ito, S., and Corfas, G. (2012). A critical period for social experience-dependent oligodendrocyte maturation and myelination. *Science* 337, 1357–1360. doi: 10.1126/science.1220845

Malenka, R. C., and Bear, M. F. (2004). LTP and LTD: an embarrassment of riches. *Neuron* 44, 5–21. doi: 10.1016/j.neuron.2004.09.012

Mann, K., Kiefer, F., Spanagel, R., and Littleton, J. (2008). Acamprosate: recent findings and future research directions. *Alcohol. Clin. Exp. Res.* 32, 1105–1110. doi: 10.1111/j.1530-0277.2008.00690.x

Manning, L., Heckscher, E. S., Purice, M. D., Roberts, J., Bennett, A. L., Kroll, J. R., et al. (2012). A resource for manipulating gene expression and analyzing cis-regulatory modules in the *Drosophila* CNS. *Cell Rep.* 2, 1002–1013. doi: 10.1016/j.celrep.2012.09.009

Mantz, J., Laudenbach, V., Lecharny, J. B., Henzel, D., and Desmonts, J. M. (1994). Riluzole, a novel antiglutamate, blocks GABA uptake by striatal synaptosomes. *Eur. J. Pharmacol.* 257, R7–R8. doi: 10.1016/0014-2999(94)90716-1

Marco, E. J., Hinkley, L. B., Hill, S. S., and Nagarajan, S. S. (2011). Sensory processing in autism: a review of neurophysiologic findings. *Pediatr. Res.* 69, 48R–54R. doi: 10.1203/PDR.0b013e3182130c54

Margulies, C., Tully, T., and Dubnau, J. (2005). Deconstructing memory in *Drosophila*. *Curr. Biol.* 15, R700–R713. doi: 10.1016/j.cub.2005.08.024

Marin-Padilla, M. (1972). Structural abnormalities of the cerebral cortex in human chromosomal aberrations: a Golgi study. *Brain Res.* 44, 625–629. doi: 10.1016/0006-8993(72)90324-1

Marrus, S. B., Portman, S. L., Allen, M. J., Moffat, K. G., and Diantonio, A. (2004). Differential localization of glutamate receptor subunits at the *Drosophila* neuromuscular junction. *J. Neurosci.* 24, 1406–1415. doi: 10.1523/JNEUROSCI.1575-03.2004

Masuyama, K., Zhang, Y., Rao, Y., and Wang, J. W. (2012). Mapping neural circuits with activity-dependent nuclear import of a transcription factor. *J. Neurogenet.* 26, 89–102. doi: 10.3109/01677063.2011.642910

McBride, S. M., Bell, A. J., and Jongens, T. A. (2012). Behavior in a *Drosophila* model of fragile X. *Results Probl. Cell Differ.* 54, 83–117. doi: 10.1007/978-3-642-21649-7_6

McBride, S. M., Choi, C. H., Wang, Y., Liebelt, D., Braunstein, E., Ferreiro, D., et al. (2005). Pharmacological rescue of synaptic plasticity, courtship behavior, and mushroom body defects in a *Drosophila* model of fragile X syndrome. *Neuron* 45, 753–764. doi: 10.1016/j.neuron.2005.01.038

McCabe, B. D., Marques, G., Haghighi, A. P., Fetter, R. D., Crotty, M. L., Haerry, T. E., et al. (2003). The BMP homolog Gbb provides a retrograde signal that regulates synaptic growth at the *Drosophila* neuromuscular junction. *Neuron* 39, 241–254. doi: 10.1016/S0896-6273(03)00426-4

McKinney, B. C., Grossman, A. W., Elisseou, N. M., and Greenough, W. T. (2005). Dendritic spine abnormalities in the occipital cortex of C57BL/6 Fmr1 knockout mice. *Am. J. Med. Genet. B Neuropsychiatr. Genet.* 136B, 98–102. doi: 10.1002/ajmg.b.30183

Meredith, R. M., Holmgren, C. D., Weidum, M., Burnashev, N., and Mansvelder, H. D. (2007). Increased threshold for spike-timing-dependent plasticity is caused by unreliable calcium signaling in mice lacking fragile X gene FMR1. *Neuron* 54, 627–638. doi: 10.1016/j.neuron.2007.04.028

Meyza, K. Z., Blanchard, D. C., Pearson, B. L., Pobbe, R. L., and Blanchard, R. J. (2012). Fractone-associated N-sulfated heparan sulfate shows reduced quantity in BTBR T+tf/J mice: a strong model of autism. *Behav. Brain Res.* 228, 247–253. doi: 10.1016/j.bbr.2011.11.004

Michalon, A., Bruns, A., Risterucci, C., Honer, M., Ballard, T. M., Ozmen, L., et al. (2014). Chronic metabotropic glutamate receptor 5 inhibition corrects local alterations of brain activity and improves cognitive performance in fragile X mice. *Biol. Psychiatry* 75, 189–197. doi: 10.1016/j.biopsych.2013.05.038

Mientjes, E. J., Nieuwenhuizen, I., Kirkpatrick, L., Zu, T., Hoogeveen-Westerveld, M., Severijnen, L., et al. (2006). The generation of a conditional Fmr1 knock out mouse model to study Fmrp function in vivo. *Neurobiol. Dis.* 21, 549–555. doi: 10.1016/j.nbd.2005.08.019

Mikuni, T., Uesaka, N., Okuno, H., Hirai, H., Deisseroth, K., Bito, H., et al. (2013). Arc/Arg3.1 is a postsynaptic mediator of activity-dependent synapse elimination in the developing cerebellum. *Neuron* 78, 1024–1035. doi: 10.1016/j.neuron.2013.04.036

Miller, L. J., Mcintosh, D. N., Mcgrath, J., Shyu, V., Lampe, M., Taylor, A. K., et al. (1999). Electrodermal responses to sensory stimuli in individuals with fragile X syndrome: a preliminary report. *Am. J. Med. Genet.* 83, 268–279. doi: 10.1002/(SICI)1096-8628(19990402)83:4<268::AID-AJMG7>3.0.CO;2-K

Mines, M. A., Yuskaitis, C. J., King, M. K., Beurel, E., and Jope, R. S. (2010). GSK3 influences social preference and anxiety-related behaviors during social interaction in a mouse model of fragile X syndrome and autism. *PLoS ONE* 5:e9706. doi: 10.1371/journal.pone.0009706

Miyashiro, K. Y., Beckel-Mitchener, A., Purk, T. P., Becker, K. G., Barret, T., Liu, L., et al. (2003). RNA cargoes associating with FMRP reveal deficits in cellular functioning in Fmr1 null mice. *Neuron* 37, 417–431. doi: 10.1016/S0896-6273(03)00034-5

Miyashita, T., Shao, Y. R., Chung, J., Pourzia, O., and Feldman, D. E. (2013). Long-term channelrhodopsin-2 (ChR2) expression can induce abnormal axonal morphology and targeting in cerebral cortex. *Front. Neural Circuits* 7:8. doi: 10.3389/fncir.2013.00008

Morrow, E. M., Yoo, S. Y., Flavell, S. W., Kim, T. K., Lin, Y., Hill, R. S., et al. (2008). Identifying autism loci and genes by tracing recent shared ancestry. *Science* 321, 218–223. doi: 10.1126/science.1157657

Moser, M. B., Moser, E. I., Forrest, E., Andersen, P., and Morris, R. G. (1995). Spatial learning with a minislab in the dorsal hippocampus. *Proc. Natl. Acad. Sci. U.S.A.* 92, 9697–9701. doi: 10.1073/pnas.92.21.9697

Muddashetty, R. S., Kelic, S., Gross, C., Xu, M., and Bassell, G. J. (2007). Dysregulated metabotropic glutamate receptor-dependent translation of AMPA receptor and postsynaptic density-95 mRNAs at synapses in a mouse model of fragile X syndrome. *J. Neurosci.* 27, 5338–5348. doi: 10.1523/JNEUROSCI.0937-07.2007

Mundy, P. (2003). Annotation: the neural basis of social impairments in autism: the role of the dorsal medial-frontal cortex and anterior cingulate system. *J. Child Psychol. Psychiatry* 44, 793–809. doi: 10.1111/1469-7610.00165

Murdoch, J. D., and State, M. W. (2013). Recent developments in the genetics of autism spectrum disorders. *Curr. Opin. Genet. Dev.* 23, 310–315. doi: 10.1016/j.gde.2013.02.003

Murray, M. J. (2010). Attention-deficit/hyperactivity disorder in the context of autism spectrum disorders. *Curr. Psychiatry Rep.* 12, 382–388. doi: 10.1007/s11920-010-0145-3

Musumeci, S. A., Hagerman, R. J., Ferri, R., Bosco, P., Dalla Bernardina, B., Tassinari, C. A., et al. (1999). Epilepsy and EEG findings in males with fragile X syndrome. *Epilepsia* 40, 1092–1099. doi: 10.1111/j.1528-1157.1999.tb00824.x

Mutoh, H., Akemann, W., and Knopfel, T. (2012). Genetically engineered fluorescent voltage reporters. *ACS Chem. Neurosci.* 3, 585–592. doi: 10.1021/cn300041b

Nahm, M., Lee, M. J., Parkinson, W., Lee, M., Kim, H., Kim, Y. J., et al. (2013). Spartin regulates synaptic growth and neuronal survival by inhibiting BMP-mediated microtubule stabilization. *Neuron* 77, 680–695. doi: 10.1016/j.neuron.2012.12.015

Napoli, I., Mercaldo, V., Boyl, P. P., Eleuteri, B., Zalfa, F., De Rubeis, S., et al. (2008). The fragile X syndrome protein represses activity-dependent translation through CYFIP1, a new 4E-BP. *Cell* 134, 1042–1054. doi: 10.1016/j.cell.2008.07.031

Narayanan, U., Nalavadi, V., Nakamoto, M., Pallas, D. C., Ceman, S., Bassell, G. J., et al. (2007). FMRP phosphorylation reveals an immediate-early signaling pathway triggered by group I mGluR and mediated by PP2A. *J. Neurosci.* 27, 14349–14357. doi: 10.1523/JNEUROSCI.2969-07.2007

Nataraj, K., and Turrigiano, G. (2011). Regional and temporal specificity of intrinsic plasticity mechanisms in rodent primary visual cortex. *J. Neurosci.* 31, 17932–17940. doi: 10.1523/JNEUROSCI.4455-11.2011

Nelson, C. A. III, Zeanah, C. H., Fox, N. A., Marshall, P. J., Smyke, A. T., and Guthrie, D. (2007). Cognitive recovery in socially deprived young children: the Bucharest Early Intervention Project. *Science* 318, 1937–1940. doi: 10.1126/science.1143921

Nelson, S. B., and Turrigiano, G. G. (2008). Strength through diversity. *Neuron* 60, 477–482. doi: 10.1016/j.neuron.2008.10.020

Nielsen, E. B., Suzdak, P. D., Andersen, K. E., Knutsen, L. J., Sonnewald, U., and Braestrup, C. (1991). Characterization of tiagabine (NO-328), a new potent and selective GABA uptake inhibitor. *Eur. J. Pharmacol.* 196, 257–266. doi: 10.1016/0014-2999(91)90438-V

Niere, F., Wilkerson, J. R., and Huber, K. M. (2012). Evidence for a fragile X mental retardation protein-mediated translational switch in metabotropic glutamate receptor-triggered Arc translation and long-term depression. *J. Neurosci.* 32, 5924–5936. doi: 10.1523/JNEUROSCI.4650-11.2012

Nitabach, M. N., Wu, Y., Sheeba, V., Lemon, W. C., Strumbos, J., Zelensky, P. K., et al. (2006). Electrical hyperexcitation of lateral ventral pacemaker neurons desynchronizes downstream circadian oscillators in the fly circadian circuit and induces multiple behavioral periods. *J. Neurosci.* 26, 479–489. doi: 10.1523/JNEUROSCI.3915-05.2006

Nosyreva, E. D., and Huber, K. M. (2006). Metabotropic receptor-dependent long-term depression persists in the absence of protein synthesis in the mouse model of fragile X syndrome. *J. Neurophysiol.* 95, 3291–3295. doi: 10.1152/jn.01316.2005

Olmos-Serrano, J. L., Paluszkiewicz, S. M., Martin, B. S., Kaufmann, W. E., Corbin, J. G., and Huntsman, M. M. (2010). Defective GABAergic neurotransmission and pharmacological rescue of neuronal hyperexcitability in the amygdala in a mouse model of fragile X syndrome. *J. Neurosci.* 30, 9929–9938. doi: 10.1523/JNEUROSCI.1714-10.2010

Osterweil, E. K., Krueger, D. D., Reinhold, K., and Bear, M. F. (2010). Hypersensitivity to mGluR5 and ERK1/2 leads to excessive protein synthesis in the hippocampus of a mouse model of fragile X syndrome. *J. Neurosci.* 30, 15616–15627. doi: 10.1523/JNEUROSCI.3888-10.2010

Ostrovsky, A., Cachero, S., and Jefferis, G. (2013). Clonal analysis of olfaction in *Drosophila*: generation of flies with mosaic labeling. *Cold Spring Harb. Protoc.* 2013, 335–341. doi: 10.1101/pdb.prot071712

Pacey, L. K., Heximer, S. P., and Hampson, D. R. (2009). Increased GABA(B) receptor-mediated signaling reduces the susceptibility of fragile X knockout mice to audiogenic seizures. *Mol. Pharmacol.* 76, 18–24. doi: 10.1124/mol.109.056127

Pacey, L. K., Xuan, I. C., Guan, S., Sussman, D., Henkelman, R. M., Chen, Y., et al. (2013). Delayed myelination in a mouse model of fragile X syndrome. *Hum. Mol. Genet.* 22, 3920–3930. doi: 10.1093/hmg/ddt246

Packard, M., Koo, E. S., Gorczyca, M., Sharpe, J., Cumberledge, S., and Budnik, V. (2002). The *Drosophila* Wnt, wingless, provides an essential signal for pre- and postsynaptic differentiation. *Cell* 111, 319–330. doi: 10.1016/S0092-8674(02)01047-4

Packer, A. M., Roska, B., and Hausser, M. (2013). Targeting neurons and photons for optogenetics. *Nat. Neurosci.* 16, 805–815. doi: 10.1038/nn.3427

Paluszkiewicz, S. M., Martin, B. S., and Huntsman, M. M. (2011). Fragile X syndrome: the GABAergic system and circuit dysfunction. *Dev. Neurosci.* 33, 349–364. doi: 10.1159/000329420

Pan, F., and Gan, W. B. (2008). Two-photon imaging of dendritic spine development in the mouse cortex. *Dev. Neurobiol.* 68, 771–778. doi: 10.1002/dneu.20630

Pan, L., and Broadie, K. S. (2007). *Drosophila* fragile X mental retardation protein and metabotropic glutamate receptor A convergently regulate the synaptic ratio of ionotropic glutamate receptor subclasses. *J. Neurosci.* 27, 12378–12389. doi: 10.1523/JNEUROSCI.2970-07.2007

Pan, L., Woodruff, E. III, Liang, P., and Broadie, K. (2008). Mechanistic relationships between *Drosophila* fragile X mental retardation protein and metabotropic glutamate receptor A signaling. *Mol. Cell. Neurosci.* 37, 747–760. doi: 10.1016/j.mcn.2008.01.003

Paradis, S., Sweeney, S. T., and Davis, G. W. (2001). Homeostatic control of presynaptic release is triggered by postsynaptic membrane depolarization. *Neuron* 30, 737–749. doi: 10.1016/S0896-6273(01)00326-9

Park, S., Park, J. M., Kim, S., Kim, J. A., Shepherd, J. D., Smith-Hicks, C. L., et al. (2008). Elongation factor 2 and fragile X mental retardation protein control the dynamic translation of Arc/Arg3.1 essential for mGluR-LTD. *Neuron* 59, 70–83. doi: 10.1016/j.neuron.2008.05.023

Parnas, M., Lin, A. C., Huetteroth, W., and Miesenbock, G. (2013). Odor discrimination in *Drosophila*: from neural population codes to behavior. *Neuron* 79, 932–944. doi: 10.1016/j.neuron.2013.08.006

Patel, A. B., Hays, S. A., Bureau, I., Huber, K. M., and Gibson, J. R. (2013). A target cell-specific role for presynaptic Fmr1 in regulating glutamate release onto neocortical fast-spiking inhibitory neurons. *J. Neurosci.* 33, 2593–2604. doi: 10.1523/JNEUROSCI.2447-12.2013

Patterson, M. A., Lagier, S., and Carleton, A. (2013). Odor representations in the olfactory bulb evolve after the first breath and persist as an odor afterimage. *Proc. Natl. Acad. Sci. U.S.A.* 110, E3340–E3349. doi: 10.1073/pnas.1303873110

Paz, J. T., Davidson, T. J., Frechette, E. S., Delord, B., Parada, I., Peng, K., et al. (2013). Closed-loop optogenetic control of thalamus as a tool for interrupting seizures after cortical injury. *Nat. Neurosci.* 16, 64–70. doi: 10.1038/nn.3269

Peabody, N. C., Pohl, J. B., Diao, F., Vreede, A. P., Sandstrom, D. J., Wang, H., et al. (2009). Characterization of the decision network for wing expansion in

Drosophila using targeted expression of the TRPM8 channel. *J. Neurosci.* 29, 3343–3353. doi: 10.1523/JNEUROSCI.4241-08.2009

Pech, U., Pooryasin, A., Birman, S., and Fiala, A. (2013). Localization of the contacts between Kenyon cells and aminergic neurons in the *Drosophila melanogaster* brain using SplitGFP reconstitution. *J. Comp. Neurol.* 521, 3992–4026. doi: 10.1002/cne.23388

Penzes, P., Cahill, M. E., Jones, K. A., Vanleeuwen, J. E., and Woolfrey, K. M. (2011). Dendritic spine pathology in neuropsychiatric disorders. *Nat. Neurosci.* 14, 285–293. doi: 10.1038/nn.2741

Perisse, E., Yin, Y., Lin, A. C., Lin, S., Huetteroth, W., and Waddell, S. (2013). Different Kenyon cell populations drive learned approach and avoidance in *Drosophila*. *Neuron* 79, 945–956. doi: 10.1016/j.neuron.2013.07.045

Persico, A. M., and Bourgeron, T. (2006). Searching for ways out of the autism maze: genetic, epigenetic and environmental clues. *Trends Neurosci.* 29, 349–358. doi: 10.1016/j.tins.2006.05.010

Pfeiffer, B. E., and Huber, K. M. (2007). Fragile X mental retardation protein induces synapse loss through acute postsynaptic translational regulation. *J. Neurosci.* 27, 3120–3130. doi: 10.1523/JNEUROSCI.0054-07.2007

Pfeiffer, B. E., Zang, T., Wilkerson, J. R., Taniguchi, M., Maksimova, M. A., Smith, L. N., et al. (2010). Fragile X mental retardation protein is required for synapse elimination by the activity-dependent transcription factor MEF2. *Neuron* 66, 191–197. doi: 10.1016/j.neuron.2010.03.017

Pop, A. S., Gomez-Mancilla, B., Neri, G., Willemsen, R., and Gasparini, F. (2013). Fragile X syndrome: a preclinical review on metabotropic glutamate receptor 5 (mGluR5) antagonists and drug development. *Psychopharmacology (Berl.).* doi: 10.1007/s00213-013-3330-3 [Epub ahead of print].

Popescu, M. V., and Polley, D. B. (2010). Monaural deprivation disrupts development of binaural selectivity in auditory midbrain and cortex. *Neuron* 65, 718–731. doi: 10.1016/j.neuron.2010.02.019

Powell, E. M., Campbell, D. B., Stanwood, G. D., Davis, C., Noebels, J. L., and Levitt, P. (2003). Genetic disruption of cortical interneuron development causes region- and GABA cell type-specific deficits, epilepsy, and behavioral dysfunction. *J. Neurosci.* 23, 622–631.

Powell, S. B., Sejnowski, T. J., and Behrens, M. M. (2012). Behavioral and neurochemical consequences of cortical oxidative stress on parvalbumin-interneuron maturation in rodent models of schizophrenia. *Neuropharmacology* 62, 1322–1331. doi: 10.1016/j.neuropharm.2011.01.049

Prieto-Godino, L. L., Diegelmann, S., and Bate, M. (2012). Embryonic origin of olfactory circuitry in *Drosophila*: contact and activity-mediated interactions pattern connectivity in the antennal lobe. *PLoS Biol.* 10:e1001400. doi: 10.1371/journal.pbio.1001400

Pulipparacharuvil, S., Renthal, W., Hale, C. F., Taniguchi, M., Xiao, G., Kumar, A., et al. (2008). Cocaine regulates MEF2 to control synaptic and behavioral plasticity. *Neuron* 59, 621–633. doi: 10.1016/j.neuron.2008.06.020

Pulver, S. R., Pashkovski, S. L., Hornstein, N. J., Garrity, P. A., and Griffith, L. C. (2009). Temporal dynamics of neuronal activation by channelrhodopsin-2 and TRPA1 determine behavioral output in *Drosophila* larvae. *J. Neurophysiol.* 101, 3075–3088. doi: 10.1152/jn.00071.2009

Puram, S. V., and Bonni, A. (2013). Cell-intrinsic drivers of dendrite morphogenesis. *Development* 140, 4657–4671. doi: 10.1242/dev.087676

Purpura, D. P. (1974). Dendritic spine "dysgenesis" and mental retardation. *Science* 186, 1126–1128. doi: 10.1126/science.186.4169.1126

Ramiro-Cortes, Y., and Israely, I. (2013). Long lasting protein synthesis- and activity-dependent spine shrinkage and elimination after synaptic depression. *PLoS ONE* 8:e71155. doi: 10.1371/journal.pone.0071155

Ramocki, M. B., and Zoghbi, H. Y. (2008). Failure of neuronal homeostasis results in common neuropsychiatric phenotypes. *Nature* 455, 912–918. doi: 10.1038/nature07457

Reddy, D. S., and Rogawski, M. A. (2010). Ganaxolone suppression of behavioral and electrographic seizures in the mouse amygdala kindling model. *Epilepsy Res.* 89, 254–260. doi: 10.1016/j.eplepsyres.2010.01.009

Reichow, B., and Volkmar, F. R. (2010). Social skills interventions for individuals with autism: evaluation for evidence-based practices within a best evidence synthesis framework. *J. Autism Dev. Disord.* 40, 149–166. doi: 10.1007/s10803-009-0842-0

Ren, Y., Kirkpatrick, C. A., Rawson, J. M., Sun, M., and Selleck, S. B. (2009). Cell type-specific requirements for heparan sulfate biosynthesis at the *Drosophila* neuromuscular junction: effects on synapse function, membrane trafficking, and mitochondrial localization. *J. Neurosci.* 29, 8539–8550. doi: 10.1523/JNEUROSCI.5587-08.2009

Repicky, S., and Broadie, K. (2009). Metabotropic glutamate receptor-mediated use-dependent down-regulation of synaptic excitability involves the fragile X mental retardation protein. *J. Neurophysiol.* 101, 672–687. doi: 10.1152/jn.90953.2008

Rice, D., and Barone, S. Jr. (2000). Critical periods of vulnerability for the developing nervous system: evidence from humans and animal models. *Environ. Health Perspect.* 108(Suppl. 3), 511–533.

Rippon, G., Brock, J., Brown, C., and Boucher, J. (2007). Disordered connectivity in the autistic brain: challenges for the "new psychophysiology". *Int. J. Psychophysiol.* 63, 164–172. doi: 10.1016/j.ijpsycho.2006.03.012

Rivera, S., Khrestchatisky, M., Kaczmarek, L., Rosenberg, G. A., and Jaworski, D. M. (2010). Metzincin proteases and their inhibitors: foes or friends in nervous system physiology? *J. Neurosci.* 30, 15337–15357. doi: 10.1523/JNEUROSCI.3467-10.2010

Rochefort, N. L., Garaschuk, O., Milos, R. I., Narushima, M., Marandi, N., Pichler, B., et al. (2009). Sparsification of neuronal activity in the visual cortex at eye-opening. *Proc. Natl. Acad. Sci. U.S.A.* 106, 15049–15054. doi: 10.1073/pnas.0907660106

Rohrbough, J., O'Dowd, D. K., Baines, R. A., and Broadie, K. (2003). Cellular bases of behavioral plasticity: establishing and modifying synaptic circuits in the *Drosophila* genetic system. *J. Neurobiol.* 54, 254–271. doi: 10.1002/neu.10171

Roos, J., Hummel, T., Ng, N., Klambt, C., and Davis, G. W. (2000). *Drosophila* Futsch regulates synaptic microtubule organization and is necessary for synaptic growth. *Neuron* 26, 371–382. doi: 10.1016/S0896-6273(00)81170-8

Rotschafer, S., and Razak, K. (2013). Altered auditory processing in a mouse model of fragile X syndrome. *Brain Res.* 1506, 12–24. doi: 10.1016/j.brainres.2013.02.038

Rubenstein, J. L., and Merzenich, M. M. (2003). Model of autism: increased ratio of excitation/inhibition in key neural systems. *Genes Brain Behav.* 2, 255–267. doi: 10.1034/j.1601-183X.2003.00037.x

Salzberg, B. M., Davila, H. V., and Cohen, L. B. (1973). Optical recording of impulses in individual neurones of an invertebrate central nervous system. *Nature* 246, 508–509. doi: 10.1038/246508a0

Sanders, S. J., Murtha, M. T., Gupta, A. R., Murdoch, J. D., Raubeson, M. J., Willsey, A. J., et al. (2012). De novo mutations revealed by whole-exome sequencing are strongly associated with autism. *Nature* 485, 237–241. doi: 10.1038/nature10945

Sanes, J. R., and Lichtman, J. W. (1999). Development of the vertebrate neuromuscular junction. *Annu. Rev. Neurosci.* 22, 389–442. doi: 10.1146/annurev.neuro.22.1.389

Santini, E., Huynh, T. N., Macaskill, A. F., Carter, A. G., Pierre, P., Ruggero, D., et al. (2013). Exaggerated translation causes synaptic and behavioural aberrations associated with autism. *Nature* 493, 411–415. doi: 10.1038/nature11782

Scattoni, M. L., Ricceri, L., and Crawley, J. N. (2011). Unusual repertoire of vocalizations in adult BTBR T+tf/J mice during three types of social encounters. *Genes Brain Behav.* 10, 44–56. doi: 10.1111/j.1601-183X.2010.00623.x

Schlaug, G., Jancke, L., Huang, Y., and Steinmetz, H. (1995). In vivo evidence of structural brain asymmetry in musicians. *Science* 267, 699–701. doi: 10.1126/science.7839149

Schroll, C., Riemensperger, T., Bucher, D., Ehmer, J., Voller, T., Erbguth, K., et al. (2006). Light-induced activation of distinct modulatory neurons triggers appetitive or aversive learning in *Drosophila* larvae. *Curr. Biol.* 16, 1741–1747. doi: 10.1016/j.cub.2006.07.023

Schuster, C. M. (2006). Glutamatergic synapses of *Drosophila* neuromuscular junctions: a high-resolution model for the analysis of experience-dependent potentiation. *Cell Tissue Res.* 326, 287–299. doi: 10.1007/s00441-006-0290-5

Selby, L., Zhang, C., and Sun, Q. Q. (2007). Major defects in neocortical GABAergic inhibitory circuits in mice lacking the fragile X mental retardation protein. *Neurosci. Lett.* 412, 227–232. doi: 10.1016/j.neulet.2006.11.062

Shakiryanova, D., Klose, M. K., Zhou, Y., Gu, T., Deitcher, D. L., Atwood, H. L., et al. (2007). Presynaptic ryanodine receptor-activated calmodulin kinase II increases vesicle mobility and potentiates neuropeptide release. *J. Neurosci.* 27, 7799–7806. doi: 10.1523/JNEUROSCI.1879-07.2007

Sheng, M., and Kim, M. J. (2002). Postsynaptic signaling and plasticity mechanisms. *Science* 298, 776–780. doi: 10.1126/science.1075333

Shimomura, O., Johnson, F. H., and Saiga, Y. (1962). Extraction, purification and properties of aequorin, a bioluminescent protein from the luminous hydromedusan, *Aequorea*. *J. Cell. Comp. Physiol.* 59, 223–239. doi: 10.1002/jcp.10305 90302

Siegel, F., Heimel, J. A., Peters, J., and Lohmann, C. (2012). Peripheral and central inputs shape network dynamics in the developing visual cortex in vivo. *Curr. Biol.* 22, 253–258. doi: 10.1016/j.cub.2011.12.026

Siegel, F., and Lohmann, C. (2013). Simultaneous imaging of structural plasticity and calcium dynamics in developing dendrites and axons. *Cold Spring Harb. Protoc.* 2013. doi: 10.1101/pdb.prot078592

Siegel, M. S., and Isacoff, E. Y. (1997). A genetically encoded optical probe of membrane voltage. *Neuron* 19, 735–741. doi: 10.1016/S0896-6273(00)80955-1

Sigrist, S. J., Reiff, D. F., Thiel, P. R., Steinert, J. R., and Schuster, C. M. (2003). Experience-dependent strengthening of *Drosophila* neuromuscular junctions. *J. Neurosci.* 23, 6546–6556.

Siller, S. S., and Broadie, K. (2011). Neural circuit architecture defects in a *Drosophila* model of fragile X syndrome are alleviated by minocycline treatment and genetic removal of matrix metalloproteinase. *Dis. Model. Mech.* 4, 673–685. doi: 10.1242/dmm.008045

Simmons, D. R., Robertson, A. E., Mckay, L. S., Toal, E., Mcaleer, P., and Pollick, F. E. (2009). Vision in autism spectrum disorders. *Vis. Res.* 49, 2705–2739. doi: 10.1016/j.visres.2009.08.005

Singh, A. P., Vijayraghavan, K., and Rodrigues, V. (2010). Dendritic refinement of an identified neuron in the *Drosophila* CNS is regulated by neuronal activity and Wnt signaling. *Development* 137, 1351–1360. doi: 10.1242/dev.044131

Spencer, C. M., Alekseyenko, O., Hamilton, S. M., Thomas, A. M., Serysheva, E., Yuva-Paylor, L. A., et al. (2011). Modifying behavioral phenotypes in Fmr1KO mice: genetic background differences reveal autistic-like responses. *Autism Res.* 4, 40–56. doi: 10.1002/aur.168

Spitzer, N. C. (2006). Electrical activity in early neuronal development. *Nature* 444, 707–712. doi: 10.1038/nature05300

State, M. W., and Sestan, N. (2012). Neuroscience. The emerging biology of autism spectrum disorders. *Science* 337, 1301–1303. doi: 10.1126/science.1224989

Steward, O., Bakker, C. E., Willems, P. J., and Oostra, B. A. (1998). No evidence for disruption of normal patterns of mRNA localization in dendrites or dendritic transport of recently synthesized mRNA in FMR1 knockout mice, a model for human fragile-X mental retardation syndrome. *Neuroreport* 9, 477–481. doi: 10.1097/00001756-199802160-00022

Stoger, R., Genereux, D. P., Hagerman, R. J., Hagerman, P. J., Tassone, F., and Laird, C. D. (2011). Testing the FMR1 promoter for mosaicism in DNA methylation among CpG sites, strands, and cells in FMR1-expressing males with fragile X syndrome. *PLoS ONE* 6:e23648. doi: 10.1371/journal.pone.0023648

Strumbos, J. G., Brown, M. R., Kronengold, J., Polley, D. B., and Kaczmarek, L. K. (2010). Fragile X mental retardation protein is required for rapid experience-dependent regulation of the potassium channel Kv3.1b. *J. Neurosci.* 30, 10263–10271. doi: 10.1523/JNEUROSCI.1125-10.2010

Su, T., Fan, H. X., Jiang, T., Sun, W. W., Den, W. Y., Gao, M. M., et al. (2011). Early continuous inhibition of group 1 mGlu signaling partially rescues dendritic spine abnormalities in the Fmr1 knockout mouse model for fragile X syndrome. *Psychopharmacology (Berl.)* 215, 291–300. doi: 10.1007/s00213-010-2130-2

Sukhotinsky, I., Chan, A. M., Ahmed, O. J., Rao, V. R., Gradinaru, V., Ramakrishnan, C., et al. (2013). Optogenetic delay of status epilepticus onset in an in vivo rodent epilepsy model. *PLoS ONE* 8:e62013. doi: 10.1371/journal.pone.0062013

Sweeney, S. T., Broadie, K., Keane, J., Niemann, H., and O'Kane, C. J. (1995). Targeted expression of tetanus toxin light chain in *Drosophila* specifically eliminates synaptic transmission and causes behavioral defects. *Neuron* 14, 341–351. doi: 10.1016/0896-6273(95)90290-2

Takemura, S. Y., Bharioke, A., Lu, Z., Nern, A., Vitaladevuni, S., Rivlin, P. K., et al. (2013). A visual motion detection circuit suggested by *Drosophila* connectomics. *Nature* 500, 175–181. doi: 10.1038/nature12450

Tanaka, N. K., Endo, K., and Ito, K. (2012). Organization of antennal lobe-associated neurons in adult *Drosophila* melanogaster brain. *J. Comp. Neurol.* 520, 4067–4130. doi: 10.1002/cne.23142

Tessier, C. R., and Broadie, K. (2008). *Drosophila* fragile X mental retardation protein developmentally regulates activity-dependent axon pruning. *Development* 135, 1547–1557. doi: 10.1242/dev.015867

Tessier, C. R., and Broadie, K. (2009). Activity-dependent modulation of neural circuit synaptic connectivity. *Front. Mol. Neurosci.* 2:8. doi: 10.3389/neuro.02.008.2009

Tessier, C. R., and Broadie, K. (2011). The fragile X mental retardation protein developmentally regulates the strength and fidelity of calcium signaling in *Drosophila* mushroom body neurons. *Neurobiol. Dis.* 41, 147–159. doi: 10.1016/j.nbd.2010.09.002

Tessier, C. R., and Broadie, K. (2012). Molecular and genetic analysis of the *Drosophila* model of fragile X syndrome. *Results Probl. Cell Differ.* 54, 119–156. doi: 10.1007/978-3-642-21649-7_7

Testa-Silva, G., Loebel, A., Giugliano, M., De Kock, C. P., Mansvelder, H. D., and Meredith, R. M. (2012). Hyperconnectivity and slow synapses during early development of medial prefrontal cortex in a mouse model for mental retardation and autism. *Cereb. Cortex* 22, 1333–1342. doi: 10.1093/cercor/bhr224

Thomas, U., and Sigrist, S. J. (2012). Glutamate receptors in synaptic assembly and plasticity: case studies on fly NMJs. *Adv. Exp. Med. Biol.* 970, 3–28. doi: 10.1007/978-3-7091-0932-8_1

Thompson, W. J. (1985). Activity and synapse elimination at the neuromuscular junction. *Cell. Mol. Neurobiol.* 5, 167–182. doi: 10.1007/BF00711091

Timmermans, W., Xiong, H., Hoogenraad, C. C., and Krugers, H. J. (2013). Stress and excitatory synapses: from health to disease. *Neuroscience* 248, 626–636. doi: 10.1016/j.neuroscience.2013.05.043

Toro, R., Konyukh, M., Delorme, R., Leblond, C., Chaste, P., Fauchereau, F., et al. (2010). Key role for gene dosage and synaptic homeostasis in autism spectrum disorders. *Trends Genet.* 26, 363–372. doi: 10.1016/j.tig.2010.05.007

Trachtenberg, J. T., Chen, B. E., Knott, G. W., Feng, G., Sanes, J. R., Welker, E., et al. (2002). Long-term in vivo imaging of experience-dependent synaptic plasticity in adult cortex. *Nature* 420, 788–794. doi: 10.1038/nature01273

Tripodi, M., Evers, J. F., Mauss, A., Bate, M., and Landgraf, M. (2008). Structural homeostasis: compensatory adjustments of dendritic arbor geometry in response to variations of synaptic input. *PLoS Biol.* 6:e260. doi: 10.1371/journal.pbio.0060260

Tsai, P. I., Wang, M., Kao, H. H., Cheng, Y. J., Lin, Y. J., Chen, R. H., et al. (2012). Activity-dependent retrograde laminin A signaling regulates synapse growth at *Drosophila* neuromuscular junctions. *Proc. Natl. Acad. Sci. U.S.A.* 109, 17699–17704. doi: 10.1073/pnas.1206416109

Tsien, R. Y., Rink, T. J., and Poenie, M. (1985). Measurement of cytosolic free Ca^{2+} in individual small cells using fluorescence microscopy with dual excitation wavelengths. *Cell Calcium* 6, 145–157. doi: 10.1016/0143-4160(85)90041-7

Turrigiano, G. G., and Nelson, S. B. (2004). Homeostatic plasticity in the developing nervous system. *Nat. Rev. Neurosci.* 5, 97–107. doi: 10.1038/nrn1327

Tye, K. M., Mirzabekov, J. J., Warden, M. R., Ferenczi, E. A., Tsai, H. C., Finkelstein, J., et al. (2013). Dopamine neurons modulate neural encoding and expression of depression-related behaviour. *Nature* 493, 537–541. doi: 10.1038/nature11740

Tye, K. M., Prakash, R., Kim, S. Y., Fenno, L. E., Grosenick, L., Zarabi, H., et al. (2011). Amygdala circuitry mediating reversible and bidirectional control of anxiety. *Nature* 471, 358–362. doi: 10.1038/nature09820

Utari, A., Chonchaiya, W., Rivera, S. M., Schneider, A., Hagerman, R. J., Faradz, S. M., et al. (2010). Side effects of minocycline treatment in patients with fragile X syndrome and exploration of outcome measures. *Am. J. Intellect. Dev. Disabil.* 115, 433–443. doi: 10.1352/1944-7558-115.5.433

van Alphen, B., Yap, M. H., Kirszenblat, L., Kottler, B., and Van Swinderen, B. (2013). A dynamic deep sleep stage in *Drosophila*. *J. Neurosci.* 33, 6917–6927. doi: 10.1523/JNEUROSCI.0061-13.2013

Van den Oever, M. C., Rotaru, D. C., Heinsbroek, J. A., Gouwenberg, Y., Deisseroth, K., Stuber, G. D., et al. (2013). Ventromedial prefrontal cortex pyramidal cells have a temporal dynamic role in recall and extinction of cocaine-associated memory. *J. Neurosci.* 33, 18225–18233. doi: 10.1523/JNEUROSCI.2412-13.2013

Verkerk, A. J., Pieretti, M., Sutcliffe, J. S., Fu, Y. H., Kuhl, D. P., Pizzuti, A., et al. (1991). Identification of a gene (FMR-1) containing a CGG repeat coincident with a breakpoint cluster region exhibiting length variation in fragile X syndrome. *Cell* 65, 905–914. doi: 10.1016/0092-8674(91)90397-H

Vickers, C. A., Stephens, B., Bowen, J., Arbuthnott, G. W., Grant, S. G., and Ingham, C. A. (2006). Neurone specific regulation of dendritic spines in vivo by post synaptic density 95 protein (PSD-95). *Brain Res.* 1090, 89–98. doi: 10.1016/j.brainres.2006.03.075

Viswanath, V., Story, G. M., Peier, A. M., Petrus, M. J., Lee, V. M., Hwang, S. W., et al. (2003). Opposite thermosensor in fruitfly and mouse. *Nature* 423, 822–823. doi: 10.1038/423822a

Vonhoff, F., Kuehn, C., Blumenstock, S., Sanyal, S., and Duch, C. (2013). Temporal coherency between receptor expression, neural activity and AP-1-dependent transcription regulates *Drosophila* motoneuron dendrite development. *Development* 140, 606–616. doi: 10.1242/dev.089235

Walsh, M. K., and Lichtman, J. W. (2003). In vivo time-lapse imaging of synaptic takeover associated with naturally occurring synapse elimination. *Neuron* 37, 67–73. doi: 10.1016/S0896-6273(02)01142-X

Wang, D. O., Martin, K. C., and Zukin, R. S. (2010a). Spatially restricting gene expression by local translation at synapses. *Trends Neurosci.* 33, 173–182. doi: 10.1016/j.tins.2010.01.005

Wang, L. W., Berry-Kravis, E., and Hagerman, R. J. (2010b). Fragile X: leading the way for targeted treatments in autism. *Neurotherapeutics* 7, 264–274. doi: 10.1016/j.nurt.2010.05.005

Wang, H., Dictenberg, J. B., Ku, L., Li, W., Bassell, G. J., and Feng, Y. (2008a). Dynamic association of the fragile X mental retardation protein as a messenger ribonucleoprotein between microtubules and polyribosomes. *Mol. Biol. Cell* 19, 105–114. doi: 10.1091/mbc.E07-06-0583

Wang, H., Wu, L. J., Zhang, F., and Zhuo, M. (2008b). Roles of calcium-stimulated adenylyl cyclase and calmodulin-dependent protein kinase IV in the regulation of FMRP by group I metabotropic glutamate receptors. *J. Neurosci.* 28, 4385–4397. doi: 10.1523/JNEUROSCI.0646-08.2008

Wang, X., Zhu, S., Drozda, M., Zhang, W., Stavrovskaya, I. G., Cattaneo, E., et al. (2003). Minocycline inhibits caspase-independent and -dependent mitochondrial cell death pathways in models of Huntington's disease. *Proc. Natl. Acad. Sci. U.S.A.* 100, 10483-10487. doi: 10.1073/pnas.1832501100

Warden, M. R., Selimbeyoglu, A., Mirzabekov, J. J., Lo, M., Thompson, K. R., Kim, S. Y., et al. (2012). A prefrontal cortex-brainstem neuronal projection that controls response to behavioural challenge. *Nature* 492, 428–432. doi: 10.1038/nature11617

Warren, Z., Mcpheeters, M. L., Sathe, N., Foss-Feig, J. H., Glasser, A., and Veenstra-Vanderweele, J. (2011). A systematic review of early intensive intervention for autism spectrum disorders. *Pediatrics* 127, e1303–e1311. doi: 10.1542/peds.2011-2426

Wayman, G. A., Impey, S., Marks, D., Saneyoshi, T., Grant, W. F., Derkach, V., et al. (2006). Activity-dependent dendritic arborization mediated by CaM-kinase I activation and enhanced CREB-dependent transcription of Wnt-2. *Neuron* 50, 897–909. doi: 10.1016/j.neuron.2006.05.008

Weiler, I. J., Irwin, S. A., Klintsova, A. Y., Spencer, C. M., Brazelton, A. D., Miyashiro, K., et al. (1997). Fragile X mental retardation protein is translated near synapses in response to neurotransmitter activation. *Proc. Natl. Acad. Sci. U.S.A.* 94, 5395–5400. doi: 10.1073/pnas.94.10.5395

West, A. E., and Greenberg, M. E. (2011). Neuronal activity-regulated gene transcription in synapse development and cognitive function. *Cold Spring Harb. Perspect. Biol.* 3. doi: 10.1101/cshperspect.a005744

Westmark, C. J., Westmark, P. R., O'Riordan, K. J., Ray, B. C., Hervey, C. M., Salamat, M. S., et al. (2011). Reversal of fragile X phenotypes by manipulation of AbetaPP/Abeta levels in Fmr1KO mice. *PLoS ONE* 6:e26549. doi: 10.1371/journal.pone.0026549

White, B. H., Osterwalder, T. P., Yoon, K. S., Joiner, W. J., Whim, M. D., Kaczmarek, L. K., et al. (2001). Targeted attenuation of electrical activity in *Drosophila* using a genetically modified K(+) channel. *Neuron* 31, 699–711. doi: 10.1016/S0896-6273(01)00415-9

Wiesel, T. N. (1982). Postnatal development of the visual cortex and the influence of environment. *Nature* 299, 583–591. doi: 10.1038/299583a0

Wiesel, T. N., and Hubel, D. H. (1963). Effects of visual deprivation on morphology and physiology of cells in the cats lateral geniculate body. *J. Neurophysiol.* 26, 978–993.

Wiesel, T. N., and Hubel, D. H. (1965a). Comparison of the effects of unilateral and bilateral eye closure on cortical unit responses in kittens. *J. Neurophysiol.* 28, 1029–1040.

Wiesel, T. N., and Hubel, D. H. (1965b). Extent of recovery from the effects of visual deprivation in kittens. *J. Neurophysiol.* 28, 1060–1072.

Willemsen, R., Bontekoe, C. J., Severijnen, L. A., and Oostra, B. A. (2002). Timing of the absence of FMR1 expression in full mutation chorionic villi. *Hum. Genet.* 110, 601–605. doi: 10.1007/s00439-002-0723-5

Williams, S. C., and Deisseroth, K. (2013). Optogenetics. *Proc. Natl. Acad. Sci. U.S.A.* 110, 16287. doi: 10.1073/pnas.1317033110

Wondolowski, J., and Dickman, D. (2013). Emerging links between homeostatic synaptic plasticity and neurological disease. *Front. Cell. Neurosci.* 7:223. doi: 10.3389/fncel.2013.00223

Wong, D. C., Lovick, J. K., Ngo, K. T., Borisuthirattana, W., Omoto, J. J., and Hartenstein, V. (2013). Postembryonic lineages of the *Drosophila* brain: II. Identification of lineage projection patterns based on MARCM clones. *Dev. Biol.* 384, 258–289. doi: 10.1016/j.ydbio.2013.07.009

Woo, C. C., and Leon, M. (2013). Environmental enrichment as an effective treatment for autism: a randomized controlled trial. *Behav. Neurosci.* 127, 487–497. doi: 10.1037/a0033010

Wu, G. Y., Deisseroth, K., and Tsien, R. W. (2001). Spaced stimuli stabilize MAPK pathway activation and its effects on dendritic morphology. *Nat. Neurosci.* 4, 151–158. doi: 10.1038/83976

Yan, Q. J., Rammal, M., Tranfaglia, M., and Bauchwitz, R. P. (2005). Suppression of two major Fragile X Syndrome mouse model phenotypes by the mGluR5 antagonist MPEP. *Neuropharmacology* 49, 1053–1066. doi: 10.1016/j.neuropharm.2005.06.004

Yasuda, R., Nimchinsky, E. A., Scheuss, V., Pologruto, T. A., Oertner, T. G., Sabatini, B. L., et al. (2004). Imaging calcium concentration dynamics in small neuronal compartments. *Sci STKE* 2004, pl5. doi: 10.1126/stke.2192004pl5

Ye, Q., and Miao, Q. L. (2013). Experience-dependent development of perineuronal nets and chondroitin sulfate proteoglycan receptors in mouse visual cortex. *Matrix Biol.* 32, 352–363. doi: 10.1016/j.matbio.2013.04.001

Yuste, R., and Bonhoeffer, T. (2001). Morphological changes in dendritic spines associated with long-term synaptic plasticity. *Annu. Rev. Neurosci.* 24, 1071–1089. doi: 10.1146/annurev.neuro.24.1.1071

Yuste, R., and Bonhoeffer, T. (2004). Genesis of dendritic spines: insights from ultrastructural and imaging studies. *Nat. Rev. Neurosci.* 5, 24–34. doi: 10.1038/nrn1300.

Zalfa, F., Eleuteri, B., Dickson, K. S., Mercaldo, V., De Rubeis, S., Di Penta, A., et al. (2007). A new function for the fragile X mental retardation protein in regulation of PSD-95 mRNA stability. *Nat. Neurosci.* 10, 578–587. doi: 10.1038/nn1893

Zalfa, F., Giorgi, M., Primerano, B., Moro, A., Di Penta, A., Reis, S., et al. (2003). The fragile X syndrome protein FMRP associates with BC1 RNA and regulates the translation of specific mRNAs at synapses. *Cell* 112, 317–327. doi: 10.1016/S0092-8674(03)00079-5

Zang, T., Maksimova, M. A., Cowan, C. W., Bassel-Duby, R., Olson, E. N., and Huber, K. M. (2013). Postsynaptic FMRP bidirectionally regulates excitatory synapses as a function of developmental age and MEF2 activity. *Mol. Cell. Neurosci.* 56, 39–49. doi: 10.1016/j.mcn.2013.03.002

Zars, T., Fischer, M., Schulz, R., and Heisenberg, M. (2000). Localization of a short-term memory in *Drosophila*. *Science* 288, 672–675. doi: 10.1126/science.288.5466.672

Zhang, F., Wang, L. P., Brauner, M., Liewald, J. F., Kay, K., Watzke, N., et al. (2007). Multimodal fast optical interrogation of neural circuitry. *Nature* 446, 633–639. doi: 10.1038/nature05744

Zhang, Y. P., Holbro, N., and Oertner, T. G. (2008). Optical induction of plasticity at single synapses reveals input-specific accumulation of alphaCaMKII. *Proc. Natl. Acad. Sci. U.S.A.* 105, 12039–12044. doi: 10.1073/pnas.0802940105

Zhang, Y. Q., Bailey, A. M., Matthies, H. J., Renden, R. B., Smith, M. A., Speese, S. D., et al. (2001). *Drosophila* fragile X-related gene regulates the MAP1B homolog Futsch to control synaptic structure and function. *Cell* 107, 591–603. doi: 10.1016/S0092-8674(01)00589-X

Zhong, Y., and Wu, C. F. (2004). Neuronal activity and adenylyl cyclase in environment-dependent plasticity of axonal outgrowth in *Drosophila*. *J. Neurosci.* 24, 1439–1445. doi: 10.1523/JNEUROSCI.0740-02.2004

Zhou, Z., Hong, E. J., Cohen, S., Zhao, W. N., Ho, H. Y., Schmidt, L., et al. (2006). Brain-specific phosphorylation of MeCP2 regulates activity-dependent Bdnf transcription, dendritic growth, and spine maturation. *Neuron* 52, 255–269. doi: 10.1016/j.neuron.2006.09.037

Zingerevich, C., Greiss-Hess, L., Lemons-Chitwood, K., Harris, S. W., Hessl, D., Cook, K., et al. (2009). Motor abilities of children diagnosed with fragile X syndrome with and without autism. *J. Intellect. Disabil. Res.* 53, 11–18. doi: 10.1111/j.1365-2788.2008.01107.x

Zito, K., Parnas, D., Fetter, R. D., Isacoff, E. Y., and Goodman, C. S. (1999). Watching a synapse grow: noninvasive confocal imaging of synaptic growth in *Drosophila*. *Neuron* 22, 719–729. doi: 10.1016/S0896-6273(00)80731-X

Ziv, N. E., and Smith, S. J. (1996). Evidence for a role of dendritic filopodia in synaptogenesis and spine formation. *Neuron* 17, 91–102. doi: 10.1016/S0896-6273(00)80283-4

Zoghbi, H. Y., and Bear, M. F. (2012). Synaptic dysfunction in neurodevelopmental disorders associated with autism and intellectual disabilities. *Cold Spring Harb. Perspect. Biol.* 4. doi: 10.1101/cshperspect.a009886

Zuo, Y., Yang, G., Kwon, E., and Gan, W. B. (2005). Long-term sensory deprivation prevents dendritic spine loss in primary somatosensory cortex. *Nature* 436, 261–265. doi: 10.1038/nature03715

Zwaigenbaum, L., Bryson, S., and Garon, N. (2013). Early identification of autism spectrum disorders. *Behav. Brain Res.* 251, 133–146. doi: 10.1016/j.bbr.2013.04.004

Zwart, M. F., Randlett, O., Evers, J. F., and Landgraf, M. (2013). Dendritic growth gated by a steroid hormone receptor underlies increases in activity in the developing *Drosophila* locomotor system. *Proc. Natl. Acad. Sci. U.S.A.* 110, E3878–E3887. doi: 10.1073/pnas.1311711110

3

The free radical scavenger Trolox dampens neuronal hyperexcitability, reinstates synaptic plasticity and improves hypoxia tolerance in a mouse model of Rett syndrome

***Oliwia A. Janc*[1,2] *and Michael Müller*[1,2] ***

[2] *Center for Nanoscale Microscopy and Molecular Physiology of the Brain, Georg-August-Universität Göttingen, Göttingen, Germany*
Zentrum für Physiologie und Pathophysiologie, Institut für Neuro- und Sinnesphysiologie, Universitätsmedizin, Georg-August-Universität Göttingen, Göttingen, Germany

Correspondence:
Michael Müller, Zentrum Physiologie und Pathophysiologie, Universität Göttingen, Humboldtallee 23, D-37073 Göttingen, Germany
e-mail: mmuelle7@gwdg.de

Rett syndrome (RS) causes severe cognitive impairment, loss of speech, epilepsy, and breathing disturbances with intermittent hypoxia. Also mitochondria are affected; a subunit of respiratory complex III is dysregulated, the inner mitochondrial membrane is leaking protons, and brain ATP levels seem reduced. Our recent assessment of mitochondrial function in MeCP2 (methyl-CpG-binding protein 2)-deficient mouse ($Mecp2^{-/y}$) hippocampus confirmed early metabolic alterations, an increased oxidative burden, and a more vulnerable cellular redox balance. As these changes may contribute to the manifestation of symptoms and disease progression, we now evaluated whether free radical scavengers are capable of improving neuronal and mitochondrial function in RS. Acute hippocampal slices of adult mice were incubated with the vitamin E derivative Trolox for 3–5 h. In $Mecp2^{-/y}$ slices this treatment dampened neuronal hyperexcitability, improved synaptic short-term plasticity, and fully restored synaptic long-term potentiation (LTP). Furthermore, Trolox specifically attenuated the increased hypoxia susceptibility of $Mecp2^{-/y}$ slices. Also, the anticonvulsive effects of Trolox were assessed, but the severity of 4-aminopyridine provoked seizure-like discharges was not significantly affected. Adverse side effects of Trolox on mitochondria can be excluded, but clear indications for an improvement of mitochondrial function were not found. Since several ion-channels and neurotransmitter receptors are redox modulated, the mitochondrial alterations and the associated oxidative burden may contribute to the neuronal dysfunction in RS. We confirmed in $Mecp2^{-/y}$ hippocampus that Trolox dampens neuronal hyperexcitability, reinstates synaptic plasticity, and improves the hypoxia tolerance. Therefore, radical scavengers are promising compounds for the treatment of neuronal dysfunction in RS and deserve further detailed evaluation.

Keywords: oxidative stress, redox signaling, reactive oxygen species (ROS), mitochondrial metabolism, free radical scavenger, neurodevelopmental disorder, synaptic dysfunction, vitamin E

INTRODUCTION

Rett syndrome (RS) is a neurodevelopmental disorder that almost exclusively affects girls. It arises from spontaneous mutations in an X-chromosomal gene encoding the transcriptional modulator MeCP2 (methyl-CpG-binding protein 2; Hagberg et al., 1983; Amir et al., 1999; Chahrour et al., 2008) and is associated with severe disabilities. In RS, an initially normal development for the first 6–18 months of life is followed by motor dysfunction, cognitive impairment, loss of speech, epilepsy, and severe breathing disturbances with intermittent systemic hypoxia (Hagberg et al., 1983; Julu et al., 2001; Steffenburg et al., 2001; Percy, 2002; Chahrour and Zoghbi, 2007; Stettner et al., 2008; Katz et al., 2009). These symptoms result from an impaired synaptic maturation and plasticity as well as a general dysfunction of MeCP2-deficient neuronal networks. Yet, despite the severity of symptoms, pronounced neurodegeneration does not occur in RS (Armstrong et al., 1995; Guy et al., 2007).

There is substantial evidence that also mitochondria are impaired in RS. Typical morphological alterations of mitochondria are membrane changes, granular inclusions, vacuolizations, and a swollen appearance (Ruch et al., 1989; Eeg-Olofsson et al., 1990; Cornford et al., 1994; Belichenko et al., 2009). Alterations of mitochondrial function include decreased levels of succinate-cytochrome c reductase and cytochrome c oxidase, a proton leak across the inner mitochondrial membrane, and a reduced respiratory capacity (Coker and Melnyk, 1991; Kriaucionis et al., 2006; Gibson et al., 2010; Li et al., 2013). Furthermore, lowered blood serum levels of vitamin E (Formichi et al., 1998) and a reduced activity of the reactive oxygen species (ROS)-detoxifying enzyme superoxide dismutase (SOD) are evident (Sierra et al., 2001). These deficiencies in cellular ROS-scavenging capabilities combined with impaired mitochondrial function could well contribute to the intensified protein- and lipid-oxidation that is detectable in patient blood samples (Sierra et al., 2001; De Felice et al., 2009), and which provided convincing evidence that RS is associated with oxidative stress [see: (De Felice et al., 2012b)].

Following these indications we have recently analyzed mitochondrial function in the hippocampus of male *Mecp2* knock-out mice (*Mecp2*$^{-/y}$). In acute tissue slices of adult mice we confirmed an increased basal mitochondrial respiration and less intensely polarized mitochondria. As mitochondrial respiration is already intensified after the 1st postnatal week, these alterations represent early defects in RS that may facilitate disease progression (Großer et al., 2012). Using the genetically encoded optical redox sensor roGFP1 (Dooley et al., 2004; Hanson et al., 2004; Funke et al., 2011), we also confirmed a more oxidized and more vulnerable cellular redox balance in neonatal *Mecp2*$^{-/y}$ hippocampus (Großer et al., 2012). Furthermore, incubating organotypic slices with the radical scavenger Trolox improved cellular redox conditions, which identifies radical scavenger treatment as a potential pharmacotherapy in RS. This is also supported by a report that a diet rich in ω-3 polyunsaturated fatty acids successfully decreases the severity of the clinical appearance and lowers the levels of various oxidative stress markers in Rett patients (De Felice et al., 2012a). It is therefore tempting to hypothesize that the chronic oxidative stress in RS underlies at least some of the typical symptoms and contributes to disease progression.

In the present study, we therefore evaluated the pharmacotherapeutic potential of the radical scavenger Trolox, a water soluble vitamin E derivative, in RS. Vitamin E and its derivatives prevent the peroxidation of unsaturated lipids in cell membranes and lipoproteins (Wang and Quinn, 1999; Slemmer et al., 2008). Since vitamin E levels are decreased in the blood serum of Rett patients (Formichi et al., 1998), supplementation with vitamin E and/or its derivatives is a logical approach. In detail, we elucidated the potential merit of Trolox in acute hippocampal tissue slices of adult wildtype (WT) and *Mecp2*$^{-/y}$ mice. Our focus was on a potential improvement of synaptic function and plasticity, hypoxia tolerance, and mitochondrial function in the tissue of already symptomatic animals. For several of the tested parameters, which are affected in RS, we found an improvement – often to those conditions typical for WT mice. We therefore conclude that radical scavenger treatment is a promising pharmacotherapeutic approach in RS which deserves further detailed analyses.

MATERIALS AND METHODS

PREPARATION

As a mouse model for RS, we continued to use mice lacking the *MECP2* gene [B6.129P2(C)-*Mecp*$^{2tm-1-1Bird}$ (Guy et al., 2001)]. Heterozygous female mice were obtained from Jackson Laboratories and bred with WT males (C57BL/6J) to generate heterozygous females, hemizygous males, and WT mice of either gender. All experiments were performed on acute tissue slices obtained from adult hemizygous males (*Mecp2*$^{-/y}$) around postnatal day 40–50. At this stage, all *Mecp2*$^{-/y}$ animals showed characteristic RS symptoms, including a ~40% reduction in body weight, smaller brain size, low motor activity, very frequent hind-limb clasping, obvious breathing disturbances (Guy et al., 2001), as well as frequent seizures during anesthesia. Only male mice were used for the experiments due their earlier and more severe phenotype and in particular to ensure a consistent and complete MeCP2-deficiency in the analyzed brain tissue.

Deeply ether anesthetized mice were decapitated, the brain was rapidly removed from the skull and placed in chilled artificial cerebrospinal fluid (ACSF) for 1–2 min. Acute neocortical/hippocampal tissue slices (400 μm thick transverse slices) were cut from the forebrain using a vibroslicer (Campden Instruments, 752M Vibroslice). The slices were then separated in the sagittal midline and depending on the very type of experiment they were either directly transferred to an interface recording chamber or to a separate submersion-style storage chamber. In any case, slices were left undisturbed for at least 90 min before the experiments were started.

SOLUTIONS

All chemicals were obtained from Sigma–Aldrich, unless stated otherwise. ACSF was composed of (in mM): 130 NaCl, 3.5 KCl, 1.25 NaH_2PO_4, 24 $NaHCO_3$, 1.2 $CaCl_2$, 1.2 $MgSO_4$, and 10 dextrose; it was aerated constantly with 95% O_2 - 5% CO_2 (carbogen) to adjust pH to 7.4. The free radical scavenger Trolox [(+/−)-6-hydroxy-2,5,7,8-tetramethylchromane-2-carboxylic acid] and the convulsant 4-aminopyridine (4-AP) were directly added to the ACSF in their final concentrations. Cyanide (CN^-, sodium salt) was dissolved as an aqueous 1 M stock solution and stored at −20°C; CN^- working dilutions were prepared freshly immediately before use. FCCP [carbonyl cyanide 4-(trifluoromethoxy) phenylhydrazone, Tocris] and Rh123 were dissolved in dimethyl sulfoxide (DMSO) as 10 mM and 20 mg/ml stocks, respectively, and stored at 4°C; final DMSO concentrations were ≤0.05%.

HYPOXIA PROTOCOL AND ELECTROPHYSIOLOGICAL RECORDINGS

Electrophysiological recordings were performed in an Oslo style interface recording chamber. It was kept at a temperature of either 31–32°C (synaptic function and plasticity) or 35–36°C (hypoxia and seizures), continuously aerated with carbogen (400 ml/min), and perfused with oxygenated ACSF (3-4 ml/min). Severe hypoxia was induced by switching the recording chamber's gas supply from carbogen to 95% N_2 − 5% CO_2 (carbogen aeration of the ACSF was continued), and it triggered hypoxia-induced spreading depression (HSD) -like depolarizations within a few minutes. O_2 was resubmitted 30 s after the onset of HSD, within that time the extracellular DC potential shift had fully reached its nadir. Extracellular recording electrodes were pulled from thin-walled borosilicate glass (GC150TF-10, Harvard Apparatus) on a horizontal electrode puller (Model P-97, Sutter Instruments). They were filled with ACSF, and their tips were trimmed to a resistance of ~5 MΩ.

Field excitatory postsynaptic potentials (fEPSPs) were elicited by 0.1 ms unipolar stimuli (S88 stimulator with PSIU6 stimulus isolation units, Grass Instruments), and delivered via steel microwire electrodes (50 μm diameter, AM-Systems) to the Schaffer collaterals. The resulting orthodromic responses and the extracellular DC potential shifts associated with HSD were measured in *st. radiatum* of the cornu ammonis 1 (CA1) subfield. Seizure-like events (SLEs) were monitored in *st. pyramidale* of the CA3 region. All electrophysiological data were recorded with a locally constructed extracellular DC potential amplifier (Hepp et al., 2005) and sampled using an Axon Instruments Digitizer 1322A and PClamp 9.2 software (Molecular Devices). HSD was sampled at 2.5 kHz, evoked potentials and SLEs were sampled at 20 kHz.

Synaptic plasticity was analyzed by paired-pulse protocols and LTP-inducing protocols. For paired-pulse facilitation (PPF), stimulus intensity was adjusted to obtain half-maximum responses and the inter-stimulus interval was varied in between 25 and 200 ms. LTP was induced in the presence of normal extracellular Ca^{2+} concentration (1.2 mM) by applying stimuli of corresponding intensity at a rate of 100 Hz. These stimuli were delivered in three trains of 1 s duration each and separated by 5 min intervals.

OPTICAL RECORDINGS

Imaging of flavin adenine dinucleotide (FAD) and nicotinamide adenine dinucleotide (NADH) autofluorescence as well as mitochondrial membrane potential ($\Delta\Psi_m$) was performed on the tissue level, using a computer-controlled digital imaging system. It was composed of a polychromatic xenon-light source (Polychrome II, Till Photonics) and a sensitive CCD camera (Imago QE, PCO Imaging). This camera type is equipped with a 2/3 inch CCD chip (1376×1040 pixels; 6.45 μm × 6.45 μm on chip pixel size), and it exhibits a 62% quantum efficiency at 500 nm.

For the imaging of slices a submersion-style chamber (30–32°C) and a 40x water immersion objective (Zeiss Achroplan, 0.8 NA) were used; the slices were kept in place by a nylon-wired platinum grid. To rate mitochondrial metabolism, FAD and NADH autofluorescence were monitored in a ratiometric approach by alternate excitation at 445 nm (FAD) and 360 nm (NADH); autofluorescence was recorded using a 450 nm beam-splitter and a 510/80 nm bandpass filter (Duchen and Biscoe, 1992; Foster et al., 2006; Gerich et al., 2006). 4×4 pixel binning was applied to increase the detection sensitivity of the CCD camera. Rh123, a marker of $\Delta\Psi_m$ (Emaus et al., 1986; Duchen, 1999; Foster et al., 2006), was excited at 480 nm and its emission was recorded in 2×2 pixel binning mode, using a 505 nm beam-splitter and a 535/35 nm bandpass filter. Slices were bulk loaded with Rh123 (5 μM, 15 min) in a miniaturized staining chamber (Funke et al., 2007; Großer et al., 2012). Rh123 was used in quenching mode. Accordingly, mitochondrial depolarization is indicated by an increase in Rh123 fluorescence due to its release from mitochondria into the cytosol. To minimize the risk of phototoxicity that may arise especially from short-wavelength (near-UV) illumination, the imaging experiments – which in part lasted up to 1 h – were performed at low frames rates, acquiring images every 5 s only. Furthermore, the illumination was minimized to those exposure times yielding sufficiently stable CCD camera readings (NADH 70 ms, FAD 40 ms, Rh123 5 ms).

Fluorescence intensities were averaged within defined regions of interest (size ~50 × 50 μm) placed in the middle of *st. radiatum* (see **Figure 4D**), since synaptic function was characterized in this layer as well. The intensity changes observed were referred to pre-treatment baselines; background correction was not performed. As intended by this approach, all optical analyses yield information from a tissue volume rather than single cells and thus represent a mixed signal from neurons and glia. Cellular boundaries or organelle structures could not be identified in the low-magnification epifluorescence recordings of tissue autofluorescence or tissue Rh123 fluorescence.

STATISTICS

Since the electrophysiological and optical experiments lasted only ~1 h, we used up to six slices from each brain. Nevertheless, to ensure independence of observations, every series of experiments was run on at least four different mice of each genotype. All numerical values are reported as mean ± standard deviation; the number of experiments (n) refers to the number of slices analyzed. Statistical significance of the changes observed was tested by two-tailed, unpaired Student's *t*-tests and a significance level of $P = 0.05$. In the diagrams, statistically significant changes are indicated by asterisks ($^{*}P < 0.05$; $^{**}P < 0.01$; $^{***}P < 0.001$), and the corresponding *P* values are reported in the text.

RESULTS

To rate the potential merits of a treatment of MeCP2-deficient neuronal networks with free radical scavengers, we preincubated acute hippocampal tissue slices of adult WT and *Mecp2*$^{-/y}$ mice with 1 mM Trolox for at least 3 h (range 3–5 h). The effects on synaptic function and synaptic plasticity, neuronal excitability, hypoxia susceptibility as well as mitochondrial function were then assessed in the continued presence of Trolox. To be able to screen for a potential reversal of typical RS symptoms, these analyses were performed at an age, at which male Rett mice already show clear phenotypic symptoms, i.e., around postnatal day p40–50.

MODULATION OF NEURONAL EXCITABILITY AND SYNAPTIC FUNCTION

Basal synaptic function was rated based on the recording of orthodromically evoked excitatory field potentials (fEPSP) in *st. radiatum* of the CA1 subfield. The fEPSP amplitudes were normalized to the fiber volley (presynaptic compound action potential) to account for differences among the individual slices and variations in electrode positioning. Under control conditions, *Mecp2*$^{-/y}$ slices ($n = 37$) showed significantly (~44%) higher fEPSP/fiber volley ratios than WT slices ($n = 50$) at all stimulation intensities tested, which indicates an increased postsynaptic responsiveness and neuronal hyperexcitability (**Figure 1A**). The fiber volley itself and the general shape of the input–output curves did, however, not differ among genotypes; neither could multiple population spikes as a clear sign of pronounced hyperexcitability be observed on a regular basis.

Trolox treatment of slices (1 mM, 3–5 h) abolished the genotypic differences in fEPSP/fiber volley ratios, by specifically decreasing the responses in *Mecp2*$^{-/y}$ slices ($n = 43$) to those levels observed in untreated and treated WT slices. Obvious changes in the shape of the input-output curves were not observed upon Trolox treatment (**Figure 1A**). In WT, Trolox did not induce any significant changes in the fEPSP/fiber volley ratio ($n = 44$).

Synaptic plasticity is markedly impaired in Rett mice (Asaka et al., 2006; Moretti et al., 2006; Guy et al., 2007; Fischer et al., 2009). Therefore, we also analyzed the effects of Trolox on

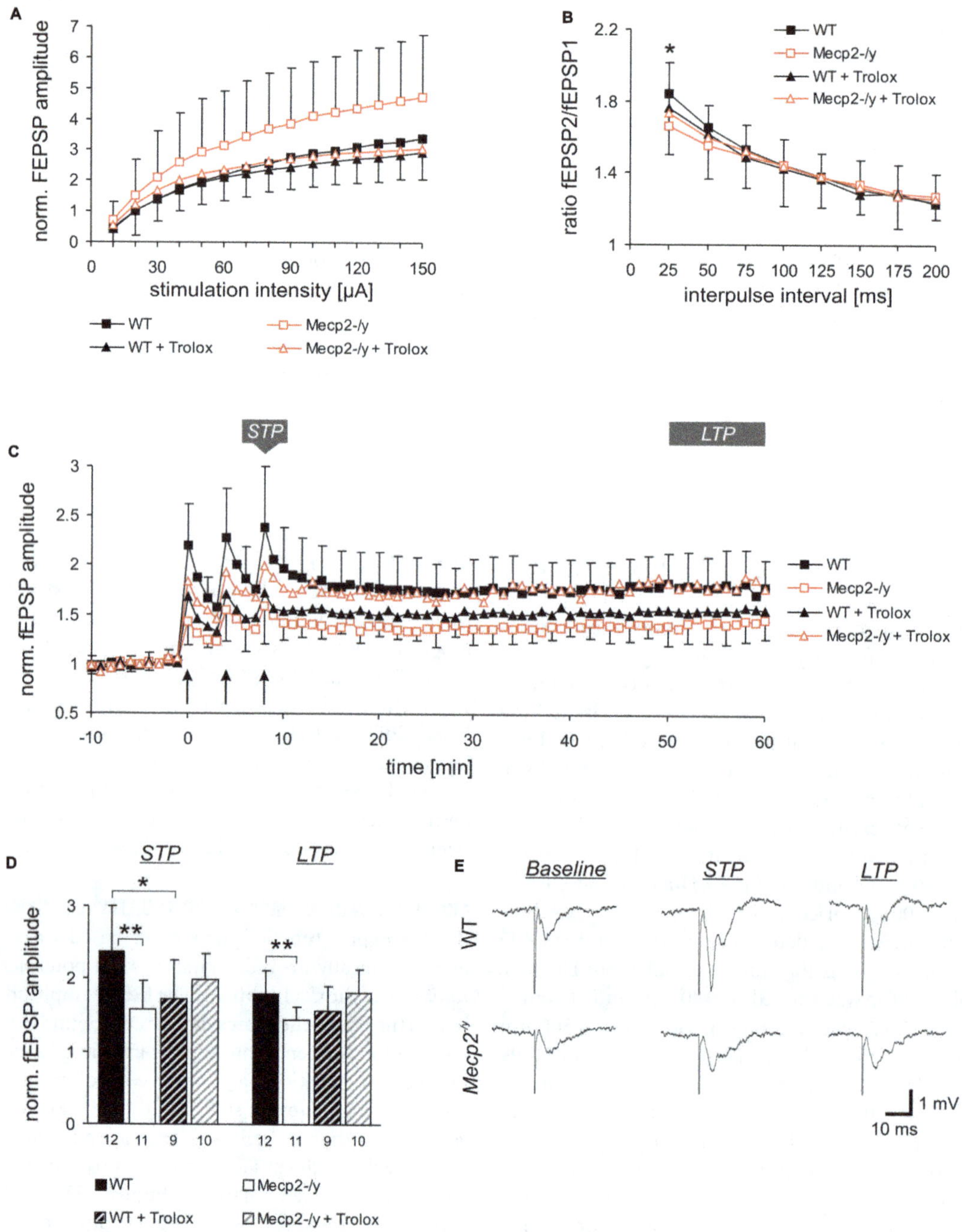

FIGURE 1 | Trolox dampens neuronal hyperexcitability and reinstates LTP in *Mecp2*$^{-/y}$ hippocampus. **(A)** Input-output curves showing a significantly increased excitability in *Mecp2*$^{-/y}$ slices as compared to WT at all stimulation intensities (10–20 µA $P < 0.05$; 30–60 µA $P < 0.01$, 70–150 µA $P < 0.001$). Trolox (1 mM, 3–5h) abolished this genotypic difference. The plotted fEPSP amplitudes are normalized to the fiber volley of the respective slice. Displayed are the averages of 37–50 slices, and error bars represent standard deviations; for clarity they are shown for *Mecp2*$^{-/y}$ and *Mecp2*$^{-/y}$ plus Trolox only. **(B)** Paired-pulse facilitation (PPF), a measure of short-term plasticity, was less pronounced in *Mecp2*$^{-/y}$ than in WT slices for the shortest interpulse-interval tested. Trolox abolished this genotypic difference, but otherwise did not mediate any noticeable effects. Plotted are the averages of 35–52 slices; asterisks indicate statistically significant changes among WT and *Mecp2*$^{-/y}$ slices (*$P < 0.05$). **(C)** STP and LTP were less intense in *Mecp2*$^{-/y}$ slices. Trolox improved both types of plasticity in *Mecp2*$^{-/y}$ slices and LTP recovered to levels seen in untreated WT slices. In WT, Trolox dampened the extent of LTP to conditions typically found in untreated *Mecp2*$^{-/y}$ slices. Averages of 9–12 slices are shown. Error bars are included for every second data point of WT and *Mecp2*$^{-/y}$ slices only. LTP was induced by three consecutive trains of 100 Hz stimuli, lasting 1 s each (see arrow marks). **(D)** Comparison of the extent STP and LTP induced in the different groups. The number of slices analyzed is indicated at the bottom of the bars. Asterisks indicate statistically significant changes as compared to WT (**$P < 0.01$). **(E)** Sample traces of fEPSPs recorded for both genotypes in ACSF under baseline conditions, immediately after the 3rd high-frequency stimulation (STP), and 1 h after inducing potentiation (LTP). Stimulus artifacts are truncated.

various types of synaptic modulation. Synaptic short-term plasticity was assessed as PPF based on twin-pulse stimulation (**Figure 1B**). Stimulation intensity was adjusted to evoke half-maximum response amplitudes and the interpulse-interval was varied between 25 and 200 ms. Whereas this potentiated the amplitude of the 2nd fEPSP in WT slices to 184.0 ± 34.4% ($n = 52$) of control, *Mecp2*$^{-/y}$ slices showed a significantly less pronounced fEPSP facilitation to only 165.9 ± 35.7% ($n = 35$; $P = 0.020$) for the shortest interpulse interval tested (25 ms, **Figure 1B**). Trolox treatment abolished this moderate genotypic difference in short-term plasticity at the 25 ms interval, but otherwise did not induce any significant changes in WT ($n = 47$) and *Mecp2*$^{-/y}$ slices ($n = 39$).

Furthermore, we assessed the modulation of short-term potentiation (STP) and LTP by Trolox. STP and LTP were induced by high-frequency stimulation (**Figure 1C**). Right after the 3rd stimulus train, fEPSPs were potentiated to 238.2 ± 62.1% ($n = 12$) of their baseline amplitudes in WT slices, but in *Mecp2*$^{-/y}$ the extent of STP averaged only 158.7 ± 38.0% ($n = 11$, $P = 0.001$). One hour after LTP induction (range 50–60 min), fEPSPs were still potentiated to 179.4 ± 31.0% in WT slices, but showed a less intense degree of LTP in *Mecp2*$^{-/y}$ (143.3 ± 18.5%, $P = 0.006$; **Figures 1C–E**).

Trolox treatment improved the extent of both, STP and LTP in *Mecp2*$^{-/y}$ slices. After the 3rd stimulus train fEPSPs were potentiated to 199.3 ± 35.2% and after 1 h they measured 181.1 ± 32.2% ($n = 10$). In WT, a stimulating effect of Trolox was not observed. Instead, the extent of STP slightly declined to 172.4 ± 53.7% ($n = 9$, $P = 0.020$) and LTP showed a tendency of being somewhat less pronounced in the presence of Trolox (155.8 ± 33.2%, $P = 0.102$; **Figures 1C–E**) than in untreated WT slices.

ANTICONVULSIVE POTENTIAL OF TROLOX

Rett patients show an increased incidence of epileptic seizures (Hagberg et al., 1983; Steffenburg et al., 2001) and increased neuronal excitability is also evident in MeCP2-deficient mice (Medrihan et al., 2008; Fischer et al., 2009; Calfa et al., 2011; McLeod et al., 2013; Toloe et al., 2014). Since the Trolox-mediated decrease in fEPSP/fiber-volley ratio in *Mecp2*$^{-/y}$ slices confirms successful dampening of neuronal hyperexcitability, we also tested for potential anticonvulsive effects of this free radical scavenger.

Seizure activity was provoked by 4-AP (Rutecki et al., 1987), and the resulting SLEs were recorded extracellularly in *st. pyramidale* of the CA3 subfield, as hyperexcitability in Rett mouse hippocampus arises particularly in this region (Calfa et al., 2011). In about two-thirds of the slices tested, 4-AP (100 μM, 35 min treatment) triggered SLEs which discharged at frequencies of 20–27/min (**Figure 2A**). In WT, SLEs arose within 9.3 ± 2.1 min of 4-AP application and during the last 5 min of treatment, an average number of 135.5 ± 87.3 discharges occurred. The duration of the individual SLEs was quite variable, averaging 362 ± 255 ms ($n = 11$, **Figures 2B,C**). In *Mecp2*$^{-/y}$ slices, similar parameters were recorded; SLEs started within 9.2 ± 2.3 min of 4-AP treatment and 105.3 ± 77.8 discharges were registered during the last 5 min; the individual SLEs exhibited an average duration of 429 ± 193 ms ($n = 12$; **Figures 2B,C**). Trolox treatment (1 mM, 3–5 h) showed a solid tendency to postpone the onset of SLEs in WT slices only ($n = 11$, $P = 0.058$); the frequency of discharges was not significantly affected (**Figure 2B**). Also the duration of the individual SLEs only showed a tendency to decrease upon Trolox treatment in both WT ($n = 11$) and *Mecp2*$^{-/y}$ slices ($n = 9$), yet the level of significance was not reached (**Figure 2C**).

TROLOX TREATMENT NORMALIZES THE HYPOXIA SUSCEPTIBILITY

Previously we reported that MeCP2-deficient hippocampus shows an increased susceptibility to hypoxia. As a consequence, the onset of the synchronized response to severe hypoxia – known as HSD – is significantly hastened in adult *Mecp2*$^{-/y}$ hippocampal slices. Accordingly, MeCP2-deficient neurons tolerate only a shorter duration of O_2 shortage and/or chemically induced anoxia before neuronal membrane potentials collapse and neural function ceases (Fischer et al., 2009; Kron and Müller, 2010).

For a comparison of hypoxic responses, HSD was induced in WT and *Mecp2*$^{-/y}$ slices with and without Trolox treatment. Similar to what was seen earlier, untreated *Mecp2*$^{-/y}$ slices generated HSD within 1.8 ± 0.5 min upon O_2 withdrawal ($n = 32$), i.e., 28% earlier than WT slices in which HSD occurred after 2.5 ± 0.8 min of severe hypoxia ($n = 37$, $P < 0.001$; **Figure 3A**). The amplitude and duration of the HSD-associated extracellular DC potential shift did not differ among genotypes (**Figure 3B**). Upon Trolox treatment (1 mM, 3–5 h; Trolox recirculated in the interface chamber) HSD occurred markedly delayed in *Mecp2*$^{-/y}$ slices, i.e., after 2.5 ± 0.7 min ($n = 36$, $P < 0.001$), and its time to onset did no longer differ from WT slices. Interestingly, in WT slices, Trolox did not postpone the occurrence of HSD ($n = 37$; **Figure 3**).

MODULATION OF MITOCHONDRIAL FUNCTION

To decide whether Trolox also modulates mitochondrial function, we assessed mitochondrial metabolism by imaging FAD and NADH autofluorescence (Duchen and Biscoe, 1992; Hepp et al., 2005; Foster et al., 2006), and mitochondrial membrane potential ($\Delta\Psi_m$) by recording Rh123 fluorescence (Emaus et al., 1986; Duchen, 1999). These imaging experiments were performed on the tissue level in *st. radiatum* of the CA1 subfield (see **Figure 4D**), as also synaptic function was analyzed in this very layer.

As we reported earlier, the ratio of FAD/NADH autofluorescence is slightly increased (i.e., more oxidized) in *Mecp2*$^{-/y}$ hippocampus, indicating an intensified basal mitochondrial respiration (Großer et al., 2012). Also in the current experiments, the FAD/NADH ratio was increased slightly by an average of 10.9% in *Mecp2*$^{-/y}$ slices ($n = 17$, $P = 0.011$) as compared to WT ($n = 19$; **Figures 4A,B**). Trolox (1 mM, 3–5 h) did not mediate any statistically significant changes in these metabolic parameters of either WT or *Mecp2*$^{-/y}$ slices; the observed fading of the moderate genotypic differences in FAD/NADH ratio (**Figure 4B**) therefore seems to arise from data variability rather than a defined effect of Trolox.

In addition to basal metabolism we also defined the impact of pharmacological inhibition of the respiratory chain. Application of low and high doses of CN^- (100 μM, 1 mM), caused the expected dose-dependent decreases in FAD/NADH ratio (up to −29.9 ± 2.5%, $n = 19$ in WT; up to −30.8 ± 2.6%, $n = 17$ in *Mecp2*$^{-/y}$), which were indistinguishable among untreated slices (**Figures 4A,C**). Trolox (1 mM, 3–5 h) slightly but significantly

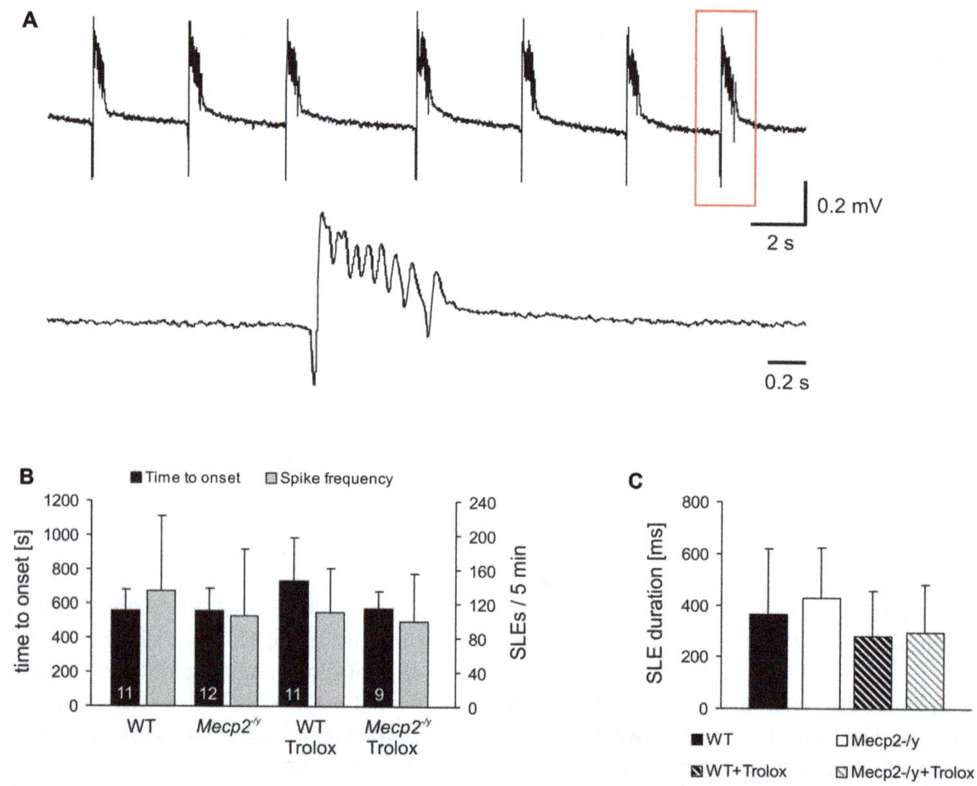

FIGURE 2 | Trolox only shows a general tendency to dampen seizure susceptibility. (A) Seizure-like discharges (SLEs) recorded from an untreated *Mecp2*$^{-/y}$ slice in CA3 *st. pyramidale*. The lower trace shows a SLE (red box) at a stretched time scale. **(B)** Summary of the times to onset and the number of SLEs recorded in the two genotypes. Only in WT Trolox tended to postpone the onset of discharges as compared to untreated slices. The number of slices analyzed is indicated and applies to panel C as well. **(C)** Statistically significant differences in the duration of the individual SLEs among the genotypes were not observed. Trolox only tended to somewhat reduce the duration of the individual discharges in WT and *Mecp2*$^{-/y}$ slices.

dampened the inhibitory effects of both low ($P = 0.008$) and high ($P = 0.021$) CN^- concentrations in *Mecp2*$^{-/y}$ slices, by an average of 13.5 and 10.1%, respectively ($n = 19$, **Figure 4C**), suggesting that it may reduce the susceptibility of mitochondrial metabolism against (chemical) anoxia. In WT slices, such dampening effects of Trolox did not occur ($n = 15$).

Our earlier experiments also suggested a partly depolarized $\Delta\Psi_m$ in *Mecp2*$^{-/y}$ hippocampus (Großer et al., 2012). Performing corresponding experiments confirmed less intense $\Delta\Psi_m$ responses in *Mecp2*$^{-/y}$ slices ($n = 20$, $P = 0.030$) upon mitochondrial uncoupling by 5 μM FCCP than in WT ($n = 20$; **Figures 4E,F**), and hence a less negative $\Delta\Psi_m$. Upon Trolox treatment, both WT ($n = 15$) and *Mecp2*$^{-/y}$ slices ($n = 17$) tended to show slightly more intense Rh123 responses to FCCP; as a result, the genotypic difference became smaller and was no longer statistically significant (**Figure 4F**).

Cyanide-mediated inhibition of mitochondrial respiration evoked marked increases in Rh123 fluorescence, indicating strong mitochondrial depolarization (**Figures 4E,G**). For better comparability, these Rh123 changes were normalized to the complete mitochondrial depolarization induced by FCCP. Genotypic differences were, however, not observed in the responses of WT and *Mecp2*$^{-/y}$ slices to low and high CN^- doses ($n = 20$ each; **Figure 4G**). Neither did Trolox significantly modulate the extent of the CN^--induced mitochondrial depolarization. Only in the case of high CN^- concentrations, the Rh123 responses tended to be slightly higher in Trolox-treated *Mecp2*$^{-/y}$ slices ($n = 17$, $P = 0.059$).

DISCUSSION

Presently, there is no cure for RS, but a number of pharmacotherapeutic strategies ameliorate certain aspects of the complex clinical presentation [see: (Chapleau et al., 2013)]. Some of these treatments aim to prevent oxidative stress by improving cellular redox balance. Curcumine-feeding of female Rett mice dampens the intensified ROS generation in mesenteric artery and reinstates normal vasculature function (Panighini et al., 2013). Initial verification of antioxidant treatment in Rett patients confirms that oral supplementation with ω-3 polyunsaturated fatty acids successfully decreases the clinical severity score by improving motor function, non-verbal communication and breathing (De Felice et al., 2012a).

Here we analyzed to what degree the radical scavenger Trolox ameliorates neuronal function in the MeCP2-deficient mouse hippocampal network. Our choice of a vitamin E derivative was based on the high scavenging efficiency of this class of compounds, and Trolox in particular was selected due to its water solubility. Vitamin E derivatives outrun any destructive interactions of hydroperoxyl radicals with polyunsaturated fatty acids by

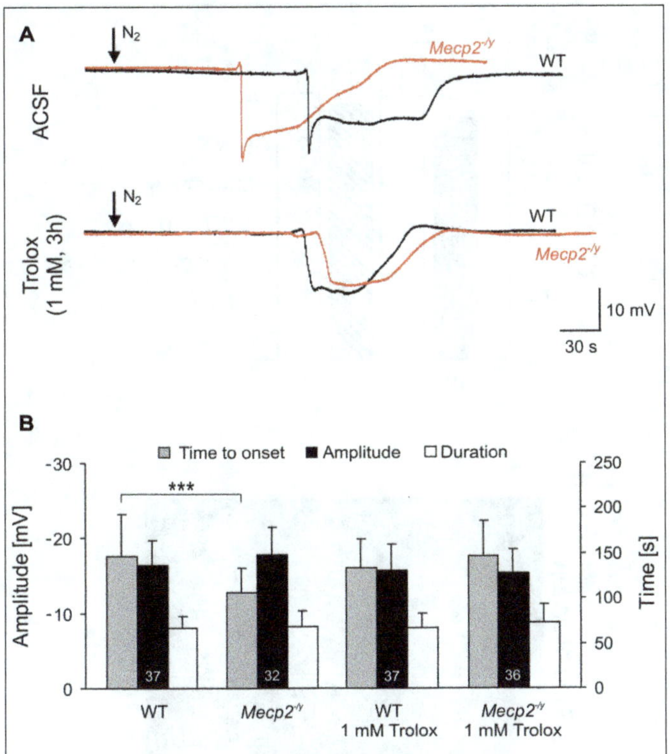

FIGURE 3 | Trolox improves the hypoxia tolerance of *Mecp2$^{-/y}$* hippocampus. (A) Extracellular DC potential deflections associated with HSD. Note that upon O_2 withdrawal, HSD occurs earlier in *Mecp2$^{-/y}$* than in WT slices. Incubation of slices with Trolox (1 mM, 3–5 h) selectively postponed HSD onset in *Mecp2$^{-/y}$* slices to values typically observed in WT. The time point of O_2 withdrawal is indicated by the arrows; oxygenation was restored 30 s upon HSD onset. Recordings were performed in CA1 *st. radiatum*. **(B)** Statistical comparison of the characteristic parameters of the HSD-associated DC potential shift, i.e., amplitude of the negative DC shift (plotted versus the left-hand ordinate in mV) as well as its time to onset and duration (both plotted versus the right-hand ordinate in s). Trolox postponed the onset of HSD in *Mecp2$^{-/y}$* slices, but did not affect the other parameters or its properties in WT. The number of slices analyzed is reported; genotypic differences are indicated by asterisks (***$P < 0.001$).

scavenging these radicals at ~1.000-fold faster kinetics and thereby break lipid peroxidation chain reactions (Buettner, 1993; Traber and Stevens, 2011; Alberto et al., 2013). Furthermore, they also react with singlet oxygen as well as superoxide, and decrease the cell endogenous H_2O_2 formation (Brigelius-Flohé and Traber, 1999; Peus et al., 2001). Most importantly, vitamin E is not degraded in the scavenging process but is rather "recycled" to its reduced state by, e.g., vitamin C (Buettner, 1993; Traber and Stevens, 2011), which further optimizes its efficiency.

Indeed, in isolated tissue of already symptomatic Rett mice, acute 3–5 h Trolox treatment clearly dampened neuronal hyperexcitability, improved synaptic plasticity, and increased the tolerance to severe hypoxia. As shown previously this free radical scavenger also decreases the elevated (more oxidized) redox baselines in *Mecp2$^{-/y}$* hippocampal slice cultures and dampens the exaggerated redox responses to oxidant challenge (Großer et al., 2012). Less clear effects of Trolox were, however, observed on mitochondria and seizure-like activity.

In detail, in the hippocampal network, Trolox improved basal synaptic function by selectively dampening neuronal hyperexcitability in *Mecp2$^{-/y}$* but not in WT slices. As a result, the normalized fEPSPs reached amplitudes typical of untreated WT slices. Mechanistically, a modulation of neuronal network function by changes in cellular redox balance is difficult to predict, since various pivotal ion-channels and transmitter receptors are modulated to different degrees and may even respond oppositely. For example oxidant challenge blocks NMDA and $GABA_A$ receptors (Aizenman et al., 1989; Sah et al., 2002) but activates voltage-gated Na^+ channels and ryanodine receptors (Hammarström and Gage, 2000; Hidalgo et al., 2004; Gerich et al., 2009). Since we did not perform detailed pharmacological trials, the molecular origin of hyperexcitability in *Mecp2$^{-/y}$* mice is unclear. Yet, independent of its mechanism, the normalization of excitability by Trolox may well be of importance in view of the pronounced seizure susceptibility associated with RS and it may also contribute to the postponed onset of HSD in Trolox-treated *Mecp2$^{-/y}$* slices.

Trolox also improved various aspects of synaptic plasticity which is an important finding in view of the severe cognitive impairment in RS. PPF was not primarily affected, but the genotypic differences among WT and *Mecp2$^{-/y}$* slices under control conditions, were no longer present upon Trolox treatment. More importantly the extent of STP was improved by Trolox and LTP was fully restored to its normal extent. As especially long-term plasticity improved, it seems that in particular postsynaptic structures were modulated by the radical scavenger treatment. LTP induction at Schaffer collateral/CA1 synapses is NMDA-receptor dependent (Bliss and Collingridge, 1993). It is therefore tempting to speculate that the more oxidizing conditions in *Mecp2$^{-/y}$* hippocampus partially inactivate the oxidation-sensitive NMDA receptors (Aizenman et al., 1989) and thus contribute to the less stable LTP seen in Rett mouse hippocampus (Asaka et al., 2006; Moretti et al., 2006; Guy et al., 2007). Along this line, the Trolox-mediated normalization of redox balance may have restored normal NMDA receptor function and thus LTP.

In WT slices, however, the extent of STP was dampened by Trolox and also LTP tended to be depressed. In this aspect the modulation of synaptic plasticity by Trolox differs from its effects on basal synaptic function, where no effects on WT were observed. A reasonable explanation for these findings is the strict dependence of LTP on exact cellular redox balance. Oxidant stress may interfere with LTP maintenance without affecting STP or PPF (Pellmar et al., 1991). Yet, also reducing shifts due to overexpression of extracellular SOD3 or administration of superoxide scavengers impair hippocampal LTP (Klann et al., 1998; Thiels et al., 2000). It therefore seems that ROS do not only oppose the induction of stable LTP but to some degree are essential for synaptic plasticity (Massaad and Klann, 2011). This emphasizes the importance of a well-balanced cellular redox equilibrium and hence optimized dosage of redox-modulators such as radical scavengers. We tested only a single concentration of Trolox (1 mM), and observed improved LTP in *Mecp2$^{-/y}$* slices, but its partial depression in WT. Accordingly, a more careful titration of redox conditions may be required to ensure that LTP improves in *Mecp2$^{-/y}$* slices without dampening synaptic plasticity in WT.

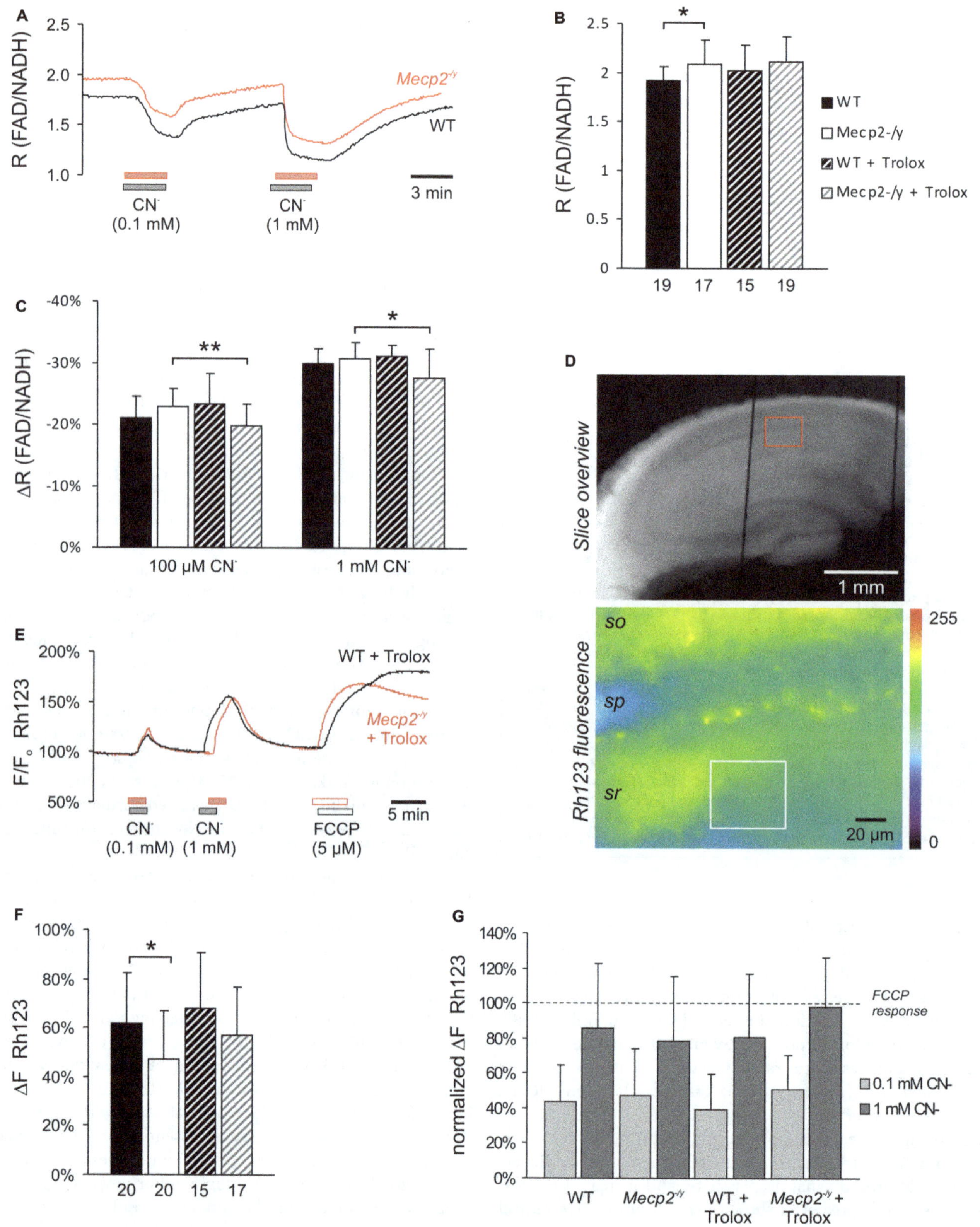

FIGURE 4 | Trolox only slightly affects mitochondria. (A) Sample traces of the decreases in FAD/NADH ratio induced by CN^- in untreated WT and *Mecp2*$^{-/y}$ slices. To clarify the baseline difference among genotypes, the traces were superimposed. Gray and red bars indicate the time points and duration of drug application to the WT and *Mecp2*$^{-/y}$ slice, respectively. **(B)** The FAD/NADH baseline ratio is moderately increased in *Mecp2*$^{-/y}$ slices, indicating intensified mitochondrial respiration. Trolox (1 mM, 3–5 h) did not

(Continued)

FIGURE 4 | Continued
affect basal respiration. Autofluorescence was analyzed in CA1 *st. radiatum*. Bar shading and patterns are identical for panels **B, C, F** (*$P < 0.05$). **(C)** Mitochondrial targeting by CN^- (3 min) arrests the respiratory chain, and thereby decreases the FAD/NADH ratio. Trolox slightly dampened these effects of CN^- in *Mecp2*$^{-/y}$ slices but not in WT (** $P < 0.01$). **(D)** Rh123-labeled slice viewed under white-light illumination and 485 nm excitation. The overview image was taken with a 5x objective, and it also shows two of the vertical-oriented nylon strings immobilizing the slice. The red box indicates the zoomed field of view used for the Rh123 recordings. Fluorescence analyses were performed with a 40x objective and represent an integrated glial/neuronal signal of a tissue volume. Cell boundaries or mitochondrial structures are not identifiable, only the pyramidal cell layer is somewhat less intensely labeled. The white box indicates a typical region of interest analyzed (*so st. oriens; sp st. pyramidale; sr st. radiatum*). **(E)** Superimposed sample traces of the relative Rh123 fluorescence changes (F/F_0) evoked by CN^- and FCCP in a Trolox-treated WT and *Mecp2*$^{-/y}$ slice. Drug treatment of the WT and *Mecp2*$^{-/y}$ slice is indicated by gray and red bars, respectively. **(F)** Uncoupling-mediated increases in Rh123 fluorescence indicating massive mitochondrial depolarization. Untreated *Mecp2*$^{-/y}$ slices showed less pronounced Rh123 increases upon FCCP treatment (5 μM, 5 min), suggesting a less negative $\Delta\Psi_m$ Trolox dampened this genotypic difference. Data were analyzed in CA1 *st. radiatum*. **(G)** Summary of the CN^--evoked increases in Rh123 fluorescence. Plotted data are normalized to the respective effects of FCCP, i.e., the maximum depolarization induced at the end of the experiment in each slice.

Despite a selective dampening of neuronal excitability in *Mecp2*$^{-/y}$ slices by Trolox, we did not observe a marked reduction in seizure susceptibility. Only in WT, the onset of SLEs tended to be postponed and the duration of the individual SLEs only tended to be decreased by Trolox in both WT and *Mecp2*$^{-/y}$ slices. Even though the latter occurred in both genotypes, it may be of some profit by dampening the severity of seizures once such abnormal discharges are triggered. It should be considered, however, that the K^+ channel inhibitor 4-AP is a rather strong convulsive stimulus. Nevertheless, as a pronounced seizure susceptibility is associated with RS, and even constitutes a potential cause for sudden death (Hagberg et al., 1983; Steffenburg et al., 2001), it is an important finding that the Trolox-mediated normalization of synaptic plasticity in *Mecp2*$^{-/y}$ hippocampus is not associated with negative side effects such as increased neuronal excitability and/or increased seizure susceptibility.

Trolox also abolished the increased susceptibility of *Mecp2*$^{-/y}$ hippocampus to the lack of O_2. The hastened onset of HSD in *Mecp2*$^{-/y}$ slices was selectively reverted to WT conditions, whereas WT slices were not affected. Hence, the normalized hypoxia susceptibility constitutes another protective effect that was induced by Trolox selectively in *Mecp2*$^{-/y}$ slices. Treatments decreasing neuronal excitability postpone the onset of spreading depression while increased excitability favors its occurrence [see (Somjen, 2001)]. Therefore, the postponement of HSD in *Mecp2*$^{-/y}$ slices by Trolox is very likely a result of the observed selective dampening of neuronal excitability, i.e., fEPSP/fiber volley ratios. In contrast, Trolox-treated WT slices did not show any alterations in neuronal excitability nor HSD onset. Also increased ROS levels (Grinberg et al., 2012), changes in thiol redox balance (Hepp et al., 2005; Hepp and Müller, 2008), and mitochondrial inhibition (Gerich et al., 2006) modulate the induction threshold of spreading depression. Hence, the postponement of HSD in Trolox-treated *Mecp2*$^{-/y}$ slices may also partly be due to the stabilized redox balance or a slightly improved mitochondrial anoxia tolerance that is suggested by the milder CN^- effects in Trolox-treated *Mecp2*$^{-/y}$ slices. In view of the highly irregular breathing and the associated intermittent systemic hypoxia in RS (Julu et al., 2001; Stettner et al., 2008; Katz et al., 2009), the Trolox-mediated increase in hypoxia tolerance is clearly of potential merit, as it may prevent additional complications especially in anoxia vulnerable neuronal networks such as the hippocampus and cortex.

Mitochondria are a primary cellular source of ROS (Boveris and Chance, 1973; Adam-Vizi, 2005), and mitochondrial alterations in RS underlie the increased oxidative burden and altered cellular redox homeostasis (Großer et al., 2012). However, mitochondria are also potential targets for oxidative damage, and respond with morphological and functional changes including altered intracellular trafficking (Petronilli et al., 1994; Gerich et al., 2009; Qi et al., 2011; Lenaz and Genova, 2012). We therefore screened whether Trolox may modulate mitochondrial function directly, but a noticeable improvement of mitochondrial function was not observed. The genotypic baseline differences in FAD/NADH ratio were not significantly affected by Trolox. During 1 mM CN^- treatment, it mediated only a moderate dampening effect on the anoxic drop in FAD/NADH ratio, which may suggest an increased anoxia tolerance of mitochondrial respiration, yet any corresponding effects on $\Delta\Psi_m$ were not observed. Also the trend to slightly increased Rh123 responses in both WT and *Mecp2*$^{-/y}$ slices during uncoupling or the tendency of somewhat increased Rh123 responses to high CN^- concentrations in *Mecp2*$^{-/y}$ slices may suggest some improvement of $\Delta\Psi_m$, but as stated, the level of significance was not reached. It therefore seems that the protective effects of vitamin E reported for rat liver mitochondria, i.e., partial normalization of the increased state 3 and state 4 respiration upon acute lipid peroxidation (Ham and Liebler, 1997), do not apply to hippocampal mitochondria and the chronic oxidative stress associated with RS. Yet, at least our data confirm that Trolox does not mediate any adverse side effects on mitochondrial function in WT and especially in *Mecp2*$^{-/y}$ slices.

CONCLUSION

The free radical scavenger treatment performed in our study verifies the potential merit of Trolox for targeting the aberrant redox conditions that manifest in MeCP2-deficient networks. In isolated *Mecp2*$^{-/y}$ hippocampal tissue of symptomatic mice we confirmed an improvement of various aspects of neuronal network function, including synaptic plasticity, neuronal excitability, and hypoxia tolerance. At the same time we ruled out potentially adverse side effects on mitochondrial metabolism and seizure susceptibility.

Of course, the hippocampus shows a tight coupling of neural function, metabolism and cellular redox balance, as it is highly vulnerable (Schmidt-Kastner and Freund, 1991), exhibits a clear basal ROS production (Bindokas et al., 1996) and its CA1 neurons are particularly sensitive to oxidative stress (Wilde et al., 1997; Wang et al., 2007). Therefore, Trolox now should undergo further detailed tests to clarify, how other, less vulnerable brain areas respond to radical scavengers and/or modulation of cellular redox homeostasis. This should also include more complex preparations up to *in vivo* treatment of Rett mice to carefully define the merits but also limitations of these compounds. In RS mitochondrial dysfunction and redox imbalance manifest early in life, and may contribute to disease progression. It is therefore crucial to start radical scavenger treatment at presymptomatic stages to define potential changes in disease progression and the manifestation of typical symptoms. Only then, these compounds may unveil their full pharmacotherapeutic potential for the treatment of RS.

ACKNOWLEDGMENTS

We are grateful to Belinda Kempkes for excellent technical assistance. This study was supported by the Cluster of Excellence and DFG Research Center *Nanoscale Microscopy and Molecular Physiology of the Brain* (*CNMPB*) and the International Rett Syndrome Foundation (IRSF; *grant #2817*).

REFERENCES

Adam-Vizi, V. (2005). Production of reactive oxygen species in brain mitochondria: contribution by electron transport chain and non-electron transport chain sources. *Antioxid. Redox. Signal.* 7, 1140–1149. doi: 10.1089/ars.2005.7.1140

Aizenman, E., Lipton, S. A., and Loring, R. H. (1989). Selective modulation of NMDA responses by reduction and oxidation. *Neuron* 2, 1257–1263. doi: 10.1016/0896-6273(89)90310-3

Alberto, M. E., Russo, N., Grand, A., and Galano, A. (2013). A physicochemical examination of the free radical scavenging activity of Trolox: mechanism, kinetics and influence of the environment. *Phys. Chem. Chem. Phys.* 15, 4642–4650. doi: 10.1039/c3cp43319f

Amir, R. E., Van Den Veyver, I. B., Wan, M., Tran, C. Q., Francke, U., and Zoghbi, H. Y. (1999). Rett syndrome is caused by mutations in X-linked MECP2, encoding methyl-CpG-binding protein 2. *Nat. Genet.* 23, 185–188. doi: 10.1038/13810

Armstrong, D., Dunn, J. K., Antalffy, B., and Trivedi, R. (1995). Selective dendritic alterations in the cortex of Rett syndrome. *J. Neuropathol. Exp. Neurol.* 54, 195–201. doi: 10.1097/00005072-199503000-00006

Asaka, Y., Jugloff, D. G., Zhang, L., Eubanks, J. H., and Fitzsimonds, R. M. (2006). Hippocampal synaptic plasticity is impaired in the Mecp2-null mouse model of Rett syndrome. *Neurobiol. Dis.* 21, 217–227. doi: 10.1016/j.nbd.2005.07.005

Belichenko, P. V., Wright, E. E., Belichenko, N. P., Masliah, E., Li, H. H., Mobley, W. C., et al. (2009). Widespread changes in dendritic and axonal morphology in Mecp2-mutant mouse models of Rett syndrome: evidence for disruption of neuronal networks. *J. Comp. Neurol.* 514, 240–258. doi: 10.1002/cne.22009

Bindokas, V. P., Jordan, J., Lee, C. C., and Miller, R. J. (1996). Superoxide production in rat hippocampal neurons: selective imaging with hydroethidine. *J. Neurosci.* 16, 1324–1336.

Bliss, T. V., and Collingridge, G. L. (1993). A synaptic model of memory: long-term potentiation in the hippocampus. *Nature* 361, 31–39. doi: 10.1038/361031a0

Boveris, A., and Chance, B. (1973). The mitochondrial generation of hydrogen peroxide. General properties and effect of hyperbaric oxygen. *Biochem. J.* 134, 707–716.

Brigelius-Flohé, R., and Traber, M. G. (1999). Vitamin E: function and metabolism. *FASEB J.* 13, 1145–1155.

Buettner, G. R. (1993). The pecking order of free radicals and antioxidants: lipid peroxidation, alpha-tocopherol, and ascorbate. *Arch. Biochem. Biophys.* 300, 535–543. doi: 10.1006/abbi.1993.1074

Calfa, G., Hablitz, J. J., and Pozzo-Miller, L. (2011). Network hyperexcitability in hippocampal slices from Mecp2 mutant mice revealed by voltage-sensitive dye imaging. *J. Neurophysiol.* 105, 1768–1784. doi: 10.1152/jn.00800.2010

Chahrour, M., Jung, S. Y., Shaw, C., Zhou, X., Wong, S. T., Qin, J., et al. (2008). MeCP2, a key contributor to neurological disease, activates and represses transcription. *Science* 320, 1224–1229. doi: 10.1126/science.1153252

Chahrour, M., and Zoghbi, H. Y. (2007). The story of Rett syndrome: from clinic to neurobiology. *Neuron* 56, 422–437. doi: 10.1016/j.neuron.2007.10.001

Chapleau, C. A., Lane, J., Pozzo-Miller, L., and Percy, A. K. (2013). Evaluation of current pharmacological treatment options in the management of Rett syndrome: from the present to future therapeutic alternatives. *Curr. Clin. Pharmacol.* 8, 358–369. doi: 10.2174/15748847113086660069

Coker, S. B., and Melnyk, A. R. (1991). Rett syndrome and mitochondrial enzyme deficiencies. *J. Child Neurol.* 6, 164–166. doi: 10.1177/088307389100600216

Cornford, M. E., Philippart, M., Jacobs, B., Scheibel, A. B., and Vinters, H. V. (1994). Neuropathology of Rett syndrome: case report with neuronal and mitochondrial abnormalities in the brain. *J. Child Neurol.* 9, 424–431. doi: 10.1177/088307389400900419

De Felice, C., Ciccoli, L., Leoncini, S., Signorini, C., Rossi, M., Vannuccini, L., et al. (2009). Systemic oxidative stress in classic Rett syndrome. *Free Radic. Biol. Med.* 47, 440–448. doi: 10.1016/j.freeradbiomed.2009.05.016

De Felice, C., Signorini, C., Durand, T., Ciccoli, L., Leoncini, S., D'Esposito, M., et al. (2012a). Partial rescue of Rett syndrome by omega-3 polyunsaturated fatty acids (PUFAs) oil. *Genes Nutr.* 7, 447–458. doi: 10.1007/s12263-012-0285-7

De Felice, C., Signorini, C., Leoncini, S., Pecorelli, A., Durand, T., Valacchi, G., et al. (2012b). The role of oxidative stress in Rett syndrome: an overview. *Ann. N. Y. Acad. Sci.* 1259, 121–135. doi: 10.1111/j.1749-6632.2012.06611.x

Dooley, C. T., Dore, T. M., Hanson, G. T., Jackson, W. C., Remington, S. J., and Tsien, R. Y. (2004). Imaging dynamic redox changes in mammalian cells with green fluorescent protein indicators. *J. Biol. Chem.* 279, 22284–22293. doi: 10.1074/jbc.M312847200

Duchen, M. R. (1999). Contributions of mitochondria to animal physiology: from homeostatic sensor to calcium signalling and cell death. *J. Physiol.* 516, 1–17. doi: 10.1111/j.1469-7793.1999.001aa.x

Duchen, M. R., and Biscoe, T. J. (1992). Mitochondrial function in type I cells isolated from rabbit arterial chemoreceptors. *J. Physiol.* 450, 13–31.

Eeg-Olofsson, O., Al-Zuhair, A. G., Teebi, A. S., Daoud, A. S., Zaki, M., Besisso, M. S., et al. (1990). Rett syndrome: a mitochondrial disease? *J. Child. Neurol.* 5, 210–214. doi: 10.1177/088307389000500311

Emaus, R. K., Grunwald, R., and Lemasters, J. J. (1986). Rhodamine 123 as a probe of transmembrane potential in isolated rat-liver mitochondria: spectral and metabolic properties. *Biochim. Biophys. Acta* 850, 436–448. doi: 10.1016/0005-2728(86)90112-X

Fischer, M., Reuter, J., Gerich, F. J., Hildebrandt, B., Hägele, S., Katschinski, D., et al. (2009). Enhanced hypoxia susceptibility in hippocampal slices from a mouse model of Rett syndrome. *J. Neurophysiol.* 101, 1016–1032. doi: 10.1152/jn.91124.2008

Formichi, P., Battisti, C., Dotti, M. T., Hayek, G., Zappella, M., and Federico, A. (1998). Vitamin E serum levels in Rett syndrome. *J. Neurol. Sci.* 156, 227–230. doi: 10.1016/S0022-510X(98)00035-5

Foster, K. A., Galeffi, F., Gerich, F. J., Turner, D. A., and Müller, M. (2006). Optical and pharmacological tools to investigate the role of mitochondria during oxidative stress and neurodegeneration. *Prog. Neurobiol.* 79, 136–171. doi: 10.1016/j.pneurobio.2006.07.001

Funke, F., Dutschmann, M., and Müller, M. (2007). Imaging of respiratory-related population activity with single-cell resolution. *Am. J. Physiol. Cell Physiol.* 292, C508–C516. doi: 10.1152/ajpcell.00253.2006

Funke, F., Gerich, F. J., and Müller, M. (2011). Dynamic, semi-quantitative imaging of intracellular ROS levels and redox status in rat hippocampal neurons. *Neuroimage* 54, 2590–2602. doi: 10.1016/j.neuroimage.2010.11.031

Gerich, F. J., Funke, F., Hildebrandt, B., Faßhauer, M., and Müller, M. (2009). H_2O_2-mediated modulation of cytosolic signaling and organelle function in rat hippocampus. *Pflügers Arch.* 458, 937–952. doi: 10.1007/s00424-009-0672-0

Gerich, F. J., Hepp, S., Probst, I., and Müller, M. (2006). Mitochondrial inhibition prior to oxygen-withdrawal facilitates the occurrence of hypoxia-induced spreading depression in rat hippocampal slices. *J. Neurophysiol.* 96, 492–504. doi: 10.1152/jn.01015.2005

Gibson, J. H., Slobedman, B., Harikrishnan, K. N., Williamson, S. L., Minchenko, D., El-Osta, A., et al. (2010). Downstream targets of methyl CpG binding protein 2 and their abnormal expression in the frontal cortex of the human Rett syndrome brain. *BMC Neurosci.* 11:53. doi: 10.1186/1471-2202-11-53

Grinberg, Y. Y., Van Drongelen, W., and Kraig, R. P. (2012). Insulin-like growth factor-1 lowers spreading depression susceptibility and reduces oxidative stress. *J. Neurochem.* 122, 221–229. doi: 10.1111/j.1471-4159.2012.07763.x

Großer, E., Hirt, U., Janc, O. A., Menzfeld, C., Fischer, M., Kempkes, B., et al. (2012). Oxidative burden and mitochondrial dysfunction in a mouse model of Rett syndrome. *Neurobiol. Dis.* 48, 102–114. doi: 10.1016/j.nbd.2012.06.007

Guy, J., Gan, J., Selfridge, J., Cobb, S., and Bird, A. (2007). Reversal of neurological defects in a mouse model of Rett syndrome. *Science* 315, 1143–1147. doi: 10.1126/science.1138389

Guy, J., Hendrich, B., Holmes, M., Martin, J. E., and Bird, A. (2001). A mouse Mecp2-null mutation causes neurological symptoms that mimic Rett syndrome. *Nat. Genet.* 27, 322–326. doi: 10.1038/85899

Hagberg, B., Aicardi, J., Dias, K., and Ramos, O. (1983). A progressive syndrome of autism, dementia, ataxia, and loss of purposeful hand use in girls: Rett's syndrome: report of 35 cases. *Ann. Neurol.* 14, 471–479. doi: 10.1002/ana.410140412

Ham, A. J., and Liebler, D. C. (1997). Antioxidant reactions of vitamin E in the perfused rat liver: product distribution and effect of dietary vitamin E supplementation. *Arch. Biochem. Biophys.* 339, 157–164. doi: 10.1006/abbi.1996.9856

Hammarström, A. K., and Gage, P. W. (2000). Oxygen-sensing persistent sodium channels in rat hippocampus. *J. Physiol.* 529, 107–118. doi: 10.1111/j.1469-7793.2000.00107.x

Hanson, G. T., Aggeler, R., Oglesbee, D., Cannon, M., Capaldi, R. A., Tsien, R. Y., et al. (2004). Investigating mitochondrial redox potential with redox-sensitive green fluorescent protein indicators. *J. Biol. Chem.* 279, 13044–13053. doi: 10.1074/jbc.M312846200

Hepp, S., Gerich, F. J., and Müller, M. (2005). Sulfhydryl oxidation reduces hippocampal susceptibility to hypoxia-induced spreading depression by activating BK-channels. *J. Neurophysiol.* 94, 1091–1103. doi: 10.1152/jn.00291.2005

Hepp, S., and Müller, M. (2008). Sulfhydryl oxidation: a potential strategy to achieve neuroprotection during severe hypoxia? *Neuroscience* 152, 903–912. doi: 10.1016/j.neuroscience.2008.01.029

Hidalgo, C., Bull, R., Behrens, M. I., and Donoso, P. (2004). Redox regulation of RyR-mediated Ca^{2+} release in muscle and neurons. *Biol. Res.* 37, 539–552. doi: 10.4067/S0716-97602004000400007

Julu, P. O., Kerr, A. M., Apartopoulos, F., Al-Rawas, S., Engerstrom, I. W., Engerstrom, L., et al. (2001). Characterisation of breathing and associated central autonomic dysfunction in the Rett disorder. *Arch. Dis. Child.* 85, 29–37. doi: 10.1136/adc.85.1.29

Katz, D. M., Dutschmann, M., Ramirez, J. M., and Hilaire, G. (2009). Breathing disorders in Rett syndrome: progressive neurochemical dysfunction in the respiratory network after birth. *Respir. Physiol. Neurobiol.* 168, 101–108. doi: 10.1016/j.resp.2009.04.017

Klann, E., Roberson, E. D., Knapp, L. T., and Sweatt, J. D. (1998). A role for superoxide in protein kinase C activation and induction of long-term potentiation. *J. Biol. Chem.* 273, 4516–4522. doi: 10.1074/jbc.273.8.4516

Kriaucionis, S., Paterson, A., Curtis, J., Guy, J., Macleod, N., and Bird, A. (2006). Gene expression analysis exposes mitochondrial abnormalities in a mouse model of Rett syndrome. *Mol. Cell. Biol.* 26, 5033–5042. doi: 10.11 28/MCB.01665-05

Kron, M., and Müller, M. (2010). Impaired hippocampal Ca^{2+} homeostasis and concomitant K^+ channel dysfunction in a mouse model of Rett syndrome during anoxia. *Neuroscience* 171, 300–315. doi: 10.1016/j.neuroscience.2010.08.031

Lenaz, G., and Genova, M. L. (2012). Supramolecular organisation of the mitochondrial respiratory chain: a new challenge for the mechanism and control of oxidative phosphorylation. *Adv. Exp. Med. Biol.* 748, 107–144. doi: 10.1007/978-1-4614-3573-0_5

Li, Y., Wang, H., Muffat, J., Cheng, A. W., Orlando, D. A., Loven, J., et al. (2013). Global transcriptional and translational repression in human-embryonic-stem-cell-derived Rett syndrome neurons. *Cell Stem Cell* 13, 446–458. doi: 10.1016/j.stem.2013.09.001

Massaad, C. A., and Klann, E. (2011). Reactive oxygen species in the regulation of synaptic plasticity and memory. *Antioxid. Redox. Signal.* 14, 2013–2054. doi: 10.1089/ars.2010.3208

McLeod, F., Ganley, R., Williams, L., Selfridge, J., Bird, A., and Cobb, S. R. (2013). Reduced seizure threshold and altered network oscillatory properties in a mouse model of Rett syndrome. *Neuroscience* 231, 195–205. doi: 10.1016/j.neuroscience.2012.11.058

Medrihan, L., Tantalaki, E., Aramuni, G., Sargsyan, V., Dudanova, I., Missler, M., et al. (2008). Early Defects of GABAergic Synapses in the Brain Stem of a MeCP2 Mouse Model of Rett Syndrome. *J. Neurophysiol.* 99, 112–121. doi: 10.1152/jn.00826.2007

Moretti, P., Levenson, J. M., Battaglia, F., Atkinson, R., Teague, R., Antalffy, B., et al. (2006). Learning and memory and synaptic plasticity are impaired in a mouse model of Rett syndrome. *J. Neurosci.* 26, 319–327. doi: 10.1523/JNEUROSCI.2623-05.2006

Panighini, A., Duranti, E., Santini, F., Maffei, M., Pizzorusso, T., Funel, N., et al. (2013). Vascular dysfunction in a mouse model of rett syndrome and effects of curcumin treatment. *PLoS ONE* 8:e64863. doi: 10.1371/journal.pone.0064863

Pellmar, T. C., Hollinden, G. E., and Sarvey, J. M. (1991). Free radicals accelerate the decay of long-term potentiation in field CA1 of guinea-pig hippocampus. *Neuroscience* 44, 353–359. doi: 10.1016/0306-4522(91)90060-2

Percy, A. K. (2002). Rett syndrome. Current status and new vistas. *Neurol. Clin.* 20, 1125–1141. doi: 10.1016/S0733-8619(02)00022-1

Petronilli, V., Costantini, P., Scorrano, L., Colonna, R., Passamonti, S., and Bernardi, P. (1994). The voltage sensor of the mitochondrial permeability transition pore is tuned by the oxidation-reduction state of vicinal thiols. Increase of the gating potential by oxidants and its reversal by reducing agents. *J. Biol. Chem.* 269, 16638–16642.

Peus, D., Meves, A., Pott, M., Beyerle, A., and Pittelkow, M. R. (2001). Vitamin E analog modulates UVB-induced signaling pathway activation and enhances cell survival. *Free Radic. Biol. Med.* 30, 425–432. doi: 10.1016/S0891-5849(00)00488-3

Qi, X., Disatnik, M. H., Shen, N., Sobel, R. A., and Mochly-Rosen, D. (2011). Aberrant mitochondrial fission in neurons induced by protein kinase Cδ under oxidative stress conditions in vivo. *Mol. Biol. Cell* 22, 256–265. doi: 10.1091/mbc.E10-06-0551

Ruch, A., Kurczynski, T. W., and Velasco, M. E. (1989). Mitochondrial alterations in Rett syndrome. *Pediatr. Neurol.* 5, 320–323. doi: 10.1016/0887-8994(89)90027-1

Rutecki, P. A., Lebeda, F. J., and Johnston, D. (1987). 4-Aminopyridine produces epileptiform activity in hippocampus and enhances synaptic excitation and inhibition. *J. Neurophysiol.* 57, 1911–1924.

Sah, R., Galeffi, F., Ahrens, R., Jordan, G., and Schwartz-Bloom, R. D. (2002). Modulation of the $GABA_A$-gated chloride channel by reactive oxygen species. *J. Neurochem.* 80, 383–391.doi: 10.1046/j.0022-3042.2001.00706.x

Schmidt-Kastner, R., and Freund, T. F. (1991). Selective vulnerability of the hippocampus in brain ischemia. *Neuroscience* 40, 599–636. doi: 10.1016/0306-4522(91)90001-5

Sierra, C., Vilaseca, M. A., Brandi, N., Artuch, R., Mira, A., Nieto, M., et al. (2001). Oxidative stress in Rett syndrome. *Brain Dev.* 23(Suppl. 1), S236–S239. doi: 10.1016/S0387-7604(01)00369-2

Slemmer, J. E., Shacka, J. J., Sweeney, M. I., and Weber, J. T. (2008). Antioxidants and free radical scavengers for the treatment of stroke, traumatic brain injury and aging. *Curr. Med. Chem* 15, 404–414. doi: 10.2174/092986708783497337

Somjen, G. G. (2001). Mechanisms of spreading depression and hypoxic spreading depression-like depolarization. *Physiol. Rev.* 81, 1065–1096.

Steffenburg, U., Hagberg, G., and Hagberg, B. (2001). Epilepsy in a representative series of Rett syndrome. *Acta Paediatr.* 90, 34–39. doi: 10.1111/j.1651-2227.2001.tb00252.x

Stettner, G. M., Huppke, P., Gärtner, J., Richter, D. W., and Dutschmann, M. (2008). Disturbances of breathing in Rett syndrome: results from patients and animal models. *Adv. Exp. Biol. Med.* 605, 503–507. doi: 10.1007/978-0-387-73693-8_88

Thiels, E., Urban, N. N., Gonzalez-Burgos, G. R., Kanterewicz, B. I., Barrionuevo, G., Chu, C. T., et al. (2000). Impairment of long-term potentiation and associative memory in mice that overexpress extracellular superoxide dismutase. *J. Neurosci.* 20, 7631–7639.

Toloe, J., Mollajew, R., Kügler, S., and Mironov, S. L. (2014). Metabolic differences in hippocampal 'Rett' neurons revealed by ATP imaging. *Mol. Cell. Neurosci.* 59, 47–56. doi: 10.1016/j.mcn.2013.12.008 [Epub ahead of print].

Traber, M. G., and Stevens, J. F. (2011). Vitamins C and E: beneficial effects from a mechanistic perspective. *Free Radic. Biol. Med.* 51, 1000–1013. doi: 10.1016/j.freeradbiomed.2011.05.017

Wang, X., Pal, R., Chen, X. W., Kumar, K. N., Kim, O. J., and Michaelis, E. K. (2007). Genome-wide transcriptome profiling of region-specific vulnerability to oxidative stress in the hippocampus. *Genomics* 90, 201–212. doi: 10.1016/j.ygeno.2007.03.007

Wang, X., and Quinn, P. J. (1999). Vitamin E and its function in membranes. *Prog. Lipid Res.* 38, 309–336. doi: 10.1016/S0163-7827(99)00008-9

Wilde, G. J., Pringle, A. K., Wright, P., and Iannotti, F. (1997). Differential vulnerability of the CA1 and CA3 subfields of the hippocampus to superoxide and hydroxyl radicals in vitro. *J. Neurochem.* 69, 883–886. doi: 10.1046/j.1471-4159.1997.69020883.x

4

MeCP2 post-translational modifications: A mechanism to control its involvement in synaptic plasticity and homeostasis?

Elisa Bellini[1], Giulio Pavesi[2], Isabella Barbiero[3], Anna Bergo[3], Chetan Chandola[3], Mohammad S. Nawaz[3], Laura Rusconi[3], Gilda Stefanelli[3], Marta Strollo[3], Maria M. Valente[1], Charlotte Kilstrup-Nielsen[3†] and Nicoletta Landsberger[1,3*†]

[1] *Division of Neuroscience, San Raffaele Rett Research Center, San Raffaele Scientific Institute, Milan, Italy*
[2] *Department of Biosciences, University of Milan, Milan, Italy*
[3] *Section of Biomedical Research, Laboratory of Genetic and Epigenetic Control of Gene Expression, Department of Theoretic and Applied Sciences, University of Insubria, Busto Arsizio, Italy*

Correspondence:
Nicoletta Landsberger, Laboratory of Genetic and Epigenetic Control of Gene Expression, Department of Theoretic and Applied Biosciences, Via Manara 7, Busto Arsizio 21052, Italy
e-mail: landsben@uninsubria.it

† Co-corresponding authors.

Although Rett syndrome (RTT) represents one of the most frequent forms of severe intellectual disability in females worldwide, we still have an inadequate knowledge of the many roles played by MeCP2 (whose mutations are responsible for most cases of RTT) and their relevance for RTT pathobiology. Several studies support a role of MeCP2 in the regulation of synaptic plasticity and homeostasis. At the molecular level, MeCP2 is described as a repressor capable of inhibiting gene transcription through chromatin compaction. Indeed, it interacts with several chromatin remodeling factors, such as HDAC-containing complexes and ATRX. Other studies have inferred that MeCP2 functions also as an activator; a role in regulating mRNA splicing and in modulating protein synthesis has also been proposed. Further, MeCP2 avidly binds both 5-methyl- and 5-hydroxymethyl-cytosine. Recent evidence suggests that it is the highly disorganized structure of MeCP2, together with its post-translational modifications (PTMs) that generate and regulate this functional versatility. Indeed, several reports have demonstrated that differential phosphorylation of MeCP2 is a key mechanism by which the methyl binding protein modulates its affinity for its partners, gene expression and cellular adaptations to stimuli and neuronal plasticity. As logic consequence, generation of phospho-defective *Mecp2* knock-in mice has permitted associating alterations in neuronal morphology, circuit formation, and mouse behavioral phenotypes with specific phosphorylation events. MeCP2 undergoes various other PTMs, including acetylation, ubiquitination and sumoylation, whose functional roles remain largely unexplored. These results, together with the genome-wide distribution of MeCP2 and its capability to substitute histone H1, recall the complex regulation of histones and suggest the relevance of quickly gaining a deeper comprehension of MeCP2 PTMs, the respective writers and readers and the consequent functional outcomes.

Keywords: chromatin, MeCP2, mouse models, phosphorylation, post-translational modifications, Rett syndrome, synaptic plasticity

INTRODUCTION

Rett syndrome (RTT) is a devastating disorder that, because of its incidence, is considered one of the main causes of severe intellectual disability in girls (Percy and Lane, 2005). Typical RTT patients appear to develop normally throughout the first 6–18 months of life when neurological development arrests and a regression phase occurs leading to the loss of previously acquired skills. During and after the regression phase, patients develop a host of typical symptoms including the substitution of purposeful hand use with continuous stereotypic hand movements, loss of language skills, the appearance of autistic features, gait abnormalities, breathing irregularities, seizures, scoliosis, hypotonia, and autonomic dysfunctions (Neul et al., 2010).

Back in 1999, the Methyl-CpG binding Protein 2 (*MECP2)* gene was discovered as the genetic cause of Rett syndrome (Amir et al., 1999); since then, hundreds of different mutations of the gene have been associated with RTT and less frequently with other forms of intellectual disabilities, such as autism, schizophrenia, mental retardation and Angelman-like syndrome

Abbreviations: MeCP2, methyl-CpG binding protein 2; RTT, Rett syndrome; PTM, post-translational modification; MBD, methyl-DNA binding domain; TRD, transcriptional repression domain; ID, intervening domain; NTD, N-terminal domain; CTD, C-terminal domain; 5hmC, 5-hydroxymethyl cytosine; pMeCP2, phosphorylated MeCP2; ChIP, chromatin immunoprecipitation; KI, knock-in; MS, mass spectrometry; LTP, long-term potentiation; Ub, ubiquitination; Met, methylation, SUMO, sumoylation; Ac, acetylation; O-GlcNAc, O-glycosylation.

(Chahrour and Zoghbi, 2007). Lately, duplication and triplication of the gene have also been identified as the genetic cause of the recently classified *MECP2* duplication syndrome that usually affects boys (Van Esch, 2011). The production of several mouse models, carrying different *Mecp2* alterations and phenotypically copying many typical features of the human disease, has indeed provided the formal genetic proof of the involvement of *MECP2* in RTT (Ricceri et al., 2008). Importantly, mouse models of *Mecp2* functions have also permitted to demonstrate that phenotypic rescue is possible at least in mice, suggesting that the *MECP2*-related conditions might be reversible (Guy et al., 2007). These studies have dramatically boosted the research of MeCP2 functions, and have yielded a wealth of evidence proving that MeCP2 functions are required for the maturation and maintenance of proper dendritic arborization and spine formation. Thus, RTT pathogenic mechanisms appear to converge at the synaptic level, disrupting synaptic transmission and plasticity.

At a molecular level, there exist more contradictory data. In fact, MeCP2 appears as a multifunctional protein, mainly but not exclusively involved in regulating gene expression. It appears that the structure of MeCP2 together with a series of differential post-translational modifications (PTMs) might justify this functional versatility, possibly occurring through the capacity of the methyl-binding protein to interact with several diverse protein partners (Klose and Bird, 2004). Thus, in this review we will briefly summarize the animal models of *Mecp2* that have been instrumental for studying Rett syndrome. We will then describe relevant evidence substantiating the functional importance of MeCP2 in synaptic and neuronal plasticity regulation. Since we are certain that the development of well-targeted therapies requires a better comprehension of the functional role(s) of MeCP2, their regulation and their relevance in the pathobiology of RTT, we will analyze in depth the current knowledge of MeCP2 structure and molecular functions and provide bioinformatics and experimental data testifying already established and putative PTMs of MeCP2. Functional studies and animal models used to characterize some of these PTMs will be surveyed, highlighting the major weaknesses in the field and which, in our mind, should be the future challenges for a better comprehension of MeCP2 activities.

Mecp2 MOUSE MODELS RECAPITULATE WELL THE HUMAN *MECP2*-RELATED PATHOLOGIES

The generation of several mouse models carrying different *Mecp2* alterations and generally recapitulating many RTT features has provided a major breakthrough for RTT research (Ricceri et al., 2008). In particular, the mostly used *Mecp2*-null males (*Mecp2*$^{-/y}$) have no apparent phenotype until 3–8 weeks of age, when they start showing gross abnormalities, such as locomotor defects, hindlimb clasping, hypotonia, reduced spontaneous movements, tremors, breathing irregularities and often seizures. Symptoms worsen over time, and the animals die within 6–10 weeks of age. Heterozygous female mice (*Mecp2*$^{-/+}$) are viable, fertile and appear normal up to 4–6 months of life, when they start manifesting RTT-like symptoms. Other models with less severe genetic lesions, often mimicking human mutations, have subsequently been generated, and are nicely reviewed in Ricceri et al. (2008). Knock-in mice, used to address the role of specific events of MeCP2 phosphorylation, are discussed in Section MeCP2 Phosphorylation: Where We Stand and Where We Might Go.

The *Mecp2*$^{308/y}$ mice, expressing a hypomorphic MeCP2 pathogenic derivative, have also been widely utilized. The mutation causes a deletion of the C-terminal portion, but spares the two most relevant functional domains, i.e., the methyl-binding domain and the transcriptional repression domain (see Section MeCP2 Functions Depend on the Highly Structured Methyl-binding Domain Embedded in a Disorganized Protein). Even though the overall phenotype is milder, the *Mecp2*$^{308/y}$ mouse model shares most of the features characterizing the knock-out animals, including learning and memory deficits (Shahbazian et al., 2002).

Conditional knock-out mice have also been generated and characterized, in order to understand better the etiology of RTT and the role of *Mecp2* in discrete brain regions or cell types. As reviewed in Na et al. (2013), the inactivation of *Mecp2* in single brain areas or neuronal subtypes generally leads only to a subset of the typical RTT features. Importantly, despite the fact that all *Mecp2* mutations investigated so far affect brain functions, they are not associated with neuronal loss. Consistently, a major breakthrough in the field came in 2007, when Dr. Bird and his collaborators demonstrated that *Mecp2*-reactivation in symptomatic adult mice (either *Mecp2*$^{-/y}$ or *Mecp2*$^{-/+}$) results in a robust rescue of the general conditions of the animals, including survival and breathing, while mobility, clasping, and tremors were less reversed. Altogether, these studies demonstrated that Mecp2-related disorders are reversible and, at least in mice, they can be treated even at late stages of disease progression (Guy et al., 2007). Importantly, these results have been confirmed by several other subsequent studies (Luikenhuis et al., 2004; Giacometti et al., 2007; Jugloff et al., 2008; Garg et al., 2013).

In spite of these recent enormous advances, we highlight that the knowledge regarding the temporal steps through which the consequences of dysfunctional MeCP2 start to manifest is still limited. In fact, most of the studies have been performed in the so-called pre-symptomatic (3–6 weeks of age) or symptomatic (adult) animals. However, recent experimental results have demonstrated that the inactivation of *Mecp2* at different post-natal ages (from late juvenile to adult) always causes the appearance of RTT-like phenotypes and premature death (McGraw et al., 2011; Cheval et al., 2012; Nguyen et al., 2012). These results demonstrate that MeCP2 functions are essential to maintain neurons in a fully functional state. Conversely, it has recently been shown that subtle but consistent impairments are present even at early post-natal stages, when typical symptoms are not yet overt, both in human heterozygous patients and hemizygous null mice. Furthermore, hemizygous *MECP2* male patients display a severe pathological condition as early as at birth (Schüle et al., 2008). Thus, considering that very few studies investigated the possible roles of Mecp2 during embryonic development (Picker et al., 2006; Santos et al., 2007; De Filippis et al., 2010), we underline the necessity to foster the comprehension of MeCP2 functions also during brain development.

MeCP2 ALTERATIONS LEAD TO A SYNAPTIC PHENOTYPE

Once the relevance of MeCP2 had been demonstrated for the central nervous system, it became imperative to define the expression pattern of the protein during brain development and the associated neuro-pathological abnormalities.

Concerning MeCP2 protein levels, it is generally accepted that its expression in brain mirrors neuronal maturation. That is, MeCP2 increases when neurons develop dendritic arbors, project axons and establish connectivity (Kishi and Macklis, 2004; Neul and Zoghbi, 2004). Interestingly, MeCP2 has been shown to be present in an experimental model that prevents synapse formation, albeit at lower level than normal, suggesting that the abundance of MeCP2, rather than its presence, depends on synapse formation (Neul and Zoghbi, 2004).

Altered MeCP2 expression and activity do not affect the gross structure of the brain, and no obvious signs of degeneration, gliosis or inflammation have been reported in RTT patients (Chahrour and Zoghbi, 2007). The most conspicuous morphological abnormalities in post-mortem RTT patients are reduced brain size and weight, with more subtle alterations, such as reduced dendritic arborization, defects in spine density and morphology, and an increase in neuronal packing, in turn leading to augmented cellular density (Bauman et al., 1995; Belichenko et al., 2009b). Abnormalities in the expression of molecules, such as NMDA, AMPA and GABA receptors, that are crucial for both excitatory and inhibitory synaptic transmission, have also been detected (Johnston et al., 2005). Mouse models of RTT have demonstrated similar defects. In particular, two elegant works from Belichenko et al. (2009a,b) have shown that most of the parameters analyzed were altered in dendrites of *Mecp2*-mutant mice of both genders. In particular, and most strikingly, dendrites were swelled, spine density was altered (generally reduced, but increased in few brain areas), and a smaller head and a longer neck characterized the spines. Overlapping results were obtained observing hippocampal neurons of female RTT patients (Chapleau et al., 2009). Furthermore, neurons generated *in vitro* from induced pluripotent stem cells (iPSCs) derived from RTT patients' fibroblasts showed lower dendritic spine density than control neurons (Moutri et al., 2010).

Taken together, all these findings have led to the hypothesis that the neurological deficits of RTT patients arise because of a failure in synaptic and circuit development and/or maintenance. Accordingly, a number of studies have shown that *Mecp2*-null hippocampal slices are characterized by significantly reduced spontaneous excitatory synaptic transmission, deficits in long-term potentiation (LTP), and long-term depression (LTD). Furthermore, 2-photon time lapse imaging has shown that, at the onset of the disease, *Mecp2*-null somatosensory cortices display remarkable alterations in the dynamics of dendritic spines; on the contrary, when maturation of the connectivity is complete, no differences in spine dynamics are evident in *Mecp2*-mutant mice with respect to their wild-type controls (Landi et al., 2011). Accordingly, it has also been demonstrated that dendritic spine density of hippocampal CA1 pyramidal neurons is lower only at postnatal day 7 (P7), while it does not differ at P15 or later, when symptoms are already well-established (Chapleau et al., 2012). These data support a role of Mecp2 during early development of dendritic spines and suggest that, at least in the *Mecp2*-null mouse model used in these studies, compensatory mechanisms that normalize spine density might occur later on in development. However, it is important to observe that a different study, performed using two diverse *Mecp2*-null lines, reported lower dendritic spine density in hippocampal neurons of animals of 3 weeks of age (Belichenko et al., 2009a). We believe that in the future it will be relevant to address these topics using models of the disease, which are less severe and mimick pathogenic human mutations. Furthermore, similar studies should include both genders: in fact, considering that RTT predominantly affects girls, it is reasonable to assume that heterozygous females represent the appropriate genetic mouse model of Rett syndrome, whereas *Mecp2*-null male mice can be considered a suitable model for addressing the biological function of the *Mecp2* gene.

Finally, evidence is accumulating that overexpression of MeCP2 also affects neuronal plasticity: indeed, decreased dendritic branching and spine density, enhanced excitatory synaptic transmission and altered glutamatergic transmission have been associated with mouse models of the so-called *MECP2* duplication syndrome. Enhanced hippocampal LTP responses have been demonstrated in Mecp2 overexpression mouse lines with respect to their littermate controls (Na et al., 2013).

To conclude, a wealth of evidence now substantiates the functional importance of MeCP2 in the regulation of dendritic structure, synaptic plasticity and homeostasis, therefore providing a rationale for the learning and memory deficits that are constitutively seen in RTT patients and in the mouse models of the disease.

MeCP2 FUNCTIONS DEPEND ON THE HIGHLY STRUCTURED METHYL-BINDING DOMAIN EMBEDDED IN A DISORGANIZED PROTEIN

Starting from the previous observations, we believe that the development of clinical applications implies the urgency of improving our understanding of the functional roles of MeCP2, their regulation, and the protein domains involved. Thus, we will now review the state of art of MeCP2 structure and function.

MeCP2 has originally been described as an abundant and ubiquitously expressed nuclear protein that binds selectively methylated DNA (Lewis et al., 1992). In this first work, the primary structure of the human protein was defined as a polypeptide 486 residues long, containing two main domains, namely, a methyl-CpG binding domain (MBD) and a transcription repression domain (TRD). Nowadays, we know that alternative splicing, occurring both in human and mouse, generates two main isoforms of the protein (MeCP2_e1 and MeCP2_e2; **Figure 1A**; Chahrour and Zoghbi, 2007). Considering that (i) the primary structure of MeCP2 is highly conserved among vertebrates, (ii) the two principal isoforms differ exclusively in the very first N-terminal residues, and (iii) RTT mutations generally refer to the MeCP2_e2 isoform, in this review, we will mainly refer to the human MeCP2_e2 isoform (486 residues; **Figure 1A**). However, it is important to recall that MeCP2_e1 is the predominant isoform in brain. Furthermore, since MeCP2 PTMs have been investigated almost exclusively in rodents, in the future, it will be important to address which of the identified PTMs are maintained in the

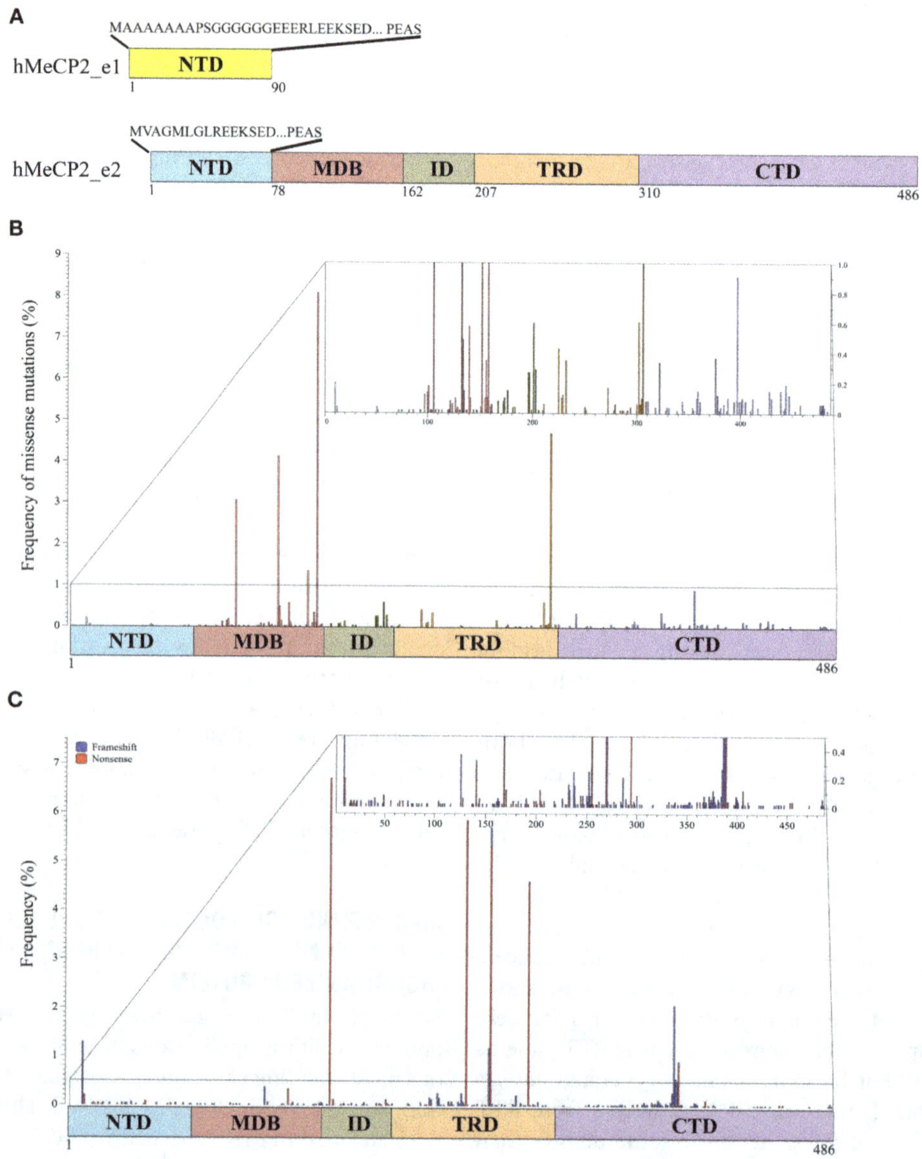

FIGURE 1 | MeCP2 isoforms and pathogenic mutations. (A) Two MeCP2 isoforms, MeCP2_e1 and MeCP2_e2, are generated by alternative splicing originating two distinct N-terminal regions. MeCP2_e1 is 498 amino acids long and contains a N-terminal domain (NTD, yellow) of 90 amino acids of which the first 21 are distinct, whereas MeCP2_e2, formed by 486 amino acids, has 9 unique amino acids in its NTD (blue). MeCP2 is constituted by five sub-domains: NTD, MBD (methyl-CpG binding domain), ID (intervening domain), TRD (transcriptional repression domain, CTD (C-terminal domain); below the MeCP2_e2 isoform is shown the amino acid numbers of the different domains. **(B)** Schematic illustration showing the localization and the frequency of pathogenic missense mutations within MeCP2. The small inset shows in details the mutation frequency between 0 and 1%. The colors of the vertical bars correspond to the color code of the distinct MeCP2 subdomains. **(C)** Localization and frequency of non-sense and truncating *MECP2* mutations. Frameshift mutations are shown in blue and non-sense mutations in red. The small inset shows in details the mutation frequency between 0 and 1%.

human protein and whether human MeCP2 is characterized by additional events of modification.

As of today, MeCP2 has been subdivided into five main structural domains corresponding to the N-terminal domain (NTD), the MBD, the intervening domain (ID), the TRD and the C-terminal domain (CTD; **Figure 1A**). The MBD was originally defined as the minimum continuous ensemble of MeCP2 residues necessary and sufficient for selective binding to methylated CpG-dinucleotides (Nan et al., 1997). Its relevance for MeCP2 functions is highlighted by the fact that almost half of the known disease-causing missense mutations in *MECP2* occurs within this domain, including three of the eight most frequent RTT mutations (**Figure 1B**; for a complete updated database of *MECP2* mutations see www.Mecp2.chw.edu.au). *In vitro* studies have confirmed the relevance of MeCP2 binding to methylated DNA, suggesting that most, if not all, missense mutations within the methyl-binding domain impair the selectivity of MeCP2 for methylated DNA (Yusufzai and Wolffe, 2000). The X-ray structure of the MBD alone or associated with methylated DNA unexpectedly revealed that the MBD recognizes the hydration of the major groove, in which methylated DNA resides, rather than cytosine methylation *per se* (Ho et al., 2008). Importantly, these studies have been extended by the recent demonstration that the MBD of MeCP2 avidly binds both 5-methyl cytosine (5mC) and 5-hydroxymethyl cytosine (5hmC). This property has not been observed for the other members of the MBD family (MBD1-4). Interestingly, the pathogenic R133C MeCP2 mutant retains most of its binding to methylated DNA, but has lost affinity for 5hmC. Since small changes in the MBD structure seemed to influence the DNA binding properties of MeCP2, the authors proposed that PTMs affecting MeCP2 might alter its substrate specificity and, thus, its downstream functions (Mellen et al., 2012). In possible accordance with this hypothesis, the MBD has been found to be phosphorylated, methylated and acetylated (see more ahead and **Figures 2, 3** and Supplementary Table 1). Interestingly, two lysine residues (K130 and K135) surrounding R133 have been found to be ubiquitinated (Gonzales et al., 2012). Although we do not yet know whether these residues are mono- or polyubiquitinated, several pieces of evidence prove that ubiquitin is a bulky modifier with possible direct steric effects on any modified protein, influencing conformational flexibility and protein-protein interactions. These studies thus suggest that ubiquitination might be a mechanism for a direct and rapid control of MeCP2 activities and interactions (Chernorudskiy and Gainullin, 2013). In the future, it would be interesting to address whether acetylated K130 and K133 affect the binding of MeCP2 to modified DNA.

The TRD was originally defined as the smallest region of MeCP2 required for transcriptional repression in functional assays (Lewis et al., 1992). No structural information is available for this domain or for the other remaining parts of MeCP2. The lack of structural information can easily be explained by Circular Dichroism studies and theoretical predictions demonstrating that almost 60% of MeCP2 is unstructured (Adams et al., 2007). Thus, MeCP2 is now recognized as an "intrinsically disordered protein" that might acquire local secondary structures upon binding to other macromolecules. Accordingly, MeCP2 is capable of multiple protein–protein interactions (Ausió et al., 2014; Bedogni et al., 2014) and appears to enter into a stable association with its cofactors only when bound to DNA. Thus, MeCP2 seems to act as a multifunctional factor that sustains interactions with specific partners depending on the architecture of its target DNA sequences (Klose and Bird, 2004). Recent findings, which will be discussed in details further on, suggest that also MeCP2 PTMs affect its protein-protein interactions. It is relevant that several of the modifications identified so far cluster in the transcriptional repression domain (**Figure 2**).

Protease digestion has been used to define the remaining NTD, ID and CTD domains (Adams et al., 2007); importantly, by analyzing the MeCP2 mutation database, we found that almost 25% of residues in the CTD and ID have been associated with pathogenic missense mutations, therefore suggesting their relevance for MeCP2 functions (**Figure 1B**; Bedogni et al., 2014). Although these two domains maintain a highly disorganized structure, the ID domain has been involved in several protein-protein interactions and diverse phosphorylation events (Bedogni et al., 2014 and **Figure 2**). On the contrary, to the best of our knowledge, the CTD has been found associated exclusively with Sdccag1, a mediator of nuclear export (Long et al., 2011). However, this domain, which is crucial for the binding of MeCP2 to chromatin, is subject to various modifications (Nikitina et al., 2007; Bedogni et al., 2014).

To summarize we can state that: (i) the highly disorganized structure of MeCP2 endows the protein with multiple functions; (ii) the structured MBD gives the protein its unique capability of interacting with both methylated and hydroxymethylated DNA; (iii) PTMs of MeCP2 are likely to affect directly its binding to DNA and protein partners, therefore contributing to the versatility of MeCP2.

MeCP2: THE COMPLEXITY OF A FUNDAMENTAL MULTIFUNCTIONAL PROTEIN

Adrian Bird and collaborators originally identified MeCP2 as a nuclear factor capable of binding DNA with at least one symmetrically methylated CpG-dinucleotide (Lewis et al., 1992) and repressing transcription mainly through its TRD (Nan et al., 1997). In this pioneering work the authors proposed that the extent of MeCP2 repression depends on its abundance in the nucleus, and that MeCP2 is capable of displacing histone H1 from chromatin to access its binding sites (Nan et al., 1997). A subsequent work demonstrated that MeCP2 uses its CTD to stabilize and asymmetrically protect linker DNA, thus mimicking the association of histone H1 with chromatin (Chandler et al., 1999). The capability of MeCP2 to play the role of an architectural chromatin protein was further supported by a report showing that MeCP2 is a potent chromatin-condensing factor, functioning directly without other corepressor or enzymatic activities (Georgel et al., 2003). The authors demonstrated that depending on its molar ratio to nucleosomes, MeCP2 assembles novel secondary and tertiary chromatin structures regardless of DNA methylation; these effects on large scale chromatin organization represent a good explanation for its ability to repress *in vivo* transcription at a distance.

A further link between the repressive activity of MeCP2 and chromatin compaction was established by demonstrating that the TRD binds to corepressor complexes (Sin3A and NCoR) with histone deacetylase activities, and that transcriptional repression of methylated DNA *in vivo* is partially relieved by the deacetylase inhibitor trichostatin A (Jones et al., 1998; Georgel et al., 2003). Importantly, through the years other chromatin-related partners of MeCP2 have been identified, such as Brahma, ATRX, CoREST, c-Ski, and H3K9 histone methyltransferase (Nan et al., 1998; Chahrour and Zoghbi, 2007; Bedogni et al., 2014).

All these results fit very well with more recent results demonstrating that in mature neurons, where MeCP2 abundance corresponds roughly to one molecule every second nucleosome, the protein is genome-wide bound, tracks methylated DNA, serves as an alternative linker histone, and organizes a specialized chromatin structure, thus dampening overall transcriptional noise (Skene et al., 2010; Guy et al., 2011). The effect on global genomic architecture is outlined by a selective increase in histone acetylation, H1 levels and transcription of repetitive elements and L1 retrotransposons in *Mecp2*-null neurons, but not in glia,

A

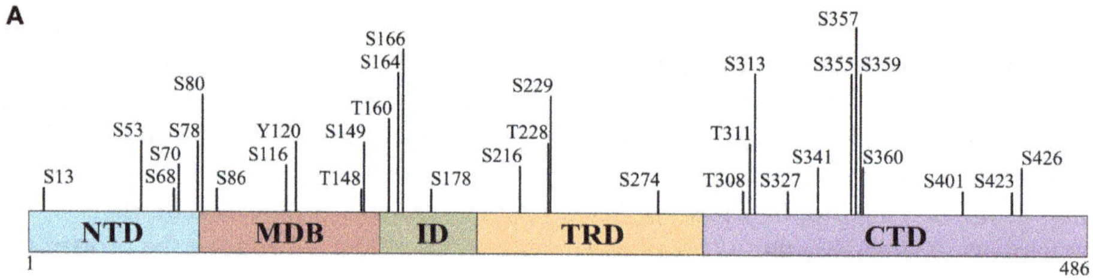

B

Domain	Residue	In silico prediction		Experimental evidence (see Table 2)
		P-value	Significance	
NTD	S13	0.885 (only in _e1 isoform)	✓	✓
	S53	0.979	✓	✓
	T64	0.513 (only in Human)	✓	✗
	S65	0.954	✓	✗
	G67	0.911 (only in Mouse)	✓	✗
	S68	0.760 (in Human isoforms) 0.926 (in Mouse isoforms)	✓	✓
	S70	0.068 (in Human isoforms) 0.225 (in Mouse isoforms)	✗	✓
	S78	0.032		✓
MBD	S80	0.994	✓	✓
	S86	0.996	✓	✓
	Y95	0.930	✓	✗
	S113	0.995	✓	✗
	S116	0.987	✓	✓
	Y120	0.650	✓	✓
	Y123	0.778	✓	✗
	S134	0.817	✓	✗
	T148	0.456	✗	✓
	S149	0.924	✓	✓
	T160	0.860	✓	✓
ID	S164	0.996	✓	✓
	S166	0.997	✓	✓
	S178	0.998	✓	✓
	T184	0.888	✓	✗
	S194	0.534 (only in Mouse)	✓	✗
	T196	0.897 (in Human isoforms) 0.822 (in Mouse isoforms)	✓	✗
	T203	0.666 (only in Human)	✓	✗
	S204	0.949 (in Human isoforms) 0.895 (in Mouse isoforms)	✓	✗
TRD	S216	0.975 (in Human isoforms) 0.986 (in Mouse isoforms)	✓	✓
	T228	0.505 (only in Human)	✓	✓
	S229	0.883 (in Human isoforms) 0.673 (in Mouse isoforms)	✓	✓
	T241	0.781 (in Human isoforms) 0.759 (in Mouse isoforms)	✓	✗
	S274	0.870	✓	✓
	S291	0.969	✓	✗
	S292	0.512 (in Human isoforms) 0.684 (in Mouse isoforms)	✓	✗
	S295	0.988 (in Human isoforms) 0.994 (in Mouse isoforms)	✓	✗
	T308	0.427	✗	✓
CTD	T311	0.743	✓	✓
	S313	0.980	✓	✓
	T327	0.218	✗	✓
	S332	0.994	✓	✗
	T338	0.526	✓	✗
	S341	0.870	✓	✓
	S346	0.998	✓	✗
	S349	0.990	✓	✓
	S350	0.997	✓	✗
	S355	0.937	✓	✓
	S356	0.991	✓	✗
	S357	0.990	✓	✓
	S359	0.925	✓	✓
	S360	0.993	✓	✓
	S375	0.993 (in Human isoforms) 0.922 (in Mouse isoforms)	✓	✗
	P385	0.534 (only in Mouse)	✓	✗
	S395	0.997	✓	✗
	S396	0.861 (only in Human)	✓	✗
	S401	0.996 (in Human isoforms) 0.993 (in Mouse isoforms)	✓	✓
	S410	0.622 (only in Mouse)	✓	✗
	S411	0.688 (in Human isoforms) 0.501 (in Mouse isoforms)	✓	✗
	S423	0.985	✓	✓
	S426	0.718	✓	✓
	A444	0.866 (only in Mouse)	✓	✗
	T445	0.736 (only in Mouse)	✓	✗
	Y450	0.875 (in Human isoforms) 0.758 (in Mouse isoforms)	✓	✗
	S463	0.953	✓	✗

FIGURE 2 | The phosphorylation signature of MeCP2. (A) All experimentally determined phosphorylation sites of MeCP2. The numbering corresponds to the hMeCP2_e2 isoform. **(B)** The probability score of phosphorylation sites within MeCP2 identified *in silico* by GPs 2.0 and NetPhos 2.0 confronted with experimentally determined sites; only residues identified as phosphorylation sites *in silico* with $P > 0.5$ are listed. Further details including references of experimentally determined sites are listed in supplementary Table 1.

where the protein is much less abundant (Moutri et al., 2010; Skene et al., 2010). Thus, the lack of functional MeCP2 in mature neurons might lead to a disorganized chromatin structure that impairs synaptic plasticity by preventing proper neuronal responses to stimuli. Cohen et al. (2011) have then recently reinforced the possibility that MeCP2 does not regulate the expression of specific genes, but rather functions as a histone-like factor, globally bound across the genome.

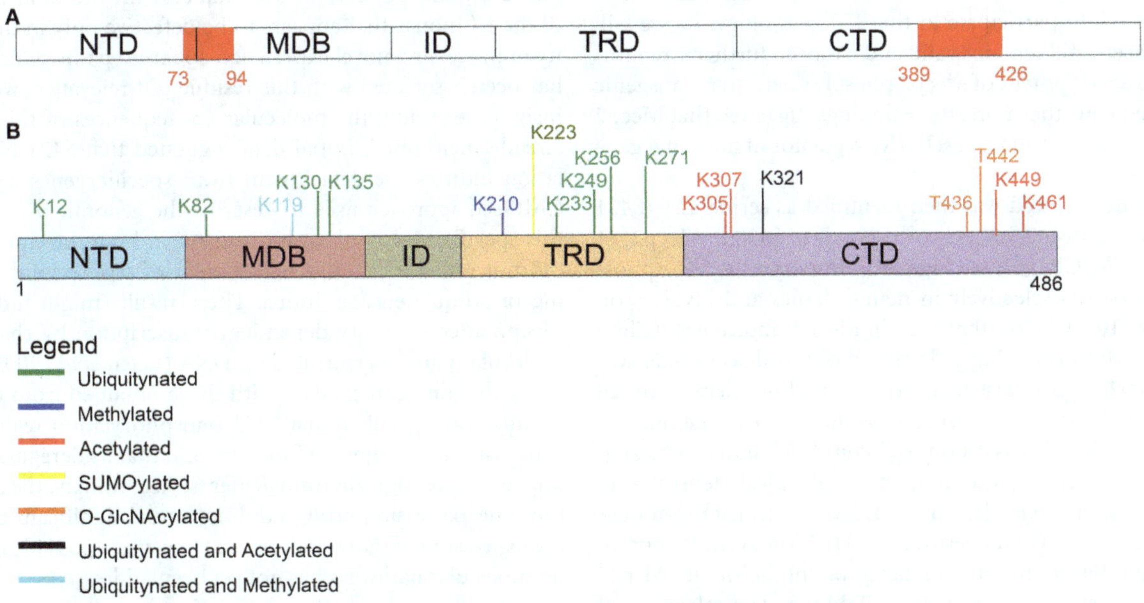

FIGURE 3 | Post-translational modifications other than phosphorylation affecting MeCP2. (A) Two PEST motives, enriched in proline, glutamate, serine, and threonine residues, are present within MeCP2 possibly regulating its stability and phosphorylation. **(B)** Schematic representation of the different types of post-translational modifications (PTM) affecting MeCP2 and the involved amino acids.

MeCP2 functions have been further expanded in the last years and a role in facilitating gene expression has also been suggested. In particular, the analysis of gene expression patterns in the hypothalamus of mice that either lack or overexpress Mecp2, led Huda Zoghbi and her colleagues to propose that MeCP2 predominantly activates transcription (Chahrour et al., 2008). The authors suggested that the association of MeCP2 with the transcriptional activator CREB1 might explain these results. Similarly, in a recent paper Rudolf Jaenisch and his collaborators demonstrated that the reduced size of *Mecp2*-null neurons affects total RNA levels per cell. By analyzing global transcriptional profiles starting from an identical number of cells, thus avoiding the usual normalization to total input RNA (Li et al., 2013), they found more down-regulated than up-regulated genes, leading to the conclusion that one of the key functions of MeCP2 is to facilitate global transcription. So far, the "per cell" perspective has been used only in one report (Li et al., 2013) and we still need to understand whether the discrepancy between the studies can be justified by the different approaches. Further, we suggest, as described in a recent publication, that higher-level bioinformatics, identifying statistically significant deregulated molecular pathways (rather than single genes), might allow the identification of the biological processes affected by dysfunctional MeCP2 (Bedogni et al., 2014).

In addition to all of this, it is important to recall that MeCP2 has also been proposed to play a role in regulating mRNA splicing and in modulating protein synthesis. In fact, Mecp2 was first found to interact with the RNA-binding protein Y box-binding protein 1 (YB1) and to regulate splicing of reporter minigenes. Supporting these data *in vivo*, aberrant alternative splicing patterns were also observed in a mouse model of RTT (Young et al., 2006; Maunakea et al., 2013). The involvement of MeCP2 in mRNA biogenesis has been further proven by the interaction of Mecp2 with Prpf3 (pre-mRNA processing factor 3), a spliceosome associated protein (Long et al., 2011). Eventually, a severe defect in protein synthesis in *Mecp2* mutant mice was for the first time demonstrated by Ricciardi et al. (2011). This deficiency, which is a common defect in autism spectrum disorders, was ascribed to a dysfunctional AKT/mTOR pathway. The relevance of these findings has subsequently been strengthened by the demonstration that pharmacological or genetic enhancement of protein synthesis ameliorates *Mecp2*-defective neurons (Li et al., 2013).

Thus, considering the structural flexibility of MeCP2 and the possibility of PTMs affecting its structure and/or interactions with protein partners, we believe that a better comprehension of MeCP2 functions might be obtained through the study of its diversely modified isoforms and their networking capabilities. Therefore, we will progress critically surveying the actual knowledge on MeCP2 phosphorylation that so far certainly represents the best characterized PTM of the methyl-binding protein.

MeCP2 PHOSPHORYLATION: WHERE WE STAND AND WHERE WE MIGHT GO

The history of MeCP2 phosphorylation (pMeCP2) began in 2003 when two independent studies demonstrated that neuronal activation triggers a calcium-dependent phosphorylation of Mecp2 and the consequent release of the methyl-binding protein from *Bdnf* promoter III, thereby facilitating transcription (Chen et al., 2003; Martinowich et al., 2003). Several were the breaking news of these publications although some of them still remain debated.

To begin with, these studies proposed for the first time that Mecp2 is involved in the control of neuronal activity-dependent gene regulation through its PTMs, and that the deregulation of this process might participate in the RTT pathology. As we will see, this concept still remains valid and has been further strengthened by the development of Mecp2 phospho-defective transgenic mice (**Table 1**). Furthermore, these findings suggested that Mecp2 might work as a dynamic and selective regulator of neuronal gene expression.

The residue involved was then identified as serine 421 (S421 refers to mouse Mecp2_e2 and corresponds to S438 in Mecp2_e1 and S423 in hMeCP2_e2; see **Figure 2**); importantly, S421 phosphorylation occurs selectively in neural tissues and involves on the average 10–30% of the overall Mecp2 molecules (Zhou et al., 2006). By expressing a S421A phospho-defective derivative of Mecp2 in primary neurons, the authors demonstrated that this PTM affects dendritic growth, whereas the importance of S421 phosphorylation for circuit development was suggested by a defective patterning of distal apical dendrites in the brain of a phospho-defective S421A knock-in (KI) mouse line ($Mecp2^{S421A/y}$, Cohen et al., 2011). Moreover, a shift in excitation-inhibition balance in favor of inhibition in Mecp2 S421A cortical slices was measured (**Table 1**). The relevance of S421 phosphorylation is emphasized by the fact that a similar shift has already been described in *Mecp2* knock-out mice. However, and possibly in accordance with the mild phenotype of the KI mouse that appears to be defective only in the capability of processing novel experience, so far no pathogenic mutation has been associated with this residue. Of relevance, we still lack insights regarding the molecular consequences of this PTM. As already mentioned, initial data suggested that S421 phosphorylation induces the detachment from specific genes. However, a ChIP-seq approach used to describe the genomic distribution of this specific Mecp2 phospho-isoform in brain of knock-in mice did not reveal a selective detachment of pMecp2 either in resting or stimulated conditions. These results might indicate that Mecp2 affects activity-dependent transcription by changing the molecular partners recruited on DNA (Chen et al., 2003).

By merging clinical data with those obtained from the S421A KI mice, we speculate that S421 phosphorylation regulates only some aspects of cognitive function, and that its deregulation leads only to subtle cognitive impairments. Accordingly, the analysis of the gene expression profiles did not reveal significant changes in the expression of individual genes. However, a possible mild effect on molecular pathways has not yet been addressed.

Importantly, S421 phosphorylation has also been associated with drug sensitivity and mood regulation. In fact, the research of stimuli affecting MeCP2 phosphorylation has led not only

Table 1 | Phosphorylation-defective *Mecp2* mouse models.

	Animal phenotype	Synaptic physiology	Molecular Phenotype	Importance
***Mecp2*^{S80A}**; Tao et al., 2009	Normal lifespan; RTT-like phenotype; -62% locomotor activity in dark cycle running wheel assays.		Decreased binding to chromatin on specific gene promoters.	S80 phosphorylation regulates MeCP2 function in resting neurons.
***Mecp2*^{T308A}**; Ebert et al., 2013	Normal body weight; Reduced brain weight; More seizures and lower seizure threshold; Locomotor defects.		T308A mutation does not alter MeCP2 stability, binding to DNA and basal interaction with NCoR complex; Decrease in membrane depolarization-induced *Npas4* and *Bdnf* expression.	Loss of phosphorylation-dependent interaction of MeCP2 with NCoR contributes to the development of some neurological defects observed in RTT.
***Mecp2*^{S421A}**; Cohen et al., 2011	No visible differences compared to their wild type littermates; No locomotor defects; Behavioral abnormalities outlined with sociability and preference for social novelty assays.	Increased dendritic complexity; Increased mIPSC amplitude.	No detectable effect on gene transcription.	S421 phosphorylation has a role in synaptic connections development within the cerebral cortex.
***Mecp2*$^{S421A;S424A}$**; Tao et al., 2009; Li et al., 2011	Normal lifespan; No RTT-like phenotype; +145% locomotor activity in dark cycle running wheel assays; Fear-conditioning test and Morris water maze test suggest an altered hippocampus function.	Stronger LTP induced at both the Schaffer collateral-CA1 synapse and the mossy fiber-CA3 synapse, compared to wild type; Increased excitatory synaptogenesis in both the hippocampal and cortical neurons.	Hippocampal $Mecp2^{S421A;S424A}$ neurons show an increase in *Bmp4* and *Bdnf* transcription and a decrease in *Mef2c* and *Grm1* transcription.	S421 phosphorylation is a neuronal-activity induced event.

to demonstrate that hippocampus-dependent behavioral training leads to a robust increase in Mecp2 S421 phosphorylation (Li et al., 2011), but also that a single acute injection of cocaine or amphetamine elicits a transient increase in pS421 Mecp2 in the caudate putamen and nucleus accumbens (Deng et al., 2010; Mao et al., 2011). Having hypothesized that cellular and behavioral adaptations to these drugs might be affected by pS421, the authors have very recently produced the first data demonstrating that phosphorylation of MeCP2 at Ser421 functionally limits cellular sensitivity and synaptic response to repeated psychostimulant exposure in the mesocorticolimbic circuitry (Deng et al., 2014). A role for MeCP2 phosphorylation in the context of chronic opioid consumption and withdrawal has also been suggested: in fact, morphine withdrawal induces pS421Mecp2 in selected brain areas, such as lateral septum and the nucleus accumbens shell (Ciccarelli et al., 2013). Eventually, S421 phosphorylation in the nucleus accumbens and lateral habenula has been associated with depressive-like behaviors: in fact, administration of the antidepressant imipramine induces pS421Mecp2 and studies with knock-in mice showed that this induction is required for a proper response to the antidepressant (Hutchinson et al., 2012).

Mass spectrometry (MS) analysis identified that neuronal activity induces also S424 phosphorylation in mouse brain (isoform 2; Tao et al., 2009). A KI mouse line, in which the phosphorylation at both residues of the endogenous protein is abolished, was also generated ($Mecp2^{S421A;S424A/y}$; Li et al., 2011). Before reviewing the results obtained, it is worth mentioning that MS failed to identify S424 phosphorylation in rat brain, therefore questioning the possible involvement of this PTM in RTT. At the molecular level, these two mutations did not affect the expression and intracellular localization of Mecp2; phenotypically, the obtained mice did not show any overt difference with respect to the wild-type animals. By exploiting conventional behavioral tests, the authors found a higher performance for some hippocampal functions, such as spatial memory, than in wild-type littermates. In accordance with enhanced hippocampus-dependent learning and memory, LTP was found significantly stronger in $Mecp2^{S421A;S424A/y}$ hippocampal slices with respect to the controls, together with an increase in excitatory synaptogenesis in both cortical and hippocampal cultured neurons. ChIP analyses permitted to hypothesize that the concomitant loss of these two phosphorylation sites enhances the binding of Mecp2 to its target gene promoters; importantly, the transcriptional outcome depends on the bound sequence, reinforcing the possibility that MeCP2 can function both as an activator and a repressor of transcription.

Summarizing the results obtained, both publications testify that MeCP2 phosphorylation impacts the development and function of the nervous system. Furthermore, they suggest that MeCP2 functions are regulated by several PTMs and their combination. Future studies need to address whether a crosstalk between MeCP2 PTMs exists, and moreover, the current contradiction concerning S424 phosphorylation needs to be solved. In fact, Michael Greenberg reported as unpublished results that they were unable to detect increased phosphorylation of Mecp2 S424 in response to neural activity both *in vitro* and *in vivo* (Cohen et al., 2011). Thus, it is unclear whether the S424A mutation in knock-in mice affects a phosphorylation site of Mecp2 or influences the molecular properties of the protein through an alternative mechanism. Although the production of a single $Mecp2^{S424A/y}$ KI line might be informative, we are not confident it would be convenient, also considering that so far this residue has never been associated with RTT.

By surveying MeCP2 phosphorylation in rat/mouse brains and in human HeLa cells, Tao et al. (2009) found that S80 phosphorylation is the most conserved phosphorylation site of MeCP2. S80 appears as the most abundantly phosphorylated residue under resting conditions whereas neuronal activity induces its dephosphorylation. $Mecp2^{S80A/y}$ knock-in mice are slightly overweight and show decreased locomotor activity (Tao et al., 2009). Functionally, S80 phosphorylation does not affect the overall subcellular localization of MeCP2, but seems to increase its affinity for chromatin. However, these *in vitro* studies, together with microarray analyses, were performed with exogenously expressed MeCP2 derivatives, expressed at levels slightly above those of the endogenous protein. Although no further data were produced with this *Mecp2* transgenic line, available information lead us to suggest that S80 phosphorylation does not have any impact on global transcription and that, probably, this MeCP2 phosphoisoform is globally bound to chromatin, therefore resembling the distribution of MeCP2 and the pS421 isoform.

A more recent work used phospho-tryptic maps to confirm that Mecp2 is phosphorylated at many sites in cultured activated and resting neurons (Ebert et al., 2013). In this study, the activity-dependent phosphorylation of Mecp2_e2 occurs on residues S86, S274, T308, and S421 (for an easier comprehension of the state of art, all the so-far-identified MeCP2 phospho-sites are summarized in **Figure 2** and Supplementary Table 1). Considering that the nearby R306 residue is mutated in RTT, and that its pathogenic R306C mutation disrupts the ability of MeCP2 to interact with the corepressor complex NCoR (Lyst et al., 2013), the authors focused their attention on T308 phosphorylation and found that it abolishes the interaction of MeCP2 with the corepressor, thereby reducing MeCP2-mediated transcriptional repression. The phospho-defective $Mecp2^{T308A/y}$ KI mice demonstrated that mutant MeCP2 maintains its global distribution on chromatin, but that activity dependent induction of MeCP2 target genes is deficient. Importantly, the brains of these mice weigh significantly less, the animals display motor system defects, and have a lower seizure threshold compared to wild-type mice. Since all these symptoms recapitulate the manifestation of several *Mecp2* mouse models, this is a groundbreaking piece of work highlighting not only the relevance of MeCP2 phosphorylation but also its role as a transcriptional silencer through its interaction with the corepressor complex NCoR/HDAC.

Eventually, the laboratory of Janine La Salle used SH-SY5Y cells stably expressing FLAG-tagged mouse MeCP2_e1 to identify MeCP2 PTMs by tandem mass spectrometry and, interestingly, found them to cluster mainly in the MBD and TRD domains (Gonzales et al., 2012). Regarding phosphorylation, six sites were identified, partly overlapping with previous data (**Figure 2**). The successful production of two phospho-specific antisera, against pS80 and pS229, permitted to confirm that these modifications are independent of one another, and can coexist on the same molecule of MeCP2 (Tao et al., 2009). Whereas both Mecp2 phospho-isoforms were found in brain and were characterized by the same subnuclear distribution as total Mecp2, pS229Mecp2 showed enriched binding to a tested promoter with respect to total Mecp2. Moreover, it was observed that pS80Mecp2 and pS229Mecp2 have a preferential association with distinct combinations of MeCP2 cofactors compared to total MeCP2, confirming the hypothesis that MeCP2 changes its partners and mechanisms of action through its PTMs. Accordingly, the phosphorylation of S80 seems to affect the interaction of MeCP2 with RNA and the RNA-binding protein YB-1 (Gonzales et al., 2012).

Summarizing, most data suggest that MeCP2 is a multifunctional protein that "transiently" performs its function(s) depending on its differential phosphorylation. Accordingly, although S421 phosphorylation remains for the time being the most widely characterized PTM and pT308 results as the most functionally relevant, several other sites of phosphorylation have been mapped, and their modification is often spatially regulated by specific stimuli. Almost no information is available so far on these PTMs and their regulation during brain development; furthermore, since a role of MeCP2 outside of the nervous system, particularly in glia and microglia, has recently been demonstrated as important for MECP2-related disorders, future studies should also investigate MeCP2 phosphorylation in these cells. MeCP2 phosphorylation has been hypothesized to affect its binding to target DNA sequences: however, no data seem to support this hypothesis in neurons, and none of the phosphorylation events characterized so far globally affect MeCP2 binding to chromatin. It is highly plausible then that the identification and/or characterization of novel phospho-residues of MeCP2 will lead to the discovery of PTMs that generally or selectively influence its binding to chromatin. Furthermore, they should help providing a better comprehension of MeCP2 in physiological and pathological conditions. To this purpose, we suggest that studies should focus first on sites that are conserved by evolution and/or have been found mutated in patients. Thus, we employed two different tools to predict phosphorylation sites (GPs 2.0, Xue et al., 2008; and NetPhos 2.0, Blom et al., 1999), at the same time screening the existent proteomic literature to reveal which residues have already been found modified in cell lines or *in vivo*. The results are summarized in **Figure 2**. Algorithms for the prediction of PTMs in proteins are usually based on machine learning approaches, and associate with the predictions a reliability score ranking the residues according to their likelihood of being modified. The two algorithms we employed yielded highly consistent results. All in all, the strong correlation between experimentally verified phosphorylated sites and their ranking in the predictions leads us to conjecture that sites with high prediction scores but not yet validated, usually considered as "false positives," might indeed be very likely candidates for phosphorylation, and worth of further experimental investigation.

Eventually, a thorough characterization of MeCP2 phosphorylation should also address which are the signaling pathways involved, and the respective kinases and phosphatases. No phosphatases have been described yet: on the contrary, a few studies (Chen et al., 2003; Martinowich et al., 2003; Zhou et al., 2006; Bracaglia et al., 2009; Tao et al., 2009; Khoshnan and Patterson, 2012; Ciccarelli et al., 2013) have suggested kinases that either directly or indirectly affect MeCP2 phosphorylation. Since the data obtained so far do not appear as conclusive, and we consider bioinformatics approaches not yet reliable enough to obtain informative data on this aspect (data not shown), we have decided not to address further this issue in this work.

MeCP2 POST-TRANSLATIONAL MODIFICATIONS OTHER THAN PHOSPHORYLATION AND CONCLUSIONS

The heterogeneity of MeCP2 posttranslational modifications, together with its genome-wide distribution (Skene et al., 2010), its capacity to mediate the formation of a highly compacted chromatin structure *in vitro* (Georgel et al., 2003) and to substitute histone H1 *in vivo* (Skene et al., 2010) have led some authors to suggest that, when highly abundant, the protein might behave as a specialized histone-like chromatin organizing factor. Thus, in analogy with the histone code, it is highly conceivable, as already hinted along this review, that MeCP2 PTMs affect its binding to specific epigenetic marks as well as its interactions with protein partners and therefore the resulting biological functions. In accordance with this hypothesis, there are a few studies demonstrating the existence on MeCP2 of PTMs different from phosphorylation on MeCP2. Thus, in this last section we will briefly survey the information existing so far. Available data are still very limited, no animal models have been generated and, often, functional studies have not been performed in neurons. Future studies will certainly have to fill this gap of knowledge.

In detail, Gonzales et al. (2012) used SH-SY5Y cells stably expressing epitope-tagged MeCP2_e1 to analyze its PTMs by tandem mass spectrometry with 90% coverage. Importantly, apart from the already mentioned phosphorylation events, 10 ubiquitination sites were identified (**Figure 3** and **Table 2**), with lysine 271 occurring as the most frequently modified site. Although, no functional role has been yet provided for these PTMs, all of them but two reside in the MBD or TRD domains leading to the hypothesis that they might affect the binding of MeCP2 to chromatin or its regulatory properties. These studies have been performed in cultured cell lines and with exogenously expressed MeCP2: however, their relevance might be underlined by the fact that three of these sites have been associated to missense mutations in RTT (**Table 2**). Eventually, by surveying literature we found that lysine 130 had already been found ubiquitinated (Wagner et al., 2011). The functional significance of ubiquitination is dual: generally, it is associated with the rapid degradation of modified proteins; however, such modification can also have a role in signaling or trafficking. Interestingly, Ausiò and his collaborators have identified two strong, conserved PEST motives in the primary sequence of MeCP2 (**Figure 3**). PEST motives are sequences enriched in proline, glutamate, serine, and threonine residues, and often predispose proteins to rapid proteolytic degradation (Thambirajah et al., 2009). The PEST structure gets destabilized upon phosphorylation leading to the degradation of the modified protein. Interestingly, although no connection to protein stability has been established so far, the two best-defined phosphorylation events (S80 and S421) reside in the PEST domains. In addition to phosphorylation, authors have identified several potential ubiquitination sites at lysine residues

Table 2 | Post-translational modifications within MeCP2 other than phosphorylation.

Residue	Mutation in RTT	PTM	Cell line/Tissue assayed	References
K12	K12N (0.04%)	Ub	SH-SY5Y neuroblast. cells	Gonzales et al., 2012
K82	K82fs (0.02%) K82R (0.02%)	Ub	SH-SY5Y neuroblast. cells	Gonzales et al., 2012
K119	–	Ub	SH-SY5Y neuroblast. cells	Gonzales et al., 2012
	–	Met	293 T	Jung et al., 2008
K130	–	Ub	HEK-293T SH-SY5Y neuroblast. cells	Wagner et al., 2011; Gonzales et al., 2012
K135	K135E (0.15%)	Ub	SH-SY5Y neuroblast. cells	Gonzales et al., 2012
R162	R162fs (0.06%)	Met	Kidney (7945, 7947) Lung (7946, 7948) Mice brain	www.PhosphoSite.org (Hornbeck et al., 2012), CST curation sets 7945, 7946, 7947, 7948, (Guo et al., 2014)
K210	K210I (0.02%)	Met	293 T	Jung et al., 2008
K223	K223NfsX3 (0.02%)	SUMO	Primary cortical neurons	Cheng et al., 2014
K233	K233fs (0.02%)	Ub	SH-SY5Y neuroblast. cells	Gonzales et al., 2012
K249	–	Ub	SH-SY5Y neuroblast. cells	Gonzales et al., 2012
K256	K256SfsX17 (0.02%)	Ub	SH-SY5Y neuroblast. cells	Gonzales et al., 2012
K271	–	Ub	SH-SY5Y neuroblast. cells	Gonzales et al., 2012
K305	K305fs (0.02%) K305E (0.02%) K305R (0.08%)	Ac	SH-SY5Y neuroblast. cells	Gonzales et al., 2012
K307	–	Ac	SH-SY5Y neuroblast. cells	Gonzales et al., 2012
K321	K321Sfs*13 (0.02%)	Ac	SH-SY5Y neuroblast. cells	Gonzales et al., 2012
		Ub	SH-SY5Y neuroblast. cells	Gonzales et al., 2012
T436	–	O-GlcNAc	Murine synaptosomes (Trinidad et al., 2012) Rat brain (Wang et al., 2010)	Wang et al., 2010; Trinidad et al., 2012
T442	T442fs (0.02%) T442A (0.02%)	O-GlcNAc	Rat brain	Wang et al., 2010
K449	–	Ac	MV4-11 (Choudhary et al., 2009) HCT 116 (CST)	(Choudhary et al., 2009) www.PhosphoSite.org (Hornbeck et al., 2012), CST curation sets 9796, 9797
K461	–	Ac	HEK-293 cells and primary cortical neurons	(Zocchi and Sassone-Corsi, 2012)

flanking the PEST domains. The hypothesis that the two PEST domains have a major role in fine-tuning MeCP2 levels and that PTMs associated with the modification of these domains regulate the activity of MeCP2 is a challenging one. However, no further data have been provided to support it and evidence for the ubiquitination of these residues is still lacking.

More recently, MeCP2 has been found modified by the covalent linkage of small ubiquitin-like modifier (SUMO) to several lysines. In particular, the sumoylation of lysine 223 is required for the recruitment of HDAC1/2 complexes and mutation of K223 abolishes its gene silencing properties in primary cortical neurons (Cheng et al., 2014). Furthermore, this mutation impacts proper excitatory synaptogenesis *in vitro* and *in vivo* suggesting the relevance of sumoylation for MeCP2 functions.

In addition, Mecp2 has been found acetylated in several residues (Choudhary et al., 2009; Gonzales et al., 2012; Zocchi and Sassone-Corsi, 2012); in particular, acetylation of K464 of Mecp2_e1 has been identified in cultured cortical neurons. The authors have demonstrated that this modification is mediated by p300 and erased by the nicotinamide-adenine dinucleotide dependent histone deacetylase SIRT1. Chromatin immunoprecipitation experiments performed in *Sirt1*-null mice have led to hypothesize that K464 acetylation affects Mecp2 binding to DNA. However, in this work only the BDNF promoter has been tested.

Finally, MeCP2 has been found methylated in 293T cells (Jung et al., 2008) and O-glycosylated in 293T cells and rat brain (Rexach et al., 2010). For convenience, we provide a table summarizing the residues of MeCP2 that have been found involved in PTMs different from phosphorylation (SI **Table 2**). In this table, as well as in SI **Table 1**, we show the cell line/tissue in which the PTM was identified, the corresponding references, and the possible association of the residue involved with Rett syndrome. Few modified residues of MeCP2 have been linked to pathological conditions and with a very low incidence: thus, so far it is impossible to draw any genotype-phenotype correlation.

To conclude, the studies reviewed strengthen the hypothesis that a complex combinatorial pattern of PTMs functions as a regulatory platform of the methyl-binding protein. Once again the RTT field is awaiting the discovery of the functional consequences of these PTMs and their combinations. Their role in regulating synaptic plasticity is of special interest since deficits in MeCP2 has a strong impact on synaptic functions. Finally, the identification of their possible "readers," as well as of effecting enzymes ("writers") and their possible involvement in MECP2 related disorders represent urgent challenges.

AUTHOR CONTRIBUTIONS

Nicoletta Landsberger wrote the manuscript with the assistance of Charlotte Kilstrup-Nielsen; Elisa Bellini generated the figures and the tables; Giulio Pavesi performed the *in silico* analyses; Isabella Barbiero, Anna Bergo, Chetan Chandola, Mohammad S. Nawaz, Laura Rusconi, Gilda Stefanelli, Marta Strollo, and Maria M. Valente contributed equally in the conception and drafting of the manuscript.

ACKNOWLEGDEMENTS

This research was supported by Associazione Italiana per la Ricerca sul Cancro (AIRC, Grant IG-10319), Telethon (Grant GGP10032), Foundation Jerome Lejeune, Ministero della Salute (Ricerca finalizzata 2008), International Rett Syndrome Foundation (Grant 2922), and the Italian parents' association ProRETT Ricerca.

REFERENCES

Adams, V. H., McBryant, S. J., Wade, P. A., Woodcock, C. L., and Hansen, J. C. (2007). Intrinsic disorder and autonomous domain function in the multifunctional nuclear protein, MeCP2. *J. Biol. Chem.* 282, 15057–15064. doi: 10.1074/jbc.M700855200

Amir, R. E., Van den Veyver, I. B., Wan, M., Tran, C. Q., Francke, U., and Zoghbi, H. Y. (1999). Rett syndrome is caused by mutations in X-linked MECP2, encoding methyl-CpG-binding protein 2. *Nat. Genet.* 23, 185–188. doi: 10.1038/13810

Ausió, J., Paz, A. M., and Esteller, M. (2014). MeCP2: the long trip from a chromatin protein to neurological disorders. *Trends Mol. Med.* doi: 10.1016/j.molmed.2014.03.004. [Epub ahead of print].

Bauman, M. L., Kemper, T. L., and Arin, D. M. (1995). Pervasive neuroanatomic abnormalities of the brain in three cases of Rett's syndrome. *Neurology* 45, 1581–1586. doi: 10.1212/WNL.45.8.1581

Beausoleil, S. A., Jedrychowski, M., Schwartz, D., Elias, J. E., Villén, J., Li, J., et al. (2004). Large-scale characterization of HeLa cell nuclear phosphoproteins. *Proc. Natl. Acad. Sci. U.S.A.* 101, 12130–12135. doi: 10.1073/pnas.0404720101

Bedogni, F., Riccardo, R., Galli, F., Cobolli Gigli, C., Gandaglia, A., Kilstrup-Nielsen, C., et al. (2014). Rett syndrome and the urge of novel approaches to study MeCP2 functions and mechanisms of action. *Neurosci. Biobehav. Rev.* doi: 10.1016/j.neubiorev.2014.01.011. [Epub ahead of print].

Belichenko, N. P., Belichenko, P. V., and Mobley, W. C. (2009b). Evidence for both neuronal cell autonomous and nonautonomous effects of methyl-CpG binding protein 2 in the cerebral cortex of female mice with Mecp2 mutation. *Neurobiol. Dis.* 34, 71–77. doi: 10.1016/j.nbd.2008.12.016

Belichenko, P. V., Wright, E. E., Belichenko, N. P., Masliah, E., Li, H. H., Mobley, W. C., et al. (2009a). Widespread changes in dendritic and axonal morphology in Mecp2-mutant mouse models of Rett syndrome: evidence for disruption of neuronal networks. *J. Comp. Neurol.* 514, 240–258. doi: 10.1002/cne.22009

Bennetzen, M. V., Larsen, D. H., Bunkenborg, J., Bartek, J., Lukas, J., and Andersen, J. S. (2010). Site-specific phosphorylation dynamics of the nuclear proteome during the DNA damage response. *Mol. Cell. Proteomics* 9, 1314–1323. doi: 10.1074/mcp.M900616-MCP200

Blom, N., Gammeltoft, S., and Brunak, S. (1999). Sequence and structure-based prediction of eukaryotic protein phosphorylation sites. *J. Mol. Biol.* 294, 1351–1362. doi: 10.1006/jmbi.1999.3310

Bracaglia, G., Conca, B., Bergo, A., Rusconi, L., Zhou, Z., and Greenberg, M. E. (2009). Methyl-CpG binding protein 2 is phosphorylated by homeodomain-interacting protein kinase 2 and contributes to apoptosis. *EMBO Rep.* 10, 1327–1333. doi: 10.1038/embor.2009.217

Carrascal, M., Ovelleiro, D., Casas, V., Gay, M., and Abian, J. (2008). Phosphorylation analysis of primary human T lymphocytes using sequential IMAC and titanium oxide enrichment. *J. Proteome Res.* 7, 5167–5176. doi: 10.1021/pr800500r

Chahrour, M., and Zoghbi, H. Y. (2007). The story of Rett syndrome: from clinic to neurobiology. *Neuron* 56, 422–437. doi: 10.1016/j.neuron.2007.10.001

Chandler, S. P., Guschin, D., Landsberger, N., and Wolffe, A. P. (1999). The methyl-CpG binding transcriptional repressor MeCP2 stably associates with nucleosomal DNA. *Biochemistry* 38, 7008–7018. doi: 10.1021/bi990224y

Chapleau, C. A., Boggio, E. M., Calfa, G., Percy, A. K., Giustetto, M., and Pozzo-Miller, L. (2012). Hippocampal CA1 pyramidal neurons of Mecp2 mutant mice show a dendritic spine phenotype only in the presymptomatic stage. *Neural Plast.* 976164. doi: 10.1155/2012/976164

Chapleau, C. A., Calfa, G. D., Lane, M. C., Albertson, A. J., Larimore, J. L., Kudo, S., et al. (2009). Dendritic spine pathologies in hippocampal pyramidal neurons from Rett syndrome brain and after expression of Rett-associated MECP2 mutations. *Neurobiol. Dis.* 35, 219–233. doi: 10.1016/j.nbd.2009.05.001

Chahrour, M., Jung, S. Y., Shaw, C., Zhou, X., Wong, S. T., Qin, J., et al. (2008). MeCP2, a key contributor to neurological disease, activates and represses transcription. *Science* 320, 1224–1229. doi: 10.1126/science.1153252

Chen, R. Q., Yang, Q. K., Lu, B. W., Yi, W., Cantin, G., Chen, Y. L., et al. (2009). CDC25B mediates rapamycin-induced oncogenic responses in cancer cells. *Cancer Res.* 69, 2663–2668. doi: 10.1158/0008-5472.CAN-08-3222

Chen, W. G., Chang, Q., Lin, Y., Meissner, A., West, A., Griffith, E. C., et al. (2003). Depression of BDNF transcription involves calcium-dependent phosphorylation of MeCP2. *Science* 302, 885–889. doi: 10.1126/science.1086446

Cheng, J., Huang, M., Zhu, Y., Xin, Y. J., Zhao, Y. K., Huang, J., et al. (2014). SUMOylation of MeCP2 is essential for transcriptional repression and hippocampal synapse development. *J. Nurochem.* 128, 798–806. doi: 10.1111/jnc.12523

Chernorudskiy, A. L., and Gainullin, M. R. (2013). Ubiquitin system: direct effects join the signaling. *Sci. Signal.* 6:pe22. doi: 10.1126/scisignal.2004251

Cheval, H., Guy, J., Merusi, C., De Sousa, D., Selfridge, J., and Bird, A. (2012). Postnatal inactivation reveals enhanced requirement for MeCP2 at distinct age windows. *Hum. Mol. Genet.* 21, 3806–3814. doi: 10.1093/hmg/dds208

Choudhary, C., Kumar, C., Gnad, F., Nielsen, M. L., Rehman, M., Walther, T. C., et al. (2009). Lysine acetylation targets protein complexes and co-regulates major cellular functions. *Science* 325, 834–840. doi: 10.1126/science.1175371

Christensen, G. L., Kelstrup, C. D., Lyngsø, C., Sarwar, U., Bøgebo, R., Sheikh, S. P., et al. (2010). Quantitative phosphoproteomics dissection of seven-transmembrane receptor signaling using full and biased agonists. *Mol. Cell. Proteomics* 9, 1540–1553. doi: 10.1074/mcp.M900550-MCP200

Ciccarelli, A., Calza, A., Santoru, F., Grasso, F., Concas, A., Sassoè-Pognetto, M., et al. (2013). Morphine withdrawal produces ERK-dependent and ERK-independent epigenetic marks in neurons of the nucleus accumbens and lateral septum. *J. Neuropharm.* 70, 168–179. doi: 10.1016/j.neuropharm.2012.12.010

Cohen, S., Gabel, H. W., Hemberg, M., Hutchinson, A. N., Sadacca, L. A., Ebert, D. H., et al. (2011). Genome-wide activitydependent MeCP2 phosphorylation regulates nervous system development and function. *Neuron* 72, 72–85. doi: 10.1016/j.neuron.2011.08.022

Courcelles, M., Frémin, C., Voisin, L., Lemieux, S., Meloche, S., and Thibault, P. (2013). Phosphoproteome dynamics reveal novel ERK1/2 MAP kinase substrates with broad spectrum of functions. *Mol. Syst. Biol.* 9:669. doi: 10.1038/msb.2013.25

De Filippis, B., Ricceri, L., and Laviola, G. (2010). Early postnatal behavioral changes in the Mecp2-308 truncation mouse model of Rett syndrome. *Genes Brain Behav.* 9, 213–223. doi: 10.1111/j.1601-183X.2009.00551.x

Demirkan, G., Yu, K., Boylan, J. M., Salomon, A. R., and Gruppuso, P. A. (2011). Phosphoproteomic profiling of *in vivo* signaling in liver by the mammalian target of rapamycin complex 1 (mTORC1). *PLoS ONE* 6:e21729. doi: 10.1371/journal.pone.0021729

Deng, J. V., Rodriguiz, R. M., Hutchinson, A. N., Kim, L. H., Wetsel, W. C., and West, A. E. (2010). MeCP2 in the nucleus accumbens contributes to neural and behavioral responses to psychostimulants. *Nat. Neurosci.* 13, 1128–1136. doi: 10.1038/nn.2614

Deng, J. V., Wan, Y., Wang, X., Cohen, S., Wetsel, W. C., Greenberg, M. E., et al. (2014). MeCP2 phosphorylation limits psychostimulant-induced behavioral and neuronal plasticity. *J. Neurosci.* 34, 4519–4527. doi: 10.1523/JNEUROSCI.2821-13.2014

Dephoure, N., Zhou, C., Villén, J., Beausoleil, S. A., Elledge, S. J., and Gygi, S. P. (2008). A quantitative atlas of mitotic phosphorylation. *Proc. Natl. Acad. Sci. U.S.A.* 105, 10762–10767. doi: 10.1073/pnas.0805139105

Ebert, D. H., Gabel, H. W., Robinson, N. D., Kastan, N. R., Hu, L. S., Cohen, S., et al. (2013). Activity-dependent phosphorylation of MECP2 threonine 308 regulates interaction with NcoR. *Nature* 499, 341–345. doi: 10.1038/nature12348

Garg, S. K., Lioy, D. T., Cheval, H., McGann, J. C., Bissonnette, J. M., Murtha, M. J., et al. (2013). Systemic delivery of MeCP2 rescues behavioral and cellular deficits in female mouse models of Rett syndrome. *J. Neurosci.* 33, 13612–13620. doi: 10.1523/JNEUROSCI.1854-13.2013

Georgel, P. T., Horowitz-Scherer, R. A., Adkins, N., Woodcock, C. L., Wade, P. A., and Hansen, J. C. (2003). Chromatin compaction by human MeCP2. Assembly of novel secondary chromatin structures in the absence of DNA methylation. *J. Biol. Chem.* 278, 32181–32188. doi: 10.1074/jbc.M305308200

Giacometti, E., Luikenhuis, S., Beard, C., and Jaenisch, R. (2007). Partial rescue of MeCP2 deficiency by postnatal activation of MeCP2. *Proc. Natl. Acad. Sci. U.S.A.* 104, 1931–1936. doi: 10.1073/pnas.0610593104

Gonzales, M. L., Adams, S., Dunaway, K. W., and LaSalle, J. M. (2012). Phosphorylation of distinct sites in MeCP2 modifies cofactor associations and the dynamics of transcriptional regulation. *Mol. Cell. Biol.* 32, 2894–2903. doi: 10.1128/MCB.06728-11

Goswami, T., Li, X., Smith, A. M., Luderowski, E. M., Vincent, J. J., Rush, J., et al. (2012). Comparative phosphoproteomic analysis of neonatal and adult murine brain. *Proteomics* 12, 2185–2189. doi: 10.1002/pmic.201200003

Grimsrud, P. A., Carson, J. J., Hebert, A. S., Hubler, S. L., Niemi, N. M., Pagliarini, D. J., et al. (2012). A quantitative map of the liver mitochondrial phosphoproteome reveals posttranslational control of ketogenesis. *Cell Metab.*16, 672–683. doi: 10.1016/j.cmet.2012.10.004

Guo, A., Gu, H., Zhou, J., Mulhern, D., Wang, Y., Lee, K. A., et al. (2014). Immunoaffinity enrichment and mass spectrometry analysis of protein methylation. *Mol. Cell. Proteomics* 13, 372–387. doi: 10.1074/mcp.O113.027870

Guy, J., Cheval, H., Selfridge, J., and Bird, A. (2011). The role of MeCP2 in the brain. *Annu. Rev. Cell Dev. Biol.* 27, 631–652. doi: 10.1146/annurev-cellbio-092910-154121

Guy, J., Gan, J., Selfridge, J., Cobb, S., and Bird, A. (2007). Reversal of neurological defects in a mouse model of Rett syndrome. *Science* 315, 1143–1147. doi: 10.1126/science.1138389

Herskowitz, J. H., Seyfried, N. T., Duong, D. M., Xia, Q., Rees, H. D., Gearing, M., et al. (2010). Phosphoproteomic analysis reveals site-specific changes in GFAP and NDRG2 phosphorylation in frontotemporal lobar degeneration. *J. Proteome Res.* 9, 6368–6379. doi: 10.1021/pr100666c

Ho, K. L., McNae, I. W., Schmiedeberg, L., Klose, R. J., Bird, A. P., and Walkinshaw, M. D. (2008). MeCP2 binding to DNA depends upon hydration at methyl-CpG. *Mol. Cell* 29, 525–531. doi: 10.1016/j.molcel.2007.12.028

Hornbeck, P. V., Kornhauser, J. M., Tkachev, S., Zhang, B., Skrzypek, E., Murray, B., et al. (2012). PhosphoSitePlus: a comprehensive resource for investigating the structure and function of experimentally determined post-translational modifications in man and mouse. *Nucleic Acids Res.* 40, D261–D270. doi: 10.1093/nar/gkr1122

Hsu, P. P., Kang, S. A., Rameseder, J., Zhang, Y., Ottina, K. A., Lim, D., et al. (2011). The mTOR-regulated phosphoproteome reveals a mechanism of mTORC1-mediated inhibition of growth factor signaling. *Science* 332, 1317–1322. doi: 10.1126/science.1199498

Hutchinson, A. N., Deng, J.-V., Cohen, S., and West, A. E. (2012). Phosphorylation of MeCP2 at Ser421 contributes to chronic antidepressant action. *J. Neurosci.* 32, 321–337. doi: 10.1523/JNEUROSCI.2156-12.2012

Huttlin, E. L., Jedrychowski, M. P., Elias, J. E., Goswami, T., Rad, R., Beausoleil, S. A., et al. (2010). A tissue-specific atlas of mouse protein phosphorylation and expression. *Cell* 143, 1174–1189. doi: 10.1016/j.cell.2010.12.001

Iliuk, A. B., Martin, V. A., Alicie, B. M., Geahlen, R. L., and Tao, W. A. (2010). In-depth analyses of kinase-dependent tyrosine phosphoproteomes based on metal ion-functionalized soluble nanopolymers. *Mol. Cell. Proteomics* 9, 2162–2172. doi: 10.1074/mcp.M110.000091

Johnston, M. V., Blue, M. E., and Naidu, S. (2005). Rett syndrome and neuronal development. *J. Child Neurol.* 20, 759–763. doi: 10.1177/08830738050200082601

Jones, P. L., Veenstra, G. J., Wade, P. A., Vermaak, D., Kass, S. U., Landsberger, N., et al. (1998). Methylated DNA and MeCP2 recruit histone deacetylase to repress transcription. *Nat. Genet.* 19, 187–191. doi: 10.1038/561

Jugloff, D. G. M., Vandamme, K., Logan, R., Visanji, N. P., Brotchie, J. M., and Eubanks, J. H. (2008). Targeted delivery of an MeCP2 transgene to forebrain neurons improves the behavior of female MeCP2-deficient mice. *Hum. Mol. Genet.* 17, 1386–1396. doi: 10.1093/hmg/ddn026

Jung, S. Y., Li, Y., Wang, Y., Chen, Y., Zhao, Y., and Qin, J. (2008). Complications in the assignment of 14 and 28 Da mass shift detected by mass spectrometry as *in vivo* methylation from endogenous proteins. *Anal. Chem.* 80, 1721–1729. doi: 10.1021/ac7021025

Khoshnan, A., and Patterson, P. H. (2012). Elevated IKKα accelerates the differentiation of human neuronal progenitor cells and induces MeCP2-dependent BDNF expression. *PLoS ONE* 7:e41794. doi: 10.1371/journal.pone.0041794

Kishi, N., and Macklis, J. D. (2004). MECP2 is progressively expressed in post-migratory neurons and is involved in neuronal maturation rather than cell fate decisions. *Mol. Cell. Neurosci.* 27, 306–321. doi: 10.1016/j.mcn.2004.07.006

Klose, R. J., and Bird, A. P. (2004). MeCP2 behaves as an elongated monomer that does not stably associate with the Sin3a chromatin remodeling complex. *J. Biol. Chem.* 279, 46490–46496. doi: 10.1074/jbc.M408284200

Landi, S., Putignano, E., Boggio, E. M., Giustetto, M., Pizzorusso, T., and Ratto, G. M. (2011). The short-time structural plasticity of dendritic spines is altered in a model of Rett syndrome. *Sci. Rep.* 1, 45–51. doi: 10.1038/srep00045

Lewis, J. D., Meehan, R. R., Henzel, W. J., Maurer-Fogy, I., Jeppesen, P., Klein, F., et al. (1992). Purification, sequence, and cellular localization of a novel chromosomal protein that binds to methylated DNA. *Cell* 69, 905–914. doi: 10.1016/0092-8674(92)90610-O

Li, H., Zhong, X., Chau, K. F., Williams, E. C., and Chang, Q. (2011). Loss of activity-induced phosphorylation of MeCP2 enhances synaptogenesis, LTP and spatial memory. *Nat. Neurosci.* 14, 1001–1008. doi: 10.1038/nn.2866

Li, Y., Wang, H., Muffat, J., Cheng, A. W., Orlando, D. A., Lovén, J., et al. (2013). Global transcriptional and translational repression in human-emmbryonic-stem-cell-derived Rett syndrome neurons. *Cell Stem Cell* 13, 446–458. doi: 10.1016/j.stem.2013.09.001

Long, S. W., Ooi, J. Y., Yau, P. M., and Jones, P. L. (2011). A brain-derived MeCP2 complex supports a role for MeCP2 in RNA processing. *Biosci. Rep.* 31, 333–343. doi: 10.1042/BSR20100124

Luikenhuis, S., Giacometti, E., Beard, C. F., and Jaenisch, R. (2004). Expression of MeCP2 in postmitotic neurons rescues Rett syndrome in mice. *Proc. Natl. Acad. Sci. U.S.A.* 101, 6033–6038. doi: 10.1073/pnas.0401626101

Lyst, M. J., Ekiert, R., Ebert, D. H., Merusi, C., Nowak, J., Selfridge, J., et al. (2013). Rett syndrome mutations abolish the interaction of MeCP2 with the NCoR/SMRT co-repressor. *Nat. Neurosci.* 167, 898–902. doi: 10.1038/nn.3434

Mao, L. M., Horton, E., Guo, M. L., Xue, B., Jin, D. Z., Fibuch, E. E., et al. (2011). Cocaine increases phosphorylation of MeCP2 in the rat striatum *in vivo*: a differential role of NMDA receptors. *Neurochem. Int.* 56, 610–617. doi: 10.1016/j.neuint.2011.04.013

Martinowich, K., Hattori, D., Wu, H., Fouse, S., He, F., Hu, Y., et al. (2003). DNA methylation-related chromatin remodeling in activity-dependent BDNF gene regulation. *Science* 302, 890–893. doi: 10.1126/science.1090842

Maunakea, A. K., Chepelev, I., Cui, K., and Zhao, K. (2013). Intragenic DNA methylation modulates alternative splicing by recruiting MeCP2 to promote exon recognition. *Cell Res.* 23, 1256–1269. doi: 10.1038/cr.2013.110

Mayya, V., Lundgren, D. H., Hwang, S. I., Rezaul, K., Wu, L., Eng, J. K., et al. (2009). Quantitative phosphoproteomic analysis of T cell receptor signaling reveals system-wide modulation of protein-protein interactions. *Sci. Signal.* 2:ra46. doi: 10.1126/scisignal.2000007

McGraw, C. M., Samaco, R. C., and Zoghbi, H. Y. (2011). Adult neural function requires MeCP2. *Science* 333:186. doi: 10.1126/science.1206593

Mellen, M., Ayata, P., Dewell, S., Kriaucionis, S., and Heintz, N. (2012). MeCP2 binds to 5hmC enriched within active genes and accessible chromatin in the nervous system. *Cell* 151, 1417–1430. doi: 10.1016/j.cell.2012.11.022

Moutri, A. R., Marchetto, M. C., Coufal, N. G., Oefner, R., Yeo, G., Nakashima, K., et al. (2010). L1 retrotransposition in neurons is modulated by MeCP2. *Nature* 468, 443–446. doi: 10.1038/nature09544

Na, E. S., Nelson, E. D., Kavalali, E. T., and Monteggia, L. M. (2013). The impact of MeCP2 loss- or gain-of-function on synaptic plasticity. *Neuropsychopharmacology* 38, 212–219. doi: 10.1038/npp.2012.116

Nan, X., Campoy, F. J., and Bird, A. (1997). MeCP2 is a transcriptional repressor with abundant binding sites in genomic chromatin. *Cell* 88, 471–481. doi: 10.1016/S0092-8674(00)81887-5

Nan, X., Ng, H. H., Johnson, C. A., Laherty, C. D., Turner, B. M., Eisenman, R. N., et al. (1998). Transcriptional repression by the methyl-CpG binding protein MeCP2 involves a histone deacetylase complex. *Nature* 393, 386–399. doi: 10.1038/30764

Neul, J., Kaufmann, W. E., Glaze, D. G., Christodoulou, J., Clarke, A. J., Bahi-Buisson, N., et al. (2010). Rett syndrome: revised diagnostic criteria and nomenclature. *Ann. Neurol.* 68, 944–950. doi: 10.1002/ana.22124

Neul, J. L., and Zoghbi, H. Y. (2004). Rett syndrome: a prototypical neurodevelopmental disorder. *Neuroscientist* 10, 118–128. doi: 10.1177/1073858403260995

Nguyen, M. V., Du, F., Felice, C. A., Shan, X., Nigam, A., Mandel, G., et al. (2012). MeCP2 is critical for maintaining mature neuronal networks and global brain anatomy during late stages of postnatal brain development and in the mature adult brain. *J. Neurosci.* 32, 10021–10034. doi: 10.1523/JNEUROSCI.1316-12.2012

Nikitina, T., Shi, X., Ghosh, R. P., Howitz-Scherer, R. A., Hansen, J. C., and Woodcock, C. L. (2007). Multiple modes of interactions between the methylated DNA binding protein MeCP2 and chromatin. *Mol. Cell. Biol.* 27, 864–877. doi: 10.1128/MCB.01593-06

Olsen, J. V., Vermeulen, M., Santamaria, A., Kumar, C., Miller, M. L., Jensen, L. J., et al. (2010). Quantitative phosphoproteomics reveals widespread full phosphorylation site occupancy during mitosis. *Sci. Signal.* 3:ra3. doi: 10.1126/scisignal.2000475

Percy, A. K., and Lane, J. B. (2005). Rett syndrome: model of neurodevelopmental disorders. *J. Child Neurol.* 20, 718–721. doi: 10.1177/08830738050200090301

Phanstiel, D. H., Brumbaugh, J., Wenger, C. D., Tian, S., Probasco, M. D., Bailey, D. J., et al. (2011). Proteomic and phosphoproteomic comparison of human ES and iPS cells. *Nat. Methods* 8, 821–827. doi: 10.1038/nmeth.1699

Picker, J. D., Yang, R., Ricceri, L., and Berger-Sweeney, J. (2006). An altered neonatal behavioral phenotype in Mecp2 mutant mice. *Neuroreport* 17, 541–544. doi: 10.1097/01.wnr.0000208995.38695.2f

Raijmakers, R., Kraiczek, K., de Jong, A. P., Mohammed, S., and Heck, A. J. (2010). Exploring the human leukocyte phosphoproteome using a microfluidic reversed-phase-TiO2-reversed-phase high-performance liquid chromatography phosphochip coupled to a quadrupole time-of-flight mass spectrometer. *Anal. Chem.* 82, 824–832. doi: 10.1021/ac901764g

Rexach, J. E., Rogers, C. J., Yu, S. H., Tao, J., Sun, Y. E., and Hsieh-Wilson, L. C. (2010). Quantification of O-glycosylation stoichiometry and dynamics using resolvable mass tags. *Nat. Chem. Biol.* 6, 645–651. doi: 10.1038/nchembio.412

Ricceri, L., De Filippis, B., and Laviola, G. (2008). Mouse models of Rett syndrome: from behavioural phenotyping to preclinical evaluation of new therapeutic approaches. *Behav. Pharmacol.* 19, 501–517. doi: 10.1097/FBP.0b013e32830c3645

Ricciardi, S., Boggio, E. M., Grosso, S., Lonetti, G., Forlani, G., Stefanelli, G., et al. (2011). Reduced AKT/mTOR signaling and protein synthesis dysregulation in a Rett syndrome animal model. *Hum. Mol. Genet.* 20, 1182–1196. doi: 10.1093/hmg/ddq563

Rigbolt, K. T., Prokhorova, T. A., Akimov, V., Henningsen, J., Johansen, P. T., Blagoev, B., et al. (2011). System-wide temporal characterization of the proteome and phosphoproteome of human embryonic stem cell differentiation. *Sci. Signal.* 4:rs3. doi: 10.1126/scisignal.2001570

Rinschen, M. M., Yu, M. J., Wang, G., Boia, E. S., Hoffert, J. D., Pisitkun, T., et al. (2010). Quantitative phosphoproteomic analysis reveals vasopressin V2-receptor-dependent signaling pathways in renal collecting duct cells. *Proc. Natl. Acad. Sci. U.S.A.* 107, 3882–3887. doi: 10.1073/pnas.0910646107

Santos, M., Silva-Fernandes, A., Oliviera, P., Sousa, N., and Maciel, P. (2007). Evidence for abnormal early development in a mouse model of Rett syndrome. *Genes Brain Behav.* 6, 277–286. doi: 10.1111/j.1601-183X.2006.00258.x

Schüle, B., Armstrong, D. D., Vogel, H., Oviedo, A., and Francke, U. (2008). Severe congenital encephalopathy caused by MECP2 null mutations in males: central hypoxia and reduced neuronal dendritic structure. *Clin. Genet.* 74, 116–126. doi: 10.1111/j.1399-0004.2008.01005.x

Shahbazian, M. D., Antalffy, B., Armstrong, D. L., and Zoghbi, H. Y. (2002). Insight into Rett syndrome: MeCP2 levels display tissue- and cell-specific differences and correlate with neuronal maturation. *Hum. Mol. Genet.* 11, 115–124. doi: 10.1093/hmg/11.2.115

Shiromizu, T., Adachi, J., Watanabe, S., Murakami, T., Kuga, T., Muraoka, S., et al. (2013). Identification of missing proteins in the neXtProt database and unregistered phosphopeptides in the PhosphoSitePlus database as part of the Chromosome-centric human proteome project. *J. Proteome Res.* 12, 2414–2421. doi: 10.1021/pr300825v

Skene, P. J., Illingworth, R. S., Webb, S., Kerr, A. R., James, K. D., Turner, D. J., et al. (2010). Neuronal MeCP2 is expressed at near histone-octamer levels and globally alters the chromatin state. *Mol. Cell* 37, 457–468. doi: 10.1016/j.molcel.2010.01.030

Tao, J., Hu, K., Chang, Q., Wu, H., Sherman, N. E., Martinowich, K., et al. (2009). Phosphorylation of MeCP2 at Serine 80 regulates its chromatin association and neurological function. *Proc. Natl. Acad. Sci. U.S.A.* 106, 4882–4887. doi: 10.1073/pnas.0811648106

Thambirajah, A. A., Eubanks, J. H., and Ausio', J. (2009). MeCP2 post-translational regulation through PEST domains: two novel hyptheses. *Bioessays* 31, 561–569. doi: 10.1002/bies.200800220

Trinidad, J. C., Barkan, D. T., Gulledge, B. F., Thalhammer, A., Sali, A., Schoepfer, R., et al. (2012). Global identification and characterization of both O-GlcNAcylation and phosphorylation at the murine synapse. *Mol. Cell. Proteomics* 11, 215–229. doi: 10.1074/mcp.O112.018366

Tweedie-Cullen, R. Y., Reck, J. M., and Mansuy, I. M. (2009). Comprehensive mapping of post-translational modifications on synaptic, nuclear, and histone proteins in the adult mouse brain. *J. Proteome Res.* 8, 4966–4982. doi: 10.1021/pr9003739

Van Esch, H. (2011). MECP2 duplication syndrome. *Mol. Syndromol.* 2, 128–113.

Wagner, S. A., Beli, P., Weiner, B. T., Nielsen, M. L., Cox, J., Mann, M., et al. (2011). A proteome-wide, quantitative survey of *in vivo* ubiquitylation sites reveals widespread regulatory roles. *Mol. Cell. Proteomics* 10, M111.013284.

Wang, Y. T., Tsai, C. F., Hong, T. C., Tsou, C. C., Lin, P. Y., Pan, S. H., et al. (2010). An informatics-assisted label-free quantitation strategy that depicts phosphoproteomic profiles in lung cancer cell invasion. *J. Proteome Res.* 9, 5582–5597. doi: 10.1021/pr100394u

Weber, C., Schreiber, T. B., and Daub, H. (2012). Dual phosphoproteomics and chemical proteomics analysis of erlotinib and gefitinib interference in acute myeloid leukemia cells. *J. Proteomics* 75, 1343–1356. doi: 10.1016/j.jprot.2011.11.004

Wiśniewski, J. R., Nagaraj, N., Zougman, A., Gnad, F., and Mann, M. (2010). Brain phosphoproteome obtained by a FASP-based method reveals plasma membrane protein topology. *J. Proteome Res.* 9, 3280–3289. doi: 10.1021/pr1002214

Wu, X., Tian, L., Li, J., Zhang, Y., Han, V., Li, Y., et al. (2012). Investigation of receptor interacting protein (RIP3)-dependent protein phosphorylation by quantitative phosphoproteomics. *Mol. Cell. Proteomics* 11, 1640–1651. doi: 10.1074/mcp.M112.019091

Xue, Y., Ren, J., Gao, X., Jin, C., Wen, L., and Yao, X. (2008). GPS 2.0, a tool to predict kinase-specific phosphorylation sites in hierarchy. *Mol. Cell. Proteomics* 7, 1598–1608. doi: 10.1074/mcp.M700574-MCP200

Yang, F., Stenoien, D. L., Strittmatter, E. F., Wang, J., Ding, L., Lipton, M. S., et al. (2006). Phosphoproteome profiling of human skin fibroblast cells in response to low- and high-dose irradiation. *J. Proteome Res.* 5, 1252–1260. doi: 10.1021/pr060028v

Young, J. I., Hong, E. P., Castle, J. C., Crespo-Barreto, J., Bowman, A. B., Rose, M. F., et al. (2006). Regulation of RNA splicing by the methylation-dependent transcriptional repressor methyl-CpG binding protein 2. *Proc. Natl. Acad. Sci. U.S.A.* 102, 17551–17558. doi: 10.1073/pnas.0507856102

Yu, Y., Yoon, S. O., Poulogiannis, G., Yang, Q., Ma, X. M., Villén, J., et al. (2011). Phosphoproteomic analysis identifies Grb10 as an mTORC1 substrate that negatively regulates insulin signaling. *Science* 332, 1322–1326. doi: 10.1126/science.1199484

Yusufzai, T. M., and Wolffe, A. P. (2000). Functional consequences of Rett syndrome mutations on human MeCP2. *Nucleic Acids Res* 28, 4172–4179. doi: 10.1093/nar/28.21.4172

Zanivan, S., Gnad, F., Wickström, S. A., Geiger, T., Macek, B., Cox, J., et al. (2008). Solid tumor proteome and phosphoproteome analysis by high resolution mass spectrometry. *J. Proteome Res.* 7, 5314–5326. doi: 10.1021/pr800599n

Zhou, H., Di Palma, S., Preisinger, C., Peng, M., Polat, A. N., Heck, A. J., et al. (2013). Toward a comprehensive characterization of a human cancer cell phosphoproteome. *J. Proteome Res.* 12, 260–271. doi: 10.1021/pr300630k

Zhou, Z., Hong, E. J., Cohen, S., Zhao, W. N., Ho, H. Y. H., Schmidt, L., et al. (2006). Brain-specific phosphorylation of MeCP2 regulates activity dependent Bdnf transcription, dendritic growth, and spine maturation. *Neuron* 52, 255–269. doi: 10.1016/j.neuron.2006.09.037

Zocchi, L., and Sassone-Corsi, P. (2012). SIRT1-mediated deacetylation of MeCP2 contributes to BDNF expression. *Epigenetics* 7, 695–700. doi: 10.4161/epi.20733

5

Convergence of circuit dysfunction in ASD: A common bridge between diverse genetic and environmental risk factors and common clinical electrophysiology

Russell G. Port[1], Michael J. Gandal[2], Timothy P. L. Roberts[3], Steven J. Siegel[1] and Gregory C. Carlson[1]*

[1] Department of Psychiatry, Perelman School of Medicine, University of Pennsylvania, Philadelphia, PA, USA
[2] Semel Institute for Neuroscience and Human Behavior, University of California at Los Angeles, Los Angeles, CA, USA
[3] Bioengineering Graduate Group, University of Pennsylvania, Philadelphia, PA, USA
[4] Department of Radiology, Lurie Family Foundations MEG Imaging Center, The Children's Hospital of Philadelphia, Philadelphia, PA, USA

***Correspondence:**
Gregory C. Carlson, Department of Psychiatry, Perelman School of Medicine, University of Pennsylvania, 125 S. 31 St., Philadelphia, PA 19104, USA
e-mail: gregc@mail.med.upenn.edu

Most recent estimates indicate that 1 in 68 children are affected by an autism spectrum disorder (ASD). Though decades of research have uncovered much about these disorders, the pathological mechanism remains unknown. Hampering efforts is the seeming inability to integrate findings over the micro to macro scales of study, from changes in molecular, synaptic and cellular function to large-scale brain dysfunction impacting sensory, communicative, motor and cognitive activity. In this review, we describe how studies focusing on neuronal circuit function provide unique context for identifying common neurobiological disease mechanisms of ASD. We discuss how recent EEG and MEG studies in subjects with ASD have repeatedly shown alterations in ensemble population recordings (both in simple evoked related potential latencies and specific frequency subcomponents). Because these disease-associated electrophysiological abnormalities have been recapitulated in rodent models, studying circuit differences in these models may provide access to abnormal circuit function found in ASD. We then identify emerging *in vivo* and *ex vivo* techniques, focusing on how these assays can characterize circuit level dysfunction and determine if these abnormalities underlie abnormal clinical electrophysiology. Such circuit level study in animal models may help us understand how diverse genetic and environmental risks can produce a common set of EEG, MEG and anatomical abnormalities found in ASD.

Keywords: ASD, circuit, gamma, VSDi, translational, EEG, MEG, neurophysiology

THE PROMISE OF TRANSLATIONAL PHENOTYPES IN ASD

Autism spectrum disorders (ASD) have an estimated prevalence of 1 in 68 children, potentially reaching as high as 1 in 42 males (Developmental Disabilities Monitoring Network Surveillance Year 2010 Principal Investigators; Centers for Disease Control and Prevention (CDC), 2014). Although the criterion for ASD has recently been updated, it is still considered a disorder of social impairments and restricted/repetitive behaviors (American Psychiatric Association, 2013). Findings of multiple weak or rare and often non-specific genetic or environmental etiologies of ASD have made it difficult to identify the common neurobiological mechanisms underlying behavioral features that define ASD. Despite this genetic and phenotypic heterogeneity, research over the last decade using Electroencephalography (EEG) and Magnetoencephalography (MEG) (E/MEG) has identified consistent differences in ASD electrophysiology, indicating common neural circuit disruptions (Wilson et al., 2007; Roberts et al., 2008; Gandal et al., 2010; Rojas et al., 2011; Edgar et al., 2013). Unfortunately the neuronal underpinnings of these electrophysiological biomarkers of ASD are not understood. The goal of this review is to describe emerging approaches in animal models to identify the circuit mechanisms that underlie these clinical E/MEG findings. To do so we first summarize the current literature of observed alterations to neural circuits in ASD, with a focus on mechanisms that may underlie the E/MEG phenotypes found in human subjects. Second, we propose that it is at the mesoscopic circuit level, particularly local circuit function that leads to high frequency activity, where many diverse alterations must integrate to produce the symptomatology of ASD. Finally, we highlight emerging techniques in assaying neural circuit abnormalities that may identify the clinical differences found in high frequency cortical activity. Thus we hope to identify how the basic science of oscillatory activity and connectivity in the brain, combined with known E/MEG phenotypes of ASD, can provide the basis for new testable hypotheses of ASD.

THE CHALLENGE OF INTEGRATING MULTIPLE PATHOGENIC MECHANISMS: NO SMOKING GUN

Studies over the last 40 years have revealed a multitude of alterations in ASD, ranging from genetic risk factors, to differences in whole brain connectivity (Pardo and Eberhart, 2007). As genetic screening began to investigate the inheritance profile of ASD, it was hypothesized that ASD may be operating on the polygenetic interaction of three genes, and that this interaction could be revealed in a sample of 60 pairs of ASD affected siblings (Piven, 1997). Within 8 years this estimate of underlying genetic profile of ASD had increased to involve 15 genes, along with strong indication of environmental factors (e.g., prenatal insults) (Santangelo and Tsatsanis, 2005). This trajectory of etiological complexity continues. Despite the presence of a disorder that impacts well over 1 in a 100 individuals, there is not a single gene or set of genes that strongly or exclusively generate ASD, and we have been unable to extrapolate any individual putative genetic deficits to neurological abnormalities that produce symptoms of ASD. Nevertheless, to produce the constellation of symptoms that define ASD, different genetic and other alterations involved in the production of ASD likely act further downstream to converge on common effectors that produces the symptomatology of ASD. Finding such a common factor at the neuronal level for ASD or related endophenotypes is a clear goal in the field of ASD research, yet success has been limited.

MULTIPLE SYNAPTIC RECEPTORS AND NEUROTRANSMITTERS ARE AFFECTED IN ASD, WITH NO SINGLE COHERENT EFFECT

Given this significant genetic heterogeneity, recent work has focused on identifying common networks and molecular pathways that may integrate multiple diverse disease risk factors (Parikshak et al., 2013). For example, a large number of ASD candidate genes are involved in developing, maintaining, or modulating synaptic connectivity. A genetic alteration repeatedly found in ASD is the duplication of the 15q11–13 locus, which is estimated to be presented in as high as 3% of the idiopathic ASD population (Meguro-Horike et al., 2011). This region is known to contain many genes that encode for GABA related proteins, such as postsynaptic GABA receptors. Separately, others have found that both $GABA_A$ (Fatemi et al., 2009b) and $GABA_B$ (Fatemi et al., 2009a) receptors levels are significantly decreased in postmortem brain samples from subjects with ASD. On the synthesis side of GABA signaling, GAD65 and 67 expression is decreased around 50% (Fatemi et al., 2002). Recent brain imaging studies have corroborated GABAergic post-mortem results, demonstrating decreased cortical GABA levels (Harada et al., 2011; Rojas et al., 2014), with some regional heterogeneity across the cortex (Gaetz et al., 2014).

γ-Aminobutyric acid signaling is not the only neurotransmitter system affected in ASD; glutamatergic signaling is also affected, with the expression of multiple genes and proteins regulating this signaling pathway (e.g., EAAT and AMPA isotypes) increased in cerebellar cortex of subjects with autism (Purcell et al., 2001). This finding of increased glutamatergic expression fits with recent *in vivo* findings using magnetic resonance spectroscopy (Brown et al., 2013), although the exact meaning of these results are unclear. Lastly the GluR6, a kainate receptor subunit, has been strongly linked to ASD risk (Jamain et al., 2002; Shuang et al., 2004; Strutz-Seebohm et al., 2006). This, when combined with glutamatergic phenotypes in mouse models that recapitulate key aspects of ASD, has led to hypotheses that altered glutamate transmission may contribute to the core phenotypes of ASD (Carlson, 2012).

As glutamate and GABA receptors comprise the majority of ligand-gated ion channels in the CNS, these genetic findings support the general neurophysiological hypothesis that a disruption of excitation/inhibition (E/I) balance contributes to the disorder (Rubenstein and Merzenich, 2003). Such proposed imbalance has been a common theme in multiple psychiatric and neurologic disorders, including Alzheimer's disease, schizophrenia and epilepsy (Eichler and Meier, 2008). Yet, though there may be similarities between those disorders and ASD, there are differences in the development and symptoms of these diseases that must be explained by specific neurobiological mechanisms to explain the divergent symptoms. While this idea is limited in specificity; if E/I imbalance is one of the underlying principle components of ASD, an immediate consequence such an alteration would be perturbed circuit activity underlying oscillatory activity in the brain. Oscillations across the frequency spectrum are evidenced and theorized to be dependent on the strength and kinetics of inhibitory and excitatory synaptic interactions at the mesocircuit level (Buzsáki and Wang, 2012). While again, this is not specific to ASD, other disorders such as schizophrenia (Kwon et al., 1999) and bipolar disorder (Maharajh et al., 2007) also show alterations to oscillatory function. What may distinguish ASD is the exact circuitry involved, the developmental timing of the disruption or the set of neurophysiological abnormalities due to specific genetic and environmental factors. For instance, preclinical work has shown that altered high frequency activity due to E/I imbalance generated in prefrontal regions but not visual cortex, is sufficient for the production of social and fear-related, but not locomotive impairments (Yizhar et al., 2011). Furthermore, this was limited to specifically CAMKII but not PV expressing neurons. In humans, oscillatory activity in specific regions have been shown to scale with impairment measures of autism specific behaviors or social ability in various conditions including, response to auditory stimuli (Rojas et al., 2011), resting (Cornew et al., 2012) or prestimulus (Edgar et al., 2013). Specificity may come from the overlap of the genetic risks for multiple psychiatric disorders (Cross-Disorder Group of the Psychiatric Genomics Consortium; Genetic Risk Outcome of Psychosis (GROUP) Consortium, 2013). It is proposed that the genetic risks are not specific to disorders, but rather domains of symptomatology instead. For instance pre-frontal E/I imbalance, due to the genetic risks common to ASD and schizophrenia, may lead to social impairments that are shared between the disorders.

NEUROMODULATORS AFFECTED IN ASD

Strengthening the concept that there are multiple synaptic paths to a common circuit dysregulation in ASD, is the evidence that neuromodulatory systems are also disrupted. Looking through the lens of E/I imbalance, neuromodulators can act at the synapse directly or on the firing properties of a cell to alter the strength, kinetics and firing probability of cells involved in circuit E/I balance and thus impacting neural functioning in ASD. In fact some of the earliest examined neurological abnormalities in ASD involved neuromodulatory systems (Boullin et al., 1970; Modahl et al., 1998), several of which are now known to be involved in emotional and social regulation. Peptide and monoaminergic transmitters appear aberrant in ASD, in particular the oxytocin and serotoninergic systems. These neuromodulators are of interest, because of oxytocin's role in social behavior and bonding (Lieberwirth and Wang, 2014) partnered with a potential for treatment efficacy (Gordon et al., 2013; Tyzio et al., 2014), and the current use of pharmacological agents aimed at the serotoniergic system for treatment of ASD symptomatology. Both of these systems can impact cell excitability in an anatomical and cell-type specific manner. Oxytocin signaling is thought to be reduced in ASD (Modahl et al., 1998) and has been an intense focus for therapeutic intervention (Weisman et al., 2012; Gordon et al., 2013) and recent research at the circuit level (Owen et al., 2013). Individuals with ASD also exhibit hyperserotonemia, potentially arising from mutations in SLC6A4 and MAOA candidate genes (Harrington et al., 2013). The affect of the such genes may be two fold, serotonin plays an important role in the development of cortical and sub-cortical tissues, not only as a neurotransmitter but also earlier during development (Whitaker-Azmitia, 2001). The serotonin system remains altered in ASD during the juvenile period with an altered developmental trajectory of serotonin synthesis (Chugani et al., 1999). Interestingly in adults, if the levels of the precursor of serotonin is lowered via specific dietary manipulations, ASD symptomatology is exacerbated, again pointing to serotonin's role in ASD (McDougle et al., 1996). This role of serotonin has been replicated in animal models, rats prenatally treated with 5-methoxytryptamine (5-MT), an agonist of serotonin receptors, demonstrate ASD like symptomatology and alterations to regions known to be involved in social activity and peptides release (such as oxytocin) (McNamara et al., 2008).

Acetylcholine (ACH) has also been focus of research with regards to pathology and treatment in ASD. Multiple studies show altered ACH related findings, such as decreased Positron emission tomography (PET) binding, altered post mortem immunoreactivity for receptors and mRNA, and decreased relative choline levels in *in vivo* in ASD (Deutsch et al., 2010). Interestingly, increasing levels of ACH specifically in striatal regions allows for the recovery of social and cognitive flexibility in an animal model that is thought to recapitulate those aspects of ASD (Karvat and Kimchi, 2014).

Another major neuromodulator linked to ASD is dopamine. Several studies have shown that dopamine is increase in frontal cortex (Chugani, 2012), and multiple genetic studies have linked dopamine associated genes with ASD (Nguyen et al., 2014). Consistent for a role of dopamine signaling in ASD, is their importance in mediating repetitive and stereotyped behaviors. Both from human genetic findings (Staal, 2014) and mice models (Chartoff et al., 2001). While oxytocin continues to be examined as a potential treatment, current drugs targeting these and other systems have not been found to be effective in treating core symptoms of ASD (Warren et al., 2011), suggesting that these modulatory system contribute to, but do not drive the disorder.

This non-exhaustive summary of alterations to the neurotransmitter and neuro-modulator systems suggests targets for treatment, yet also indicate that no single target will be broadly effective. Single perturbations are not consistently present throughout all cases of ASD, and furthermore such alterations are usually found in differing combinations; yet ultimately they synergize to produce the symptomatology known as ASD. Thus, hypothesis such as E/I balance suggests common neuronal circuit differences that could be targeted to repair circuit function in ASD.

IMMUNE SYSTEM DYSFUNCTION

Maternal infections, fever and antibiotic treatment, as well as post-natal infections, are associated with an increased likelihood of the child being diagnosed with ASD (Hsiao, 2013). This relationship can be modeled in animals via injections of various components of pathogens, which lead to the discovery that the immune response driven by cytokines that can produce this link (Garay and McAllister, 2010). Of note, is the evidence from several studies that autoimmune diseases and/or allergies are at a greater prevalence in ASD (Hsiao, 2013). In fact it has been demonstrated that maternal antibodies reactive to fetal tissue are linked to ASD (Fox et al., 2012). These brain targeting antibodies also are found in patients with ASD, and certain sub-types correlate with specific ASD behavioral symptoms (Goines et al., 2011). At the cellular level, evidence of immune system involvement is found in ASD, with increased activation and number of migroglial cells both in patients with ASD and animal models that recapitulate ASD via genetic or environmental insults (Hsiao, 2013). The major histocompatibility complex (MHC) locus, a region of the genetic code which contains genes for immune system functioning, is of particular note to circuit function in ASD. Multiple genes and haplotypes in the MHC local are linked to higher incidence of autism (Needleman and McAllister, 2012). These MHC genes are important for neuronal development, connectivity, and circuit function (see Section Cellular Assessment of Circuit Activity: Targeting the Neurophysiology of Local Circuit Dysfunction in ASD).

STRUCTURAL AND CONNECTIVITY ALTERATIONS ARE PRESENT IN ASD

Sub-cellular and synaptic alterations are not the only alterations found in ASD. At the level of local cytoarchitecture, post-mortem studies of individuals with ASD have shown increases in the density of minicolumns in multiple cortical regions, while each column itself is narrower, primarily due to decreases in peripheral neuropil compartments (Casanova et al., 2010). These cytoarchitectural changes are in concert with increased rates of macrocephaly in individuals with ASD, for which increases in brain volume are disproportionately greater for local cortical white matter connections (Herbert, 2005). Such local increases in anatomical connectivity, observed in ASD as an increase in local white matter tracts, may exist alongside decreases in long-range connectivity (Jou et al., 2011). Of note, alterations in long range connectivity have been correlated with electrophysiological deficits in bottom-up sensory processing (Roberts et al., 2009). Thus, ASD are associated with alterations across function, modulation, and structure. While there are likely causal relationships between alteration in any of these components (activity during development leading to structural changes or vice versa), the heterogeneity of any of these findings within and outside ASD also suggest that they can combine to produce a common set of neurological abnormalities. Assaying the combined and potentially differing impact of these diverse potential etiologies is limited in human patients and technically difficult in model systems.

EEG AND MEG STUDIES PRESENT COMMON CLINICAL NEUROPHYSIOLOGICAL DIFFERENCES IN ASD

In contrast to the divergent assortment of complex combinatorial risks found for ASD, clinical electrophysiology has identified specific resting, event related potential, and spectral changes that suggest common neural circuit function abnormalities (**Figure 1**). In particular spectro-temporal processing of auditory stimuli in ASD demonstrates deficits in gamma-band activity (30–50 Hz) (Wilson et al., 2007; Rojas et al., 2008; Gandal et al., 2010; Edgar et al., 2013). These alterations in stimulus-produced responses occur alongside aberrant resting state profile in ASD (Orekhova et al., 2007; Cornew et al., 2012). As such, coherent alterations have been identified in ASD, which point to common neurobiological underpinning. Because of the complexity of the neurophysiology underlying these clinical electrophysiological findings, there are many points where differing etiologies could perturb these measures. This poses the critical question: How is the ensemble neuronal activity that generates the EEG and MEG signals perturbed in ASD?

ASD RELATED E/MEG ENDOPHENOTYPES ARE REPLICATED IN MULTIPLE MODELS RELATED TO ASD AND POINT TO LOCAL CIRCUIT CHANGE

The alterations detected via E/MEG in auditory event related potentials and gamma-band abnormalities have been a focus of translational research, since auditory processing in mice, rats and humans is remarkably well conserved (**Figure 1**). Event related potentials themselves have shown an increased latency in both MEG and EEG in ASD and representative animal models respectively. These findings indicate differences in the speed of auditory processing as information is passed via auditory nuclei to the cortex (**Figures 1A,C**). Auditory responses to stimuli can also be separated into their spectral subcomponents, which exhibit a strong phase-locked gamma band activity between 30–50 Hz (**Figures 1B,E**). This ability of a subject to produce an alignment of gamma-band phases over multiple trials with respect to the stimuli can be viewed as the local circuit's reliability. The less able the system is to respond to an input with an appropriate and controlled response, the more dysfunctional the system will be. This is especially important when the responses are basic sensory responses that need to be combined into meaningful stimuli. This quality of phase-locked activity between trials (reflected as ITC in **Figure 1**) is decreased in ASD individuals compared to typically developing age-matched subjects (TD). This finding has been replicated across research groups (Rojas et al., 2008; Gandal et al., 2010). Similarly, evoked gamma-band power in response to analogous auditory stimuli is also decreased in ASD, and animal models that recapitulate key phenotypes of ASD (**Figure 1D**; Gandal et al., 2010, 2012a; Saunders et al., 2012), suggesting neuronal mechanisms are shared between ASD and these models of the disorder. While ITC and evoked power are very similar entities, they remain crucially separate (**Box 1**).

> **BOX 1 | ITC vs. evoked power, similar yet not redundant.**
>
> Changes seen in ITC and evoked activity are related, since both are referring to phase and time locked activity, though ITC is questioning "what fraction of signals are in phase", and evoked power asks "of those time and phase locked, what is the amplitude of the response". If there are no in-phase signals then ITC would equal 0, and evoked power would also be 0. If responses were perfectly in phase ITC would equal 1 (its maximum possible value), and evoked power would be the amplitude of the resulting wave. Yet, because ITC is only a measure of trial-to-trial phase reliability and not the amplitude of power generated by the stimulus, ITC can be independently disrupted. Such a case could occur when a manipulation could increase the ability cells to more temporally accurately fire, but the total amount of cells firing is reduced.

In contrast to the loss of phase reliability across repeated stimuli, other findings in the gamma band are an increase in baseline spectral activity in ASD and increased stimulus related non-phase locked activity (often called "induced" activity (Wilson et al., 2007; Edgar et al., 2013 respectively)). Increases in gamma activity related to an event or stimuli that is not phase locked has traditionally been presumed to be involved in higher cognitive processing of the signal (Tallon-Baudry and Bertrand, 1999), but a feature in ASD is that the increase in induced activity appears coupled to a reduction in evoked activity, suggesting that in ASD there is a reduction in the ability of the brain to respond reliably to a event/stimulus and it is this loss phase-locked activity that may be increasing induced activity (Wilson et al., 2007).

From the multiple putative neuronal differences indicated in ASD it should not be surprising that gamma-band activity is impacted. The generation of high frequency oscillatory activity during ensemble activity requires low latency feedback between inhibitory and excitatory neurons, in the case of 40 Hz activity one cycle of activity must comprise 25 ms. Gamma-band activity is also sensitive to behavioral states and their associated neuromodulators (Schadow et al., 2009; Kim et al., 2014). Finally, unlike the event related potential latencies, changes in gamma-frequency may be due primarily to local changes in circuit connectivity (Kopell et al., 2000; Cardin et al., 2009; Wang and Carlén, 2012). Because of gamma's dependence on local circuit function, many mechanisms of gamma can be assayed in brain slices. Thus, focusing on gamma-band changes in ASD and rodent models that share EEG validity with ASD (Gandal et al., 2010, 2012a,c; Saunders et al., 2012) may provide a path to directly assay mechanisms of gamma-band dysfunction using the enhanced access of *in vitro* preparations.

PROMISE OF CIRCUIT LEVEL FOCUSED EXAMINATION OF ASD: POTENTIAL FOR TRANSLATION BETWEEN MODEL SYSTEMS AND INQUIRY AT MULTIPLE SCALES

Mesoscopic level examination of circuits, and in particular microcircuits, maybe be the ideal area for investigation, because they integrate multiple sub-cellular to systems alterations. Not only is ensemble activity sensitive to genetic (Carlson et al., 2011),

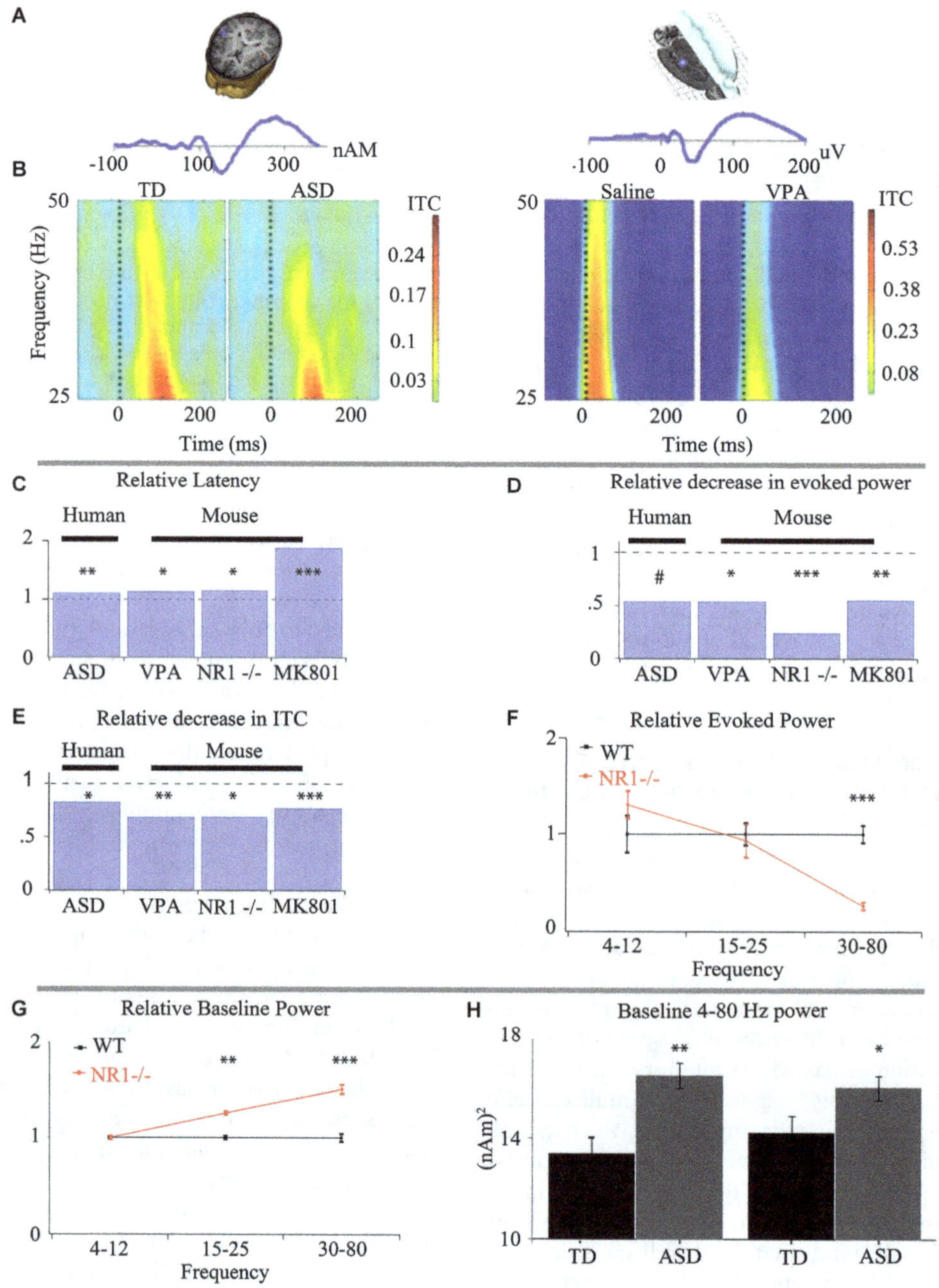

FIGURE 1 | Intermediate phenotypes seen in human subjects are translatable to animal models that recapitulate differing aspects of ASD. **(A)** Representative dipole/electrode placement (top) and ERP trace (bottom) for control human (left) and mouse (right) appear qualitatively similar. **(B)** Time-frequency plots of phase-locking factor for humans (left panel) and mouse (right panel) exhibit direct translatability. Note the decrease in phase locking in gamma frequencies in both ASD and an environmental insult based model of ASD. **(C)** Event-related potential latencies are delayed both in children with ASD and animal models of ASD utilizing prenatal insult, genetic insult and pharmacological treatment. Similar deficits in gamma-band responses are seen between children with ASD and numerous animal models of ASD with varying biological mechanisms for both evoked power **(D)** and inter-trial coherence/phase-locking factor (ITC/PLF) **(E)**. **(F)** The observed alterations to the spectral response are specific to gamma-band frequencies when examined in an animal model recapitulating keep aspects of ASD. **(G)** As proof of the predictive validity of translational electrophysiology, increases in baseline activity, first observed in animal models utilizing a genetic basis **(G)**, have been demonstrated in children with ASD **(H)**. *** $P < 0.001$, ** $P < 0.01$, * $P < 0.05$, # $P < 0.1$ Figure adapted from Gandal et al. (2010)—**(A–E)**, Gandal et al. (2012a)—**(C–E)**, Gandal et al. (2012c)—**(C–F)**, Saunders et al. (2012)—**(C–E)**; **(H)** courtesy of J.C. Edgar, adapted from Edgar et al. (2013).

pharmacological (Saunders et al., 2012) and cellular manipulation (Cardin et al., 2009; Sohal et al., 2009; Billingslea et al., 2014), but it can provide insight into the human pathogenic markers of ASD. Identifying an intermediate phenotype at the population activity level may allow the translational bridging of basic, pre-clinical, and human-subject research. Furthermore it provides additional bridging of the molecular to behavioral domains.

Differences in circuit function activity in model systems may be easier to interpret in terms of changes in clinical electrophysiology found in EEG. There has been success modeling social and behavioral deficits as markers of ASD-like symptomatology (Silverman et al., 2010), yet questions remain of how to fully model and validate the behavioral disturbances seen in ASD and reliably link them with neurophysiological differences. Recapitulating ensemble electrophysiological activity that is seen in patients with ASD can provide mechanistic bridge between the construct validity of a model and its behavioral phenotypes. Gandal et al. (2010) demonstrated that the electrophysiological abnormalities seen in children with ASD were recapitulated in a prenatal insult based mouse model of ASD (**Figure 1**), and these changes correlated with synaptic protein expression and behavior. Similarly analogous changes have been seen in response to pharmacological treatment (Saunders et al., 2012) and genetic manipulations (Gandal et al., 2012a). Thus, with increasing evidence in animal models for recapitulation of EMEG phenotypes of ASD it becomes important to ask what are the underlying neurophysiological differences that mediate observed changes in cortical ensemble activity that in turn lead to disrupted E/MEG activity in ASD.

To make the link between circuit function and E/MEG differences three areas of inquiry show promise: (1) direct cellular modulation of local circuit properties; (2) assays of ensemble activity linking circuit dysfunction to E/MEG phenotypes; and (3) measures of functional connectivity. Below we discuss each of these approaches.

CURRENT CIRCUIT LEVEL RESEARCH IN ASD: CURRENT METHODOLOGIES FOR FUTURE ADVANCES

CELLULAR ASSESSMENT OF CIRCUIT ACTIVITY: TARGETING THE NEUROPHYSIOLOGY OF LOCAL CIRCUIT DYSFUNCTION IN ASD

Recent basic science research at the microcircuit level has had particular relevance to ASD. While there is a wealth of data looking at synaptic or cellular firing properties in putative models of autism, there are few studies that directly assay modulation of circuit activity. An exception is *in vitro* work in the hippocampus that looked at the role of the peptide Oxytocin. Oxytocin, is a neuromodulatory peptide known to be important in social bonding, prosocial behavior and social recognition (Lieberwirth and Wang, 2014) and is reduced in patients with ASD (Modahl et al., 1998), making it an area of interest regarding therapeutics (Weisman et al., 2012; Gordon et al., 2013; Tyzio et al., 2014). At the single cell level Oxytocin was known to increase excitability (Raggenbass et al., 1989). It was therefore surprising that in response to a compound synaptic potential, where both local inhibitory and principle cells are activated by synaptic input, oxytocin signaling was shown to regulate the fidelity of stimulus produced firing and reducing baseline neural activity (Owen et al., 2013). This was because the most prominent affect of oxytocin was to increase spontaneous activity in the inhibitory neurons and thus increase baseline GABA related inhibitory tone of the system. By increasing spontaneous inhibitory activity, the feedforward inhibitory signaling evoked by afferent stimuli was reduced. Thus a more faithful transmission of signaling and better signal-to-noise ratio was achieved (Owen et al., 2013; **Figure 2**). Such increase in reliability may scale at the ensemble level to produce a greater trial-to-trial phase reliability detected in EEG or MEG signal that is measured as increased ITC. Analysis at this cellular circuit level in models relevant to ASD may similarly identify underlying changes in reliability that could be linked to reduced ITC in patients. Importantly, such a role for oxytocin would be opaque, without studying the interactions of excitatory and inhibitory cells within their microcircuit context.

Studying microcircuits can also be used to study changes in the number or strength of synaptic interconnections. Using a model of prenatal exposure to the antiepileptic drug valproic acid, which is associated with a ~7 fold increased risk for autism, Rinaldi et al. (2008) patch-clamped multiple connected cells in cortical slices to measure connectivity between neurons. Consistent with interpretations of hyper local connectivity from post-mortem anatomical data, in valproic exposed animals they showed local circuit hyper-connectivity and hyperactive cortical local networks.

Mesoscopic level dysfunction can also be detected due to immune system based insults. Alterations to the retinogeniculate pathways, as well as more local cytoarchitectural alterations in hippocampus, cortex and retina, are well documented in mice with MHC class I proteins perturbations (Elmer and McAllister, 2012). Such architectural modifications are not the only effect MHC class I related alterations, perturbations to in circuit function with regards to plasticity, and critical periods in several animal models also exist (Boulanger, 2009). These changes in plasticity can arise from changes to the intrinsic cellular properties of neurons, such as increases in excitability and frequency of mEPSCs (Boulanger, 2009). Following this trend, mice with MHC related alterations can show altered E/I balance in cortex and short term plasticity modifications in cerebellum (Elmer and McAllister, 2012). Plasticity over the longer term is also aberrant in these animal models were altered LTD/LTP is exhibited (Elmer and McAllister, 2012).

Using monogenetic insults that mimic syndromes similar to ASD, plasticity has also been found to be perturbed in multiple animal models. In a mouse model of fragile X disorder, a disorder closely linked to ASD, mice demonstrated increased LTP (Huber et al., 2002). Plasticity alterations have been found in an model of Angelman syndrome, where again LTP and LTD were perturbed (Yashiro et al., 2009). Moreover, these mice also demonstrated altered visual cortex plasticity with decrease ocular dominance following monocular derivation (Yashiro et al., 2009). Alterations to visual cortex plasticity, was also demonstrated in a mouse model of Rett's syndrome, with a MeCP2 mutation extending the period within which alterations could occur (Tropea et al., 2009). Interestingly, when traditional measures of spine phenotypes and protein production were recovered so

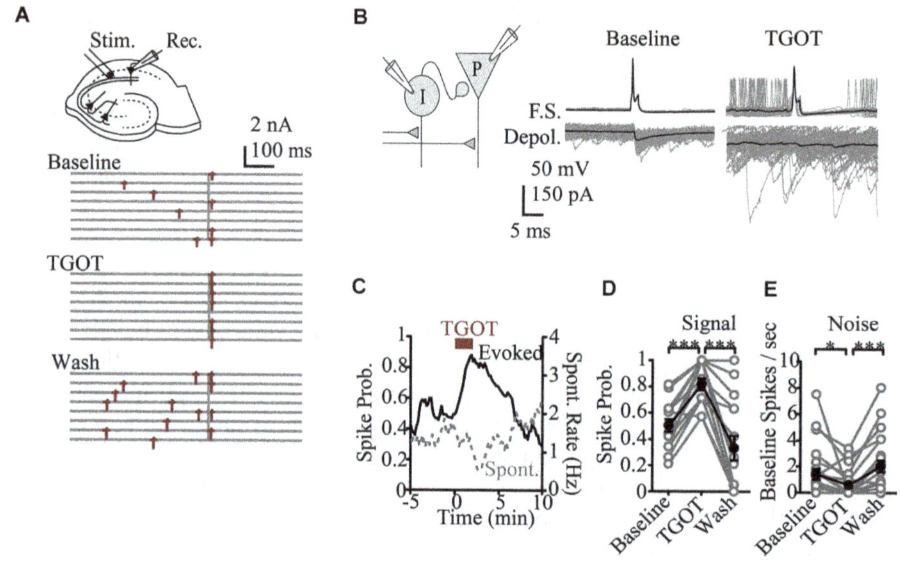

FIGURE 2 | Effects of oxytocin at the circuit level. (A) Representative response to Shaffer Collateral stimulation (vertical bar) of a CA1 pyramidal cell (red—spike, TGOT—Thr^4,Gly^7-oxytocin—specific agonist for oxytocin receptors) **(B)** Responses of presynaptic interneurons (gray—sweeps, black—average) to TGOT, note effect is to increase baseline and reduce stimulus evoked firing. **(C)** Time course of spike probability for both evoked spikes (black) and spontaneous events (gray) from pyramidal neurons. Spike probability in response to stimulation **(D)** and at baseline **(E)**. Figure courtesy of R.W. Tsien, adapted from Owen et al. (2013). *** $P < 0.001$, ** $P < 0.01$, * $P < 0.05$, # $P < 0.1$.

was ocular dominance in a similar model of fragile X as used by Huber et al. (2002) and Dölen et al. (2007). Such ocular dominance can be measured as an ensemble activity by analyzing visual event related potentials. This demonstrates both monogenetic models and immune system dysfunction can produce measured circuit level dysfunction, and therefore may have promise in identifying common features of circuit related disorder in ASD.

ENSEMBLE ACTIVITY

Ultimately, to produce changes measured at an EEG electrode, micro-circuit changes need to be expressed by large numbers of neurons producing ensemble activity. Using voltage sensitive dye imaging (VSDi), that can measure voltage changes across all the excitable membrane (**Box 2**), this ensemble activity can be studied directly in slices. Comparable changes as predicted by cellular studies, have been found in other models of ASD and ASD-related syndromes. For instance mice lacking MeCP2, which model Rett Syndrome, have been shown to be hyperexcitable, and possibly hyperconnected, within hippocampal circuits using VSDi, shedding light on previous dichotomous results of single cell recordings (Calfa et al., 2011).

While it appears that circuit-level study of animal models that recapitulate key aspects of ASD are finding common alterations, there has yet to be one study or set of studies that takes one model of ASD and examines it from the cellular through to the EEG level, thus directly linking the cellular to the ensemble and on to intermediate phenotypes and behavior.

While experiments *in vitro* using animal models that recreate key aspects of ASD have demonstrated promise, work targeting ensemble activity that generate abnormal oscillatory activity in ASD could provide vital cues. By extrapolating the interaction of known cellular components and their connectivity, and modeling them as circuits *in silico*, pioneers in the field of neuronal oscillations made great strides in identifying the types of circuit activity that can generate specific patterns of oscillations recorded by EEG. Original *in vitro* work combined field, intracellular recordings and modeling to identify the neurophysiological elements that support such ensemble activity (Traub et al., 1996, 1999; Ermentrout and Kopell, 1998). These groups identified intracellular and specific cellular qualities that could generate gamma-band activity, which included potassium channel subtypes, spike conductance trajectories and a strong role for both glutamatergic and GABAergic signaling (Buzsáki and Wang, 2012). One repeated finding was that gamma-band activity occurring around 40 Hz band is strongly dependent on GABA receptor activity (Whittington et al., 2000). Thus, in diseases much of the focus on gamma-band abnormalities has been the role of inhibition.

Studying gamma band activity at the local ensemble level takes advantage of the fact that gamma-band (30–100 Hz) activity measured by E/MEG are produced by synchronous neuronal activity arising from these local cortical interactions (Buzsáki and Wang, 2012; Buzsáki et al., 2012). By assaying and modulating ensemble activity, researchers have been able to identify the cell types involved and begin to validate their impact on EEG using modern measures and modulation of ensemble activity. As such the E/MEG detected phenotypes of ASD can be teased apart, potentially leady to a common substrate.

BOX 2 | *In vitro* techniques to study spatial and temporal qualities of cortical gamma-band abnormalities.

Voltage sensitive dye imaging allows for the direct assay of membrane voltage. Because of most of the excitable membrane available for VSDI in the brain is found in dendrites (for review see Chemla and Chavane, 2010) the VSDI signals are biased towards the membrane that is most involved in generating the cortical cellular dipoles recorded at the MEG or EEG sensors (Buzsáki et al., 2012). When used to study the population level, the summed membrane responses can measure the kinetics of the membrane response and this can be associated with differences in EEG responses at the *in vivo* level (Carlson et al., 2011) as well as being amenable to direct examination via time frequency analysis (**Figure 3**).

Similar to how sensory-elicited changes in cortical population responses are reflected in E/MEG power (**Figure 1**), *in vitro* studies can use the population responses driven by electrically evoked afferent activity to more directly study the interplay between excitatory input and the coupled oscillations of excitatory and inhibitory neurons. In areas such as the neocortex and area CA3, which support spontaneous population gamma events *in vitro* (Köhling et al., 2000; Csicsvari et al., 2003; Cunningham et al., 2004), afferent stimulation will generate an increase in membrane potential as well as power when frequency is analyzed (**Figure 3**; Prechtl et al., 1997). Thus, these more complex local interactions can reveal the same time-frequency components measured from repeated sensory stimulation in human subjects, including evoked, ITC and induced power, as well as the spectral background population activity. In EEG/MEG these different components can be mapped to specific dipoles. When these components are identified *in vitro* using VSDi, they also can similarly be mapped back to specific lamina and the extent of functional coupling among horizontal components measured (**Figure 3**). This level of laminar specificity may be important for identifying the cortical circuit components that are disrupted in ASD. In auditory cortex it has been demonstrated that higher frequency gamma oscillations (50–80 Hz) occur primarily in layer 4, with a high dependence on NMDA signaling (Ainsworth et al., 2011). On the other hand lower frequencies of gamma oscillations (30–45 Hz) arose from layer 2 and 3 are highly reliant on gap junctions (Ainsworth et al., 2011). Using cortical slice preparations from validated models of EEG phenotypes, it appears possible to map E/MEG endophenotypes of ASD to specific lamina (**Figure 3E**). As these laminae are characterized by specific developmental origin, cell types and connectivity, identifying the laminae involved in producing specific EEG phenotypes can help detect the developmental and cellular etiology underlying the E/MEG phenotypes.

TARGETING SPECIFIC CELLULAR COMPONENTS TO UNDERSTAND THEIR IMPACT ON ENSEMBLE ACTIVITY

Post-mortem studies and transgenic models where genetic changes are limited to specific cell types anatomical areas have suggested that changes primarily limited specific cell types and brain areas may underlie ASD related symptoms and clinical electrophysiological abnormalities. Using optogenetics to optically excite or inhibit specific cell types involved in oscillatory activity has shown great promise to directly test these hypotheses. The prominent role of parvalbumin (PV) fast spiking cells in generating high-frequency oscillations was demonstrated by specifically expressing the photoactivated Cl^- pump halorhodopsin *in vivo* (Sohal et al., 2009). The reduction in gamma-band activity when PV cells were disabled is consistent with the role of GABA receptors in high-frequency activity. This study was in line with evidence of the role of PV cells in disorders such as schizophrenia, which demonstrate both disruptions in PV cell immunoreactivity (Zhang and Reynolds, 2002) and gamma-band function (Sun et al., 2011). Optogenetics has also been used to link *in vivo* cortical E/I balance, gamma-band oscillations and social behavior by directly increasing excitation in the medial prefrontal cortex (Yizhar et al., 2011). Though there are limited indications that PV cells are disrupted in autism (Lawrence et al., 2010) connectivity involving these and other inhibitory cells types may be abnormal, which may lead to multiple changes in cell type excitability (Zikopoulos and Barbas, 2013). The problem therefore remains that within ASD, differing cell types, synaptic disruptions or connectivity may contribute to similar oscillatory dysfunction. Because optogenetics can be used to excite and inhibit different genetically targeted cell types or anatomical areas, it is well suited to probe the differential contributions of cellular and synaptic dysfunction that may lead to changes in oscillatory activity. In particular where the specific disruption in the E/I balance or connectivity may lead to increased excitation in one cell type and reduced excitation in another, the use of ontogenetic probes with different excitation wavelengths and kinetics can potentially mimic or more fully reverse those conditions (Yizhar et al., 2011).

ASSESSING FUNCTIONAL CONNECTIVITY WITHIN THE CORTEX

Circuit based findings could also aid in testing other hypotheses of ASD. Connectivity, and in particular regulation of functional connectivity is very apt to be studied using circuit/ensemble based techniques as demonstrated in Wilson et al. (2012). Moreover Gray et al. (1989) demonstrated the ability to examine ensemble functional connectivity within cortex, akin to what is detected with EEG but with more precision. Here recording sites located in non-overlapping receptive fields of visual cortex with similar preferred orientation, synchronized maximally for a stimuli that were continuous between recording site's respective receptive fields. Ensemble functional connectivity remains of consequence because along with changes in cellular and receptor properties, alterations in cortical connectivity have been reported in subjects with ASD (Belmonte et al., 2004). High-density electrode arrays or VSDI recordings *in vitro* from cortical slices and *in vivo* from cortical surface can be used to assay the functional connectivity that is associated with local coherence in E/MEG. An immediate area of investigation could directly identify how connectivity is mediated (e.g., directly via axon connectivity or via unmasking of surround inhibition), using *in vitro* pharmacological tools and differing ionic composition (Ang et al., 2005). Ultimately it could provide functional analysis of layer specific connectivity; while directly imaging the surface *in vivo* can precisely map the extent of activity in animals modeling ASD.

Changes in functional connectivity can be incredibly sensitive to alterations to even molecular constituents. For example knocking out the potassium channel KV3.2 in mice reduces high frequency, but not low frequency correlated activity within cortical locations. In these KV3.2 −/− mice, the lack of high frequency

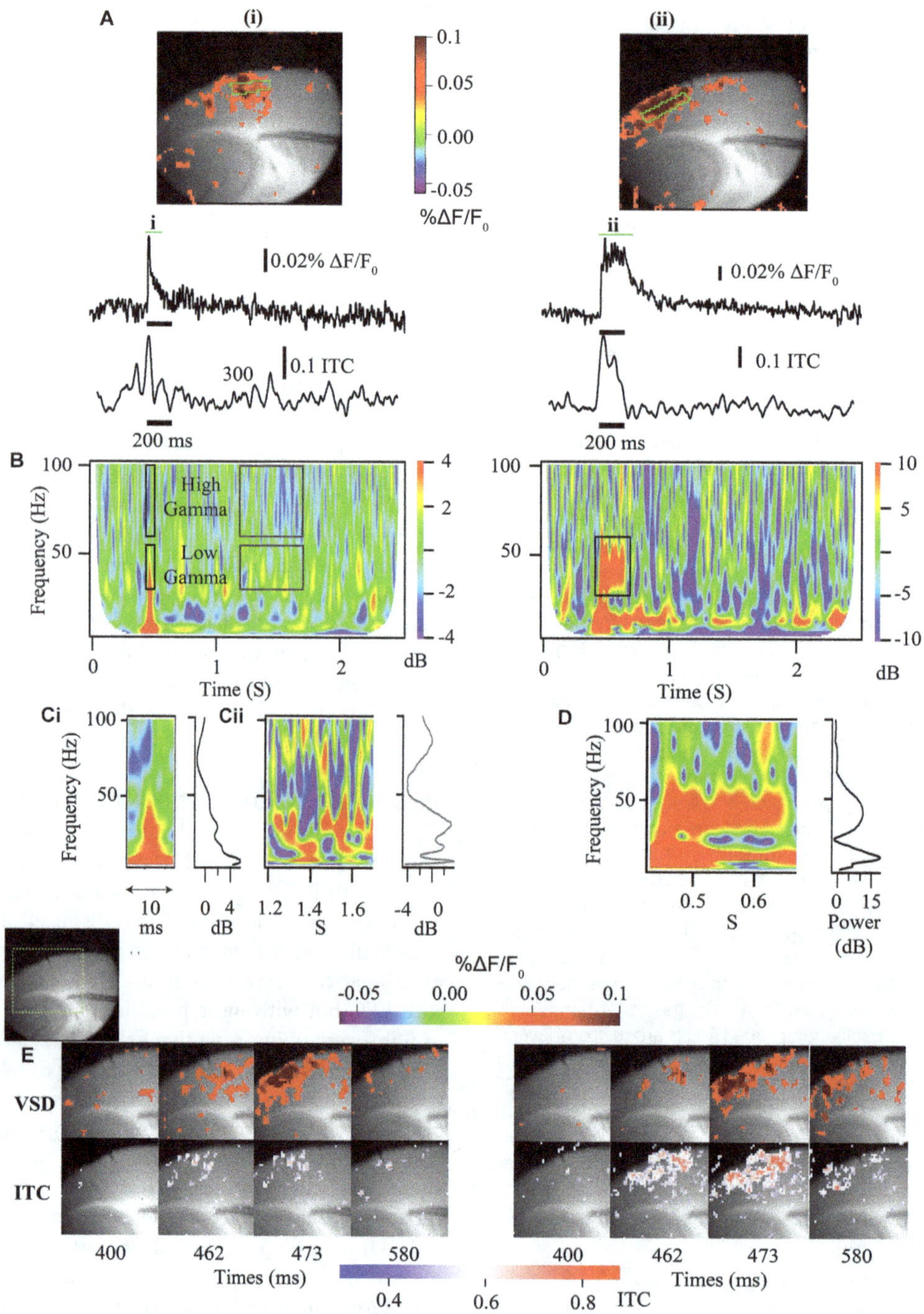

FIGURE 3 | Voltage sensitive dye imaging signals are amenable to time-frequency decomposition. (A) Auditory cortex VSDi responses to single stimulation (left) and burst stimulation at 40 Hz of white matter input tracts (right). Top—2D representation of evoked response [green square—ROIs used below]. Middle—VSDi florescence traces of the ROI depicted in above for single stimulation (left) and burst stimulation (right). Bottom—30–50 Hz ITC calculated for same ROI. **(B)** Time frequency plots for single stimulation (left) and burst stimulation (right). Note that the single stimulation time frequency plot can be separated not only into high and low gamma, but also stimulus related (black boxes) and baseline activity (gray boxes). For the burst stimulated time frequency plot a large increase in power occurs around the frequency that is stimulated at (black box). **(C)** Parsed stimulus related activity **(i)** and baseline activity **(ii)** for the single stimulation paradigm demonstrated in **(B)** [left—time frequency plot, right—image profile of time frequency plot]. Note local peak of activity at 40 Hz in image line profile for both stimulus related activity and baseline. **(D)** Parsed period of stimulation [left—time frequency plot, right—image profile of time frequency plot] for the 40 Hz burst stimulation paradigm demonstrated in **(B)**. Note large increase in 40 Hz power. **(E)** Series of stills from a region of interest (green dashed box in gray scale image shows relative location) in response to a single stimulation (left) and a 40 Hz burst stimulation (right) [top frames—standard VSDi imaging measure; bottom frames—35–55 Hz band passed movie from which pixel-wise ITC has been calculated and overlaid back onto grayscale image]. Note that this analysis allows the determination of laminar and regional existence of inter-trial coherence (ITC).

coherence was not due to single site reductions in high frequency power, which were unchanged from wild type counterparts, but alterations in coherence (Harvey et al., 2012). Such changes to coherence have the potential to cause behavior abnormalities in *in vivo* systems. Operant learning has been shown to be coincident with increase in coherence between striatum and amygdala via coupling in the high frequency range (Popescu et al., 2009). While anxiety has been associated with increase in hippocampal synchrony between the hippocampus and prefrontal cortex at theta frequency (Adhikari et al., 2011). Such specificity of high-frequency coherence may be opaque to imaging modalities with lower temporal resolution, such as fMRI, or less spatial resolution for deep structures, such as E/MEG. Thus, preclinical models may be the only efficient way to studying disease specific disruption of such functional connectivity between coupled nuclei at higher frequencies.

PRE-CLINICAL EEG AND LFP RECORDINGS

In vivo population recording in mice and rats obtained using implanted electrodes to measure EEG also provide useful circuit based insights into ASD. The ability to detect analogous alterations in population activity as seen in ASD was demonstrated with the prenatal VPA insult model of ASD as well through genetic reduction in NMDA receptors (**Figure 1**; Gandal et al., 2010, 2012a). The behavioral deficits seen in this NR1 reduction model correlate with the observed increase in gamma-band power (Gandal et al., 2012c). More importantly, in this model reduction of ASD-like symptomatology was mirrored by a rectification of gamma-band activity (Gandal et al., 2012c). Such changes in baseline power prompted the examination of clinical data, where similar increases in power was found in children with ASD (Edgar et al., 2013), demonstrating directly the important of translational electrophysiology. Similar techniques are now being combined with cell-selective receptor manipulations, producing differing phenotypes, both for behavior and ensemble activity recordings (Billingslea et al., 2014). Such an approach may be useful in other models where cell or location specific genetic modifications have led to ASD related phenotypes.

CURRENT LIMITATIONS OF THIS APPROACH

Focusing on circuit level analysis of ASD pathogenic mechanisms does have its own weaknesses. For example findings of delays and reduced dynamic range in electrophysiological markers of auditory processing (M100) in ASD have been well documented (Roberts et al., 2008; **Figure 1**). Currently such phenomena are difficult for circuit level analysis to dissect as it likely involves complex system level interactions that are difficult to assay. Nevertheless, recent improvements in technique such as multielectrode recordings in rodent cortex has allowed investigators to tease out different onset latencies in auditory fields and coherence between auditory fields (Centanni et al., 2013). Such work is showing promise at illuminating the regional electrophysiological dysfunctions within the auditory fields associated with an environmental insult thought to model ASD in rodents (Engineer et al., 2014).

Another important challenge for the circuit level approach is to determine the exact role that the observed electrophysiological abnormalities play in the specific symptomatology of ASD, whether they are specific to core symptoms or more cognitive issues. This is of importance because of the appearance of similar electrophysiological findings in disorders such as schizophrenia (Uhlhaas and Singer, 2006; Gandal et al., 2012b). In schizophrenia, gamma-band alterations are correlated to negative symptomatology and treatment resistant symptoms, and have to be shown to mirror improved cognitive activity after pharmacological treatments (Gandal et al., 2012b). The exact relation of local circuit activity to behavioral outcomes across multiple disorders must be established.

The question of specificity of electrophysiological findings with regards to ASD symptomatology also arises since the aforementioned markers, such as disrupted gamma-band activity, have been found in first degree relative of patients with ASD (Rojas et al., 2008, 2011; McFadden et al., 2012). First-degree relatives of patients with ASD often exhibit a broad autism phenotype however (Losh et al., 2008), and as such may reflect this behavioral predisposition. This leads to hypothesis that electrophysiological makers such as M100 delay and gamma-band dysfunction may signal a risk for ASD or schizophrenia rather than be a sign of the disease, thus more clinical work is needed to better understand the role of high-frequency changes in activity associated with ASD. Nevertheless, this does not limit the importance of understanding the circuit mechanisms underlying these common E/MEG phenomena, rather it suggest care in interpretation and a need to dissect the connection between disordered circuit activity and behavior. Conversely, recovery of normal gamma-function appears to predict amelioration of behavioral deficits in some models of ASD (Gandal et al., 2012c), and inducing higher baseline gamma-band activity can inhibit social exploration (Yizhar et al., 2011). Such studies have not been completed in ASD patients. If such a link between E/MEG and treatment efficacy is established in patients, the significance of such circuit level studies will increase significantly.

SUMMARY: CIRCUIT-LEVEL EXAMINATION SHOWS POTENTIAL FOR UNIFYING THE CURRENT STATE OF ASD FINDINGS

Synaptic dysfunction, local and long range alterations in connectivity, as well as aberrant modulation can each contribute to altered circuit function, leading to abnormal ensemble activity and disordered brain function. Such changes in brain function likely result in the symptoms of ASD. These changes in ensemble activity and brain function are reflected in differences in EEG, MEG and other functional imaging modalities, yet the actual neurophysiologic mechanisms remain to be identified. The current and developing techniques available to investigators finally allows for the examination of circuit related alterations in ASD, which is critical to bridging cellular and molecular changes commonly studied in animal models and recent clinical electrophysiology from patients with ASD. Circuits that produce gamma-oscillations appear sensitive to changes ranging from subcellular expression to white matter tract alterations. These circuit abnormalities also appear to be a locus where different

ASD-related markers produce similar effects, thus the ASD related gamma changes are a fruitful area for translational inquiry. For instance gamma-band activity has been correlated to hallmark behavioral phenotypes (Rojas et al., 2011), and translational research has demonstrated behavioral improvement due to pharmacological treatment can mirror amelioration of gamma-band function in preclinical models (Gandal et al., 2012c), indicating such an approach can help lead to better treatments in human patients.

Other psychiatric disorders (ADHD and schizophrenia) have similar genetic underpinnings with ASD (Cross-Disorder Group of the Psychiatric Genomics Consortium; Genetic Risk Outcome of Psychosis (GROUP) Consortium, 2013). There is also similar changes in resting and evoked gamma, and a differential impact on EEG coherence between and within hemispheres in these disorders (Uhlhaas and Singer, 2006). Thus, the study of circuit dysfunction in ASD may refine the unique or common cellular character of the E/I imbalance and connectivity seen in multiple disorders. In particular further developing these measures in models and patients can provide the basis for testing the interaction of specific circuit abnormalities and cognitive and behavioral domains associated with these diseases as codified in the Research Domain Criteria by the NIMH (RDoC). As such these developing measures may provide the necessary neurophysiological foundation for understanding differences within ASD and between ASD and other psychiatric disorders. By identifying these mechanisms we can design interventions that directly target circuit function.

AUTHORS AND CONTRIBUTIONS

All authors contributed to the preparation and finalizing of this manuscript.

ACKNOWLEDGMENTS

The authors would like to thank JC Egdar and RW Tsien for their generous allowance and help in adapting their previous published data. This work was supported by Conte Centre Grant 5P50MH096891-02, and a pre-doctoral fellowship from Autism Science Foundation to Russell G. Port.

REFERENCES

Adhikari, A., Topiwala, M. A., and Gordon, J. A. (2011). Single units in the medial prefrontal cortex with anxiety-related firing patterns are preferentially influenced by ventral hippocampal activity. *Neuron* 71, 898–910. doi: 10.1016/j.neuron.2011.07.027

Ainsworth, M., Lee, S., Cunningham, M. O., Roopun, A. K., Traub, R. D., Kopell, N. J., et al. (2011). Dual γ rhythm generators control interlaminar synchrony in auditory cortex. *J. Neurosci.* 31, 17040–17051. doi: 10.1523/JNEUROSCI.2209-11.2011

American Psychiatric Association (2013). *Diagnostic and Statistical Manual of Mental Disorders.* 5th Edn. Washington, DC: American Psychiatric Publishing. Inc

Ang, C. W., Carlson, G. C., and Coulter, D. A. (2005). Hippocampal CA1 circuitry dynamically gates direct cortical inputs preferentially at theta frequencies. *J. Neurosci.* 25, 9567–9580. doi: 10.1523/jneurosci.2992-05.2005

Belmonte, M. K., Allen, G., Beckel-Mitchener, A., Boulanger, L. M., Carper, R. A., and Webb, S. J. (2004). Autism and abnormal development of brain connectivity. *J. Neurosci.* 24, 9228–9231. doi: 10.1523/jneurosci.3340-04.2004

Billingslea, E. N., Tatard-Leitman, V. M., Anguiano, J., Jutzeler, C. R., Suh, J., Saunders, J. A., et al. (2014). Parvalbumin cell ablation of NMDA-R1 causes increased resting network excitability with associated social and self-care deficits. *Neuropsychopharmacology* 39, 1603–1613. doi: 10.1038/npp.2014.7

Boulanger, L. M. (2009). Immune proteins in brain development and synaptic plasticity. *Neuron* 64, 93–109. doi: 10.1016/j.neuron.2009.09.001

Boullin, D. J., Coleman, M., and O'Brien, R. A. (1970). Abnormalities in platelet 5-hydroxytryptamine efflux in patients with infantile autism. *Nature* 226, 371–372. doi: 10.1038/226371a0

Brown, M. S., Singel, D., Hepburn, S., and Rojas, D. C. (2013). Increased glutamate concentration in the auditory cortex of persons with autism and first-degree relatives: a (1)H-MRS study. *Autism Res.* 6, 1–10. doi: 10.1002/aur.1260

Buzsáki, G., Anastassiou, C. A., and Koch, C. (2012). The origin of extracellular fields and currents–EEG, ECoG, LFP and spikes. *Nat. Rev. Neurosci.* 13, 407–420. doi: 10.1038/nrn3241

Buzsáki, G., and Wang, X.-J. (2012). Mechanisms of gamma oscillations. *Annu. Rev. Neurosci.* 35, 203–225. doi: 10.1146/annurev-neuro-062111-150444

Calfa, G., Hablitz, J. J., and Pozzo-Miller, L. (2011). Network hyperexcitability in hippocampal slices from Mecp2 mutant mice revealed by voltage-sensitive dye imaging. *J. Neurophysiol.* 105, 1768–1784. doi: 10.1152/jn.00800.2010

Cardin, J. A., Carlén, M., Meletis, K., Knoblich, U., Zhang, F., Deisseroth, K., et al. (2009). Driving fast-spiking cells induces gamma rhythm and controls sensory responses. *Nature* 459, 663–667. doi: 10.1038/nature08002

Carlson, G. C. (2012). Glutamate receptor dysfunction and drug targets across models of autism spectrum disorders. *Pharmacol. Biochem. Behav.* 100, 850–854. doi: 10.1016/j.pbb.2011.02.003

Carlson, G. C., Talbot, K., Halene, T. B., Gandal, M. J., Kazi, H. A., Schlosser, L., et al. (2011). Dysbindin-1 mutant mice implicate reduced fast-phasic inhibition as a final common disease mechanism in schizophrenia. *Proc. Natl. Acad. Sci. U S A* 108, E962–E970. doi: 10.1073/pnas.1109625108

Casanova, M. F., El-Baz, A., Vanbogaert, E., Narahari, P., and Switala, A. (2010). A topographic study of minicolumnar core width by lamina comparison between autistic subjects and controls: possible minicolumnar disruption due to an anatomical element in-common to multiple laminae. *Brain Pathol.* 20, 451–458. doi: 10.1111/j.1750-3639.2009.00319.x

Centanni, T. M., Engineer, C. T., and Kilgard, M. P. (2013). Cortical speech-evoked response patterns in multiple auditory fields are correlated with behavioral discrimination ability. *J. Neurophysiol.* 110, 177–189. doi: 10.1152/jn.00092.2013

Chartoff, E. H., Marck, B. T., Matsumoto, A. M., Dorsa, D. M., and Palmiter, R. D. (2001). Induction of stereotypy in dopamine-deficient mice requires striatal D1 receptor activation. *Proc. Natl. Acad. Sci. U S A* 98, 10451–10456. doi: 10.1073/pnas.181356498

Chemla, S., and Chavane, F. (2010). Voltage-sensitive dye imaging: technique review and models. *J. Physiol. Paris* 104, 40–50. doi: 10.1016/j.jphysparis.2009.11.009

Chugani, D. C. (2012). Neuroimaging and neurochemistry of autism. *Pediatr. Clin. North Am.* 59, 63–73, x. doi: 10.1016/j.pcl.2011.10.002

Chugani, D. C., Muzik, O., Behen, M., Rothermel, R., Janisse, J. J., Lee, J., et al. (1999). Developmental changes in brain serotonin synthesis capacity in autistic and nonautistic children. *Ann. Neurol.* 45, 287–295. doi: 10.1002/1531-8249(199903)45:3<287::aid-ana3>3.0.co;2-9

Cornew, L., Roberts, T. P. L., Blaskey, L., and Edgar, J. C. (2012). Resting-state oscillatory activity in autism spectrum disorders. *J. Autism Dev. Disord.* 42, 1884–1894. doi: 10.1007/s10803-011-1431-6

Cross-Disorder Group of the Psychiatric Genomics Consortium; Genetic Risk Outcome of Psychosis (GROUP) Consortium. (2013). Identification of risk loci with shared effects on five major psychiatric disorders: a genome-wide analysis. *Lancet* 381, 1371–1379. doi: 10.1016/s0140-6736(12)62129-1

Csicsvari, J., Jamieson, B., Wise, K. D., and Buzsáki, G. (2003). Mechanisms of gamma oscillations in the hippocampus of the behaving rat. *Neuron* 37, 311–322. doi: 10.1016/s0896-6273(02)01169-8

Cunningham, M. O., Whittington, M. A., Bibbig, A., Roopun, A., LeBeau, F. E. N., Vogt, A., et al. (2004). A role for fast rhythmic bursting neurons in cortical gamma oscillations in vitro. *Proc. Natl. Acad. Sci. U S A* 101, 7152–7157. doi: 10.1073/pnas.0402060101

Deutsch, S. I., Urbano, M. R., Neumann, S. A., Burket, J. A., and Katz, E. (2010). Cholinergic abnormalities in autism: is there a rationale for selective nicotinic agonist interventions? *Clin. Neuropharmacol.* 33, 114–120. doi: 10.1097/wnf.0b013e3181d6f7ad

Developmental Disabilities Monitoring Network Surveillance Year 2010 Principal Investigators; Centers for Disease Control and Prevention (CDC). (2014).

Prevalence of autism spectrum disorder among children aged 8 years—autism and developmental disabilities monitoring network, 11 sites, United States, 2010. *MMWR Surveill. Summ.* 63, 1–21.

Dölen, G., Osterweil, E., Rao, B. S. S., Smith, G. B., Auerbach, B. D., Chattarji, S., et al. (2007). Correction of fragile X syndrome in mice. *Neuron* 56, 955–962. doi: 10.1016/j.neuron.2007.12.001

Edgar, J. C., Khan, S. Y., Blaskey, L., Chow, V. Y., Rey, M., Gaetz, W., et al. (2013). Neuromagnetic oscillations predict evoked-response latency delays and core language deficits in autism spectrum disorders. *J. Autism Dev. Disord.* doi: 10.1007/s10803-013-1904-x. [Epub ahead of print].

Eichler, S. A., and Meier, J. C. (2008). E-I balance and human diseases - from molecules to networking. *Front. Mol. Neurosci.* 1:2. doi: 10.3389/neuro.02.002.2008

Elmer, B. M., and McAllister, A. K. (2012). Major histocompatibility complex class I proteins in brain development and plasticity. *Trends Neurosci.* 35, 660–670. doi: 10.1016/j.tins.2012.08.001

Engineer, C. T., Centanni, T. M., Im, K. W., Borland, M. S., Moreno, N. A., Carraway, R. S., et al. (2014). Degraded auditory processing in a rat model of autism limits the speech representation in non-primary auditory cortex. *Dev. Neurobiol.* 74, 972–986. doi: 10.1002/dneu.22175

Ermentrout, G. B., and Kopell, N. (1998). Fine structure of neural spiking and synchronization in the presence of conduction delays. *Proc. Natl. Acad. Sci. U S A* 95, 1259–1264. doi: 10.1073/pnas.95.3.1259

Fatemi, S. H., Folsom, T. D., Reutiman, T. J., and Thuras, P. D. (2009a). Expression of GABA(B) receptors is altered in brains of subjects with autism. *Cerebellum* 8, 64–69. doi: 10.1007/s12311-008-0075-3

Fatemi, S. H., Halt, A. R., Stary, J. M., Kanodia, R., Schulz, S. C., and Realmuto, G. R. (2002). Glutamic acid decarboxylase 65 and 67 kDa proteins are reduced in autistic parietal and cerebellar cortices. *Biol. Psychiatry* 52, 805–810. doi: 10.1016/s0006-3223(02)01430-0

Fatemi, S. H., Reutiman, T. J., Folsom, T. D., and Thuras, P. D. (2009b). GABA(A) receptor downregulation in brains of subjects with autism. *J. Autism Dev. Disord.* 39, 223–230. doi: 10.1007/s10803-008-0646-7

Fox, E., Amaral, D., and Van de Water, J. (2012). Maternal and fetal antibrain antibodies in development and disease. *Dev. Neurobiol.* 72, 1327–1334. doi: 10.1002/dneu.22052

Gaetz, W., Bloy, L., Wang, D. J., Port, R. G., Blaskey, L., Levy, S. E., et al. (2014). GABA estimation in the brains of children on the autism spectrum: measurement precision and regional cortical variation. *Neuroimage* 86, 1–9. doi: 10.1016/j.neuroimage.2013.05.068

Gandal, M. J., Anderson, R. L., Billingslea, E. N., Carlson, G. C., Roberts, T. P. L., and Siegel, S. J. (2012a). Mice with reduced NMDA receptor expression: more consistent with autism than schizophrenia? *Genes Brain Behav.* 11, 740–750. doi: 10.1111/j.1601-183x.2012.00816.x

Gandal, M. J., Edgar, J. C., Ehrlichman, R. S., Mehta, M., Roberts, T. P. L., and Siegel, S. J. (2010). Validating γ oscillations and delayed auditory responses as translational biomarkers of autism. *Biol. Psychiatry* 68, 1100–1106. doi: 10.1016/j.biopsych.2010.09.031

Gandal, M. J., Edgar, J. C., Klook, K., and Siegel, S. J. (2012b). Gamma synchrony: towards a translational biomarker for the treatment-resistant symptoms of schizophrenia. *Neuropharmacology* 62, 1504–1518. doi: 10.1016/j.neuropharm.2011.02.007

Gandal, M. J., Sisti, J., Klook, K., Ortinski, P. I., Leitman, V., Liang, Y., et al. (2012c). GABAB-mediated rescue of altered excitatory-inhibitory balance, gamma synchrony and behavioral deficits following constitutive NMDAR-hypofunction. *Transl. Psychiatry* 2:e142. doi: 10.1038/tp.2012.69

Garay, P. A., and McAllister, A. K. (2010). Novel roles for immune molecules in neural development: implications for neurodevelopmental disorders. *Front. Synaptic Neurosci.* 2:136. doi: 10.3389/fnsyn.2010.00136

Goines, P., Haapanen, L., Boyce, R., Duncanson, P., Braunschweig, D., Delwiche, L., et al. (2011). Autoantibodies to cerebellum in children with autism associate with behavior. *Brain Behav. Immun.* 25, 514–523. doi: 10.1016/j.bbi.2010.11.017

Gordon, I., Vander Wyk, B. C., Bennett, R. H., Cordeaux, C., Lucas, M. V., Eilbott, J. A., et al. (2013). Oxytocin enhances brain function in children with autism. *Proc. Natl. Acad. Sci. U S A* 110, 20953–20958. doi: 10.1073/pnas.1312857110

Gray, C. M., König, P., Engel, A. K., and Singer, W. (1989). Oscillatory responses in cat visual cortex exhibit inter-columnar synchronization which reflects global stimulus properties. *Nature* 338, 334–337. doi: 10.1038/338334a0

Harada, M., Taki, M. M., Nose, A., Kubo, H., Mori, K., Nishitani, H., et al. (2011). Non-invasive evaluation of the GABAergic/glutamatergic system in autistic patients observed by MEGA-editing proton MR spectroscopy using a clinical 3 tesla instrument. *J. Autism Dev. Disord.* 41, 447–454. doi: 10.1007/s10803-010-1065-0

Harrington, R. A., Lee, L.-C., Crum, R. M., Zimmerman, A. W., and Hertz-Picciotto, I. (2013). Serotonin hypothesis of autism: implications for selective serotonin reuptake inhibitor use during pregnancy. *Autism Res.* 6, 149–168. doi: 10.1002/aur.1288

Harvey, M., Lau, D., Civillico, E., Rudy, B., and Contreras, D. (2012). Impaired long-range synchronization of gamma oscillations in the neocortex of a mouse lacking Kv3.2 potassium channels. *J. Neurophysiol.* 108, 827–833. doi: 10.1152/jn.00102.2012

Herbert, M. R. (2005). Large brains in autism: the challenge of pervasive abnormality. *Neuroscientist* 11, 417–440. doi: 10.1177/0091270005278866

Hsiao, E. Y. (2013). Immune dysregulation in autism spectrum disorder. *Int. Rev. Neurobiol.* 113, 269–302. doi: 10.1016/B978-0-12-418700-9.00009-5

Huber, K. M., Gallagher, S. M., Warren, S. T., and Bear, M. F. (2002). Altered synaptic plasticity in a mouse model of fragile X mental retardation. *Proc. Natl. Acad. Sci. U S A* 99, 7746–7750. doi: 10.1073/pnas.122205699

Jamain, S., Betancur, C., Quach, H., Philippe, A., Fellous, M., Giros, B., et al. (2002). Linkage and association of the glutamate receptor 6 gene with autism. *Mol. Psychiatry* 7, 302–310. doi: 10.1038/sj.mp.4000979

Jou, R. J., Mateljevic, N., Kaiser, M. D., Sugrue, D. R., Volkmar, F. R., and Pelphrey, K. A. (2011). Structural neural phenotype of autism: preliminary evidence from a diffusion tensor imaging study using tract-based spatial statistics. *AJNR Am. J. Neuroradiol.* 32, 1607–1613. doi: 10.3174/ajnr.a2558

Karvat, G., and Kimchi, T. (2014). Acetylcholine elevation relieves cognitive rigidity and social deficiency in a mouse model of autism. *Neuropsychopharmacology* 39, 831–840. doi: 10.1038/npp.2013.274

Kim, B. S., Lee, J., Bang, M., Seo, B. A., Khalid, A., Jung, M. W., et al. (2014). Differential regulation of observational fear and neural oscillations by serotonin and dopamine in the mouse anterior cingulate cortex. *Psychopharmacology (Berl)* 231, 4371–4381. doi: 10.1007/s00213-014-3581-7

Köhling, R., Vreugdenhil, M., Bracci, E., and Jefferys, J. G. (2000). Ictal epileptiform activity is facilitated by hippocampal GABAA receptor-mediated oscillations. *J. Neurosci.* 20, 6820–6829.

Kopell, N., Ermentrout, G. B., Whittington, M. A., and Traub, R. D. (2000). Gamma rhythms and beta rhythms have different synchronization properties. *Proc. Natl. Acad. Sci. U S A* 97, 1867–1872. doi: 10.1073/pnas.97.4.1867

Kwon, J. S., O'Donnell, B. F., Wallenstein, G. V., Greene, R. W., Hirayasu, Y., Nestor, P. G., et al. (1999). Gamma frequency-range abnormalities to auditory stimulation in schizophrenia. *Arch. Gen. Psychiatry* 56, 1001–1005. doi: 10.1001/archpsyc.56.11.1001

Lawrence, Y. a., Kemper, T. L., Bauman, M. L., and Blatt, G. J. (2010). Parvalbumin-, calbindin-, and calretinin-immunoreactive hippocampal inter neuron density in autism. *Acta Neurol. Scand.* 121, 99–108. doi: 10.1111/j.1600-0404.2009.01234.x

Lieberwirth, C., and Wang, Z. (2014). Social bonding: regulation by neuropeptides. *Front. Neurosci.* 8:171. doi: 10.3389/fnins.2014.00171

Losh, M., Childress, D., Lam, K., and Piven, J. (2008). Defining key features of the broad autism phenotype: a comparison across parents of multiple- and single-incidence autism families. *Am. J. Med. Genet. B Neuropsychiatr. Genet.* 147B, 424–433. doi: 10.1002/ajmg.b.30612

Maharajh, K., Abrams, D., Rojas, D. C., Teale, P., and Reite, M. L. (2007). Auditory steady state and transient gamma band activity in bipolar disorder. *Int. Congr. Ser.* 1300, 707–710. doi: 10.1016/j.ics.2006.12.073

McDougle, C. J., Naylor, S. T., Cohen, D. J., Aghajanian, G. K., Heninger, G. R., and Price, L. H. (1996). Effects of tryptophan depletion in drug-free adults with autistic disorder. *Arch. Gen. Psychiatry* 53, 993–1000. doi: 10.1001/archpsyc.1996.01830110029004

McFadden, K. L., Hepburn, S., Winterrowd, E., Schmidt, G. L., and Rojas, D. C. (2012). Abnormalities in gamma-band responses to language stimuli in first-degree relatives of children with autism spectrum disorder: an MEG study. *BMC Psychiatry* 12:213. doi: 10.1186/1471-244x-12-213

McNamara, I. M., Borella, A. W., Bialowas, L. A., and Whitaker-Azmitia, P. M. (2008). Further studies in the developmental hyperserotonemia model (DHS)

of autism: social, behavioral and peptide changes. *Brain Res.* 1189, 203–214. doi: 10.1016/j.brainres.2007.10.063

Meguro-Horike, M., Yasui, D. H., Powell, W., Schroeder, D. I., Oshimura, M., Lasalle, J. M., et al. (2011). Neuron-specific impairment of inter-chromosomal pairing and transcription in a novel model of human 15q-duplication syndrome. *Hum. Mol. Genet.* 20, 3798–3810. doi: 10.1093/hmg/ddr298

Modahl, C., Green, L., Fein, D., Morris, M., Waterhouse, L., Feinstein, C., et al. (1998). Plasma oxytocin levels in autistic children. *Biol. Psychiatry* 43, 270–277. doi: 10.1016/s0006-3223(97)00439-3

Needleman, L. A., and McAllister, A. K. (2012). The major histocompatibility complex and autism spectrum disorder. *Dev. Neurobiol.* 72, 1288–1301. doi: 10.1002/dneu.22046

Nguyen, M., Roth, A., Kyzar, E. J., Poudel, M. K., Wong, K., Stewart, A. M., et al. (2014). Decoding the contribution of dopaminergic genes and pathways to autism spectrum disorder (ASD). *Neurochem. Int.* 66, 15–26. doi: 10.1016/j.neuint.2014.01.002

Orekhova, E. V., Stroganova, T. A., Nygren, G., Tsetlin, M. M., Posikera, I. N., Gillberg, C., et al. (2007). Excess of high frequency electroencephalogram oscillations in boys with autism. *Biol. Psychiatry* 62, 1022–1029. doi: 10.1016/j.biopsych.2006.12.029

Owen, S. F., Tuncdemir, S. N., Bader, P. L., Tirko, N. N., Fishell, G., and Tsien, R. W. (2013). Oxytocin enhances hippocampal spike transmission by modulating fast-spiking interneurons. *Nature* 500, 458–462. doi: 10.1038/nature12330

Pardo, C. A., and Eberhart, C. G. (2007). The neurobiology of autism. *Brain Pathol.* 17, 434–447. doi: 10.1111/j.1750-3639.2007.00102.x

Parikshak, N. N., Luo, R., Zhang, A., Won, H., Lowe, J. K., Chandran, V., et al. (2013). Integrative functional genomic analyses implicate specific molecular pathways and circuits in autism. *Cell* 155, 1008–1021. doi: 10.1016/j.cell.2013.10.031

Piven, J. (1997). The biological basis of autism. *Curr. Opin. Neurobiol.* 7, 708–712. doi: 10.1016/S0959-4388(97)80093-1

Popescu, A. T., Popa, D., and Paré, D. (2009). Coherent gamma oscillations couple the amygdala and striatum during learning. *Nat. Neurosci.* 12, 801–817. doi: 10.1038/nn.2305

Prechtl, J. C., Cohen, L. B., Pesaran, B., Mitra, P. P., and Kleinfeld, D. (1997). Visual stimuli induce waves of electrical activity in turtle cortex. *Proc. Natl. Acad. Sci. U S A* 94, 7621–7626. doi: 10.1073/pnas.94.14.7621

Purcell, A. E., Jeon, O. H., Zimmerman, A. W., Blue, M. E., and Pevsner, J. (2001). Postmortem brain abnormalities of the glutamate neurotransmitter system in autism. *Neurology* 57, 1618–1628. doi: 10.1212/wnl.57.9.1618

Raggenbass, M., Tribollet, E., Dubois-Dauphin, M., and Dreifuss, J. J. (1989). Correlation between oxytocin neuronal sensitivity and oxytocin receptor binding: an electrophysiological and autoradiographical study comparing rat and guinea pig hippocampus. *Proc. Natl. Acad. Sci. U S A* 86, 750–754.

Rinaldi, T., Silberberg, G., and Markram, H. (2008). Hyperconnectivity of local neocortical microcircuitry induced by prenatal exposure to valproic acid. *Cereb. Cortex* 18, 763–770. doi: 10.1093/cercor/bhm117

Roberts, T. P. L., Khan, S. Y., Blaskey, L., Dell, J., Levy, S. E., Zarnow, D. M., et al. (2009). Developmental correlation of diffusion anisotropy with auditory-evoked response. *Neuroreport* 20, 1586–1591. doi: 10.1097/wnr.0b013e3283306854

Roberts, T. P. L., Schmidt, G. L., Egeth, M., Blaskey, L., Rey, M. M., Edgar, J. C., et al. (2008). Electrophysiological signatures: magnetoencephalographic studies of the neural correlates of language impairment in autism spectrum disorders. *Int. J. Psychophysiol.* 68, 149–160. doi: 10.1016/j.ijpsycho.2008.01.012

Rojas, D. C., Maharajh, K., Teale, P., and Rogers, S. J. (2008). Reduced neural synchronization of gamma-band MEG oscillations in first-degree relatives of children with autism. *BMC Psychiatry* 8:66. doi: 10.1186/1471-244x-8-66

Rojas, D. C., Singel, D., Steinmetz, S., Hepburn, S., and Brown, M. S. (2014). Decreased left perisylvian GABA concentration in children with autism and unaffected siblings. *Neuroimage* 86, 28–34. doi: 10.1016/j.neuroimage.2013.01.045

Rojas, D. C., Teale, P. D., Maharajh, K., Kronberg, E., Youngpeter, K., Wilson, L. B., et al. (2011). Transient and steady-state auditory gamma-band responses in first-degree relatives of people with autism spectrum disorder. *Mol. Autism* 2:11. doi: 10.1186/2040-2392-2-11

Rubenstein, J. L. R., and Merzenich, M. M. (2003). Model of autism: increased ratio of excitation/inhibition in key neural systems. *Genes Brain Behav.* 2, 255–267. doi: 10.1034/j.1601-183x.2003.00037.x

Santangelo, S. L., and Tsatsanis, K. (2005). What is known about autism: genes, brain and behavior. *Am. J. Pharmacogenomics* 5, 71–92. doi: 10.2165/00129785-200505020-00001

Saunders, J. A., Gandal, M. J., Roberts, T. P., and Siegel, S. J. (2012). NMDA antagonist MK801 recreates auditory electrophysiology disruption present in autism and other neurodevelopmental disorders. *Behav. Brain Res.* 234, 233–237. doi: 10.1016/j.bbr.2012.06.032

Schadow, J., Lenz, D., Dettler, N., Fründ, I., and Herrmann, C. S. (2009). Early gamma-band responses reflect anticipatory top-down modulation in the auditory cortex. *Neuroimage* 47, 651–658. doi: 10.1016/j.neuroimage.2009.04.074

Shuang, M., Liu, J., Jia, M. X., Yang, J. Z., Wu, S. P., Gong, X. H., et al. (2004). Family-based association study between autism and glutamate receptor 6 gene in Chinese Han trios. *Am. J. Med. Genet. B Neuropsychiatr. Genet.* 131B, 48–50. doi: 10.1002/ajmg.b.30025

Silverman, J. L., Yang, M., Lord, C., and Crawley, J. N. (2010). Behavioural phenotyping assays for mouse models of autism. *Nat. Rev. Neurosci.* 11, 490–502. doi: 10.1038/nrn2851

Sohal, V. S., Zhang, F., Yizhar, O., and Deisseroth, K. (2009). Parvalbumin neurons and gamma rhythms enhance cortical circuit performance. *Nature* 459, 698–702. doi: 10.1038/nature07991

Staal, W. G. (2014). Autism, DRD3 and repetitive and stereotyped behavior, an overview of the current knowledge. *Eur. Neuropsychopharmacol.* doi: 10.1016/j.euroneuro.2014.08.011. [Epub ahead of print].

Strutz-Seebohm, N., Korniychuk, G., Schwarz, R., Baltaev, R., Ureche, O. N., Mack, A. F., et al. (2006). Functional significance of the kainate receptor GluR6(M836I) mutation that is linked to autism. *Cell. Physiol. Biochem.* 18, 287–294. doi: 10.1159/000097675

Sun, Y., Farzan, F., Barr, M. S., Kirihara, K., Fitzgerald, P. B., Light, G. A., et al. (2011). γ oscillations in schizophrenia: mechanisms and clinical significance. *Brain Res.* 1413, 98–114. doi: 10.1016/j.brainres.2011.06.065

Tallon-Baudry, C., and Bertrand, O. (1999). Oscillatory gamma activity in humans and its role in object representation. *Trends Cogn. Sci.* 3, 151–162. doi: 10.1016/s1364-6613(99)01299-1

Traub, R. D., Schmitz, D., Jefferys, J. G., and Draguhn, A. (1999). High-frequency population oscillations are predicted to occur in hippocampal pyramidal neuronal networks interconnected by axoaxonal gap junctions. *Neuroscience* 92, 407–426. doi: 10.1016/s0306-4522(98)00755-6

Traub, R. D., Whittington, M. A., Colling, S. B., Buzsáki, G., and Jefferys, J. G. (1996). Analysis of gamma rhythms in the rat hippocampus in vitro and in vivo. *J. Physiol.* 493, 471–484.

Tropea, D., Giacometti, E., Wilson, N. R., Beard, C., McCurry, C., Fu, D. D., et al. (2009). Partial reversal of Rett Syndrome-like symptoms in MeCP2 mutant mice. *Proc. Natl. Acad. Sci. U S A* 106, 2029–2034. doi: 10.1073/pnas.0812394106

Tyzio, R., Nardou, R., Ferrari, D. C., Tsintsadze, T., Shahrokhi, A., Eftekhari, S., et al. (2014). Oxytocin-mediated GABA inhibition during delivery attenuates autism pathogenesis in rodent offspring. *Science* 343, 675–679. doi: 10.1126/science.1247190

Uhlhaas, P. J., and Singer, W. (2006). Neural synchrony in brain disorders: relevance for cognitive dysfunctions and pathophysiology. *Neuron* 52, 155–168. doi: 10.1016/j.neuron.2006.09.020

Wang, X., and Carlén, M. (2012). Optogenetic dissection of cortical information processing-shining light on schizophrenia. *Brain Res.* 1476, 31–37. doi: 10.1016/j.brainres.2012.04.015

Warren, Z., Veenstra-VanderWeele, J., Stone, W., Bruzek, J., Nahmias, A., Foss-Feig, J., et al. (2011). Therapies for children with autism spectrum disorders. comparative effectiveness review no. 26. *Agency Healthc. Res. Qual.* Available online at: www.effectivehealthcare.ahrq.gov/reports/final.cfm

Weisman, O., Zagoory-Sharon, O., and Feldman, R. (2012). Oxytocin administration to parent enhances infant physiological and behavioral readiness for social engagement. *Biol. Psychiatry* 72, 982–989. doi: 10.1016/j.biopsych.2012.06.011

Whitaker-Azmitia, P. M. (2001). Serotonin and brain development: role in human developmental diseases. *Brain Res. Bull.* 56, 479–485. doi: 10.1016/s0361-9230(01)00615-3

Whittington, M. A., Traub, R. D., Kopell, N., Ermentrout, B., and Buhl, E. H. (2000). Inhibition-based rhythms: experimental and mathematical observations on network dynamics. *Int. J. Psychophysiol.* 38, 315–336. doi: 10.1016/s0167-8760(00)00173-2

Wilson, T. W., Rojas, D. C., Reite, M. L., Teale, P. D., and Rogers, S. J. (2007). Children and adolescents with autism exhibit reduced MEG steady-state gamma responses. *Biol. Psychiatry* 62, 192–197. doi: 10.1016/j.biopsych.2006.07.002

Wilson, N. R., Runyan, C. a., Wang, F. L., and Sur, M. (2012). Division and subtraction by distinct cortical inhibitory networks in vivo. *Nature* 488, 343–348. doi: 10.1038/nature11347

Yashiro, K., Riday, T. T., Condon, K. H., Roberts, A. C., Bernardo, D. R., Prakash, R., et al. (2009). Ube3a is required for experience-dependent maturation of the neocortex. *Nat. Neurosci.* 12, 777–783. doi: 10.1038/nn.2327

Yizhar, O., Fenno, L. E., Prigge, M., Schneider, F., Davidson, T. J., O'Shea, D. J., et al. (2011). Neocortical excitation/inhibition balance in information processing and social dysfunction. *Nature* 477, 171–178. doi: 10.1038/nature10360

Zhang, Z. J., and Reynolds, G. P. (2002). A selective decrease in the relative density of parvalbumin-immunoreactive neurons in the hippocampus in schizophrenia. *Schizophr. Res.* 55, 1–10. doi: 10.1016/s0920-9964(01)00188-8

Zikopoulos, B., and Barbas, H. (2013). Altered neural connectivity in excitatory and inhibitory cortical circuits in autism. *Front. Hum. Neurosci.* 7:609. doi: 10.3389/fnhum.2013.00609

6

CYFIP family proteins between autism and intellectual disability: Links with Fragile X Syndrome

***Sabiha Abekhoukh*[1,2,3] *and Barbara Bardoni*[1,2,3] ***

[1] *CNRS, Institute of Molecular and Cellular Pharmacology, UMR 7275, Valbonne, France*
[2] *University of Nice Sophia-Antipolis, Nice, France*
[3] *CNRS, International Associated Laboratories–NEOGENEX, Valbonne, France*

Correspondence:
Barbara Bardoni, CNRS, Institute of Molecular and Cellular Pharmacology, UMR7275, 660 Route des Lucioles, Sophia Antipolis, 06560 Valbonne, France
e-mail: bardoni@ipmc.cnrs.fr; bardoni@unice.fr

Intellectual disability (ID) and autism spectrum disorders (ASDs) have in common alterations in some brain circuits and brain abnormalities, such as synaptic transmission and dendritic spines morphology. Recent studies have indicated a differential expression for specific categories of genes as a cause for both types of disease, while an increasing number of genes is recognized to produce both disorders. An example is the Fragile X mental retardation gene 1 (*FMR1*), whose silencing causes the Fragile X syndrome, the most common form of ID and autism, also characterized by physical hallmarks. Fragile X mental retardation protein (FMRP), the protein encoded by *FMR1,* is an RNA-binding protein with an important role in translational control. Among the interactors of FMRP, CYFIP1/2 (cytoplasmic FMRP interacting protein) proteins are good candidates for ID and autism, on the bases of their genetic implication and functional properties, even if the precise functional significance of the CYFIP/FMRP interaction is not understood yet. CYFIP1 and CYFIP2 represent a link between Rac1, the WAVE (WAS protein family member) complex and FMRP, favoring the cross talk between actin polymerization and translational control.

Keywords: autism, intellectual disability, Fragile X, CYFIP family proteins, WAVE complex, F-actin, dendritic spines

INTRODUCTION

Intellectual disability (ID) and autism spectrum disorders (ASD) are a serious public health problem. The causes of ID and autism are extremely heterogeneous, ranging from environmental to genetic and even combinations of the two. Autism is a disorder of neural development characterized by impaired social interaction and communication and by restricted and repetitive behavior. Signs all begin before a child is three years old. Autism is a pervasive developmental disorder (PDD) that involves severe deficits in a person's ability to communicate and interact with others. Children with autism often have trouble using their imagination, have a limited range of interests, and may show repetitive patterns of behavior or body movements. Different people with autism can have very different symptoms, thus health care providers consider autism as a "spectrum" disorder (ASD), a group of disorders with similar features, including autistic disorder (also called "classic" autism), Asperger syndrome and PDD not otherwise specified or atypical autism. ASD is a very common disorder (prevalence of 1:1000 newborns). Worldwide, 2–3% of the population is affected by mild to severe ID. The economic and social consequences of this disorder are very important since the majority of people with ID require long-term supportive care or service. New technologies allowed the identification of many mutations in ID patients affecting single genes. Thus, genetic alterations identified in ID are fast expanding. It is interesting to underline that mutations in the same gene can cause ID or ASD or both and interestingly more than 80% of XLID (X-Linked Intellectual Disabilities) genes are also cause of autism (Schwartz and Neri, 2012; Brentani et al., 2013; Murdoch and State, 2013). These two disorders have in common alterations in some brain circuits and brain abnormalities, such as synaptic transmission and dendritic spine morphology (Gilman et al., 2011). Remarkably, even if both ID and ASD are heterogeneous in their genetic and molecular bases, recent studies have indicated a significant enrichment for specific categories of genes as a cause for both types of disease, while an increasing number of genes is recognized to produce both disorders. Search for genes causing ID and ASD, as well as characterization of animal models for these disorders, allows to better understand the physiopathology of these diseases and to understand the functioning of the brain. During the last few years huge efforts have been made by many groups in this field, that have indicated the involvement of several categories of genes in these disorders, including genes regulating axon outgrowth, synaptogenesis, cell–cell adhesion, GTPase signaling and the actin cytoskeleton (Gilman et al., 2011; Voineagu and Eapen, 2013). On the same track, also for ID common pathways seem to emerge (e.g., Rho-GTPase and other small GTPase pathways, JNK and Ras signaling), even if the full picture is in continuous evolution (Davidovic et al., 2011; Hashimoto et al., 2011; Pavlowsky et al., 2012; Melko et al., 2013). The increasing number of genes involved in ASD allowed the generation of networks of genes involved in this disease that are spatio-temporally coexpressed (Willsey et al., 2013).

An example of disorder characterized by both ID and ASD is the Fragile X syndrome (FXS), the most common form of inherited ID (estimated prevalence of 1:4000 males and 1:8000 females) and also the most frequent known cause of autism (Auerbach et al., 2011). Silencing of the *FMR1* gene, encoding the Fragile X mental retardation protein (FMRP), causes

FXS. The clinical manifestations characterizing patients affected by FXS include moderate to severe cognitive impairment, elongated facial features, attention deficit, hyperactivity, stereotypy, seizure, impulsivity, sensory hyperarousal, anxiety, and autistic behavior (Bardoni et al., 2000). In brain the major phenotype of FXS patients and FXS animal models (mouse, *Drosophila*) is the presence of dendritic spines that are longer, thinner and denser than normal (Comery et al., 1997; Irwin et al., 2000, 2002; Schenck et al., 2003). They represent the cellular defect underpinning the neuronal dysfunctions characterizing this disorder. Interestingly, this morphological defect is associated to the alteration of different forms of synaptic plasticity in mouse brain (Dolen et al., 2010). FMRP is an RNA-binding protein that plays a role in several steps of mRNA metabolism and, in particular, in translational control at the synaptic level. The absence of FMRP may alter the processing, localization or translational regulation of mRNAs encoding pre- and post-synaptic proteins. These defects can account for the abnormal maturation of dendritic spines in FXS (Swanger and Bassell, 2011; Bardoni et al., 2012; Maurin et al., 2014).The lack of FMRP interferes with mechanisms underlying metabotropic glutamate receptor (mGluR) receptor-dependent long-term depression (LTD) – a prominent form of synaptic plasticity (Huber et al., 2002) and epileptogenesis (Chuang et al., 2005). Indeed, mGluR receptor-dependent LTD in the hippocampus is amplified in the absence of FMRP, whereas NMDA receptor-dependent LTD is not (Huber et al., 2002). mGlu5 receptor-dependent long-term potentiation (LTP) is instead reduced in the cerebral cortex of *Fmr1* null mice (Wilson and Cox, 2007). The mGlu5 receptor-dependent LTD found in animal models of FXS, unlike the one found in wild-type animals, is insensitive to inhibitors of protein synthesis (Bureau et al., 2008). One possibility is that the constitutive abnormality in the expression of synaptic proteins alters long-term responses to mGluR5 receptor activation in this syndrome. This data is consistent with the increased internalization of AMPAR in FMRP-deficient dendrites in the basal state (Nakamoto et al., 2007). Moreover, it is noteworthy that mGluR5 receptors are less associated to the Homer protein in the brain of *Fmr1* knockout mice, which is suggestive of an important alteration in receptor signaling (Giuffrida et al., 2005). Hippocampal epileptogenesis is another form of synaptic plasticity that depends on group I mGlu receptor activation and protein synthesis and is altered in *Fmr1* null mice. The increased excitability in the absence of FMRP can be reversibly blocked by 2-methyl-6-(phenylethynyl)pyridine (MPEP) a specific antagonist of mGluR5, suggesting elevated constitutive mGluR5 receptor activation in FXS. *Fmr1* mutant mice with a 50% reduction in mGluR5 expression exhibited a rescued phenotype (Dolen et al., 2010). However, other different pathways are controlled by FMRP (Davidovic et al., 2011) and up to date is has been difficult to dissect signaling defects determining ID and signaling defects relevant for autistic behavior. Two main paths however, seem to emerge as a link between the two pathologies in FXS: one is represented by the correct balance of the mGluR signaling pathway (Auerbach et al., 2011) and the other by the link with RhoGTPase activity and actin remodeling, represented by the two cytoplasmic FMRP interacting proteins CYFIP1 and CYFIP2 (Schenck et al., 2001, 2003).

CYFIP PROTEINS: THE WAVE COMPLEX AND BEYOND

CYFIP1 and CYFIP2 (also known as PIR121) are members of a gene family highly conserved during evolution (Schenck et al., 2001). They are components of the canonical WAVE regulatory complex (WRC) that, besides the WAVE protein (WAS protein family member), also contains the NAP1 (NCKAP1 or HEM1 in hematopoietic cells) subunit, the ABI1 protein (or one of its paralogous proteins, ABI2 or NESH) and BRK1 (also known as HSPC300) (Cory and Ridley, 2002; Derivery et al., 2009). The WAVE complex transduces Rac signaling via CYFIP1 to trigger Arp2/3-dependent actin nucleation (Cory and Ridley, 2002; Derivery et al., 2009). This process is important in the spatio-temporal regulation of actin dynamics to get correct cell migration, cell polarity (in particular in neurons the axonal polarity), cell adhesion and vesicle trafficking. The WASP family (Wiskott–Aldrich syndrome protein) is composed by five members: WASP, N-WASP and WAVE1, 2, and 3. All these proteins are characterized by the presence of a VCA (verprolin homology, central and acidic region) domain able to activate the Arp2/3 complex. Indeed, as shown in **Figure 1**, CYFIP1/2 interact with the small RhoGTPase Rac1. Upon this binding the subcomplex CYFIP1/2, Nckap1/ABI1 leaves the inactive WAVE holo complex. While WAVE can now interact with Arp2/3, the CYFIP1-containing subcomplex is available to interact with other proteins (**Figure 1**) and then also with FMRP. Indeed, we have shown that the FMRP/CYFIP interaction is GTP dependent (Schenck et al., 2001, 2003). Purified Rho GTPase Rac1 can bind and activate recombinant WAVE complex *in vitro* (Lebensohn and Kirschner, 2009) and the crystal structure of the WAVE complex identified a potential binding site for Rac1 in CYFIP1(Chen et al., 2010). Interestingly it has also been shown that WAVE complex activation is obtained by the cooperation of the Arf and Rac1 GTPases (Koronakis et al., 2011).

Consistent with this function, the WAVE complex has been shown to be involved in lamellipodia formation via the interaction with clathrin heavy chain (CHC), a protein known to be involved in membrane trafficking. In this new role CHC recruits the WAVE complex to the membrane, increasing the speed of protrusion and cell migration (Gautier et al., 2011). Interestingly, this mechanism is conserved from *Drosophila* until mammalian cells (Kunda et al., 2003; Gautier et al., 2011). Moreover, in another study it was shown that activated ARF1 (ADP-ribosylation factor 1) GTPase triggers the recruitement of AP-1 (Adaptor Protein-1) and clathrin on the trans-Golgi network (TGN) membranes. At the edges of the clathrin-, AP-1 coated subdomains also the CYFIP, ABI, NAP1 complex is recruted. HIP1R binding to clathrin light chains could prevent actin polymerization on the surface of clathrin coats. In a second step, activated Rac1 binds to CYFIP and activates the actin nucleation complex leading to N-WASP-dependent activation of ARP2/3 and actin polymerization toward the TGN membrane. This mechanism provides complementary but independent levels of regulation during early stages of clathrin-AP1-coated carrier biogenesis. Thus the WAVE complex, or at least a CYFIP-containing subcomplex, participates to different clathrin functions (Anitei et al., 2010). Interestingly enough, inactivation of *CYFIP1* in MCF-10A (an immortalized but not transformed mammary epithelial cell line able to form 3D acinar structures in Matrigel) produced acini with abnormal structures while cells

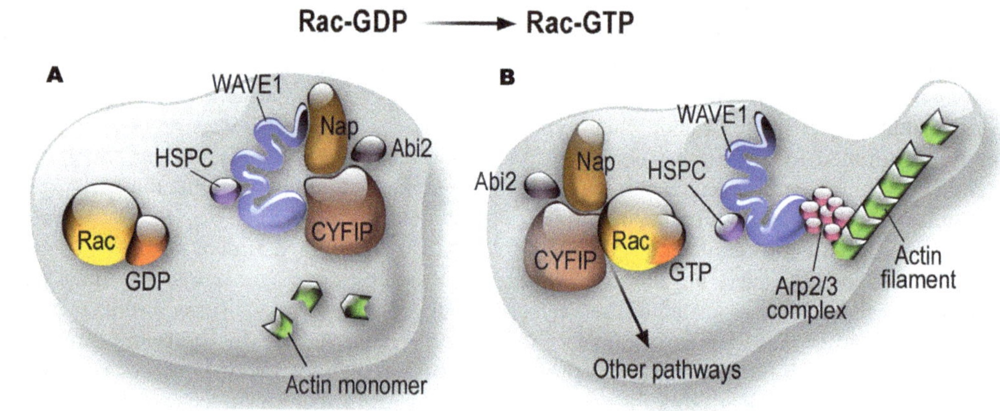

FIGURE 1 | Dynamics of CYFIP Proteins in the context of the WAVE complex and actin polymerization. (A) Structural organization of the WRC in the Rac-GDP condition; **(B)** Structural organization of the WRC in the Rac-GTP condition.

expressing normal CYFIP1 levels display a normal morphology. Knockdown of WAVE pathway components, Nckap1 and WAVE 2, generated phenotypes similar to those observed upon CYFIP1 silencing, while inactivation of *FMR1* has no impact on cell morphology. Furthermore, silencing of *CYFIP1* interferes with normal epithelial morphogenesis and cooperates with Ras to produce invasive carcinomas *in vivo* (Silva et al., 2009). A proapoptotic role was also proposed for CYFIP2 by interacting with the Insulin-like growth factor 2 mRNA-binding protein-1 (IMP-1; Mongroo et al., 2011).

Very recently, in fly a new motif, named WIRS, was identified defining a new class of ligands of the WRC including ~120 membrane proteins (e.g., protocadherins, ROBOs, netrin receptors, neuroligins, GPCRs, and channels). The WIRS peptide motif specifically interacts with the surface formed between Sra (CYFIP1/2) and Abi2 (Ortholog of Abi1 and Abi3). In *Drosophila* mutations altering this interaction result in the disruption of actin cytoskeleton organization and egg morphology leading to female sterility (Chen et al., 2014).

CYFIP1 and 2 are localized at the synapse and have been described to interact with FMRP in a GTP-dependent manner. Interestingly, while CYFIP1 interacts only with FMRP, CYFIP2 was also shown to interact with FXR1P and FXR2P, the two paralogs of FMRP belonging to the FXR (Fragile X related) genes family. These two proteins share a high level of homology with FMRP and they are supposed to have a similar function, probably partially compensating for the absence of FMRP in FXS patients (Schenck et al., 2001). CYFIP1/2 are not RNA-binding proteins and their function is thought to modify some functional properties of FMRP. Indeed the domain of CYFIP1/2 interaction with FMRP is the same that mediates homo-heterodimeryzation of the FXR family (Schenck et al., 2001). This suggested binding with CYFIP1/2 can interfere with the ability of FMRP to dimerize with its paralogs FXR1P and FXR2P. Alternatively, CYFIP1/2 could modify FMRP affinity for RNA. A role of CYFIP1 was also proposed as a component of the translational initiation complex interacting with the FMRP/BC1 complex (Napoli et al., 2008). However, the *in vivo* and *in vitro* formation of this complex is controversial (Iacoangeli et al., 2008a,b). A recent study using double FMR1/BC1 KO mice has definitively shown that FMRP and BC1 cannot belong to the same complex even if they are likely to modulate common target RNAs via independent mechanisms (Zhong et al., 2010). Furthermore, since more than 80% of the FMRP pool is located on translating polyribosomes, the role of a putative CYFIP-FMRP containing initiation complex in regulating initiation of translation is very unlikely to have an impact on FMRP function (Corbin et al., 1997; Feng et al., 1997; Khandjian et al., 2004; Stefani et al., 2004; Aschrafi et al., 2005; Darnell et al., 2011). It is also important to underline that the interaction of CYFIP1/2 via FMRP with polyribosomes was shown, suggesting that CYFIP can also modulate the main function of FMRP when it is associated to actively translating polyribosomes (Schenck et al., 2001). In this context, the link between membrane proteins and CYFIP recently described (Chen et al., 2014) may represent an interesting FMRP-dependent regulation of translation *via* external stimuli driven by CYFIP proteins to actively translating polyribosomes.

CYFIP2 mRNA was also reported to be a target of FMRP, that can modulate its expression (Darnell et al., 2011), creating a double link between the two proteins. It is well known that FMRP modulates the expression of proteins that have an effect on the cytoskeleton [e.g., *MAP1B, PP2Ac, p0071* (Brown et al., 2001; Castets et al., 2005; Nolze et al., 2013)] suggesting that the link between CYFIP1/2 and the reorganization of the cytoskeleton is two-fold: on one side *via* its participation to the WRC as a regulator of WAVE activity and on the other *via* its interaction with FMRP.

In conclusion, CYFIP role in RNA metabolism through its interaction with FMRP and/or other RNA-binding proteins, as recently proposed (De Rubeis et al., 2013), should be better determined by a large-scale study that is still lacking to date.

CYFIP ANIMAL MODELS

Drosophila

The link between CYFIP proteins and other protein/complexes and in particular with the RhoGTPase pathway, pushed us to develop an animal model in *Drosophila* allowing a first analysis of the role of CYFIP in development/maturation of the nervous system. We considered the fly to be a simplified model since only one homolog of the CYFIP family (*dCYFIP*) and only one homolog of the FXR family (*dFMR1*) are present. *dCYFIP* is specifically expressed in the nervous system and interacts biochemically and genetically with *dFMR1* and *dRac*. d*CYFIP* mutations affect axons (growth, guidance, branching) much like mutations in *dFMR1* and in Rho GTPase *dRac1*. *CYFIP*, like the fly *FMRP* and *Rac1* orthologs, plays a pivotal role in the establishment of neuronal connectivity (Schenck et al., 2001). A similar phenotype has been validated for *Cyfip2* (not yet for *Cyfip1*) in zebrafish (Pittman et al., 2010) and rat hippocampal neurons (Kawano et al., 2005). Since neuromuscular junctions (NMJs) share a number of features with central excitatory synapses in vertebrate brain and constitute the best known synaptic plasticity model in *Drosophila*, we analyzed these structures in *dCYFIP* and *dFMR1* mutant flies. In *dCYFIP* mutants, synapse terminals are shorter and display a higher number of buds than in wild-type animals, indicative of impaired synapse growth (Schenck et al., 2001). Loss of *dFMR1* (Zhang et al., 2001) produces a NMJ phenotype that is opposite to that of *dCYFIP* null flies, suggesting an opposite functional role for these two proteins. Furthermore, a co-overexpression of *dCYFIP* partly rescues the *dFMR1* overexpression phenotype (e.g., short synapses) suggesting that *dCYFIP* negatively controls *dFMR1* at the synapse. Finally, using the fly eye to test for genetic interactions, we could order the three molecules within a pathway where dRac1 controls *dCYFIP* that, in turn, regulates *dFMR1* (Schenck et al., 2003). Both the convergent phenotypes and dosage experiments clearly indicated a molecular link between *dFMR1* and the Rho GTPases pathway in neuronal remodeling. We speculated that *CYFIP* proteins may regulate *dFMR* -mediated translational control. Regulation of NMJ development by *dCYFIP* was confirmed by the study of Zhao et al. (2013) Furthermore, these authors performed a detailed analysis of synapses of *dCYFIP* mutants. Using electron microscopy they showed that synaptic vesicles (SVs) are larger in mutants. While the number of SV was unchanged between mutants and wild-type flies, the number of cisternae was elevated in mutants. These abnormalities suggest that dCYFIP may regulate endocytosis and/or vesicle recycling by inhibiting F-actin assembly (Zhao et al., 2013).

Interestingly, inactivation of *Drosophila CYFIP* resulted also in the reduced expression of Kette (Nckap1) and Scar (WAVE) as well as all the other members of the WAVE complex (Bogdan et al., 2004; Schenck et al., 2004; Qurashi et al., 2007; De Rubeis et al., 2013). Inactivation of each member of the WRC has been shown to produce a similar phenotype, in *Drosophila* as well as in cell lines, as it was was shown in HeLa cells (Gautier et al., 2011), in MEF (Dubielecka et al., 2011) and, as already mentioned, in MCF-10A cells (Silva et al., 2009). Collectively these findings demonstrate the tight regulation of the expression of the members of the WAVE complex that is conserved during evolution as well as their function. In conclusion, silencing of each member of the WAVE complex disrupts its function enabling actin polymerization, lamellipodia formation, and cell migration (Eden et al., 2002; Dang et al., 2013).

ZEBRAFISH

Observations in the fly have been confirmed in zebrafish, where two CYFIP genes are expressed. Pittman et al. (2010) studied the function of Cyfip2 during eye and brain development by analyzing a mutant (*nevermind*, also called *nev*) isolated in a screen for mutations affecting retinotectal axon pathfinding). These authors showed that Cyfip2 is required to mantain positional information by dorsonasal axons as they project through the optic tract and the tectum. The lamination of the eye is disrupted in *nev* mutants, apparently independently of the axon guidance phenotype. Interestingly, these authors addressed the question of the redundancy between *Cyfip1* and *Cyfip2*, but they were unable to show any compensation of *Cyfip1* in the absence of *Cyfip2* (Pittman et al., 2010).

MOUSE

Cyfip1-null mouse are lethal at the first steps of embryonic development. Bozdagi et al. (2012) decided to analyze haploinsufficiency of *Cyfip1*. They observed that this condition mimics key aspects of the phenotype of *Fmr1* knockout mice. Indeed, in *Cyfip1* heterozygous mice mGluR-dependent LTD was significantly increased in comparison to wild-type mice. In *Cyfip1+/−* mice mGluR-LTD was not affected in the presence of protein synthesis inhibitor (Bozdagi et al., 2012). Unfortunately, these authors did not analyze the presence of audiogenic seizures in Cyfip1 +/− mice, which is the most relevant phenotype in the FXS mouse model and is dependent on the exaggerated activation of mGluR5. Indeed, this phenotype is rescued by treating mice with MPEP (2-Methyl-6-(phenylethynyl)pyridine) an antagonist of mGluR5 (Musumeci et al., 2000; Yan et al., 2005; Thomas et al., 2012). This experiment would be very important to define common actions/pathways of CYFIP1 and FMRP in neuronal function. Behaviorally, *Cyfip1* heterozygous mice showed enhanced extinction of inhibitory avoidance, similarly to *Fmr1* KO mouse, while no differences have been observed in Y-maze and Morris water maze (to detect alterations in working memory and learning and memory ability, respectively; Bozdagi et al., 2012). On the same track, the inactivation of *Cyfip1* in neurons by siRNA generates dendritic spines that are similar to those observed by silencing *Fmr1 (*immature filopodia) even if their number does not appear to be increased (De Rubeis et al., 2013). However, these latter data are in contradiction with literature concerning the WAVE complex, since if the increased level of immaturity of spines is observed by all investigators, it appears that the reduced activity of the WAVE complex results in a reduced number and length of spines. Indeed, in agreement with previous studies in *Drosophila* NMJ (Schenck et al., 2003, 2004; Bogdan et al., 2004; Qurashi et al., 2007), cultured hippocampal neurons obtained from mice lacking WAVE-1 display a 60% reduction of the extent of neurite outgrowth when compared with wild-type as well as 20% reduction of dendritic spines density, and spines appear more immature (Soderling et al., 2007). These mice display a reduced number (−30%) of post-synaptic spines in CA1 hippocampus and these spines made abnormal synaptic contacts; furthermore, the spine head was flattened, with an abnormal content of internal membrane-bound structures (Hazai et al., 2013). In rat hippocampal neurons, inactivation of WAVE or CYFIP1 resulted in a reduced axonal outgrowth (Kawano et al., 2005), as previously shown in the fly (Schenck et al., 2003). Surprisingly, De Rubeis et al. (2013) do not comment on all discrepancies observed between their results and the literature concerning actin remodeling studies. Even more puzzlingly, they wrote "…..Active-Rac1 promotes CYFIP1 recruitment to the WAVE complex and thus actin polymerization." Indeed, as already mentioned and described by many authors, activated Rac induces the release of CYFIP/NAP/ABI from the WAVE complex that at this point becomes active since the WAVE complex is intrinsically inactive (Cory and Ridley, 2002; Eden et al., 2002; Derivery et al., 2009; **Figure 1**). In the model of De Rubeis et al. (2013) Rac activation should block the WAVE complex instead than activating it!

At this stage we can only conclude that the function of this protein is complex and its implication in different cell pathways is not easy to study. Only in the future the generation of a conditional mouse model for CYFIP1/2 will allow to answer to many questions concerning the role of this family of proteins (and the WRC in a general manner) in neuronal morphology and maturation.

GENETICS OF CYFIP1 AND 2 GENES AND ASSOCIATED GENETIC PATHOLOGIES

No point mutations associated to diseases have been described so far in these genes but some indications concerning their impact on human cognition and/or behavior are indicated by genetic abnormalities. Human *CYFIP1* is located in 15q13. Structural abnormalities involving 15q11–q13 are relatively common and many, but not all, of these rearrangements are associated with an abnormal phenotype. Paternal deletions of this region result in Prader–Willi syndrome (PWS) and maternal deletions in Angelman syndrome (AS), both characterized by ID (Cassidy et al., 2000). Interstitial duplications of maternal origin that include the critical region for PWS and AS (PWACR) produce a more variable phenotype, distinct from PWS and AS, that includes hypotonia, ataxia, seizures, developmental delay and autism or atypical autism with no or only minor dysmorphic features. Conversely, paternal duplications of the PWACR are not associated with an abnormal phenotype (Browne et al., 1997). Many different deletions/duplications have been reported to cause these syndromes: class I abnormalities are larger than those of class II since they include four genes (*NIPA1, NIPA2, CYFIP1,* and *TUBGCP5*) and the non-coding mRNA WHAMML1 (Leblond et al., 2012; **Figure 2**). Patients with class I deletions/duplications (TI) seem to have generally more severe behavioral and psychological problems than individuals with class II deletion (TII; **Figure 2**). In PWS, TI deletion also induces an increased cognitive impairment (Buiting, 2010; Peters et al., 2012). For instance in PWS patients carrying the TI deletion adaptative behavior, obsessive-compulsive behaviors, reading, and visual motor integration asseements are in general poorer if compared with PWS patients carrying a TII deletion. Some researchers have analyzed only microdeletions between BP1 and BP2 (Breakpoint 1 and breakpoint 2, respectively – see **Figure 2**). These patients do not have PWS and share several features including different degrees of learning disability, delayed motor and speech development, dysmorphisms and behavioral problems (ADHD, autism, obsessive-compulsive behavior). Two studies reported patients affected by schizophrenia (Stefansson et al., 2008; Kirov et al., 2009) and in one case by epilepsia (De Kovel et al., 2010), while another group recently published a deletion of BP1–BP2 in two young patients affected only by ID and several dysmorphic features (Madrigal et al., 2012). These results suggest that the genes located between the BP1–BP2 breakpoints are determining behavior and intellectual abilities (Bittel et al., 2006). In addition, very recently, BP1–BP2 deletions have been associated to a high risk of dyslexia and dyscalculia (Stefansson et al., 2014). The different authors proposed different conclusions concerning the implication of each gene in the observed phenotype. For instance, Bittel et al. (2006) analyzed the expression level of the four genes in eight PWS patients carrying the BP1 deletion and nine carrying the BP2 deletion and they compared the expression level of each mRNA with the phenotype, concluding that NIPA1, NIPA2, and CYFIP1 may have a greater influence on behavioral and cognitive parameters that have been taken in consideration in this study. In particular NIPA2, a selective Mg^{++} transporter, has the greatest impact, according to these authors (Bittel et al., 2006). Doornbos et al. (2009) proposed that while NIPA1 and CYFIP1 may be important in neurological development and thus play a role in ID and motor/speech delays, TUBGCP5 may have a pivotal role in behavioral abnormalities. Interestingly, TUBGCP5 is ubiquitously expressed with the highest level in subtalamic nuclei, the brain region involved in ADHD and obsessive-compulsive behavior (Doornbos et al., 2009). A reduced expression of mRNA and protein level of CYFIP1 was reported in patients affected by FXS and PWP. These patients displayed ASD, ID associated to hyperphagia and obesity without cytogenetic or methylation abnormalities at 15q11–13 (Nowiki et al., 2007). However, since a genome-wide analysis was not performed on these patients, it is difficult to assess the impact of the perturbed expression of CYFIP1 on their complex phenotype. The findings that in this study ASD occurs in 10 out of 13 patients and autism in 7 out of 13 cases seems to support the implication of CYFIP1 in autism. Conversely, Stefansson et al. (2008) supported the hypothesis that CYFIP1 is involved in schizophrenia due also to its link to FMRP. However, the opinion that "Fragile X behavioral abnormalities resemble features of schizophrenia" appears strongly arguable (Stefansson et al., 2008). Interestingly, recent findings pointed out a common physiopathological mechanism in schizophrenia, autism and ID. Indeed, these studies found an enrichement of mutations causing schizophrenia in genes involved in synaptic pathways that have been already shown to be involved in autism and ID. In some cases, their mRNA is a target of FMRP (Fromer et al., 2014; Purcell et al., 2014). This common etiology of neurodevelopmental disorders could explain also a complex and variable phenotype of deletions of the 15q11–q13 region. However, it wil be important also to perform genome-wide analysis of these patients to assess whether other mutations could contribute to their phenotype.

A submicroscopic chromosome 15q11.2 duplication segregating in a pedigree with ASD was described. By expression analysis of the genes contained in the duplicated region, *CYFIP1* was suggested to be candidate for involvement in the ASD phenotype

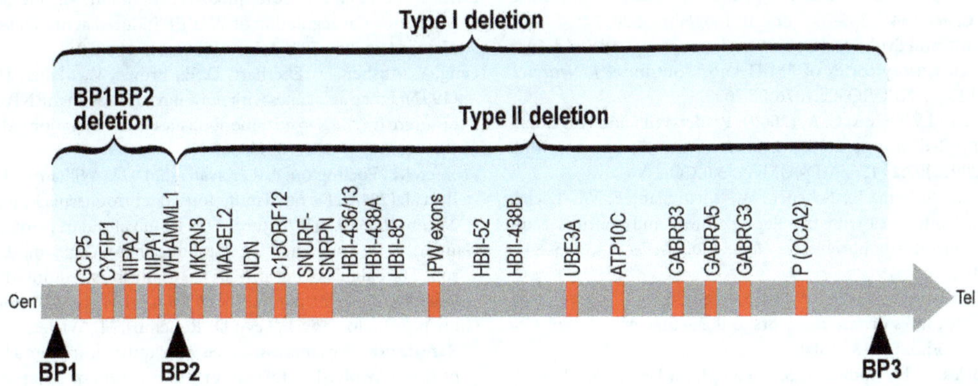

FIGURE 2 | Schematic representation of TI and TII deletions at the chromosomic region 15q11-q13. The BP1-BP2 deletion (including *CYFIP1*) is located in 15q11.2.

in this family. A 30% increase in peripheral blood mRNA levels for the four genes present in the duplicated region in patients, and RNA *in situ* hybridization on mouse embryonic and adult brain sections revealed that two of the four genes, CYFIP1 and NIPA1, were highly expressed in the developing mouse brain (Ingason et al., 2011). These findings point toward a contribution of microduplications at chromosome 15q11.2 to autism, and highlight CYFIP1 and NIPA1 as autism risk genes functioning in axonogenesis and synaptogenesis. Taking into account also its functional properties, CYFIP1 is, among the other genes located in the 15q critical region, the best candidate to produce an ASD (or ID) phenotype when its expression is perturbed. This is consistent with the gene-balance hypothesis, which posits that the same phenotype can arise from under- or over-expression of dosage sensitive proteins because they both disrupt stoichiometry of the same complex (Conrad and Antonarakis, 2007; Darnell et al., 2011) Another example of this situation is provided by findings showing that, as already mentioned, normal synaptic plasticity and cognition occur within an optimal range of metabotropic glutamate-receptor-mediated protein synthesis. In this model, as shown by results in FXS and TSC (tuberous sclerosis), deviation in either direction can cause common behavioral abnormalities (Auerbach et al., 2011).

CYFIP2 -initially identified as a p53 dependent-apoptosis inducible factor (Saller et al., 1999)- is localized on human chromosome 5q33.3. This gene was not associated to human pathologies so far. Only one case of a girl with a *de novo* deletion of 5q33.3q35.1 affected by psychomotor delay, minor facial anomalies and seizures was described, but we do not know if *CYFIP2* expression was modified by this chromosomal abnormality (Spranger et al., 2000). By homology and analogy with CYFIP1, the function of the two CYFIP proteins may be very similar, as well as their role in neuronal maturation and connectivity.

ACKNOWLEDGMENTS

The authors are grateful to Dr. E. Lalli for critical reading of the manuscript, Prof. F. Askenazy for discussion and to Frank Aguila for graphics. This study was supported by INSERM, CNRS LIA NEOGENEX, Agence Nationale de la Recherche: ANR-11-LABX-0028-01, ANR-Blanc (Molecular Biology) SVSE4-2012, and ANR-Blanc (Neuroscience) SVSE8-2012. Sabiha Abekhoukh is recipient of an ARC (Fondation ARC pour la Recherche Sur le Cancer) fellowship.

REFERENCES

Anitei, M., Stange, C., Parshina, I., Baust, T., Schenck, A., Raposo, G., et al. (2010). Protein complexes containing CYFIP/Sra/PIR121 coordinate Arf1 and Rac1 signalling during clathrin-AP-1-coated carrier biogenesis at the TGN. *Nat. Cell Bio.* 12, 330–340. doi: 10.1038/ncb2034

Aschrafi, A., Cunningham, B. A., Edelman, G. M., and Vanderklish, P. W. (2005). The fragile X mental retardation protein and group I metabotropic glutamate receptors regulate levels of mRNA granules in brain. *Proc. Natl. Acad. Sci. U.S.A.* 102, 2180–2185. doi: 10.1073/pnas.0409803102

Auerbach, B. D., Osterweil, E. K., and Bear, M. F. (2011). Mutations causing syndromic autism define an axis of synaptic pathophysiology. *Nature* 480, 63–68. doi: 10.1038/nature10658

Bardoni, B., Abekhoukh, S., Zongaro, S., and Melko, M. (2012). Intellectual disabilities, neuronal posttranscriptional RNA metabolism, and RNA-binding proteins: three actors for a complex scenario. *Prog. Brain Res.* 197, 29–51. doi: 10.1016/B978-0-444-54299-1.00003-0

Bardoni, B., Mandel, J. L., and Fisch, G. S. (2000). Fmr1 gene and fragile X syndrome. *Am. J. Med. Genet.* 97, 153–163. doi: 10.1002/1096-8628(200022)97:2<153::AID-AJMG7>3.0.CO;2-M

Bittel, D. C., Kibiryeva, N., and Butler, M. G. (2006). Expression of 4 genes between chromosome 15 breakpoints 1 and 2 and behavioral outcomes in Prader-Willi syndrome. *Pediatrics* 118, e1276–e1283. doi: 10.1542/peds.2006-0424

Bogdan, S., Grewe, O., Strunk, M., Mertens, A., and Klambt, C. (2004). Sra-1 interacts with Kette and Wasp and is required for neuronal and bristle development in *Drosophila. Development* 131, 3981–3989. doi: 10.1242/dev.01274

Bozdagi, O., Sakurai, T., Dorr, N., Pilorge, M., Takahashi, N., and Buxbaum, J. D. (2012). Haploinsufficiency of Cyfip1 produces fragile X-like phenotypes in mice. *PLoS ONE* 7:e42422. doi: 10.1371/journal.pone.0042422

Brentani, H., De Paula, C. S., Bordini, D., Rolim, D., Sato, F., Portolese, J., et al. (2013). Autism spectrum disorders: an overview on diagnosis and treatment. *Rev. Bras. Psiquiatr.* 35(Suppl. 1), S62–S72. doi: 10.1590/1516-4446-2013-S104

Brown, V., Jin, P., Ceman, S., Darnell, J. C., O'Donnell, W. T., Tenenbaum, S. A., et al. (2001). Microarray identification of FMRP-associated brain mRNAs and altered mRNA translational profiles in fragile X syndrome. *Cell* 107, 477–487. doi: 10.1016/S0092-8674(01)00568-2

Browne, C. E., Dennis, N. R., Maher, E., Long, F. L., Nicholson, J. C., Sillibourne, J., et al. (1997). Inherited interstitial duplications of proximal 15q: genotype-phenotype correlations. *Am. J. Hum. Genet.* 61, 1342–1352. doi: 10.1086/301624

Buiting, K. (2010). Prader-Willi syndrome and Angelman syndrome. *Am. J. Med. Genet. C Semin. Med. Genet.* 154C, 365–376. doi: 10.1002/ajmg.c.30273

Bureau, I., Shepherd, G. M., and Svoboda, K. (2008). Circuit and plasticity defects in the developing somatosensory cortex of FMR1 knock-out mice. *J. Neurosci.* 28, 5178–5188. doi: 10.1523/JNEUROSCI.1076-08.2008

Cassidy, S. B., Dykens, E., and Williams, C. A. (2000). Prader-Willi and Angelman syndromes: sister imprinted disorders. *Am. J. Med. Genet.* 97, 136–146. doi: 10.1002/1096-8628(200022)97:2<136::AID-AJMG5>3.0.CO;2-V

Castets, M., Schaeffer, C., Bechara, E., Schenck, A., Khandjian, E. W., Luche, S., et al. (2005). FMRP interferes with the Rac1 pathway and controls actin cytoskeleton dynamics in murine fibroblasts. *Hum. Mol. Genet.* 14, 835–844. doi: 10.1093/hmg/ddi077

Chen, B., Brinkmann, K., Chen, Z., Pak, C. W., Liao, Y., Shi, S., et al. (2014). The WAVE regulatory complex links diverse receptors to the actin cytoskeleton. *Cell* 156, 195–207. doi: 10.1016/j.cell.2013.11.048

Chen, Z., Borek, D., Padrick, S. B., Gomez, T. S., Metlagel, Z., Ismail, A. M., et al. (2010). Structure and control of the actin regulatory WAVE complex. *Nature* 468, 533–538. doi: 10.1038/nature09623

Chuang, S. C., Zhao, W., Bauchwitz, R., Yan, Q., Bianchi, R., and Wong, R. K. (2005). Prolonged epileptiform discharges induced by altered group I metabotropic glutamate receptor-mediated synaptic responses in hippocampal slices of a fragile X mouse model. *J. Neurosci.* 25, 8048–8055. doi: 10.1523/JNEUROSCI.1777-05.2005

Comery, T. A., Harris, J. B., Willems, P. J., Oostra, B. A., Irwin, S. A., Weiler, I. J., et al. (1997). Abnormal dendritic spines in fragile X knockout mice: maturation and pruning deficits. *Proc. Natl. Acad. Sci. U.S.A.* 94, 5401–5404. doi: 10.1073/pnas.94.10.5401

Conrad, B., and Antonarakis, S. E. (2007). Gene duplication: a drive for phenotypic diversity and cause of human disease. *Annu. Rev. Genomics Hum. Genet.* 8, 17–35. doi: 10.1146/annurev.genom.8.021307.110233

Corbin, F., Bouillon, M., Fortin, A., Morin, S., Rousseau, F., and Khandjian, E. W. (1997). The fragile X mental retardation protein is associated with poly(A)+ mRNA in actively translating polyribosomes. *Hum. Mol. Genet.* 6, 1465–1472. doi: 10.1093/hmg/6.9.1465

Cory, G. O., and Ridley, A. J. (2002). Cell motility: braking WAVEs. *Nature* 418, 732–733. doi: 10.1038/418732a

Dang, I., Gorelik, R., Sousa-Blin, C., Derivery, E., Guerin, C., Linkner, J., et al. (2013). Inhibitory signalling to the Arp2/3 complex steers cell migration. *Nature* 503, 281–284. doi: 10.1038/nature12611

Darnell, J. C., Van Driesche, S. J., Zhang, C., Hung, K. Y., Mele, A., Fraser, C. E., et al. (2011). FMRP stalls ribosomal translocation on mRNAs linked to synaptic function and autism. *Cell* 146, 247–261. doi: 10.1016/j.cell.2011.06.013

Davidovic, L., Navratil, V., Bonaccorso, C. M., Catania, M. V., Bardoni, B., and Dumas, M. E. (2011). A metabolomic and systems biology perspective on the brain of the fragile X syndrome mouse model. *Genome Res.* 21, 2190–2202. doi: 10.1101/gr.116764.110

De Kovel, C. G., Trucks, H., Helbig, I., Mefford, H. C., Baker, C., Leu, C., et al. (2010). Recurrent microdeletions at 15q11.2 and 16p13.11 predispose to idiopathic generalized epilepsies. *Brain* 133, 23–32. doi: 10.1093/brain/awp262

De Rubeis, S., Pasciuto, E., Li, K. W., Fernandez, E., Di Marino, D., Buzzi, A., et al. (2013). CYFIP1 coordinates mRNA translation and cytoskeleton remodeling to ensure proper dendritic spine formation. *Neuron* 79, 1169–1182. doi: 10.1016/j.neuron.2013.06.039

Derivery, E., Lombard, B., Loew, D., and Gautreau, A. (2009). The Wave complex is intrinsically inactive. *Cell Motil. Cytoskeleton* 66, 777–790. doi: 10.1002/cm.20342

Dolen, G., Carpenter, R. L., Ocain, T. D., and Bear, M. F. (2010). Mechanism-based approaches to treating fragile X. *Pharmacol. Ther.* 127, 78–93. doi: 10.1016/j.pharmthera.2010.02.008

Doornbos, M., Sikkema-Raddatz, B., Ruijvenkamp, C. A., Dijkhuizen, T., Bijlsma, E. K., Gijsbers, A. C., et al. (2009). Nine patients with a microdeletion 15q11.2 between breakpoints 1 and 2 of the Prader-Willi critical region, possibly associated with behavioural disturbances. *Eur. J. Hum. Genet.* 52, 108–115. doi: 10.1016/j.ejmg.2009.03.010

Dubielecka, P. M., Ladwein, K. I., Xiong, X., Migeotte, I., Chorzalska, A., Anderson, K. V., et al. (2011). Essential role for Abi1 in embryonic survival and WAVE2 complex integrity. *Proc. Natl. Acad. Sci. U.S.A.* 108, 7022–7027. doi: 10.1073/pnas.1016811108

Eden, S., Rohatgi, R., Podtelejnikov, A. V., Mann, M., and Kirschner, M. W. (2002). Mechanism of regulation of WAVE1-induced actin nucleation by Rac1 and Nck. *Nature* 418, 790–793. doi: 10.1038/nature00859

Feng, Y., Absher, D., Eberhart, D. E., Brown, V., Malter, H. E., and Warren, S. T. (1997). Fmrp associates with polyribosomes as an mRNP, and the I304N mutation of severe fragile X syndrome abolishes this association. *Mol. Cell.* 1, 109–118. doi: 10.1016/S1097-2765(00)80012-X

Fromer, M., Poclington, A. J., Kavanagh, D. H., Williams, H. J., Dwyer, S., Gormley, P., et al. (2014). De novo mutations in schizophrenia implicate synaptic networks. *Nature.* doi: 10.1038/nature12929 [Epub ahead of print].

Gautier, J. J., Lomakina, M. E., Bouslama-Oueghlani, L., Derivery, E., Beilinson, H., Faigle, W., et al. (2011). Clathrin is required for Scar/Wave-mediated lamellipodium formation. *J. Cell Sci.* 124, 3414–3427. doi: 10.1242/jcs.081083

Gilman, S. R., Iossifov, I., Levy, D., Ronemus, M., Wigler, M., and Vitkup, D. (2011). Rare de novo variants associated with autism implicate a large functional network of genes involved in formation and function of synapses. *Neuron* 70, 898–907. doi: 10.1016/j.neuron.2011.05.021

Giuffrida, R., Musumeci, S., D'antoni, S., Bonaccorso, C. M., Giuffrida-Stella, A. M., Oostra, B. A., et al. (2005). A reduced number of metabotropic glutamate subtype 5 receptors are associated with constitutive homer proteins in a mouse model of fragile X syndrome. *J. Neurosci.* 25, 8908–8916. doi: 10.1523/JNEUROSCI.0932-05.2005

Hashimoto, S., Boissel, S., Zarhrate, M., Rio, M., Munnich, A., Egly, J. M., et al. (2011). MED23 mutation links intellectual disability to dysregulation of immediate early gene expression. *Science* 333, 1161–1163. doi: 10.1126/science.1206638

Hazai, D., Szudoczki, R., Ding, J., Soderling, S. H., Weinberg, R. J., Sotonyi, P., et al. (2013). Ultrastructural Abnormalities in CA1 Hippocampus Caused by Deletion of the Actin Regulator WAVE-1. *PLoS ONE* 8:e75248. doi: 10.1371/journal.pone.0075248

Huber, K. M., Gallagher, S. M., Warren, S. T., and Bear, M. F. (2002). Altered synaptic plasticity in a mouse model of fragile X mental retardation., *Proc. Natl. Acad. Sci. U.S.A.* 99, 7746–7750. doi: 10.1073/pnas.122205699

Iacoangeli, A., Rozhdestvensky, T. S., Dolzhanskaya, N., Tournier, B., Schutt, J., Brosius, J., et al. (2008a). On BC1 RNA and the fragile X mental retardation protein. *Proc. Natl. Acad. Sci. U.S.A.* 105, 734–739. doi: 10.1073/pnas.0710991105

Iacoangeli, A., Rozhdestvensky, T. S., Dolzhanskaya, N., Tournier, B., Schutt, J., Brosius, J., et al. (2008b). Reply to Bagni: On BC1 RNA and the fragile X mental retardation protein. *Proc. Natl. Acad. Sci. U.S.A.* 105, E29. doi: 10.1073/pnas.0803737105

Ingason, A., Kirov, G., Giegling, I., Hansen, T., Isles, A. R., Jakobsen, K. D., et al. (2011). Maternally derived microduplications at 15q11-q13: implication of imprinted genes in psychotic illness. *Am. J. Psychiatry* 168, 408–417. doi: 10.1176/appi.ajp.2010.09111660

Irwin, S. A., Galvez, R., and Greenough, W. T. (2000). Dendritic spine structural anomalies in fragile-X mental retardation syndrome. *Cereb. Cortex* 10, 1038–1044. doi: 10.1093/cercor/10.10.1038

Irwin, S. A., Idupulapati, M., Gilbert, M. E., Harris, J. B., Chakravarti, A. B., Rogers, E. J., et al. (2002). Dendritic spine and dendritic field characteristics of layer V pyramidal neurons in the visual cortex of fragile-X knockout mice. *Am. J. Med. Genet.* 111, 140–146. doi: 10.1002/ajmg.10500

Kawano, Y., Yoshimura, T., Tsuboi, D., Kawabata, S., Kaneko-Kawano, T., Shirataki, H., et al. (2005). CRMP-2 is involved in kinesin-1-dependent transport of the Sra-1/WAVE1 complex and axon formation. *Mol. Cell. Biol.* 25, 9920–9935. doi: 10.1128/MCB.25.22.9920-9935.2005

Khandjian, E. W., Huot, M. E., Tremblay, S., Davidovic, L., Mazroui, R., and Bardoni, B. (2004). Biochemical evidence for the association of fragile X mental retardation protein with brain polyribosomal ribonucleoparticles. *Proc. Natl. Acad. Sci. U.S.A.* 101, 13357–13362. doi: 10.1073/pnas.0405398101

Kirov, G., Grozeva, D., Norton, N., Ivanov, D., Mantripragada, K. K., Holmans, P., et al. (2009). Support for the involvement of large copy number variants in the pathogenesis of schizophrenia. *Hum. Mol. Genet.* 18, 1497–1503. doi: 10.1093/hmg/ddp043

Koronakis, V., Hume, P. J., Humphreys, D., Liu, T., Horning, O., Jensen, O. N., et al. (2011). WAVE regulatory complex activation by cooperating GTPases Arf and Rac1. *Proc. Natl. Acad. Sci. U.S.A.* 108, 14449–14454. doi: 10.1073/pnas.1107666108

Kunda, P., Craig, G., Dominguez, V., and Baum, B. (2003). Abi, Sra1, and Kette control the stability and localization of SCAR/WAVE to regulate the formation of actin-based protrusions. *Curr. Biol.* 13, 1867–1875. doi: 10.1016/j.cub.2003.10.005

Lebensohn, A. M., and Kirschner, M. W. (2009). Activation of the WAVE complex by coincident signals controls actin assembly. *Mol. Cell.* 36, 512–524. doi: 10.1016/j.molcel.2009.10.024

Leblond, C. S., Heinrich, J., Delorme, R., Proepper, C., Betancur, C., Huguet, G., et al. (2012). Genetic and functional analyses of SHANK2 mutations suggest a multiple hit model of autism spectrum disorders. *PLoS Genet.* 8:e1002521. doi: 10.1371/journal.pgen.1002521

Madrigal, I., Rodriguez-Revenga, L., Xuncla, M., and Mila, M. (2012). 15q11.2 microdeletion and FMR1 premutation in a family with intellectual disabilities and autism. *Gene* 508, 92–95. doi: 10.1016/j.gene.2012.07.023

Maurin, T., Zongaro, S., and Bardoni, B. (2014). Fragile X Syndrome: From molecular pathology to therapy. *Neurosci. Biobehav. Rev.* doi: 10.1016/j.neubiorev.2014.01.006 [Epub ahead of print].

Melko, M., Nguyen, L. S., Shaw, M., Jolly, L., Bardoni, B., Gecz, J., et al. (2013). Loss of FMR2 further emphasizes the link between deregulation of immediate early response genes FOS and JUN and intellectual disability. *Hum. Mol. Genet.* 22, 2984–2991. doi: 10.1093/hmg/ddt155

Mongroo, P. S., Noubissi, F. K., Cuatrecasas, M., Kalabis, J., King, C. E., Johnstone, C. N., et al. (2011). IMP-1 displays cross-talk with K-Ras and modulates colon cancer cell survival through the novel proapoptotic protein CYFIP2. *Cancer Res.* 71, 2172–2182. doi: 10.1158/0008-5472.CAN-10-3295

Murdoch, J. D., and State, M. W. (2013). Recent developments in the genetics of autism spectrum disorders. *Curr. Opin. Genet. Dev.* 23, 310–315. doi: 10.1016/j.gde.2013.02.003

Musumeci, S. A., Bosco, P., Calabrese, G., Bakker, C., De Sarro, G. B., Elia, M., et al. (2000). Audiogenic seizures susceptibility in transgenic mice with fragile X syndrome. *Epilepsia* 41, 19–23. doi: 10.1111/j.1528-1157.2000.tb01499.x

Nakamoto, M., Nalavadi, V., Epstein, M. P., Narayanan, U., Bassell, G. J., and Warren, S. T. (2007). Fragile X mental retardation protein deficiency leads to excessive mGluR5-dependent internalization of AMPA receptors. *Proc. Natl. Acad. Sci. U.S.A.* 104, 15537–15542. doi: 10.1073/pnas.0707484104

Napoli, I., Mercaldo, V., Boyl, P. P., Eleuteri, B., Zalfa, F., De Rubeis, S., et al. (2008). The fragile X syndrome protein represses activity-dependent translation through CYFIP1, a new 4E-BP. *Cell* 134, 1042–1054. doi: 10.1016/j.cell.2008.07.031

Nolze, A., Schneider, J., Keil, R., Lederer, M., Huttelmaier, S., Kessels, M. M., et al. (2013). FMRP regulates actin filament organization via the armadillo protein p0071. *RNA* 19, 1483–1496. doi: 10.1261/rna.037945.112

Nowiki, S. T., Tassone, F., Ono, M. Y., Ferranti, J., Croquette, M. F., Goodlin_Jones, B., et al. (2007). The Prader-Willi phenotype of fragile X syndrome. *J. Dev. Behav. Pediatr.* 28, 133–138. doi: 10.1097/01.DBP.0000267563.18952.c9

Pavlowsky, A., Chelly, J., and Billuart, P. (2012). Major synaptic signaling pathways involved in intellectual disability. *Mol. Psychiatry* 17, 663. doi: 10.1038/mp.2012.79

Peters, S. U., Horowitz, L., Barbieri-Welge, R., Taylor, J. L., and Hundley, R. J. (2012). Longitudinal follow-up of autism spectrum features and sensory behaviors in Angelman syndrome by deletion class. *J. Child Psychol. Psychiatry* 53, 152–159. doi: 10.1111/j.1469-7610.2011.02455.x

Pittman, A. J., Gaynes, J. A., and Chien, C. B. (2010). nev (cyfip2) is required for retinal lamination and axon guidance in the zebrafish retinotectal system. *Dev. Biol.* 344, 784–794. doi: 10.1016/j.ydbio.2010.05.512

Purcell, S. M., Moran, J. L., Fromer, M., Rudefer, D., Solovieff, N., Roussos, P., et al. (2014). A polygenic burden of rare disruptive mutations in schizophrenia. *Nature* doi: 10.1038/nature12975 [Epub ahead of print].

Qurashi, A., Sahin, H. B., Carrera, P., Gautreau, A., Schenck, A., and Giangrande, A. (2007). HSPC300 and its role in neuronal connectivity. *Neural Dev.* 2, 18. doi: 10.1186/1749-8104-2-18

Saller, E., Tom, E., Brunori, M., Otter, M., Estreicher, A., Mack, D. H., et al. (1999). Increased apoptosis induction by 121F mutant p53. *EMBO J.* 18, 4424–4437. doi: 10.1093/emboj/18.16.4424

Schenck, A., Bardoni, B., Langmann, C., Harden, N., Mandel, J. L., and Giangrande, A. (2003). CYFIP/Sra-1 controls neuronal connectivity in *Drosophila* and links the Rac1 GTPase pathway to the fragile X protein. *Neuron* 38, 887–898. doi: 10.1016/S0896-6273(03)00354-4

Schenck, A., Bardoni, B., Moro, A., Bagni, C., and Mandel, J. L. (2001). A highly conserved protein family interacting with the fragile X mental retardation protein (FMRP) and displaying selective interactions with FMRP-related proteins FXR1P and FXR2P. *Proc. Natl. Acad. Sci. U.S.A.* 98, 8844–8849. doi: 10.1073/pnas.151231598

Schenck, A., Qurashi, A., Carrera, P., Bardoni, B., Diebold, C., Schejter, E., et al. (2004). WAVE/SCAR, a multifunctional complex coordinating different aspects of neuronal connectivity. *Dev. Biol.* 274, 260–270. doi: 10.1016/j.ydbio.2004.07.009

Schwartz, C. E., and Neri, G. (2012). Autism and intellectual disability: two sides of the same coin. *Am. J. Med. Genet. C Semin. Med. Genet.* 160C, 89–90. doi: 10.1002/ajmg.c.31329

Silva, J. M., Ezhkova, E., Silva, J., Heart, S., Castillo, M., Campos, Y., et al. (2009). Cyfip1 is a putative invasion suppressor in epithelial cancers. *Cell* 137, 1047–1061. doi: 10.1016/j.cell.2009.04.013

Soderling, S. H., Guire, E. S., Kaech, S., White, J., Zhang, F., Schutz, K., et al. (2007). A WAVE-1 and WRP signaling complex regulates spine density, synaptic plasticity, and memory. *J. Neurosci.* 27, 355–365. doi: 10.1523/JNEUROSCI.3209-06.2006

Spranger, S., Rommel, B., Jauch, A., Bodammer, R., Mehl, B., and Bullerdiek, J. (2000). Interstitial deletion of 5q33.3*q*35.1 in a girl with mild mental retardation. *Am. J. Med. Genet.* 93, 107–109. doi: 10.1002/1096-8628(20000717)93:2<107::AID-AJMG5>3.0.CO;2-8

Stefani, G., Fraser, C. E., Darnell, J. C., and Darnell, R. B. (2004). Fragile X mental retardation protein is associated with translating polyribosomes in neuronal cells. *J. Neurosci.* 24, 7272–7276. doi: 10.1523/JNEUROSCI.2306-04.2004

Stefansson, H., Rujescu, D., Cichon, S., Pietilainen, O. P., Ingason, A., Steinberg, S., et al. (2008). Large recurrent microdeletions associated with schizophrenia. *Nature* 455, 232–236. doi: 10.1038/nature07229

Stefansson, H., Meyer-Lindenberg, A., Steinberg, S., Magnusdottir, B. B., Morgen, K., Arnarsdottir, S., et al. (2014). CNVs conferring risk of autism or schizophrenia affect cognition in controls. *Nature* 505, 361–366. doi: 10.1038/nature12818

Swanger, S. A., and Bassell, G. J. (2011). Making and breaking synapses through local mRNA regulation. *Curr. Opin. Genet. Dev.* 21, 414–421. doi: 10.1016/j.gde.2011.04.002

Thomas, A. M., Bui, N., Perkins, J. R., Yuva-Paylor, L. A., and Paylor, R. (2012). Group I metabotropic glutamate receptor antagonists alter select behaviors in a mouse model for fragile X syndrome. *Psychopharmacology (Berl),* 219, 47–58. doi: 10.1007/s00213-011-2375-4

Voineagu, I., and Eapen, V. (2013). Converging pathways in autism spectrum disorders: interplay between synaptic dysfunction and immune responses. *Front. Hum. Neurosci.* 7:738. doi: 10.3389/fnhum.2013.00738

Willsey, A. J., Sanders, S. J., Li, M., Dong, S., Tebbenkamp, A. T., Muhle, R. A., et al. (2013). Coexpression networks implicate human midfetal deep cortical projection neurons in the pathogenesis of autism. *Cell* 155, 997–1007. doi: 10.1016/j.cell.2013.10.020

Wilson, B. M., and Cox, C. L. (2007). Absence of metabotropic glutamate receptor-mediated plasticity in the neocortex of fragile X mice. *Proc. Natl. Acad. Sci. U.S.A.* 104, 2454–2459. doi: 10.1073/pnas.0610875104

Yan, Q. J., Rammal, M., Tranfaglia, M., and Bauchwitz, R. P. (2005). Suppression of two major Fragile X Syndrome mouse model phenotypes by the mGluR5 antagonist MPEP. *Neuropharmacology* 49, 1053–1066. doi: 10.1016/j.neuropharm.2005.06.004

Zhang, Y. Q., Bailey, A. M., Matthies, H. J., Renden, R. B., Smith, M. A., Speese, S. D., et al. (2001). *Drosophila* fragile X-related gene regulates the MAP1B homolog Futsch to control synaptic structure and function. *Cell* 107, 591–603. doi: 10.1016/S0092-8674(01)00589-X

Zhao, L., Wang, D., Wang, Q., Rodal, A. A., and Zhang, Y. Q. (2013). *Drosophila cyfip* regulates synaptic development and endocytosis by suppressing filamentous actin assembly. *PLoS Genet.* 9:e1003450. doi: 10.1371/journal.pgen.1003450

7

Epigenetic effect of testosterone in the behavior of *C. elegans*: A clue to explain androgen-dependent autistic traits?

M. Mar Gámez-Del-Estal, Israel Contreras, Rocío Prieto-Pérez and Manuel Ruiz-Rubio *

Departamento de Genética, Universidad de Córdoba, Hospital Universitario Reina Sofía, Instituto Maimónides de Investigación Biomédica de Córdoba, Córdoba, Spain

Correspondence:
Manuel Ruiz-Rubio, Departamento de Genética, Universidad de Córdoba, Campus de Rabanales, Edificio Gregor Mendel C-5, 14071 Córdoba, Spain
e-mail: ge1rurum@uco.es

Current research indicates that the causes of autism spectrum disorders (ASDs) are multifactorial and include both genetic and environmental factors. To date, several works have associated ASDs with mutations in genes that encode proteins involved in neuronal synapses; however other factors and the way they can interact with the development of the nervous system remain largely unknown. Some studies have established a direct relationship between risk for ASDs and the exposure of the fetus to high testosterone levels during the prenatal stage. In this work, in order to explain possible mechanisms by which this androgenic hormone may interact with the nervous system, *C. elegans* was used as an experimental model. We observed that testosterone was able to alter the behavioral pattern of the worm, including the gentle touch response and the pharyngeal pumping rate. This impairment of the behavior was abolished using specific RNAi against genes orthologous to the human androgen receptor gene. The effect of testosterone was eliminated in the *nhr-69* (*ok1926*) deficient mutant, a putative ortholog of human *AR* gene, suggesting that this gene encodes a receptor able to interact with the hormone. On the other hand the testosterone effect remained in the gentle touch response during four generations in the absence of the hormone, indicating that some epigenetic mechanisms could be involved. Sodium butyrate, a histone deacetylase inhibitor, was able to abolish the effect of testosterone. In addition, the lasting effect of testosterone was eliminated after the dauer stage. These results suggest that testosterone may impair the nervous system function generating transgenerational epigenetic marks in the genome. This work may provide new paradigms for understanding biological mechanisms involved in ASDs traits.

Keywords: testosterone, *Caenorhabditis elegans*, epigenetics, gentle touch, pharyngeal pumping, nhr-69, nuclear hormone receptor, Autism spectrum disorders (ASDs)

INTRODUCTION

Autism spectrum disorders (ASDs) are diagnosed with a ratio of about four (male): one (female) across the whole spectrum (Baird et al., 2006), increasing to eight or nine to one in samples with higher functioning patients (Mandy et al., 2011). Some studies suggest that factors in neonatal development, such as those associated with male vs. female sexual development, may play a role in the etiology of some forms of this psychopathology (Baron-Cohen et al., 2003; Keller and Ruta, 2010). Thus, the prenatal environmental has been proposed as a key factor in the connection between autism and maleness. In 1973 it was observed that testosterone neonatal exposure controls male synaptic features in the rat hypothalamus (Raisman and Field, 1973). Subsequent studies have confirmed the effect of perinatal androgen hormone in the masculinization of brain morphology and function in rats, mice, and other mammalian animal models (Morrison and Rieder, 2004). In particular, the role of fetal testosterone has been highlighted as an influential hormone on cognitive and psychological brain development (Baron-Cohen et al., 2004). There are studies supporting this assumption indicating that testosterone exposure has permanent effects on brain development that may guide to male-differences, cognition and behavior respect to females (Cohen-Bendahan et al., 2005a,b; Hines, 2008; Auyeung et al., 2009; Whitehouse et al., 2012; Saenz and Alexander, 2013; Teatero and Netley, 2013). Therefore, it has been hypothesized that high levels of testosterone during early development might be a risk factor for ASDs. This idea is supported by several studies showing that testosterone levels are associated with autistic-like traits (Auyeung et al., 2009, 2010, 2012). Further, the importance of sex steroid related genes in ASDs is sustained by studies reporting associations between polymorphisms in genes involved in sex steroid synthesis/metabolism and ASDs and autistic-like traits (Chakrabarti et al., 2009; Henningsson et al., 2009; Zettergren et al., 2013). Children of mothers affected by hyperandrogenic polycystic ovary syndrome seem to have a higher risk for ASDs probably due to an unbalanced prenatal exposure to high levels of testosterone (Palomba et al., 2012). Finally, other results have shown association between the androgen receptor (*AR*) gene and ASDs (Henningsson et al., 2009).

The human *AR* gene, also known as *NR3C4* (nuclear receptor subfamily 3, group C, member 4), is a nuclear receptor activated by binding either one of the two androgenic hormones, testosterone, or dihydrotestosterone (Roy et al., 1999). The hormones bind in the cytoplasm to the receptor which then translocate into the nucleus to act upon transcription (Brinkmann, 2011). During androgen-dependent gene activation, histone demethylases are involved in the control of gene expression (Metzger et al., 2006). Specifically, phosphorylation of histone H3 at threonine 6 by protein kinase C beta-1 (PRKCB1) appears to prevent lysine-specific demethylase 1 from demethylating histone H3 at lysine 4 (H3K4) during androgen receptor-dependent gene activation (Metzger et al., 2010). The down-regulation of *PRKCB1* in the temporal lobe has been correlated with ASDs (Lintas et al., 2009). Therefore, there is a strong current of opinion that considers the involvement of epigenetic mechanisms in autism (Mbadiwe and Millis, 2013).

Although studies in patients with ASDs have contributed significantly to the understanding of the pathogenesis of these diseases, many aspects of the molecular etiological basis remain unknown. Mammalian animal models have obvious advantages in order to translate them to humans, but their neuronal wiring maps are highly complex. The nematode *Caenorhabditis elegans* is an organism that has some exceptional characteristics for studying behavior and neurological diseases (Brenner, 1974; Calahorro and Ruiz-Rubio, 2011; Bessa et al., 2013). Up to the present time, only the neuronal wiring diagram of this nematode has been determined (White et al., 1986; Jarrell et al., 2012).

Steroid hormone receptors are included in the large superfamily of nuclear hormone receptors (NHRs), a group of transcription factors that bind lipophilic hormones (e.g., steroids, retinoids, thyroid hormones, bile-acid like hormones, and fatty acids) and they control the transcription of many target genes. *C. elegans* genome contains at least 284 predicted nuclear receptor gene (Gissendanner et al., 2004). Except the DAF-12 (dauer formation 12), which is the best understood steroid hormone receptor in *C. elegans* at the functional level (Galikova et al., 2010), the other NHRs are "orphan receptors" whose ligands have not been identified yet. On the other hand, the nematode requires dietary cholesterol during all developmental stages (Shim et al., 2002) and it has been reported that the worm has an ecdysteroid-like substance (Mercer et al., 1988). A more recent work showed that *C. elegans* contained several hormonal steroids, including pregnenolone (3β -hydroxy-pregn-5-en-20-one) and other pregnane and androstane derivatives. It has been found that pregnenolone increased the worm lifespan and influenced the regulation of aging. This study suggested that steroid hormones in *C. elegans* are synthesized from cholesterol since they are not detected in adults growing in cholesterol-deprived conditions (Broue et al., 2007). Other studies have described the effect of several vertebrate steroid sex hormones and synthetic hormones on *C. elegans* reproduction (Tominaga et al., 2003; Mimoto et al., 2007). For instance, testosterone at 5 μM reduced fecundity and this effect was significantly higher after long-term exposure to this hormone (Tominaga et al., 2003).

The implication of specific genes in autism, in particular those encoding neuroligins and neurexins, has supported the use of this nematode in the study of ASDs (Calahorro et al., 2009; Hunter et al., 2010). Moreover, behaviors impaired in neuroligin (*nlg-1*) and neurexin (*nrx-1*) mutants of *C. elegans* were rescued by transgenic expression of human orthologous genes *NLGN1* (Calahorro and Ruiz-Rubio, 2012), and alpha- and beta-*NRXN1* isoforms (Calahorro and Ruiz-Rubio, 2013), respectively. These observations revealed that human neuroligin and neurexin were functional in the nematode. In addition, methylphenidate (a dopamine reuptake inhibitor) and fluoxetine (a serotonin reuptake inhibitor), two drugs widely used for the treatment of behavioral disorders in humans, were able to restore behavioral impairments related to dopamine and serotonin pathways in neuroligin deficient mutants of *C. elegans* (Izquierdo et al., 2013).

One of the advantages of studying epigenetic mechanisms caused by testosterone in *C. elegans* could be the absence of DNA methylation in this organism (Bird, 2002), given that it links the possible epigenetic mechanisms exclusively to histone modifications. In this study, we observed that testosterone alters the mechanosensory response to gentle touch and the pharyngeal pumping rate of the worm. This effect of testosterone was abolished in the *nhr-69* (*ok1926*) deficient mutant, a putative ortholog of human *AR* gene, suggesting that this gene encodes a nuclear receptor able to interact with the hormone. The testosterone effect remained in the mechanosensory response during four generations in the absence of the hormone, indicating that some epigenetic mechanisms could be involved. These results suggest that testosterone may impair the nervous system functionality through a specific receptor generating transgenerational epigenetic marks in the genome.

MATERIALS AND METHODS

STRAINS AND MAINTENANCE

All nematodes were grown and maintained at 20°C under standard conditions on Nematode Growth Medium (NGM) agar plates (Brenner, 1974). **Table 1** shows the *C. elegans* strains used in this study. OP50 *Escherichia coli* strain was obtained from the Caenorhabditis Genetic Center (University of Minnesota, Minneapolis, MN, USA). For the bacterial feeding RNA interference assay, HT115 *E. coli* strain (DE3) with plasmid pL4440 carrying ORFs from different *C. elegans* genes were used. They were obtained from Julián Cerón, at the Bellvitge Institute for Biomedical Research (IDIBELL, Barcelona, Spain) and from Peter Askjaer at the Centro Andaluz de Biología del Desarrollo (CABD, Sevilla, Spain).

BEHAVIORAL ASSAYS

All the behavioral assays experiments were carried out at 20°–24°C with L4 animals.

Gentle touch response assay

This assay was performed using an eyebrow hair attached to a toothpick. The phenotype was tested by stroking the worm ten times with the eyebrow hair alternating the anterior (just behind the pharynx) and posterior (just before the anus) part of the body.

Table 1 | *C. elegans* strains used in this study.

Strain name	Genotype	Source
N2	Wild type, DR subclone of CB original	CGC[a]
TU3335	*lin-15B(n744) X; uIs57 [unc-119p::YFP + unc-119p::sid-1 + mec-6p::mec-6]*	CGC
VC1127	*nhr-126 (gk520) V*	CGC
RB812	*fax-1 (ok624) X*	CGC
RB1578	*nhr-69 (ok1926) I*	CGC
VC1120	*nhr-17 (gk509) X*	CGC
VC469	*+/szT1[lon-2(e678)] I; nhr-25(ok645)/ szT1 X*	CGC
STE68	*nhr-49(nr2041) I*	CGC
RB1592	*nhr-64(ok1957) I*	CGC
VC40185	*nhr-226 (gk502851) V*	CGC
CRR300[b]	*nhr-69 (ok1926) I*	This study

[a] *CGC: Caenorhabditis Genomic Center.*
[b] *After outcrossing RB1578 strain with N2 wild type two times.*

A positive response causes the animal to move backward or forward respectively (Chalfie et al., 1985; Bounoutas and Chalfie, 2007).

Pharyngeal pumping assay

Pumping rates of individual worms were quantified by counting pharyngeal contractions. Individual L4 hermaphrodite grown on NGM plates seeded with OP50 were recorded, focusing on pharyngeal pumping. The video recording was followed by off-line analysis in slow motion.

TESTOSTERONE ASSAYS

Testosterone powder (Sigma-Aldrich, St. Louis, MO, USA) was diluted in 70% ethanol to obtain a stock concentration of 100 mM and was added to NGM plates to get a final concentration of 0.01, 0.1, or 1 mM. In the majority of the experiments 1 mM testosterone was used because the worms grew well and we could be sure that the hormone was not a limiting factor. Gravid adults were placed on seeded NGM control plates (with 0.7% ethanol) or seeded NGM with testosterone (1 mM testosterone; 0.7% ethanol) and allowed to lay eggs to ensure that developing embryos were exposed to testosterone. The progeny were allowed to develop to the late L4 larval stage and then assayed for gentle touch response and pharyngeal pumping rate.

BACTERIAL FEEDING RNA INTERFERENCE ASSAYS

Wild type N2 Bristol and TU3335 *C. elegans* strains were used for *RNAi* experiments (**Table 1**). HT115 *E. coli* strain (DE3) with plasmid pL4440 carrying *nhr-14* (T01B10.4), *fax-1* (F56E3.4), *nhr-111* (F44G3.9), *nhr-236* (Y38F2AL.5), or *mec-4* (T01C8.7) gene ORFs were provided by Julián Cerón at the Bellvitge Institute for Biomedical Research (IDIBELL, Barcelona, Spain). Worms were fed on standard agar plates supplemented with carbenicillin (50 mg/mL-1) and 1 mM IPTG to induce *dsRNA* production. HT115 transformed with the empty pL4440, pL4440/unc-22 constructs (from Peter Askjaer at the Centro Andaluz de Biología del Desarrollo, CABD, Sevilla, Spain), were also used as controls in the experiments.

SODIUM BUTYRATE ASSAYS

Sodium butyrate (SB) powder (Sigma-Aldrich, St. Louis, MO, USA) was dissolved in water to obtain a stock concentration of 100 mM and added to NGM plates to get a final concentration of 1 mM. Gravid adults coming from NGM testosterone plates (1 mM testosterone; 0.7% ethanol) were placed or seeded NGM plates with testosterone and SB (1 mM testosterone; 0.7% ethanol; 1 mM sodium butyrate), and allowed to lay eggs. The progeny were allowed to develop to the late L4 larval stage, and then they were assayed for gentle touch response and pharyngeal pumping rate.

DAUER STAGE ASSAYS

Gravid adults were placed on NGM control plates (0.7% ethanol) or NGM testosterone plates (1 mM testosterone; 0.7% ethanol) and allowed to lay eggs. The progeny were allowed to develop to the dauer larval stage (one month approximately). Then, dauer larval stage animals were placed on NGM plates seeded with OP50 bacteria and allowed to develop to the late L4 larval stage. Then, the animals were assayed for gentle touch response and pharyngeal pumping rate.

TRANSGENERATIONAL ASSAY

Gravid adults were placed on seeded NGM control plates (0.7% ethanol) or seeded NGM testosterone plates (1 mM testosterone; 0.7% ethanol) and allowed to lay eggs. The progeny were allowed to develop until the late L4 larval stage or to the gravid adult stage. The L4 animals were assayed for gentle touch response and pharyngeal pumping rate. The gravid adult animals were placed on seeded NGM plates without testosterone and allowed again to develop to the late L4 larval stage or to the gravid adult stage. Again, the L4 animals were assayed for gentle touch response and pharyngeal pumping rate, and the gravid adult animals were placed on seeded NGM plates without testosterone and allowed again to develop to the late L4 larval stage or to the gravid adult stage. This procedure was successively repeated to analyze the behavior in the following generations without testosterone.

STATISTICAL ANALYSIS

Comparisons shown in each experiment were done by One-Way ANOVA using Excel statistical tool.

RESULTS

INFLUENCE OF TESTOSTERONE IN GENTLE TOUCH RESPONSE AND PHARYNGEAL PUMPING RATE

When the nematode receives a tactile stimulus with an eyebrow hair in the anterior or posterior part of its body, it changes the direction of motion inducing movement back or forward respectively (Chalfie et al., 1985). Sensory cells of *C. elegans* translate mechanical inputs into ionic currents, which activate a neural circuit that drives a locomotory response (O'Hagan et al., 2005). The presence of different concentrations of testosterone induced the loss of a significant capability of the mechanosensory response with respect to the wild type strain (**Figure 1A**).

When *C. elegans* is stimulated repeatedly with an eyebrow hair (gentle touch), the stimulus fails to produce a response and the

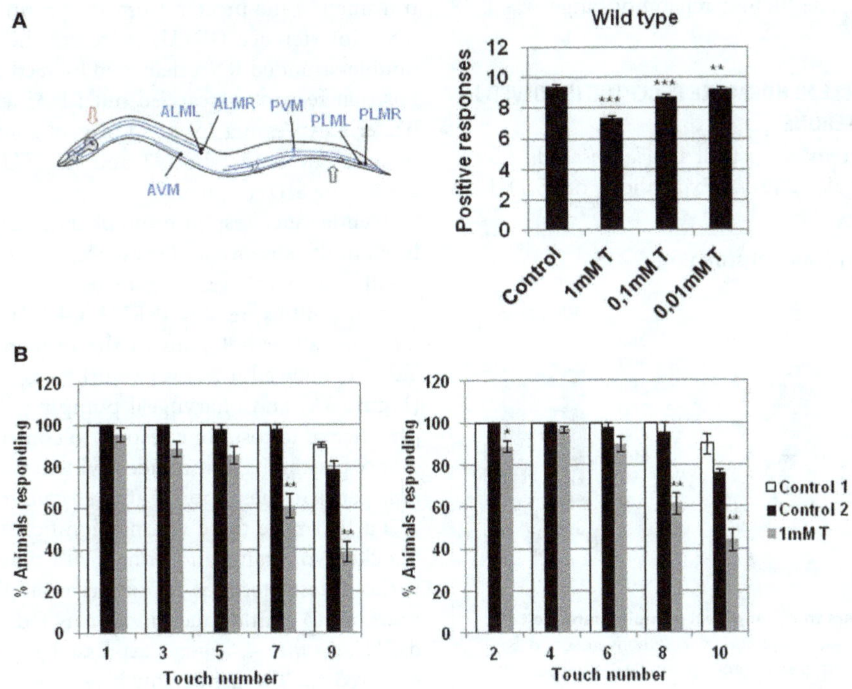

FIGURE 1 | Effect of testosterone on gentle touch response. (A) Left panel: diagram of 6 mechanosensory neurons involved in gentle touch response (blue) modified from Bounoutas and Chalfie (2007). In the gentle touch response animals were touched by stroking an eyebrow hair across the body just behind the pharynx (red arrow) for the anterior touch response, or just before the anus (black arrow) for the posterior touch response; Right panel: gentle touch response of N2 wild type strain was carried out either in the presence or absence of different concentration of testosterone (0.01, 0.1, and 1 mM). Data were analyzed as number of positive responses to ten alternative gentle touches in the anterior and the posterior part of the body. **(B)** Testosterone alters the wild type gentle touch response. In the absence of the hormone N2 wild type strain responds five times consecutively to gentle touch in the anterior and posterior part of the body. In the presence of testosterone (1 mM) the worm fails to respond significantly to the fourth and the fifth touch. Data were quantified as percentage of animals responding to ten alternative gentle touches in the anterior (left panel) and the posterior (right panel) part of the body (five each). At least three independent experiments were carried out (at least 10 L4 worms per experiment). Bars represent the mean ± SEM. Statistical significance was calculated by 1-factor-ANOVA. Statistical *p*-values in **(A)**: $^{***}p < 0.01$, $^{**}p < 0.001$ vs. "Control." Control: NGM + 0.7% ETOH; T: NGM + 0.7% ETOH + 1, 0.1, or 0.01 mM testosterone. Statistical *p*-values in **(B)**: $^{**}p < 0.01$, $^{*}p < 0.05$ *vs*. "Control 2." Control 1: NGM; Control 2: NGM + 0.7% ETOH; 1 mM T: NGM + 0.7% ETOH + 1 mM testosterone.

animal become refractory (Chalfie et al., 1985). **Figure 1B** shows that in the absence of testosterone the wild type strain responds five times consecutively to gentle touch in the anterior and posterior parts of the body, whereas in the presence of testosterone the worms failed to respond mainly to the fourth and fifth touch.

We investigate whether testosterone had an effect in other complex behavior where motor control requires the interaction of the nervous system, muscles, and environment. The pharynx muscle movements of the nematode *C. elegans* is very well characterized (Bean et al., 2004). The worm feeding depends on a neuromuscular pump that connects the mouth to the intestine. The pharyngeal muscle takes bacteria and transports them through the gut. This is achieved with a combination of two actions, pumping and isthmus peristalsis. Pumping is the best understood and consists of a cycle of contraction and relaxation that sucks in liquid with suspended particles from the environment, and then expels the liquid trapping the solid particles. Pharyngeal muscle is capable of pumping without nervous system input, but during normal rapid feeding its timing is controlled by two pharyngeal motor neuron types (Avery and Horvitz, 1989). We examined the pharyngeal pumping in the absence and presence of 1 mM testosterone and a significant reduction in the number of pumps count was observed in the presence of the hormone (**Figure 2**).

C. ELEGANS ORTHOLOGOUS GENES OF THE HUMAN ANDROGEN RECEPTOR

To test the presence of orthologous genes of the human androgen receptor gene (*AR*) in the *C. elegans* genome, we carried out a BLAST search using the human AR receptor ligand-binding domain sequence (residues from 690 to 919) as a query, and as database the protein sequences of *C. elegans* (http://blast.ncbi.nlm.nih.gov/). **Table 2** shows the results obtained from the BLAST analysis were the *C. elegans* proteins with homology are ordered respect to their E-values. The protein with the lowest E-value, that is, the best matching with the human AR receptor ligand-binding domain was NHR-69.

On the other hand the proteins obtained with the BLAST search were structurally compared with the human AR binding with testosterone (**Table 3**). The quality of the model was measured using QMEAN (Benkert et al., 2008, 2009). The QMEAN score4 measures the global score of the whole model, reflecting the predicted model reliability range from 0 to 1 with higher values for better models. The highest reliability range was 0.48 for the FAX1 protein.

CANDIDATE GENES FOR NUCLEAR HORMONE RECEPTOR INVOLVED IN THE RESPONSE TO TESTOSTERONE

Feeding RNAi is efficient in almost all *C. elegans* cells except neurons (Timmons et al., 2001). Expression of SID-1, a transmembrane protein from the worm is required for systemic RNA interference (RNAi) increases the response of neurons to double-stranded RNA delivered by feeding (Calixto et al., 2010). For that reason, we carried out RNAi feeding experiments with bacteria expressing specific ORFs of some *C. elegans nhr-* genes, in both the wild type N2 and the TU3335 strains, this latter expressing SID-1 in neurons.

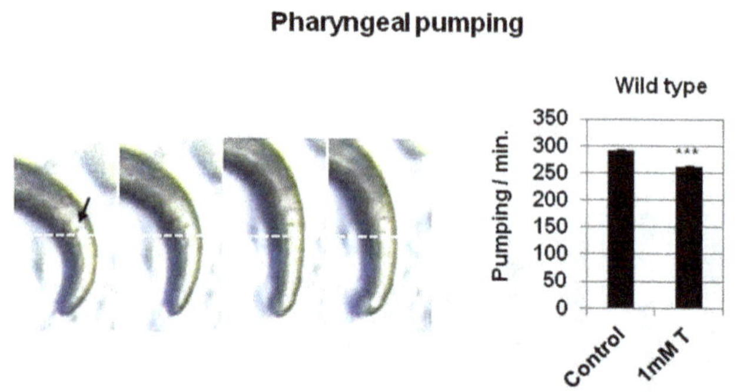

FIGURE 2 | Testosterone alters the pharyngeal pumping rate. Left panel: Pharyngeal pumping images captured by a stereomicroscope (8× magnification). White line was used as reference to measure grinder (black arrow) movement. **Right panel**: pharyngeal pumping rate analysis of N2 wild type strain in the presence or absence of 1 mM testosterone. At least three independent experiments were carried out (at least 10 L4 worms per experiment). Bars represent the mean ± SEM. Statistical significance was calculated by 1-factor-ANOVA. Statistical *p*-values: $^{***}p < 0.001$ vs. "Control." Control: NGM + 0.7% ETOH; T: NGM + 0.7% ETOH + 1 mM testosterone.

Gentle touch response and pharyngeal pumping rate were analyzed in the absence and presence of testosterone (**Figure 3**). The results showed that *C. elegans* fed with bacteria containing plasmid pL4440 expressing dsRNA ORFs from *fax-1*, *nhr-111*, and *nhr-236* (all orthologous of the human androgen receptor, see **Table 1**) showed a recovery in the response to the gentle touch (**Figure 3A**) and pharyngeal pumping (**Figure 3B**) assays in the presence of testosterone respect to control fed with bacteria with empty plasmid. This provides evidence for an *in vivo* function of *nhr-* genes in the response of *C. elegans* to testosterone.

Furthermore there was no significant difference between the knockdown strains and either wild type N2 or TU3335 strains without testosterone, an observation that contrasts with the response to gentle touch in worms fed with bacteria expressing dsRNA to *mec-4*, a gene expressed specifically in neurons and required for the gentle touch response (O'Hagan et al., 2005). These results suggest that the deficiency of *nhr-* genes in the effect of testosterone in gentle touch and pharyngeal pumping probably depends on the expression of these genes in different type of cells.

On the other hand the RNAi feeding experiment was also carry out with bacteria containing plasmid pL4440 expressing dsRNA ORFs from *nhr-14*, a *C. elegans* gene ortholog to human

Table 2 | Sequence comparison of the human androgen receptor ligand-binding domain (hAR-LBD) and the proteins in the *C. elegans* database*.

Protein symbol	Accession number	Protein size (residue number)	LBD position	Alignment position	% identity	*E*-value
NHR-69	NP_492615.2	373	98–340	133–282	24.84	3,00E-06
NHR-91	NP_001024953.1	474	222–465	248–418	23.26	3,00E-04
NHR-192	NP_505584.2	352	160–321	180–348	21.71	6,00E-04
S/T/R NHR homolog nhr-35	T34093	515	230–441	244–274	45.16	0,03
NHR-17	NP_510115.1	396	182–360	192–358	25.74	0,03
NHR-35	NP_001024366.1	486	174–378	188–307	28.57	0,039
NHR-25	NP_001024551.1	492	269–421	274–314	36.59	0,086
NHR-49	AAG15140.1	337	59–253	60–170	24.14	0,15
FAX-1	NP_001263953.1	390	233–367	235–320	23.42	0,21
NHR-47	NP_504455.1	579	385–522	208–267	25	0,55
NHR-46	NP_001023065.1	576	365–540	372–411	33.33	0,83
NHR-248	NP_507334.1	342	149–313	235–342	27.19	0,83
NHR-64	NP_001021043.2	344	101–323	128–269	20.39	1,1
NHR-10	AAO39172.1	396	197–355	200–231	37.5	1,2
NHR-119	NP_494368.2	708	213–382	213–256	27.27	2,3
NHR-219	NP_505314.1	511	289–492	300–330	29.03	3,7
NHR-226	NP_503630.1	387	165–368	174–232	28.81	3,7
NHR-126	NP_503609.2	404	184–388	193–227	28.57	8,1

**http://blast.ncbi.nlm.nih.gov/*

A selection of worm proteins with the highest identity values is shown. The results were obtained from BLAST analysis using human hAR-LBD (residues from 690 to 919) as a query.

Table 3 | Putative genes from *C. elegans* that could act as testosterone receptors.

Protein symbol	Accession number	Protein size (residue number)	Modeled residue range	QMEAN score4
FAX-1	NP_001263953.1	390	223–386	0.48
NHR-119	NP_494368.2	708	208–413	0.463
NHR-192	NP_505584.2	352	154–351	0.451
NHR-69	NP_492615.2	373	130–366	0.449
NHR-64	NP_001021043.2	344	97–344	0.442
NHR-126	NP_503609.2	404	185–381	0.426
NHR-35	NP_001024366.1	486	177–384	0.423
NHR-226	NP_503630.1	387	166–362	0.422
NHR-17	NP_510115.1	396	178–390	0.416
NHR-236	CCD66972.1	283	115–273	0.415
NHR-49	AAG15140.1	337	37–256	0.404
NHR-248	NP_507334.1	342	120–341	0.402
NHR-25	NP_001024551.1	492	265–460	0.4
NHR-91	NP_001024953.1	474	234–453	0.389
NHR-111	CAB05521.2	311	141–307	0.384
NHR-219	NP_505314.1	511	290–484	0.378
NHR-46	NP_001023065.1	576	360–574	0.352
S/T/R NHR homolog nhr-35	T34093	515	233–480	0.278
NHR-47	NP_504455.1	579	201–578	0.269

*A selection of worm proteins with the highest identity values obtained from BLAST analysis using human hAR-LBD (residues from 690 to 919) vs. protein sequences of C. elegans database (**Table 2**), were structurally modeled by comparison with human androgen receptor in complex with testosterone. Swiss-Model Proteomic Serve was implemented. QMEANscore4 reflects the predicted model reliability ranging from 0 to 1 with higher values for better models.*

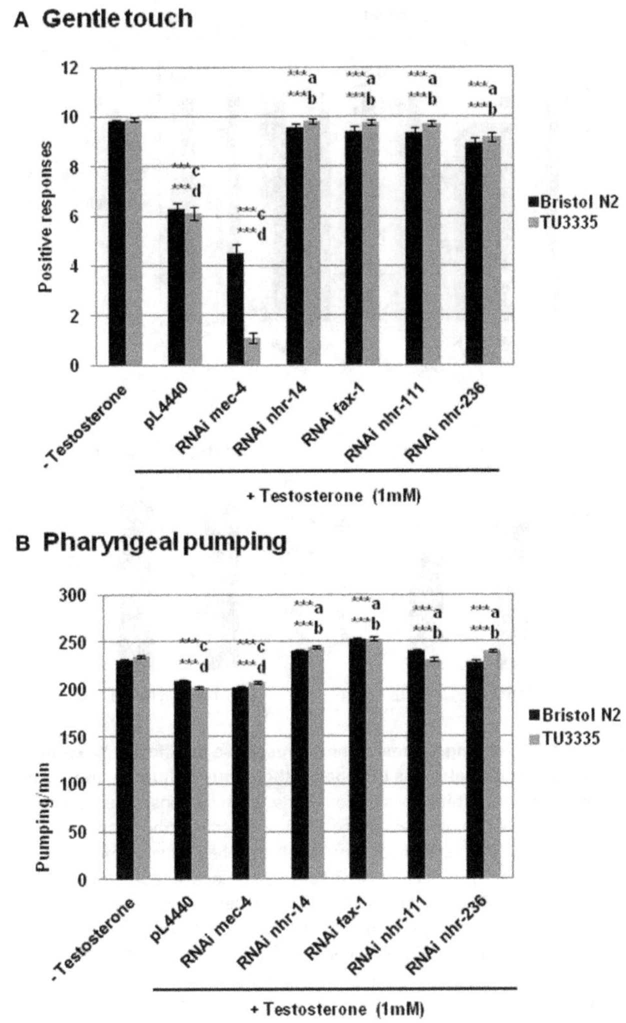

FIGURE 3 | RNAi feeding against genes from *C. elegans*. orthologous to human androgen and estrogen receptors abolishes the effect of testosterone in the behavior of *C. elegans*. Bristol N2 and TU3335 ($P_{unc-119}$*sid* − 1) strains were fed with bacteria carrying the pL4440 vector with different RNAi ORFs of *mec-4, nhr-14, fax-1, nhr-111,* and *nhr-236* genes, or with the empty vector. Gentle touch response **(A)** and pharyngeal pumping rate **(B)** were quantified in the presence or absence of 1 mM testosterone. At least three independent experiments were carried out (at least 10 L4 worms per experiment). Bars represent the mean ± SEM. Statistical significance was calculated by 1-factor-ANOVA. Statistical *p*-values: ***a,b $p < 0.001$ *vs.* "pL4440 empty vector" for N2 and TU3335 strains respectively; ***c,d $p < 0.001$ *vs.* "−Testosterone" for N2 and TU3335 strains respectively. −Testosterone: NGM + 0.7% ETOH; +Testosterone: NGM + 0.7% ETOH + 1 mM testosterone.

estrogenic receptor (Mimoto et al., 2007). The sequence of the protein encoded by this gene presents a region with specific identity to the human androgen ligand-binding domain (12.17%). The results obtained with *nhr-14* knockdown animals were similar to those of *fax-1, nhr-111,* and *nhr-236* knockdown ones (**Figure 3**). One explanation to this observation is an effect of cross-interference due to the high percentage of similarity between all these sequences. In fact, it has been demonstrate that siRNAs may cross-react with targets of limited sequence similarity (Jackson et al., 2003). Cross-interference seems to be very likely if there is 80% nucleotide identity over 200 bp (Kamath and Ahringer, 2003).

NHR-69 A PUTATIVE TESTOSTERONE RECEPTOR IN *C. ELEGANS*

With the objective of finding genes able to function as a testosterone receptor, we carried out a screening for testosterone response in different mutant strains (**Table 1**) with deletions in genes orthologous of human *AR*. **Figure 4A** shows the effect of testosterone of these mutants on gentle touch response. Only the strain having a deletion in the gene *nhr-69* did not show response to testosterone. To further confirm this observation, the mutant strain *nhr-69* (*ok1926*) was out-crossed to clean its genome of undesired mutations, and then assayed again with testosterone respect of gentle touch response and pharyngeal pumping rate. The results shown in **Figure 4B** confirmed that mutant *nhr-69* (*ok1926*) lost the capability to respond to testosterone in both behavioral assays.

TRANSGENERATIONAL EPIGENETIC INHERITANCE OF IMPAIRED GENTLE TOUCH RESPONSE INDUCED BY TESTOSTERONE

Steroid hormones can induce epigenetic chromatin modifications, including covalent changes of histone proteins, bringing

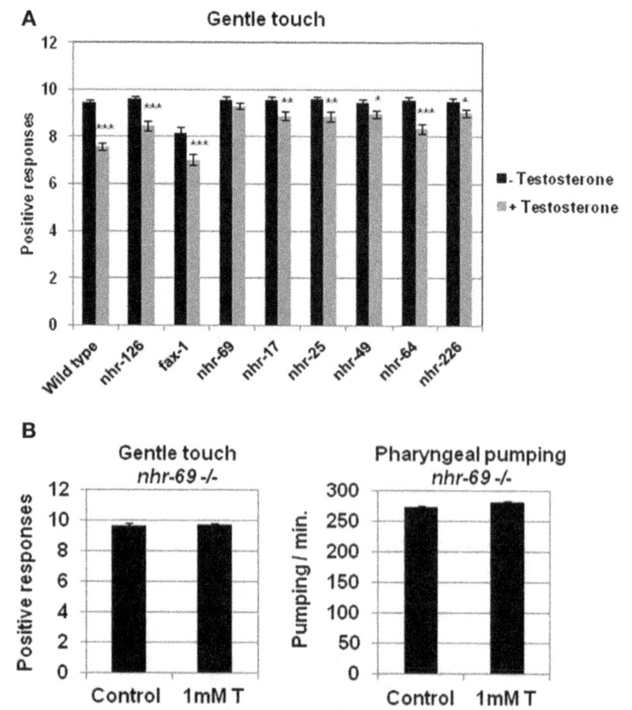

FIGURE 4 | Screening for testosterone response in different *C. elegans* strains harboring deletions in genes orthologous of human androgen receptor. (A) Quantitative assays for gentle touch response were carried out in different strain of *C. elegans* defective in genes orthologous to human AR. **(B)** Touch sensitivity (left panel) and pharyngeal pumping rate (right panel) were quantified in *nhr-69*(*ok1926*) defective mutant strain (outcrossed 2×). At least three independent experiments were carried out (at least 10 L4 worms per experiment). Bars represent the mean ± SEM. Statistical significance was calculated by 1-factor-ANOVA. Statistical *p*-values in **(A)**: $^{*}p < 0.05$, $^{**}p < 0.01$, $^{***}p < 0.001$ *vs.* "Wild type + Testosterone". -Testosterone: NGM + 0.7% ETOH; +Testosterone: NGM + 0.7% ETOH + 1 mM testosterone. Statistical *p*-values in **(B)**: not significant ($p > 0.05$) *vs.* "Control". Control: NGM + 0.7% ETOH; 1 mM T: NGM + 0.7% ETOH + 1 mM testosterone.

long-lasting adjustments in gene expression in cancer cell lines and peripheral tissues (Ruiz-Cortes et al., 2005; Zhu et al., 2008). There are evidences of epigenetic action of neonatal testosterone in brain masculinization in mice (Murray et al., 2009).

The possible epigenetic changes originated by testosterone in the worm could not be due to DNA methylation, since *C. elegans* has not a predictable DNA methyltransferase in its genome neither 5-methyl cytosine (5 mC) in its DNA (Bird, 2002). This suggests that other mechanisms has to be involved, most likely changes in chromatin histones. Indeed, it has been previously demonstrated that acute administration of sodium butyrate (SB) inhibits histone deacetylase in several organisms, including *C. elegans* (Catoire et al., 2008; Zhang et al., 2009), *Drosophila* (Tie et al., 2009), mammalian cells (Candido et al., 1978; Catoire et al., 2008) and even *Saccharomyces cerevisiae* (Yu et al., 2005) and plants (Chua et al., 2003). Therefore, to determine the possibility of the existence of epigenetic mechanisms induced by testosterone in the worm, we studied whether the histone deacetylase inhibitor SB had any effect on the results observed in the behavior associated to the steroid hormone action. Acute administration of SB resulted in marked increase in acetylation of histone H3 lysine 14 and histone H4 lysine 8 in specific tissues of mice (Itzhak et al., 2013). **Figure 5A** shows that SB (1 mM) abolishes the effect of testosterone on gentle touch response and pharyngeal pumping rate in *C. elegans*.

To determine whether the testosterone was able to induced epigenetic changes in behavior that were transgenerationally inherited, we studied its action on gentle touch response and pharyngeal pumping over several generations in the absence of the hormone. The results presented in **Figure 5B** shows that in the case of gentle touch response the effect could still extend in the four subsequent generations. However the reduction of the pharyngeal pumping rate disappeared just in the next generation.

There are mechanisms of reprogramming which are able of erasing epigenetic signatures typified by DNA methylation or histone modification (Apostolou and Hochedlinger, 2013). The life expectancy of *C. elegans* is approximately 2 weeks. However, in conditions of starvation, the developing larvae can adopt an alternative form, called the dauer stage. In this period the worm does not feed and is almost metabolically inactive (Fielenbach and Antebi, 2008). Dauer larva can survive for several months, and prolong the life span of the worm until 12 times more. The observations that the aging clock can be paused in the *C. elegans* dauer stage and reversed by environmental factors, suggest that the causes should be epigenetic mechanisms: on the one hand, blocking the gene expression in the dauer stage by epigenetic marks, and on the other hand reprogramming the metabolism and erasing these marks. For this reason it was possible that the dauer stage, could lead to the removing the epigenetic signals caused by testosterone. As seen in **Figure 5C**, when the worms were maintained on testosterone until dauer stage, and then growing on plates without the hormone, the gentle touch response and the pharyngeal pumping rate were similar to the control without testosterone.

DISCUSSION

In humans, testosterone performs critical functions from pregnancy to adolescence. An elevated level of testosterone during early human embryo development has been hypothesized to be a risk factor for ASDs. This idea is supported by several studies showing that high maternal testosterone levels are associated with autistic-like traits in the offspring. The mechanisms by which testosterone interacts with cells and carries out its effects on the development of the nervous system are poorly understood.

This study examines the effect of testosterone in two different behavioral traits of the nematode *C. elegans*, the response to gentle touch stimulation and the pharyngeal pumping rate. The presence of the hormone in the culture media induced the loss of a significant capacity of the reaction to gentle touch stimuli. In fact, it was observed that mechanic stimulation with an eyebrow hair led to a reduction in the response to the fourth and fifth touch of five consecutive touches in both the anterior and posterior parts of the body. Testosterone also induced a decrease in the pharyngeal pumping rate. These behaviors are mediated by distinct neural circuits, suggesting a broad impact of testosterone on neuronal synapse functionality. The way by which testosterone

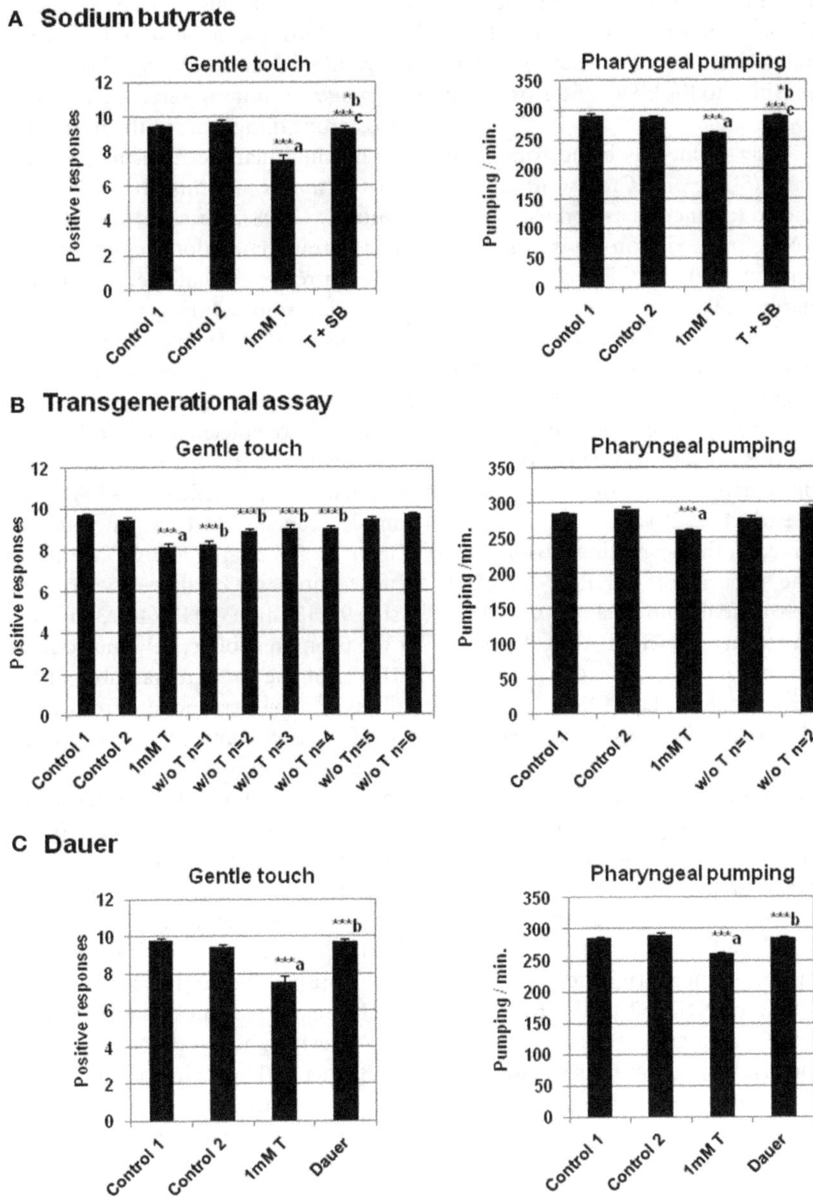

FIGURE 5 | Sodium butyrate and dauer stage abolish the effect of testosterone in gentle touch response and pharyngeal pumping rate. Transgenerational epigenetic inheritance of testosterone in *C. elegans*. **(A)** Sodium butyrate (SB) (1 mM) recues impaired gentle touch response (left panel) and pharyngeal pumping rate (right panel) in N2 wild type strain growing in the presence of 1 mM testosterone. **(B)** Transgenerational effect of the testosterone on gentle touch response (left panel) and pharyngeal pumping rate (right panel) in N2 wild type strain after several generations (n) in the absence of testosterone ("w/o T"). **(C)** Analysis of the testosterone effect on gentle touch response (left panel) and pharyngeal pumping rate (right panel) in N2 wild type strain after dauer stage (Dauer). At least three independent experiments were carried out (at least 10 L4 worms per experiment). Bars represent the mean ± SEM. Statistical significance was calculated by 1-factor-ANOVA. Statistical *p*-values in **(A)**: ***a $p < 0.001$ *vs.* "Control 1"; *b $p < 0.05$ *vs.* "Control 2". ***c $p < 0.001$ *vs.* "1 mM T". Control 1: NGM + 0.7% ETOH; Control 2: NGM + 0.7% ETOH + 1 mM sodium butyrate; 1 mM T: NGM + 0.7% ETOH + 1 mM testosterone; T + SB: NGM + 0.7% ETOH + 1 mM testosterone + 1 mM sodium butyrate. Statistical *p*-values in **(B)**: ***a $p < 0.001$ *vs.* "Control 2"; ***b $p < 0.001$ *vs.* "Control 1". Control 1: NGM; Control 2: NGM + 0.7% ETOH; 1 mM T: NGM + 0.7% ETOH + 1 mM testosterone. Statistical *p*-values in **(C)**: ***a $p < 0.001$ *vs.* "Control 2". ***b $p < 0.001$ *vs.* "1 mM T". Control 1: NGM; Control 2: NGM + 0.7% ETOH; 1 mM T: NGM + 0.7% ETOH + 1 mM testosterone.

affect the nervous system function is presumably by altering gene expression through a nuclear hormone receptor.

The genome of *C. elegans* contains at least 284 predicted nuclear receptor genes (Gissendanner et al., 2004). This number outnumbers those in mammals (~50 genes) (Zhang et al., 2004). A BLAST search with the human androgen receptor ligand-binding domain sequence against protein sequences of *C. elegans* resulted in several potential orthologous genes. Between them,

NHR-69 presented the best matching sequence with the human AR receptor ligand-binding domain. Accordingly with this finding, we observed that the strain RB1578 with a deletion in the gene *nhr-69* (*ok1926*) was insensitive to the effect of testosterone in both behavioral assays.

The gene *nhr-69* was previously defined as being conserved between *C. elegans* and humans (Shaye and Greenwald, 2011). Furthermore, NHR-69 is predicted to function as a transcription factor that could activate or repress transcription in response to a hormonal signal (Gissendanner et al., 2004). A GFP-reporter gene for *nhr-69* was expressed in pharynx, hypodermis, intestine, rectal epithelium, and uterine toroidal epithelial (Gissendanner et al., 2004). In addition a NHR-69::GFP fusion protein driven by the *nhr-69* promoter was detected in the nucleus of the E8 intestinal precursor cells in developing embryos, expression that persisted until adulthood. In adults, expression was also detected in the ASI sensory neurons (gustatory-chemosensory, thermosensory), hypodermis, and tail neurons (Park et al., 2012).

Supporting the results observed in this work, previous *in vitro* experiments demonstrated the capacity of NHR-69 to bind both progesterone and testosterone (Mimoto et al., 2007). More recently it was found that NHR-69 partners with DAF-8. A model is proposed where this interaction represses the *exp-2* gene that encodes a voltage-gated potassium channel. Low EXP-2 increases the secretion of the insulin-like peptide DAF-28 in ASI neurons (Park et al., 2012).

In respect of insulin it has been shown that pan-neuronal expression of APL-1, the *C. elegans* ortholog of the human amyloid precursor protein, disrupts several behavioral traits of the nematode. All these behaviors require activity of the transforming growth factor beta (TGF-beta) signaling pathway and reduced activity of the insulin pathway (Ewald et al., 2012). This might explain, at least indirectly, some of the effect originated by testosterone in behavior, if the binding of NHR-69 to the hormone compete the binding to DAF-8, and therefore modify insulin secretion and the activity of the insulin pathway. It is known that age-dependent neuronal defects are regulated by insulin signaling pathway (Peng et al., 2011).

We also found that the effects of testosterone on behavior were eliminated in presence of the deacetylase inhibitor SB and after dauer stage. Both experimental conditions suggest possible epigenetic mechanisms. In the case of sodium butyrate it is known that inhibits histone deacetylation in mammalian culture cells (Candido et al., 1978) and increases histone acetylation in *C. elegans* (Zhang et al., 2009). More recently was shown that an acute administration of SB resulted in a marked increase in acetylation of histone H3 at lysine 14 and histone H4 at lysine 8 in specific tissues of mice (Itzhak et al., 2013). In respect of dauer larval stage it was demonstrated that transiently passed through this stage, post-dauer adults exhibited significant changes in gene expression profiles and chromatin states when compared with control adults (Hall et al., 2010), which suggests a mechanism of DNA-chromatin reprogramming able to erase epigenetic marks.

Interestingly, we observed that the effect of testosterone in the gentle touch response was maintained, in the absence of the hormone, in the four subsequent generations after the exposition to the steroid. This observation suggests that the epigenetic effects of testosterone can be inherited transgenerationally. However, the results in the gentle touch contrast with the observed in the pharyngeal pumping rate, where the reduction rate induced by testosterone disappears in the next generation.

The molecular mechanisms underlying transgeneracional epigenetic marks are insufficiently understood (Youngson and Whitelaw, 2008). Research in *C. elegans* has illustrated several cases of transgenerational epigenetic inheritance. For example, it has been reported that modified histones incorporated into the sex chromosomes during spermatogenesis persist for several cell divisions postfertilization (Bean et al., 2004). One possible explanation for the differences between the gentle touch response and pharyngeal pumping rate after the exposure to testosterone is that the removal of epigenetic marks between generations depends on their position in the genome. Regarding this idea, a recent study demonstrates that deficiencies in genes involved in the COMPASS complex can induce transgenerational inheritance of longevity (Greer et al., 2011). The COMPASS complex, conserved from yeast to humans, catalyzes the trimethylation of histone H3 at lysine 9 (H3K4me3). H3K4me3 histone marks are usually present at the promoters of actively transcribed genes (Barth and Imhof, 2010). But the most remarkable phenomenon was that genetically wild type descendants from ancestors with a mutation in the COMPASS complex still display extended lifespan until the third generation (Greer et al., 2011). Interestingly, the number of genes showing down differential regulation was 7820 and 1740 genes in P0 and F4 generations respectively, in respect of the wild type strain. This observation suggests that the transgenerationally inherited gene misexpression profile returned to normal at the next (F5) generation, suggesting that these phenotypes may be directly linked. Thus, in this case the H3K4me3 dearth would be replenished, but only progressively, at each generation, until the chromatin state near the key mediator genes responsible for the longevity phenotype could be completely reset (Benayoun and Brunet, 2012). A similar mechanism could explain the differences between the gentle touch response and pharyngeal pumping rate phenotypes in successive generations after the exposure to testosterone.

Other potential molecular mechanism underlying the transgenerational inheritance could be activated by the production and transmission of non-coding RNAs. The introduction of double-stranded RNA (dsRNA) triggered sequence-specific genetic interference (RNAi) that was transmitted to offspring with the single sperm and maintained for three or more generations (Grishok et al., 2000; Grishok, 2013 and references therein). To this respect, genomic analysis demonstrated a connection between RNAi, chromatin and transgenerational RNAi inheritance (Gu et al., 2012). This work identified dsRNA-induced histone H3 lysine 9 trimethylation (H3K9me3) marks at several loci in animals fed with dsRNA. These H3K9me3 marks were also present in the F1 and F2 progenies, and they could spread up to 11 kb away from the dsRNA trigger region (Gu et al., 2012). On other hand, it was shown that a germline nuclear small RNA/chromatin pathway can maintain stable inheritance for many generations when triggered by a piwi-interacting RNA (piRNA)-dependent foreign RNA response (Ashe et al., 2012). There is a recent report that relates testosterone, epigenetic, and miRNA function (Morgan and Bale, 2011).

In conclusion, our results demonstrate that testosterone can influence the behavior of *C. elegans*. The hormone appears to act causing epigenetic marks that can be inherited transgenerationally. Due to the finding of a positive association between elevated levels of fetal testosterone and autistic traits in humans, these results found in the nematode may be relevant to the understanding of mechanisms by which the hormone may interact with the nervous system.

ACKNOWLEDGMENTS

We thank the Caenorhabditis Genetics Center, funded by the NIH National Center for Research Resources, for worm strains, and Julián Cerón, Peter Askjaer, and Antonio Miranda-Vizuete for sharing bacterial strains and plasmids. We are very grateful to Antonio Moreno-Herrera for critical reading and reviewing the manuscript and José Antonio Bárcena for his help in analyzing protein sequences. We also thank Fernando Calahorro and Patricia G. Izquierdo for helpful comments and advices in the laboratory. Comments from Encarna Alejandre and assistance from Isabel Caballero are sincerely acknowledged. The research work has been supported by grant number PI0197 from Consejería de Salud, Junta de Andalucía Spain, and ITC20111029 from CDTI (Centro para el Desarrollo Tecnológico Industrial), Spain.

REFERENCES

Apostolou, E., and Hochedlinger, K. (2013). Chromatin dynamics during cellular reprogramming. *Nature* 502, 462–471. doi: 10.1038/nature12749

Ashe, A., Sapetschnig, A., Weick, E. M., Mitchell, J., Bagijn, M. P., Cording, A. C., et al. (2012). piRNAs can trigger a multigenerational epigenetic memory in the germline of *C. elegans. Cell* 150, 88–99. doi: 10.1016/j.cell.2012.06.018

Auyeung, B., Ahluwalia, J., Thomson, L., Taylor, K., Hackett, G., O'Donnell, K. J., et al. (2012). Prenatal versus postnatal sex steroid hormone effects on autistic traits in children at 18 to 24 months of age. *Mol. Autism* 3, 17. doi: 10.1186/2040-2392-3-17

Auyeung, B., Baron-Cohen, S., Ashwin, E., Knickmeyer, R., Taylor, K., and Hackett, G. (2009). Fetal testosterone and autistic traits. *Br. J. Psychol.* 100, 1–22. doi: 10.1348/000712608X311731

Auyeung, B., Taylor, K., Hackett, G., and Baron-Cohen, S. (2010). Foetal testosterone and autistic traits in 18 to 24-month-old children. *Mol. Autism* 1:11. doi: 10.1186/2040-2392-1-11

Avery, L., and Horvitz, H. R. (1989). Pharyngeal pumping continues after laser killing of the pharyngeal nervous system of *C. elegans. Neuron* 3, 473–485. doi: 10.1016/0896-6273(89)90206-7

Baird, G., Simonoff, E., Pickles, A., Chandler, S., Loucas, T., Meldrum, D., et al. (2006). Prevalence of disorders of the autism spectrum in a population cohort of children in South Thames: the Special Needs and Autism Project (SNAP). *Lancet* 368, 210–215. doi: 10.1016/S0140-6736(06)69041-7

Baron-Cohen, S., Lutchmaya, S., and Knickmeyer, R. (2004). *Prenatal Testosterone in Mind.* Cambridge, MA: The MIT Press.

Baron-Cohen, S., Richler, J., Bisarya, D., Gurunathan, N., and Wheelwright, S. (2003). The systemizing quotient: an investigation of adults with Asperger syndrome or high-functioning autism, and normal sex differences. *Philos. Trans. R. Soc. Lond. B Biol. Sci.* 358, 361–374. doi: 10.1098/rstb.2002.1206

Barth, T. K., and Imhof, A. (2010). Fast signals and slow marks: the dynamics of histone modifications. *Trends Biochem. Sci.* 35, 618–626. doi: 10.1016/j.tibs.2010.05.006

Bean, C. J., Schaner, C. E., and Kelly, W. G. (2004). Meiotic pairing and imprinted X chromatin assembly in *Caenorhabditis elegans. Nat. Genet.* 36, 100–105. doi: 10.1038/ng1283

Benayoun, B. A., and Brunet, A. (2012). Epigenetic memory of longevity in *Caenorhabditis elegans. Worm* 1, 77–81. doi: 10.4161/worm.19157

Benkert, P., Kunzli, M., and Schwede, T. (2009). QMEAN server for protein model quality estimation. *Nucleic Acids Res.* 37, W510–W514. doi: 10.1093/nar/gkp322

Benkert, P., Tosatto, S. C., and Schomburg, D. (2008). QMEAN: a comprehensive scoring function for model quality assessment. *Proteins* 71, 261–277. doi: 10.1002/prot.21715

Bessa, C., Maciel, P., and Rodrigues, A. J. (2013). Using *C. elegans* to decipher the cellular and molecular mechanisms underlying neurodevelopmental disorders. *Mol. Neurobiol.* 48, 465–489. doi: 10.1007/s12035-013-8434-6

Bird, A. (2002). DNA methylation patterns and epigenetic memory. *Genes Dev.* 16, 6–21. doi: 10.1101/gad.947102

Bounoutas, A., and Chalfie, M. (2007). Touch sensitivity in *Caenorhabditis elegans. Pflugers Arch.* 454, 691–702. doi: 10.1007/s00424-006-0187-x

Brenner, S. (1974). The genetics of *Caenorhabditis elegans. Genetics* 77, 71–94.

Brinkmann, A. O. (2011). Molecular mechanisms of androgen action–a historical perspective. *Methods Mol. Biol.* 776, 3–24. doi: 10.1007/978-1-61779-243-4_1

Broue, F., Liere, P., Kenyon, C., and Baulieu, E. E. (2007). A steroid hormone that extends the lifespan of *Caenorhabditis elegans. Aging Cell* 6, 87–94. doi: 10.1111/j.1474-9726.2006.00268.x

Calahorro, F., Alejandre, E., and Ruiz-Rubio, M. (2009). Osmotic avoidance in *Caenorhabditis elegans*: synaptic function of two genes, orthologues of human NRXN1 and NLGN1, as candidates for autism. *J. Vis. Exp.* 34:e1616. doi: 10.3791/1616

Calahorro, F., and Ruiz-Rubio, M. (2011). *Caenorhabditis elegans* as an experimental tool for the study of complex neurological diseases: Parkinson's disease, Alzheimer's disease and autism spectrum disorder. *Invert. Neurosci.* 11, 73–83. doi: 10.1007/s10158-011-0126-1

Calahorro, F., and Ruiz-Rubio, M. (2012). Functional phenotypic rescue of *Caenorhabditis elegans* neuroligin-deficient mutants by the human and rat NLGN1 genes. *PLoS ONE* 7:e39277. doi: 10.1371/journal.pone.0039277

Calahorro, F., and Ruiz-Rubio, M. (2013). Human alpha- and beta-NRXN1 isoforms rescue behavioral impairments of *Caenorhabditis elegans* neurexin-deficient mutants. *Genes Brain Behav.* 12, 453–464. doi: 10.1111/gbb.12046

Calixto, A., Chelur, D., Topalidou, I., Chen, X., and Chalfie, M. (2010). Enhanced neuronal RNAi in *C. elegans* using SID-1. *Nat. Methods* 7, 554–559. doi: 10.1038/nmeth.1463

Candido, E. P., Reeves, R., and Davie, J. R. (1978). Sodium butyrate inhibits histone deacetylation in cultured cells. *Cell* 14, 105–113. doi: 10.1016/0092-8674(78)90305-7

Catoire, H., Pasco, M. Y., Abu-Baker, A., Holbert, S., Tourette, C., Brais, B., et al. (2008). Sirtuin inhibition protects from the polyalanine muscular dystrophy protein PABPN1. *Hum. Mol. Genet.* 17, 2108–2117. doi: 10.1093/hmg/ddn109

Chakrabarti, B., Dudbridge, F., Kent, L., Wheelwright, S., Hill-Cawthorne, G., Allison, C., et al. (2009). Genes related to sex steroids, neural growth, and social-emotional behavior are associated with autistic traits, empathy, and Asperger syndrome. *Autism Res.* 2, 157–177. doi: 10.1002/aur.80

Chalfie, M., Sulston, J. E., White, J. G., Southgate, E., Thomson, J. N., and Brenner, S. (1985). The neural circuit for touch sensitivity in *Caenorhabditis elegans. J. Neurosci.* 5, 956–964.

Chua, Y. L., Watson, L. A., and Gray, J. C. (2003). The transcriptional enhancer of the pea plastocyanin gene associates with the nuclear matrix and regulates gene expression through histone acetylation. *Plant Cell* 15, 1468–1479. doi: 10.1105/tpc.011825

Cohen-Bendahan, C. C., Buitelaar, J. K., van Goozen, S. H., Orlebeke, J. F., and Cohen-Kettenis, P. T. (2005a). Is there an effect of prenatal testosterone on aggression and other behavioral traits? A study comparing same-sex and opposite-sex twin girls. *Horm. Behav.* 47, 230–237. doi: 10.1016/j.yhbeh.2004.10.006

Cohen-Bendahan, C. C., van de Beek, C., and Berenbaum, S. A. (2005b). Prenatal sex hormone effects on child and adult sex-typed behavior: methods and findings. *Neurosci. Biobehav. Rev.* 29, 353–384. doi: 10.1016/j.neubiorev.2004.11.004

Ewald, C. Y., Cheng, R., Tolen, L., Shah, V., Gillani, A., Nasrin, A., et al. (2012). Pan-neuronal expression of APL-1, an APP-related protein, disrupts olfactory, gustatory, and touch plasticity in *Caenorhabditis elegans. J. Neurosci.* 32, 10156–10169. doi: 10.1523/JNEUROSCI.0495-12.2012

Fielenbach, N., and Antebi, A. (2008). *C. elegans* dauer formation and the molecular basis of plasticity. *Genes Dev.* 22, 2149–2165. doi: 10.1101/gad.1701508

Galikova, M., Klepsatel, P., Senti, G., and Flatt, T. (2010). Steroid hormone regulation of *C. elegans* and Drosophila aging and life history. *Exp. Gerontol.* 46, 141–147. doi: 10.1016/j.exger.2010.08.021

Gissendanner, C. R., Crossgrove, K., Kraus, K. A., Maina, C. V., and Sluder, A. E. (2004). Expression and function of conserved nuclear receptor genes in *Caenorhabditis elegans*. *Dev. Biol.* 266, 399–416. doi: 10.1016/j.ydbio.2003.10.014

Greer, E. L., Maures, T. J., Ucar, D., Hauswirth, A. G., Mancini, E., Lim, J. P., et al. (2011). Transgenerational epigenetic inheritance of longevity in *Caenorhabditis elegans*. *Nature* 479, 365–371. doi: 10.1038/nature10572

Grishok, A. (2013). Biology and mechanisms of short RNAs in *Caenorhabditis elegans*. *Adv. Genet.* 83, 1–69. doi: 10.1016/B978-0-12-407675-4.00001-8

Grishok, A., Tabara, H., and Mello, C. C. (2000). Genetic requirements for inheritance of RNAi in *C. elegans*. *Science* 287, 2494–2497. doi: 10.1126/science.287.5462.2494

Gu, S. G., Pak, J., Guang, S., Maniar, J. M., Kennedy, S., and Fire, A. (2012). Amplification of siRNA in *Caenorhabditis elegans* generates a transgenerational sequence-targeted histone H3 lysine 9 methylation footprint. *Nat. Genet.* 44, 157–164. doi: 10.1038/ng.1039

Hall, S. E., Beverly, M., Russ, C., Nusbaum, C., and Sengupta, P. (2010). A cellular memory of developmental history generates phenotypic diversity in *C. elegans*. *Curr. Biol.* 20, 149–155. doi: 10.1016/j.cub.2009.11.035

Henningsson, S., Jonsson, L., Ljunggren, E., Westberg, L., Gillberg, C., Rastam, M., et al. (2009). Possible association between the androgen receptor gene and autism spectrum disorder. *Psychoneuroendocrinology* 34, 752–761. doi: 10.1016/j.psyneuen.2008.12.007

Hines, M. (2008). Early androgen influences on human neural and behavioural development. *Early Hum. Dev.* 84, 805–807. doi: 10.1016/j.earlhumdev.2008.09.006

Hunter, J. W., Mullen, G. P., McManus, J. R., Heatherly, J. M., Duke, A., and Rand, J. B. (2010). Neuroligin-deficient mutants of *C. elegans* have sensory processing deficits and are hypersensitive to oxidative stress and mercury toxicity. *Dis. Model. Mech.* 3, 366–376. doi: 10.1242/dmm.003442

Itzhak, Y., Liddie, S., and Anderson, K. L. (2013). Sodium butyrate-induced histone acetylation strengthens the expression of cocaine-associated contextual memory. *Neurobiol. Learn. Mem.* 102, 34–42. doi: 10.1016/j.nlm.2013.03.007

Izquierdo, P. G., Calahorro, F., and Ruiz-Rubio, M. (2013). Neuroligin modulates the locomotory dopaminergic and serotonergic neuronal pathways of *C. elegans*. *Neurogenetics* 14, 233–242. doi: 10.1007/s10048-013-0377-6

Jackson, A. L., Bartz, S. R., Schelter, J., Kobayashi, S. V., Burchard, J., Mao, M., et al. (2003). Expression profiling reveals off-target gene regulation by RNAi. *Nat. Biotechnol.* 21, 635–637. doi: 10.1038/nbt831

Jarrell, T. A., Wang, Y., Bloniarz, A. E., Brittin, C. A., Xu, M., Thomson, J. N., et al. (2012). The connectome of a decision-making neural network. *Science* 337, 437–444. doi: 10.1126/science.1221762

Kamath, R. S., and Ahringer, J. (2003). Genome-wide RNAi screening in *Caenorhabditis elegans*. *Methods* 30, 313–321. doi: 10.1016/S1046-2023(03)00050-1

Keller, F., and Ruta, L. (2010). "The male prevalence in autism spectrum disorders: hypotheses on its neurobiological basis," in *The Neurochemical Basis of Autism: From Molecules to Minicolumns*, ed G. J. Blatt (New York, NY: Springer), 13–28.

Lintas, C., Sacco, R., Garbett, K., Mirnics, K., Militerni, R., Bravaccio, C., et al. (2009). Involvement of the PRKCB1 gene in autistic disorder: significant genetic association and reduced neocortical gene expression. *Mol. Psychiatry* 14, 705–718. doi: 10.1038/mp.2008.21

Mandy, W., Charman, T., Gilmour, J., and Skuse, D. (2011). Toward specifying pervasive developmental disorder-not otherwise specified. *Autism Res.* 4, 121–131. doi: 10.1002/aur.178

Mbadiwe, T., and Millis, R. M. (2013). Epigenetics and autism. *Autism Res. Treat.* 2013:826156. doi: 10.1155/2013/826156

Mercer, J. G., Munn, A. E., and Rees, H. H. (1988). *Caenorhabditis elegans*: occurrence and metabolism of ecdysteroids in adults and dauer larvae. *Comp. Biochem. Physiol. B* 90, 261–267. doi: 10.1016/0305-0491(88)90070-3

Metzger, E., Imhof, A., Patel, D., Kahl, P., Hoffmeyer, K., Friedrichs, N., et al. (2010). Phosphorylation of histone H3T6 by PKCbeta(I) controls demethylation at histone H3K4. *Nature* 464, 792–796. doi: 10.1038/nature08839

Metzger, E., Wissmann, M., and Schule, R. (2006). Histone demethylation and androgen-dependent transcription. *Curr. Opin. Genet. Dev.* 16, 513–517. doi: 10.1016/j.gde.2006.08.013

Mimoto, A., Fujii, M., Usami, M., Shimamura, M., Hirabayashi, N., Kaneko, T., et al. (2007). Identification of an estrogenic hormone receptor in *Caenorhabditis elegans*. *Biochem. Biophys. Res. Commun.* 364, 883–888. doi: 10.1016/j.bbrc.2007.10.089

Morgan, C. P., and Bale, T. L. (2011). Early prenatal stress epigenetically programs dysmasculinization in second-generation offspring via the paternal lineage. *J. Neurosci.* 31, 11748–11755. doi: 10.1523/JNEUROSCI.1887-11.2011

Morrison, C., and Rieder, C. L. (2004). Chromosome damage and progression into and through mitosis in vertebrates. *DNA Repair (Amst.)* 3, 1133–1139. doi: 10.1016/j.dnarep.2004.03.005

Murray, E. K., Hien, A., de Vries, G. J., and Forger, N. G. (2009). Epigenetic control of sexual differentiation of the bed nucleus of the stria terminalis. *Endocrinology* 150, 4241–4247. doi: 10.1210/en.2009-0458

O'Hagan, R., Chalfie, M., and Goodman, M. B. (2005). The MEC-4 DEG/ENaC channel of *Caenorhabditis elegans* touch receptor neurons transduces mechanical signals. *Nat. Neurosci.* 8, 43–50. doi: 10.1038/nn1362

Palomba, S., Marotta, R., Di Cello, A., Russo, T., Falbo, A., Orio, F., et al. (2012). Pervasive developmental disorders in children of hyperandrogenic women with polycystic ovary syndrome: a longitudinal case-control study. *Clin. Endocrinol. (Oxf.)* 77, 898–904. doi: 10.1111/j.1365-2265.2012.04443.x

Park, D., Jones, K. L., Lee, H., Snutch, T. P., Taubert, S., and Riddle, D. L. (2012). Repression of a potassium channel by nuclear hormone receptor and TGF-beta signaling modulates insulin signaling in *Caenorhabditis elegans*. *PLoS Genet.* 8:e1002519. doi: 10.1371/journal.pgen.1002519

Peng, C. Y., Chen, C. H., Hsu, J. M., and Pan, C. L. (2011). *C. elegans* model of neuronal aging. *Commun. Integr. Biol.* 4, 696–698. doi: 10.4161/cib.4.6.17138

Raisman, G., and Field, P. M. (1973). Sexual dimorphism in the neuropil of the preoptic area of the rat and its dependence on neonatal androgen. *Brain Res.* 54, 1–29. doi: 10.1016/0006-8993(73)90030-9

Roy, A. K., Lavrovsky, Y., Song, C. S., Chen, S., Jung, M. H., Velu, N. K., et al. (1999). Regulation of androgen action. *Vitam. Horm.* 55, 309–352. doi: 10.1016/S0083-6729(08)60938-3

Ruiz-Cortes, Z. T., Kimmins, S., Monaco, L., Burns, K. H., Sassone-Corsi, P., and Murphy, B. D. (2005). Estrogen mediates phosphorylation of histone H3 in ovarian follicle and mammary epithelial tumor cells via the mitotic kinase, Aurora B. *Mol. Endocrinol.* 19, 2991–3000. doi: 10.1210/me.2004-0441

Saenz, J., and Alexander, G. M. (2013). Postnatal testosterone levels and disorder relevant behavior in the second year of life. *Biol. Psychol.* 94, 152–159. doi: 10.1016/j.biopsycho.2013.05.011

Shaye, D. D., and Greenwald, I. (2011). OrthoList: a compendium of *C. elegans* genes with human orthologs. *PLoS ONE* 6:e20085. doi: 10.1371/journal.pone.0020085

Shim, Y. H., Chun, J. H., Lee, E. Y., and Paik, Y. K. (2002). Role of cholesterol in germ-line development of *Caenorhabditis elegans*. *Mol. Reprod. Dev.* 61, 358–366. doi: 10.1002/mrd.10099

Teatero, M. L., and Netley, C. (2013). A critical review of the research on the extreme male brain theory and digit ratio (2D:4D). *J. Autism Dev. Disord.* 43, 2664–2676. doi: 10.1007/s10803-013-1819-6

Tie, F., Banerjee, R., Stratton, C. A., Prasad-Sinha, J., Stepanik, V., Zlobin, A., et al. (2009). CBP-mediated acetylation of histone H3 lysine 27 antagonizes Drosophila polycomb silencing. *Development* 136, 3131–3141. doi: 10.1242/dev.037127

Timmons, L., Court, D. L., and Fire, A. (2001). Ingestion of bacterially expressed dsRNAs can produce specific and potent genetic interference in *Caenorhabditis elegans*. *Gene* 263, 103–112. doi: 10.1016/S0378-1119(00)00579-5

Tominaga, N., Ura, K., Kawakami, M., Kawaguchi, T., Kohra, S., Mitsui, Y., et al. (2003). *Caenorhabditis elegans* responses to specific steroid hormones. *J. Health Sci.* 49, 28–33. doi: 10.1248/jhs.49.28

White, J. G., Southgate, E., Thomson, J. N., and Brenner, S. (1986). The structure of the nervous system of the nematode *Caenorhabditis elegans*. *Philos. Trans. R. Soc. Lond. B Biol. Sci.* 314, 1–340. doi: 10.1098/rstb.1986.0056

Whitehouse, A. J., Mattes, E., Maybery, M. T., Dissanayake, C., Sawyer, M., Jones, R. M., et al. (2012). Perinatal testosterone exposure and autistic-like traits in the general population: a longitudinal pregnancy-cohort study. *J. Neurodev. Disord.* 4, 25. doi: 10.1186/1866-1955-4-25

Youngson, N. A., and Whitelaw, E. (2008). Transgenerational epigenetic effects. *Annu. Rev. Genomics Hum. Genet.* 9, 233–257. doi: 10.1146/annurev.genom.9.081307.164445

Yu, Y., Teng, Y., Liu, H., Reed, S. H., and Waters, R. (2005). UV irradiation stimulates histone acetylation and chromatin remodeling at a repressed yeast locus. *Proc. Natl. Acad. Sci. U.S.A.* 102, 8650–8655. doi: 10.1073/pnas.0501458102

Zettergren, A., Jonsson, L., Johansson, D., Melke, J., Lundstrom, S., Anckarsater, H., et al. (2013). Associations between polymorphisms in sex steroid related genes and autistic-like traits. *Psychoneuroendocrinology* 38, 2575–2584. doi: 10.1016/j.psyneuen.2013.06.004

Zhang, M., Poplawski, M., Yen, K., Cheng, H., Bloss, E., Zhu, X., et al. (2009). Role of CBP and SATB-1 in aging, dietary restriction, and insulin-like signaling. *PLoS Biol.* 7:e1000245. doi: 10.1371/journal.pbio.1000245

Zhang, Z., Burch, P. E., Cooney, A. J., Lanz, R. B., Pereira, F. A., Wu, J., et al. (2004). Genomic analysis of the nuclear receptor family: new insights into structure, regulation, and evolution from the rat genome. *Genome Res.* 14, 580–590. doi: 10.1101/gr.2160004

Zhu, X., Asa, S. L., and Ezzat, S. (2008). Fibroblast growth factor 2 and estrogen control the balance of histone 3 modifications targeting MAGE-A3 in pituitary neoplasia. *Clin. Cancer Res.* 14, 1984–1996. doi: 10.1158/1078-0432.CCR-07-2003

8

Synaptic proteins and receptors defects in autism spectrum disorders

***Jianling Chen*[1†], *Shunying Yu*[1*†], *Yingmei Fu*[1] and *Xiaohong Li*[2]**

[1] *Shanghai Key Laboratory of Psychotic Disorders, Shanghai Mental Health Center, Shanghai Jiao Tong University School of Medicine, Shanghai, China*
[2] *Department of Neurochemistry, New York State Institute for Basic Research in Developmental Disabilities, Staten Island, NY, USA*

Correspondence:
Shunying Yu, Shanghai Key Laboratory of Psychotic Disorders, Shanghai Mental Health Center, Shanghai Jiao Tong University School of Medicine, 600 Wanping Nan Road, Shanghai 200030, China
e-mail: yushuny@gmail.com

†Jianling Chen and Shunying Yu have contributed equally to this work.

Recent studies have found that hundreds of genetic variants, including common and rare variants, rare and *de novo* mutations, and common polymorphisms contribute to the occurrence of autism spectrum disorders (ASDs). The mutations in a number of genes such as neurexin, neuroligin, postsynaptic density protein 95, SH3, and multiple ankyrin repeat domains 3 (*SHANK3*), synapsin, gephyrin, cadherin, and protocadherin, thousand-and-one-amino acid 2 kinase, and contactin, have been shown to play important roles in the development and function of synapses. In addition, synaptic receptors, such as gamma-aminobutyric acid receptors and glutamate receptors, have also been associated with ASDs. This review will primarily focus on the defects of synaptic proteins and receptors associated with ASDs and their roles in the pathogenesis of ASDs via synaptic pathways.

Keywords: autism spectrum disorders, synaptic protein, GABA, PSD-95, SHANK3, TAOK2

INTRODUCTION

Autism spectrum disorders (ASDs) are a heterogeneous group of neurodevelopmental disorders characterized by social communication deficits and stereotyped behaviors with restricted interests (American Psychiatry Association [APA], 2013). Autism was first reported by Kanner (1943), who described seven boys and four girls who exhibited "extreme aloneness from the very beginning of life, not responding to anything that comes to them from the outside world." Asperger (1944) described four boys with social communication difficulties. During the past 70 years, the definition of autism has developed as understanding of the disorder increased. It was first introduced as infantile autism in the official diagnostic nomenclature in the third edition of the Diagnostic and Statistical Manual of Mental Disorders (DSM-III), was referred to as Pervasive Developmental Disorders (PDD) in DSM-IV and was defined as ASDs in the latest revision of the DSM, DSM-V (American Psychiatry Association [APA], 2013), which was published in May 2013. In DSM-V, ASDs includes disorders that were previously diagnosed separately, such as autistic disorder, Asperger's disorder, childhood disintegrative disorder, and pervasive developmental disorder not otherwise specified. The decision to merge the three disorders was taken because they could not be easily distinguished from each other. Studies have shown that more than half of adults with autism have poor or very poor outcomes (Howlin et al., 2004; Billstedt et al., 2005) in terms of independent living, educational attainment, employment, and peer relationships.

Autism was considered as a rare childhood disorder, and in the first epidemiological study conducted in the UK in 1966, Lotter (1966) reported a prevalence rate of autism of 4.5 in 10,000 children. However, the prevalence of ASDs has steadily increased in the past two decades; for example, in the USA the estimated prevalence was reported to be 19 in 10,000 children in 1992 increasing to 1 in 150 in 2002, 1 in 110 in 2006, and 1 in 88 in 2008 (Rice, 2012). ASDs are recognized as a common disorder today, with a median worldwide prevalence of 0.62% (Elsabbagh et al., 2012), and boys are affected by ASDs four times more frequently than girls. The increased prevalence of ASDs is most likely because of broadened diagnostic criteria and heightened awareness, but may also partially reflect a true increase due to environmental factors acting upon a genetically vulnerable background (King and Bearman, 2009; Lintas and Persico, 2009; Li et al., 2012).

In addition to a variable severity of the core deficits, ASDs patients also present other psychiatric and medical conditions, such as intellectual disability, epilepsy, motor control problems, attention-deficit/hyperactivity disorder, tics, anxiety, sleep disorders, and gastrointestinal problems (Simonoff et al., 2008; Lai et al., 2014).

For the past several decades, ASDs have been recognized as a complex brain disorder with high heritability, except with rare pedigrees, usually accompanied with other neurodevelopmental conditions shown to have Mendelian inheritance (Morrow et al., 2008; Novarino et al., 2012). Recent genomic and genetic studies have found that hundreds of genetic variants, including common and rare variants, contribute to the occurrence of ASDs. Rare and *de novo* mutations may pose a substantial risk for ASDs and play a substantial role in population risk, and common polymorphisms also contribute to ASDs. The role of individual alleles remains elusive and underestimated due to their small effect sizes (Murdoch and State, 2013). Many genes associated with ASDs play roles in the development and function of synapses, such as neuroligin 3 (*NLGN3*), *NLGN4X*, neurexin 1 (*NRXN1*), and SH3, and multiple ankyrin repeat domains 3 (*SHANK3*).

Post-mortem studies of ASDs patients have shown a reduction in the number of neurons in the amygdala, fusiform gyrus, and cerebellum and signs of persistent neuroinflammation (Lai et al., 2014). In addition, reduction in the density of serotonin transporters (5-HTT) was also found in the deep layers of the fusiform gyrus in autistic subjects (Oblak et al., 2013). Transcriptome analyses showed that genes involved in synaptic function were downregulated in the ASDs post-mortem brain. Moreover, the emergence of various types of genetically modified mouse models targeting ASDs-associated genes or loci in recent years have provided insights into particular aspects of ASDs. Therefore, it may be proposed that ASDs are a synaptic defect disease. In this review, we will focus on the role of synaptic-related genes in ASDs.

SYNAPTIC PROTEINS, RECEPTORS, AND AUTISM SPECTRUM DISORDERS

SYNAPTIC PROTEINS AND AUTISM SPECTRUM DISORDERS

Neurexin (NRXN)

Neurexins (*NRXN*) are a family of synaptic adhesion proteins that are located on the presynaptic membrane and bind to their postsynaptic counterpart, *NLGN*s. The *NRXN* family consists of three genes (*NRXN1*, *NRXN2*, and *NRXN3*), each of them generating a long mRNA encoding α-*NRXN* and a short mRNA encoding β-*NRXN* from two independent promoters. The intracellular domains of α-*NRXN*s and β-*NRXN*s are identical, whereas the extracellular domains are different. Specifically, the extracellular domains of α-*NRXN*s contain six laminin, nectin, and sex-hormone binding globulin (LNS) domains and three epidermal growth factor (EGF) domains, which form three repeated LNS (A)-EGF-LNS (B) structure. However, β-*NRXN*s have no EGF domain and only one LNS domain (Tabuchi and Sudhof, 2002). *NRXN*1, *NRXN*2, and *NRXN*3 are located on chromosomes 2p16.3, 11q13, and 14q31, respectively. α-*NRXN* triple knockout mice had reduced synaptic Ca^{2+} channel function, which causes impaired spontaneous and evoked neurotransmitter release (Missler et al., 2003).

Rare copy number variations and/or point mutations in *NRXN* genes have been repeatedly reported to be associated with ASDs (**Table 1**). Friedman and Luiselli (2008) first reported a 320 kb *de novo* heterozygous deletion of the *NRXN*-1α promoter and exons 1–5 in a boy with cognitive impairment, autistic features and physical dysmorphism. Later, the Autism Genome Project Consortium et al. (2007) identified a *de novo* heterozygous deletion that eliminated several *NRXN1* exons, including 1α and 1β, in two affected female siblings in one ASDs family. Several other studies have also reported deletions in *NRXN1* in ASDs patients (Kim et al., 2008; Marshall et al., 2008; Morrow et al., 2008; Glessner et al., 2009; Pinto et al., 2010; Bremer et al., 2011; Levy et al., 2011). To date, no homozygous deletions in *NRXN1* have been found, which may suggest that the dosage of *NRXN*1 is very important for neurological development. P300P, an *NRXN*1 common variant, was associated with ASDs in a Chinese ASDs patient. In addition to being associated with ASDs, *NRXN1* deletions have also been reported in other psychiatric conditions, such as schizophrenia, bipolar disorder, attention deficit hyperactivity disorder, and Tourette syndrome (International Schizophrenia Consortium, 2008; Walsh et al., 2008; Guilmatre et al., 2009; Zhang et al., 2009; Sundaram et al., 2010; Lionel et al., 2011).

A truncated mutation of *NRXN2* inherited from a father with severe language delay and a family history of schizophrenia was identified by Gauthier et al in an ASDs patient (Gauthier et al., 2011). *NRXN3* deletions have also been found in four ASD individuals: one was a *de novo* mutation, two were inherited from a non-affected mother or father, and one was inherited from a father with subclinical autism (Vaags et al., 2012).

NRXN animal models have provided evidence supporting the role of *NRXN* in ASDs pathology. *NRXN*1α KO mice showed a defect in excitatory synaptic strength, with a decrease in miniature excitatory postsynaptic current frequency and in the input–output relation of evoked postsynaptic potentials (Etherton et al., 2009). Behavioral studies have shown that *NRXN*-1 deficient mice display decreased prepulse inhibition and increased grooming behaviors but no obvious changes in social behaviors or spatial learning (Etherton et al., 2009). Studies in an α-*NRXN* triple KO mice with all three α-*NRXN*s (Nrxn1α/2α/3α) deleted have shown that α-*NRXN*s were not required for synapse formation but were essential for Ca^{2+}-triggered neurotransmitter release (Missler et al., 2003).

Contactin associated protein-2 (CNTNAP2, also known as Caspr2) is a member of the *NRXN* superfamily and is involved in neuron–glia interactions and clustering K^{+} channels in myelinated axons. Strauss et al. (2006) identified a homozygous mutation of *CNTNAP2* in Amish children with PDD, seizures, and language regression (Strauss et al., 2006; **Table 1**). Bakkaloglu et al. (2008) found 13 rare non-synonymous variants unique to ASDs patients, which suggests that ASDs patients carry more *CNTNAP2* rare variants. Several other studies have also found other common polymorphisms of *CNTNAP2* that are associated with ASDs (Alarcón et al., 2008; Arking et al., 2008; Sampath et al., 2013). Interestingly, Alarcón et al. (2008) found that *CNTNAP2* provided a strong male affection bias in ASDs.

CNTNAP2 KO mice exhibited deficits in the core ASDs behavioral domains, such as stereotypic motor movements, behavioral inflexibility, communication, and social behavior abnormalities (Peñagarikano et al., 2011).

Neuroligin (NLGN)

Neuroligins (*NLGN*) are a different type of synaptic cell adhesion proteins that are located in the postsynaptic membrane. *NLGN*s bind to their adhesive counterpart *NRXN*s and play an important role in synapse formation and function (**Figure 1**). The human *NLGN* family includes five *NLGN* genes (*NLGN*1, 2, 3, 4, 4Y), which are localized at 3q26 (*NLGN1*), 17p13 (*NLGN2*), Xq13 (*NLGN3*), Xp22.3 (*NLGN4*), and Yq11.2 (*NLGN4Y*). *NLGN*s contain a large extracellular domain that shares sequence homology with acetylcholinesterase and that is necessary for β-*NRXN* binding and synaptogenic activity, two EF-hand motifs that bind to Ca^{2+}, an *O*-glycosylation region, a transmembrane domain, and a cytoplasmic C-terminal tail that contains a PSD-95/Dlg/ZO-1 (PDZ) interaction site (Dean and Dresbach, 2006; **Figure 1**). *NLGN*s-1, -3, and -4 localize mainly to glutamate synaptic sites, whereas *NLGN*-2 localizes primarily to gamma-aminobutyric acid (GABA) synapses (Missler et al.,

Table 1 | Summary of different defects in gene encoding for synaptic proteins in autism spectrum disorders.

Synaptic gene	Loci	Type of genetic defects	Reference
NRXN1	2p16.3	*de novo* heterozygous deletion	Autism Genome Project Consortium et al. (2007)
		Deletion	Pinto et al. (2010), Bremer et al. (2011)
NRXN2	11q13	Truncated mutation	Gauthier et al. (2011)
NRXN3	14q31	*de novo* deletion	Vaags et al. (2012)
		Inherited deletion	Vaags et al. (2012)
CNTNAP2		Homozygous mutation	Strauss et al. (2006)
		Rare non-synonymous variants	Bakkaloglu et al. (2008)
		Common polymorphisms	Alarcón et al. (2008), Sampath et al. (2013)
NLGN1	3q26	Common variants (rs1488545)	Talebizadeh et al. (2004), Gauthier et al. (2005)
NLGN3	Xq13	R451C transition	Jamain et al. (2003), Földy et al. (2013)
		Common variants (DXS7132)	Talebizadeh et al. (2004)
NLGN4	Xp22.3	Frameshift mutation (1186insT)	Laumonnier et al. (2004)
		Missense mutation	Yan et al. (2005)
		Deletion (1253delAG)	Laumonnier et al. (2004)
		Common variants (DXS996)	Talebizadeh et al. (2004)
SHANK3	22q13.3	Deletion	Durand et al. (2007), Gauthier et al. (2009)
		Novel non-synonymous variants	Moessner et al. (2007)
		Missense mutation	Gauthier et al. (2009)
		de novo heterozygous insertion	Durand et al. (2007)
SHANK2		*de novo* nonsense mutation	Berkel et al. (2010), Pinto et al. (2010)
SHANK1		Inherited deletion	Sato et al. (2012), Guilmatre et al. (2013)
PSD-95		Deletion	Feyder et al. (2010)
Synapsin1	Xp11.23	Nonsense mutation (Q555X)	Fassio et al. (2011)
		Mutations (A51G, A550T, T567A)	Fassio et al. (2011)
Synapsin2	3p25.2	Nonsense mutation (p.A94fs199X)	Corradi et al. (2014)
		Missense mutation (p.Y236S, p.G464R)	Corradi et al. (2014)
Gephyrin		Hemizygous deletions	Lionel et al. (2013)
		de novo deletion	Lionel et al. (2013)
		Paternally inherited deletion	Lionel et al. (2013)
CDH13	16q23	Recurrent larger genomic deletions	Sanders et al. (2011)
PCDHA		SNP	Anitha et al. (2013)
PCDH9		CNV	Betancur et al. (2009)
PCDH10		Homozygous deletion	Betancur et al. (2009)
TAOK2	16p11.2	Novel, recurrent microdeletion	Weiss et al. (2008)
		de novo deletion	Weiss et al. (2008)
		Reciprocal microduplication	Weiss et al. (2008)
CNTN4		Disruption	Roohi et al. (2009), Guo et al. (2012)

NRXN: neurexin; CNTNAP2: contactin associated protein-2; NLGN: neuroligin; CDH: cadherin; PCDH: protocadherin; TAOK2: thousand-and-one-amino acid 2 kinase; CNTN: contactin; CNV: copy number variation; SNP: Single-nucleotide polymorphism.

2003; **Figure 1**). *In vitro* and *in vivo*, *NLGN*-1 overexpression increases excitatory synaptic responses and potentiates synaptic NMDA receptor (NMDAR)/AMPAR ratios. In contrast, *NLGN*-2 overexpression increases inhibitory synaptic responses. Accordingly, the inhibition of *NLGN*-1 expression selectively decreases the NMDAR/AMPAR ratio, whereas the deletion of *NLGN*-2 selectively decreases inhibitory synaptic responses. Furthermore, *NLGN*-1 expression selectively increases the maturation but not initiation of excitatory synapse formation in adult-born neurons (Chubykin et al., 2007; Schnell et al., 2012).

The earliest report regarding the potential association of *NLGN* genes and ASDs is Jamain et al. (2003; **Table 1**). In one ASDs

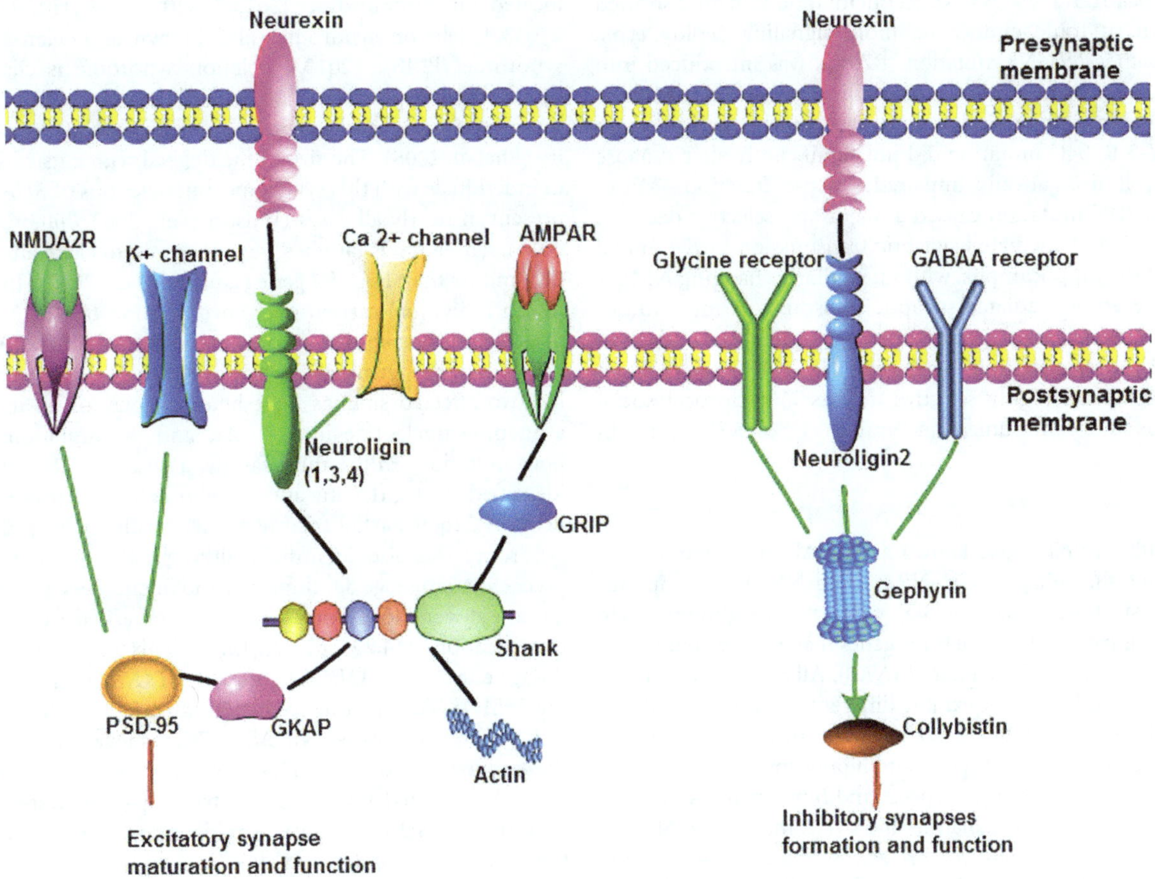

FIGURE 1 | The main synaptic proteins and receptors involved in this review in synaptogenesis and function. (1) Neuroligins(*NLGNs*) can bind to neurexins (*NRXNs*), Ca^{2+} channel and shank through their different domains to play an important role in synapse maturation and function. *NLGNs* 1, 3, and 4 localize to excitatory synaptic sites, whereas *NLGN-2* localizes primarily to inhibitory synapses. Shank are synaptic scaffold proteins that bind *NLGN–NRXN* and NMDA receptor complexes at the postsynaptic density of excitatory glutamatergic synapses. Multiple domains of shank are useful for protein–protein interaction, such as linking to actin cytoskeleton, binding to glutamate receptor-interacting protein to link with α-amino-3-hydroxy-5-methyl-4-isoxazolepropionic acid receptors. Postsynaptic density protein 95 (PSD-95) serves as a major functional bridge interconnecting the *NRXN-NLGN*-SHANK pathway. (2) Gephyrin is a key scaffold molecule of the postsynaptic membrane at inhibitory synapses. Gephyrin can interact with glycine receptor and alpha and beta subunits of the gamma-aminobutyric acid A ($GABA_A$) receptor to mediate inhibition of synapse formation and function. *NLGN* 2 can bind to protein gephyrin and activate collybistin. *NLGN* 2, gephyrin, and collybistin complexes are sufficient to inhibitory neurotransmitter receptors clustering.

multiplex family, the group found three ASDs siblings carrying one frameshift mutation (1186insT) of *NLGN4* that was inherited from the non-affected mother, creating a stop codon that led to a premature termination of the protein. In another family, a R451C transition in *NLGN3* that changed a highly conserved arginine residue into cysteine within the esterase domain was identified in two affected siblings. This point mutation was inherited from the non-affected mother. A study in a large French family found a 2 bp deletion (1253delAG) that resulted in a premature stop codon in the middle of the sequence of the normal *NLGN4* gene (Laumonnier et al., 2004). In this family, 10 males had non-specific X-linked mental retardation, two had autism, and one had pervasive developmental disorder. All affected patients had the same frameshift mutation. Missense changes in *NLGN4* were also found in Portuguese ASDs families (Yan et al., 2005). A study in a small Finnish autism sample did not find any functional mutation of *NLGN1*, *NLGN3*, *NLGN4*, or *NLNG4Y*, although three common variants (rs1488545 in *NLGN1*, DXS7132 in *NLGN3*, and DXS996 in *NLGN4*) that showed minor association with ASDs were found. Despite the evidence that *NLGN* is associated with ASDs, several studies have failed to find associations between rare mutations and common variants and ASDs (Talebizadeh et al., 2004; Vincent et al., 2004; Gauthier et al., 2005; Blasi et al., 2006; Wermter et al., 2008; Liu et al., 2013).

Several *NLGN* mutant mouse models have been developed to investigate the role of *NLGN* mutations in ASDs. Nlgn3 R451C knock-in mice, which corresponded to the human non-synonymous SNP (R451C) in *NLGN3* found in ASDs patients (Jamain et al., 2003), showed social interaction deficits and increased spatial memory and an electrophysiological phenotype consisting of increased inhibitory synaptic transmission in the somatosensory cortex (Tabuchi et al., 2007; Etherton et al., 2011a). Furthermore, researchers found that both *NLGN-3*

R451C-knockin and *NLGN*-3 knockout mutations in mice showed impairment in tonic endocannabinoid signaling (Földy et al., 2013). Another *NLGN3* mutation, R704C, was introduced into mouse *NLGN*-3 by homologous recombination, and electrophysiological and morphological studies have shown that although the *NLGN*-3 R704C mutation did not significantly alter synapse formation, it dramatically impaired synapse function. Moreover, the R704C mutation caused a major and selective decrease in AMPA receptor-mediated synaptic transmission in pyramidal neurons of the hippocampus, without similarly changing NMDA or GABA receptor-mediated synaptic transmission and without detectably altering presynaptic neurotransmitter release (Etherton et al., 2011b). Mice lacking the human *NLGN*4 (*NLGN*4-KOs) ortholog exhibited highly selective deficits in reciprocal social interactions and communication reminiscent of ASDs (Jamain et al., 2008).

Shank

Shank family proteins, also known as ProSAP, are synaptic scaffold proteins that bind *NLGN-NRXN* and NMDAR complexes at the postsynaptic density (PSD) of excitatory glutamatergic synapses (**Figure 1**). There are three genes that encode Shank proteins (*SHANK1*, *SHANK2*, and *SHANK3*). All Shank proteins are expressed in the brain but exhibit different patterns. Shank1 is expressed in most parts of the brain, except for the striatum, and it is highly expressed in the cortex and hippocampus. Shank2 and Shank3 are also present in the cortex and hippocampus. Shank2 is mostly absent from the thalamus and striatum, whereas Shank3 appears to be predominantly expressed in those regions. In the cerebellum, Shank2 is restricted to Purkinje cells, whereas Shank3 is restricted to granule cells (Sheng and Kim, 2000). *SHANK* directly or indirectly binds to *NLGNs* in the PSD. *In vitro* and *in vivo* studies highlight the important role of Shank3 for synaptic function. *SHANK3* functions as a scaffolding protein in spine morphogenesis and synaptic plasticity. Knockdown of *Shank3* in cultured hippocampal neurons leads to a reduced number and increased length of dendritic spines. When overexpressed in cultured hippocampal neurons, *Shank3* promotes the maturation and enlargement of dendritic spines (Betancur et al., 2009). Knockdown of *Shank3* in hippocampal neurons decreases spiny density, whereas transfection of *Shank3* in aspiny neurons induces the formation of dendritic spines with functional synapses (Betancur et al., 2009).

Shank contains multiple domains for protein–protein interaction, including ankyrin repeats (binding to α-fodrin to link to the actin cytoskeleton and calpain/calmodulin-mediated Ca^{2+} signaling), an SH3 domain (binding to glutamate receptor-interacting protein to link with α-amino-3-hydroxy-5-methyl-4-isoxazolepropionic acid (AMPA) receptors to the postsynaptic scaffold), a PDZ domain (binding different molecules within the PSD, including GKAP, to allow Shank to attach to PSD-95), a proline-rich region (which contains sites for Homer and cortactin), and a sterile alpha motif domain (which is involved in the polymerization of Shank molecules; Lim et al., 1999; Yoo et al., 2014; **Figure 1**).

SHANK3 was the first gene in the *SHANK* family reported to be associated with ASDs (**Table 1**). The *SHANK3* gene is located on chromosome 22q13.3 within the critical region of 22q13.3 deletion syndrome (also known as Phelan-McDermid syndrome, PMS). 22q13.3 deletion syndrome is characterized by neonatal hypotonia, global developmental delay, absent or severely delayed speech, autistic behaviors, and intellectual disability (Phelan, 2008). The size of the deleted segments varied widely in individuals with this syndrome, but deletions of *SHANK3* were present in nearly all cases (Wilson et al., 2003, 2008; Dhar et al., 2010). Three ASDs families were observed to carry alterations of 22q and/or the *SHANK3* gene (Durand et al., 2007). In one family, an individual carried a *de novo* deletion of 22q13, in which the deletion breakpoint was located in intron 8 of SHANK3 and a 142 kb of the terminal 22q13 was removed. In the second family, two affected siblings were heterozygous for an insertion of a guanine nucleotide in exon 21, and the mutation was a *de novo* mutation. In the third family, a terminal 22q deletion was identified in a girl with autism who exhibited severe language delay. A 22qter partial trisomy in her brother who had Asperger syndrome was also identified, although the boy demonstrated precocious language development and fluent speech. These unbalanced cytogenetic abnormalities were inherited from a paternal translocation, t(14;22) (p11.2;q13.33). This finding suggests a gene dosage effect of *SHANK3*. A study of *SHANK3* variants by screening *SHANK*'s exon sequence in 400 ASDs families found 10 novel non-synonymous variants in ASDs (Moessner et al., 2007). Among these mutations, one was a *de novo* mutation, and the other nine were all inherited from one unaffected parent. Rare functional mutations of *SHANK3* have been identified in two ASDs families. One was a *de novo* deletion at an intronic donor splice site, and one was a missense mutation inherited from an epileptic father (Gauthier et al., 2009). Moreover, three deleterious variants (one 6-amino acid deletion upstream of the SH3 domain, one missense variant in the PDZ domain, and one insertion/deletion of a repeated 10 bp GC sequence located 9-bp downstream from the 3′ end of exon 11) were found in Japanese ASDs families (Waga et al., 2011). It has been reported that 2.3% of ASDs patients carry deleterious mutations in *SHANK3* (Boccuto et al., 2013).

Several studies have identified *de novo* deleterious mutations of *SHANK2* in ASDs (Berkel et al., 2010; Pinto et al., 2010; Leblond et al., 2012; **Table 1**). In one study, a *de novo* nonsense mutation, seven rare inherited changes and additional variants specific to ASDs were identified by sequencing *SHANK2* in 396 ASDs patients. In a separate study, *SHANK2* was sequenced in 455 patients. When combining the results of these two studies, a significant enrichment of variants affecting conserved amino acids in 29 of 851 (3.4%) patients and 16 of 1090 (1.5%) controls was observed. In neuronal cell cultures, the variants identified in patients were associated with reduced synaptic density at dendrites compared with the variants only detected in controls (Leblond et al., 2012).

The *SHANK1* gene rare mutation has also been associated with ASDs (Sato et al., 2012; **Table 1**). An inherited deletion of 63.8 kb encompassing *SHANK1* and the *CLEC11A* gene was found in a multigenerational family. In this family, four males carrying this deletion showed high-functioning autism or a broader autism phenotype, whereas the two females carrying the same deletion were not affected by ASDs (Sato et al., 2012). *SHANK1* deletions may be associated with high-functioning autism in males (Guilmatre et al., 2013).

Genetic mouse models resembling different *SHANK* mutations have been created to investigate the role of Shank in synapse conformation and function and its contribution to autistic pathology. Shank1 mutant mice (with a deletion of exons 14 and 15, which includes most of the PDZ region, resulted in the knockout of all detectable Shank1 protein in these animals) showed decreased movement in the open field and deficits in motor learning and contextual fear conditioning. Although these animals did not show apparent repetitive behaviors and seemed to have normal levels of social interaction, they showed a general deficit in social communicative behaviors by both ultrasonic vocalizations and urine-based communicative behaviors (Hung et al., 2008; Silverman et al., 2011; Wöhr et al., 2011). Shank2 mutant mice, mimicking the human microdeletion of exons 6 and 7, which targeted the PDZ domain and knocked out of all Shank2 isoforms, also showed alterations in behavior and synaptic plasticity (Schmeisser et al., 2012; Won et al., 2012). Shank3 exons 4–9 KO mice (resulting in the loss of the longest two isoforms of Shank3) were used to mimic human SHANK3 mutation by several research groups. Although the deficits in social interaction in these models were not consistent (Bozdagi et al., 2010; Peça et al., 2011; Yang et al., 2012), all of the models showed a repetitive self-grooming phenotype (Wang et al., 2011; Yang et al., 2012).

PSD-95

Postsynaptic density protein 95 (PSD-95; also known as DLG4, SAP90), is a member of the membrane-associated guanylate kinase family of synaptic molecules and serves as a major functional bridge interconnecting the *NRXN-NLGN*-SHANK pathway (**Figure 1**). *PSD-95* contains three PDZ domains, a single interior SH3 domain, and a COOH-terminal guanylate kinase domain. The cytoplasmic domains of all three *NLGNs* bind to the third PDZ domain of PSD-95, whereas NMDA2 receptors and K^+channels bind to the first and second PDZ domains. *PSD-95* is localized at excitatory synapses and has been implicated in promoting synapse stability. *PSD-95* makes synaptic contacts more stable in older neurons than in younger neurons.

PSD-95 knockout mice exhibit reduced AMPAR function and a decreased frequency of AMPAR-mediated miniature EPSCs, suggesting that *PSD-95* may regulate synaptic maturation through postsynaptic AMPA-type glutamate receptors (GluARs).

Thus far, no rare point mutation or CNV or common variants have been reported to be associated with ASDs, but *PSD-95* deletion (*Dlg4*$^{-/-}$) mice have been shown to exhibit a complex range of behavioral and molecular abnormalities relevant to ASDs (**Table 1**). Dlg4$^{-/-}$ mice showed increased repetitive behaviors, abnormal communication and social behaviors, impaired motor coordination, increased stress reactivity, and anxiety-related responses. *Dlg4*$^{-/-}$ mice also had subtle dysmorphology of amygdala dendritic spines and altered forebrain expression of various synaptic genes (Feyder et al., 2010).

Synapsin

The synapsins are a family of presynaptic phosphoproteins that account for 9% of the vesicle protein and can regulateneurotransmitter release and neurite outgrowth (Rosahl et al., 1995). Synapsins contain a mosaic of conserved (A–C, E) and individual domains (D, F–J). They have three family members in mammals (*synapsin 1*, *synapsin 2*, and *synapsin 3*), which locate on chromosomes Xp11.23, 3p25.2, and 22q12.3, respectively. Cultured neurons from *synapsin 1,2,3(–/–)* triple knock-out mice exhibit severely dispersed synaptic vesicles and considerably reduced synaptic vesicles number (Fornasiero et al., 2012).

Mutations in *synapsin 1* (Q555X, A51G, A550T, and T567A) were found in a large French-Canadian family with epilepsy and ASDs (Fassio et al., 2011; **Table 1**). Furthermore, the nonsense Q555X mutation can reduce the phosphorylation caused by CaMKII and Mapk/Erk, which regulate synaptic vesicles trafficking and neurite outgrowth. The missense mutation of A550T and T567A can impair the targeting to nerve terminals (Fassio et al., 2011).

Synapsin 2 has also been identified as an autism predisposing gene. In a study involving 190 individuals with ASDs, researchers found one nonsense mutation (p.A94fs199X) and two missense mutations of *synapsin 2* (p.Y236S and p.G464R; Corradi et al., 2014; **Table 1**).

Synapsin knockout mice may be identified as a useful experimental model of ASDs and epilepsy. Researchers found that *synapsin* knockout mice exhibit social novelty abnormality and avoidance behavior in social approach which are reminiscent of ASDs. Specifically, *synapsin 2* deletion mice display deficits in short-term social recognition and increased repetitive self-grooming behavior. *Synapsin 1*and *synapsin 3* deletion mice display an impaired social transmission of food preference. Synapsin 1and synapsin 2 deletion mice display a decreased environmental interest (Greco et al., 2013). The results demonstrate an involvement of synapsins in the development of the behavioral traits of ASDs.

Gephyrin

Gephyrin is a key scaffold molecule of the postsynaptic membrane at inhibitory synapses (**Figure 1**). It contains three domains, G domain in N-terminal, E-domain in C-terminal, and a large linker domain of the two. Gephyrin can interact with glycine receptor and alpha and beta subunits of the $GABA_A$ receptor to mediate inhibition. *NLGN* 2 can bind to protein gephyrin through a conserved cytoplasmic motif and activate collybistin. *NLGN* 2, gephyrin, and collybistin complexes are sufficient to inhibitory neurotransmitter receptors clustering. Deletion of *NLGN* 2 in mice leads to a loss of recruitment of gephyrin at perisomatic but not dendritic sites (Poulopoulos et al., 2009; **Table 1**). Gephyrin-deficient mice die early postnatally and display loss of postsynaptic GABA(A) receptor and glycine receptors clustering, whereas glutamate receptor subunits were normally localized (Kneussel et al., 1999; Grosskreutz et al., 2003).

Exonic microdeletions in gephyrin gene have been reported a correlation with neurodevelopmental disorders including ASDs (Lionel et al., 2013). In one family, the proband with ASDs has a 357 kb *de novo* deletion in gephyrin and exhibits limited movement, slow motor development, and language delay. The second family has a 319 kb paternally inherited deletion in gephyrin and exhibits mild global developmental delay in early life, social difficulties, and repetitive behaviors. The third family has a 273 kb de novo deletion in gephyrin gene and exhibits developmental delay, cyclical seizures, and behavioral issues including anxiety, obsessive compulsive disorders, tics, and impulsive behaviors (Lionel et al., 2013).

Cadherins (CDHs) and protocadherins (PCDHs)

Cadherins (CDHs) are a family of glycosylated transmembrane proteins that mediate cell–cell adhesion, neuronal migration, spine morphology, synapse formation, and synaptic remodeling (Redies et al., 2012). Because the function of CDHs is dependent on the presence of Ca^{2+}, they are named for the Ca^{2+}-dependent cell adhesion molecule family. The CDH family is classified into classical CDHs, desmosomal cadherins, and protocadherins (PCDHs). Genome-wide association studies on a cohort of 4305 autistic subjects have shown that common variants between the *CDH9* and *CDH10* genes on chromosome 5p14.1 are associated with autism (Wang et al., 2009). Similarly, recurrent larger genomic deletions in 16q23 in *CDH13* was also observed in ASDs patients in 1124 ASDs families participating in genome-wide analyses (Sanders et al., 2011; **Table 1**). Furthermore, after the detection of 14 SNPs of protocadherin α in DNA samples of 3211 individuals with autism, 5 SNPs were showed significantly associated with autism (Anitha et al., 2013). In addition, CNVs in *PCDH9* and homozygous deletions in *PCDH10* have also been reported in ASDs (Betancur et al., 2009; **Table 1**).

In situ hybridization analysis in the embryonic and postnatal mouse demonstrated that CDH8 expression is restricted to specific developing gray matter structures. Later, a study using the PPL statistical framework identified that CDH8 is expressed in the developing human cortex of ASDs family, which implicates CDH8 in susceptibility to autism (Redies et al., 2012).

Thousand-and-one-amino acid 2 kinase (TAOK2)

Thousand-and-one-amino acid 2 kinase (TAOK2), also known as TAO2, is a serine/threonine-protein kinase that is encoded by the *TAOK2* gene in humans. It can activate mitogen-activated protein kinase (MAPK) pathways to regulate gene transcription. *TAOK2* interact with semaphorin 3A receptor neuropilin 1, which regulates basal dendrite arborization. In addition, *TAOK2* can be phosphorylated and activated by Sema3A. In cultured cortical neurons, *TAOK2* downregulation can decrease JNK phosphorylation and cause its inactivation. Furthermore, basal dendrite formation in cortical neurons caused by *TAOK2* downregulation can be rescued by active JNK1 overexpression. TAOK2 is involved in membrane blebbing, the DNA damage response, and the MAPK14/p38 MAPK stress-activated MAPK cascade. Recently, TAOK2 has been shown to play a role in basal dendrite formation (de Anda et al., 2012).

The *TAOK2* gene is located in the 16p11.2 chromosomal region. Approximately 1% of autistic subjects have been shown to have a novel, recurrent microdeletion, a *de novo* deletion of 593 kb on chromosome 16p11.2, and a reciprocal microduplication on chromosome 16p11.2 (Weiss et al., 2008), suggesting that 16p11.2 or the *TAOK2* gene is involved in susceptibility to ASDs (**Table 1**).

Contactin (CNTN)

Contactins (CNTNs) are members of the immunoglobulin superfamily. They are glycosylphosphatidylinositol-anchored neuronal membrane proteins and play important roles in axon growth and guidance and synapse formation and plasticity.

Array-based comparative genomic hybridization identified a paternally inherited chromosome 3 copy number variation in three autistic subjects. Specifically, a deletion in two siblings and a duplication in an unrelated individual were detected. Furthermore, these variations were mediated by disruptions of *CNTN4* (Roohi et al., 2009), suggesting that *CNTN4* may be involved in ASDs (**Table 1**). Recently, a study conducted in a Chinese population also came to the same conclusion (Guo et al., 2012). Although the sample sizes of these two studies were small, a CNV analysis involving 2195 autistic subjects indicated that CNTN4 deletions and duplications are associated with ASDs (Betancur et al., 2009). In a cohort of ASDs subjects, a CNV in the *CNTN5* gene was identified in one individual. In addition, a *CNTN6* deletion has also been found in an autistic family (Zuko et al., 2013).

Cntn6 knockout mice exhibited slower learning in terms of equilibrium and vestibular senses (Zuko et al., 2013), indicating that Cntn6-deficiency leads to defects in motor coordination. Other characteristics of ASDs, such as social interaction and social communication, remain to be determined in these mice. Cntn5 knockout mice exhibited decreased susceptibility to audiogenic seizures and impaired hearing, which may be related to the impairment of sensory information integration reminiscent of ASDs (Zuko et al., 2013).

SYNAPTIC RECEPTORS AND AUTISM SPECTRUM DISORDERS

GABA receptors

Gamma-aminobutyric acid is the major inhibitory neurotransmitter in the human brain and is synthesized from excitatory neurotransmitter glutamate via the action of glutamate decarboxylase (GAD) enzymes, which have two main isoforms, GAD65 and GAD67. There are two main types of GABA receptors, ionotropic $GABA_A$ receptors and metabotropic $GABA_B$ receptors. $GABA_B$ receptors are localized at pre-, post-, or extrasynaptic sites as functional heterodimers, whereas $GABA_A$ receptors are the major mediators of fast inhibitory neurotransmission in the mammalian brain.

There are three $GABA_A$ receptor genes (*GABRB3*, *GABRA5*, and *GABRG3*) localized on the human chromosome 15q11–q13, a part of the genome which is involved with genome instability, gene expression, imprinting and recombination and is one of the most complex regions in the genome (Martin et al., 2000). Duplications of the 15q11–13 locus have been observed in ASDs in several studies (Bolton et al., 2001; Kwasnicka-Crawford et al., 2007; Depienne et al., 2009). Duplication of the region containing $GABA_A$ receptor subunits may lead to excessive inhibitory neurotransmission due to gene dosage; however, an *in vitro* study using a human neuronal cell line carrying a maternal 15q duplication showed that this variant leads to reduced GABRB3 expression via impaired homologous pairing (Meguro-Horike et al., 2011), suggesting that 15q11–q13 genes are regulated epigenetically at the level of both inter- and intra-chromosomal associations and that chromosome imbalance disrupts the epigenetic regulation of genes in 15q11–q13.

Moreover, mouse models mimicking human 15q11–q13 duplication have exhibited features of autism, such as poor social interaction, behavioral inflexibility, and abnormal ultrasonic vocalizations (Nakatani et al., 2009).

$GABA_B$ receptors play an important role in maintaining excitatory-inhibitory balance in brain. In autistic brain subjects, researchers have found that the expression of $GABA_B$ receptor subunits $GABA_B$ receptor 1 (GABBR1) and $GABA_B$ receptor 2 (GABBR2) were significantly reduced (Fatemi et al., 2009). Furthermore, clinical trials show that the selective $GABA_B$ receptor agonist STX209 (arbaclofen) has a potential to improve social function and behavior in patients with fragile X syndrome and was generally well-tolerated in ASDs individuals (Berry-Kravis et al., 2012; Erickson et al., 2014).

In vitro, STX209 (arbaclofen, R-baclofen) can correct the elevated basal protein synthesis in the hippocampus of Fmr1-knockout mice, an animal model of Fragile X syndrome. *In vivo*, acute administration of STX209 can decrease mRNA translation in the cortex of Fmr1-knockout mice. Furthermore, the chronic administration of STX209 in juvenile mice can improve the increased spine density in Fmr1-knockout mice (Henderson et al., 2012). Since ASDs individuals have something in common with Fragile X syndrome, this implies that $GABA_B$ receptor agonist STX209 may also improve synaptic abnormalities in ASDs.

Consistent with the genetic evidence for the involvement of GABAergic genes in ASDs, the expression of GABAergic genes and related proteins have been reported to be reduced in the post-mortem ASDs brain. GAD65 and GAD67 proteins were reduced in the cerebellum and parietal cortex (Fatemi et al., 2002), GAD67 mRNA was reduced in cerebellar Purkinje cells (Yip et al., 2007), and $GABA_A$ receptor binding was reduced in the hippocampus (Blatt et al., 2001) and anterior and posterior cingulate cortices (Oblak et al., 2009, 2011).

Although technical difficulties still exist, researchers have attempted to measure GABA function *in vivo*, and these results support the presence of GABAergic defects in ASDs patients. Using proton magnetic resonance spectroscopy ([^{1}H]MRS; Harada et al., 2011) reported that GABA concentrations were reduced in the frontal cortex of ASDs children, whereas no differences were observed in the basal ganglia (Harada et al., 2011). Two studies using SPECT (Single Photon Emission Computed Tomography) found reductions in $GABA_A$ receptors in both ASDs adults and children (Mori et al., 2012; Mendez et al., 2013).

In addition to the genes/proteins involved directly in GABA synthesis and transmission, many other factors exert indirect effects on GABA functioning through the regulation of gene expression, receptor trafficking, and downstream signaling pathways; therefore, GABAergic dysfunction could also be a downstream consequence of mutations in the genes involved in the increase or decrease of GABA transmission. CNTNAP2, which is a part of the *NRXN* family, has been associated with autism (Gregor et al., 2011; Stein et al., 2011). CNTNAP2 knockout mice showed specific deficits in inhibitory signaling, with reduced GAD1 expression and a reduced number of GABAergic interneurons (Peñagarikano et al., 2011). Similar findings have been observed in another ASDs candidate gene model; CADPS2 knockout mice showed reduced cortical parvalbumin GABA interneurons and a reduced number of cerebellar Purkinje cells (Sadakata et al., 2007).

Glutamate receptors

Glutamate is the major excitatory neurotransmitter in the human brain. Glutamate receptors (GluARs) are composed of ionotropic glutamate receptors (iGluRs) and metabotropic glutamate receptors (mGluRs). Findings from genetic studies, post-mortem brain studies, animal models, and clinical drug trials have implicated a dysfunctional glutamatergic system in ASDs; however, hypo- and hyperfunction coexists in different forms of ASDs.

Ionotropic glutamate receptors are classified into NMDA (*N*-methyl-D-aspartate), AMPA (2-amino-3-hydroxy-5-methyl-4-isoxazolepropionic acid), and kainate receptors based on structural, pharmacological, and physiological properties. iGluRs are tetramers encoded by 18 genes. NMDARs are obligate heteromers formed as tetramers from the co-assembly of GluN1, GluN2A-GluN2D, GluN3A, and GluN3B subunits. Each NMDAR channel contains a combination of two GluN1 and two GluN2A–GluN2D subunits or two GluN1 with one GluN2 and one GluN3 subunit. AMPARs are homo- or hetero-tetramers formed from the GluA1–GluA4 subunits and are Mg^{2+}-insensitive. Kainate receptors are tetramers formed from combinations of the GluK1–GluK5 subunits.

Several genetic studies have reported that *NMDARs* genes are associated with ASDs. Two studies that sequenced ASDs patients identified rare disruptive mutations in the GluN2B (*GRIN2B*) gene (Tarabeux et al., 2011; O'Roak et al., 2012). Common polymorphisms in *GRIN2B* and *GRIN2A* have also been associated with ASDs (Barnby et al., 2005; Yoo et al., 2012). Interestingly, the NMDAR subunits have differential expression during development, with GluN2B expressed early in development, followed by GluN2A during later development and synapse maturation (Sanz-Clemente et al., 2013).

Ramanathan et al. (2004) identified a 19 mb deletion of chromosome 4q in an ASDs child, which included the AMPA 2 gene that encodes the glutamate receptor GluR2 sub-unit (Ramanathan et al., 2004). One study identified chromosome 6q21 as a candidate region for autism and found a functional SNP in glutamate receptor 6 (*GluR6* or *GRIK2*) gene associated with ASDs (Jamain et al., 2002).

A post-mortem brain study also found that ASDs patients have specific abnormalities in AMPA receptors and glutamate transporters in the cerebellum (Purcell et al., 2001). The mRNA levels of excitatory amino acid transporter 1 and glutamate receptor AMPA1 (GluA1) were significantly increased in autism subjects, and AMPAR density was decreased in the ASDs cerebellum (Purcell et al., 2001).

Parvalbumin-selective NMDAR 1 knockout (NR1 KO) mice exhibited autism-like phenotypes compared with wild-type mice; the N1 ERP latency was delayed, sociability was reduced, and mating USVs were impaired (Saunders et al., 2013).

The administration of acute PCP and ketamine, NMDAR antagonists, has been shown to mimic the symptoms of autism in humans (Carlsson, 1998). Based on this phenomenon and neuroimaging and neuroanatomical studies, Carlsson (1998) proposed that infantile autism is a hypoglutamatergic disorder. Recently, both the use of an NMDAR agonist and antagonist has been reported in ASDs patients. Daily doses of D-cycloserine, an NMDAR glycine site partial agonist, significantly improved social withdrawal (Posey et al., 2004), and daily doses of amantadine (memantine), an NMDAR non-competitive antagonist, reduced some negative symptoms of autism, such as hyperactivity (King et al., 2001; Chez et al., 2007).

mGluRs are members of the group C family of G-protein-coupled receptors. mGluRs have seven transmembrane domains that span the cell membrane. Differently to iGluRs, they are not ion channels. There are eight different types of mGluRs, namely mGluR1 to mGluR8, which are divided into three groups, group 1, group 2, and group 3. mGluR1 and mGluR5 belong to group 1 family, mGluR2, mGluR3, and mGluR4 belong to group 2 family, and mGluR6, mGluR7, and mGluR8 belong to group 3 family. They can regulate neuronal excitability, learning, and memory.

A study using high-throughput multiplex sequencing revealed significant enrichment of rare functional variants in the mGluR pathway in non-syndromic autism cases. (Kelleher et al., 2012). Most recently, in a valproate-induced rat model of autism, the expressions of mGluR2/3 protein and mGluR2 mRNA were found significantly reduced. *N*-acetylcysteine (NAC) recued social interaction and anxiety-like behaviors of the VPA-exposed rats. In addition, these effects can be blocked by intra-amygdala infusion of mGluR2/3 antagonist LY341495 (Chen et al., 2014). These results indicate that the disruption of social interaction in VPA induced rats could be restored by NAC, which may depend on the activation of mGluR2/3.

A decrease in mGluR has been found in PTEN knockout mice showing autism-like behavioral deficits (Lugo et al., 2014). By reducing 50% of mGluR5 expression, several abnormalities of Fmr1 knockout mice can be rescued. For example, density of dendritic spines on cortical pyramidal neurons and basal protein synthesis in hippocampus are increased, inhibitory avoidance extinction and audiogenic seizures are improved (Dolen et al., 2007).

CONCLUDING REMARKS

In this review, we have summarized findings about some synapse proteins and receptors linked to ASDs. Due to different sample sizes and research methods, some results need further replication in additional and larger samples. For some of the synapse protein defects described in this review, animal model studies are lacking. Furthermore, genetic mutations only have been found in some ASDs subjects. Many patients do not exhibit these types of changes. Other signaling pathways, such as MAPK/JNK, have been correlated with synapse pathways in the pathogenesis of ASDs. Therefore, an intriguing question for future work is whether other signaling pathways have crosstalk with synapse pathways during the occurrence of ASDs.

ACKNOWLEDGMENTS

The author gratefully acknowledges the support of Shanghai Jiao Tong University K.C. Wong Medical Fellowship Fund and the National Basic Research Program 973 of China (Grant No. 2012CB 517900).

REFERENCES

Alarcón, M., Abrahams, B. S., Stone, J. L., Duvall, J. A., Perederiy, J. V., Bomar, J. M., et al. (2008). Linkage, association, and gene-expression analyses identify CNTNAP2 as an autism-susceptibility gene. *Am. J. Hum. Genet.* 82, 150–159. doi: 10.1016/j.ajhg.2007.09.005

American Psychiatry Association [APA]. (2013). *Diagnostic and Statistical Manual of Mental Disorders*, 5th Edn. Arlington, VA: American Psychiatric Publishing.

Anitha, A., Thanseem, I., Nakamura, K., Yamada, K., Iwayama, Y., Toyota, T., et al. (2013). Protocadherin alpha (PCDHA) as a novel susceptibility gene for autism. *J. Psychiatry Neurosci.* 38, 192–198. doi: 10.1503/jpn.120058

Arking, D. E., Cutler, D. J., Brune, C. W., Teslovich, T. M., West, K., Ikeda, M., et al. (2008). A common genetic variant in the neurexin superfamily member CNTNAP2 increases familial risk of autism. *Am. J. Hum. Genet.* 82, 160–164. doi: 10.1016/j.ajhg.2007.09.015

Asperger, H. (1944). Die 'autistischen psychopathen' im kindesalter. *Arch. Psychiatr. Nervenkr.* 117, 76–136. doi: 10.1007/BF01837709

Autism Genome Project Consortium, Szatmari, P., Paterson, A. D., Zwaigenbaum, L., Roberts, W., Brian, J., et al. (2007). Mapping autism risk loci using genetic linkage and chromosomal rearrangements. *Nat. Genet.* 39, 319–328. doi: 10.1038/ng1985

Bakkaloglu, B., O'Roak, B. J., Louvi, A., Gupta, A. R., Abelson, J. F., Morgan, T. M., et al. (2008). Molecular cytogenetic analysis and resequencing of contactin associated protein-like 2 in autism spectrum disorders. *Am. J. Hum. Genet.* 82, 165–173. doi: 10.1016/j.ajhg.2007.09.017

Barnby, G., Abbott, A., Sykes, N., Morris, A., Weeks, D. E., Mott, R., et al. (2005). Candidate-gene screening and association analysis at the autism-susceptibility locus on chromosome 16p: evidence of association at GRIN2A and ABAT. *Am. J. Hum. Genet.* 76, 950–966. doi: 10.1086/430454

Berkel, S., Marshall, R. C., Weiss, B., Howe, J., Roeth, R., Moog, U., et al. (2010). Mutations in the SHANK2 synaptic scaffolding gene in autism spectrum disorder and mental retardation. *Nat. Genet.* 42, 489–491. doi: 10.1038/ng.589

Berry-Kravis, E. M., Hessl, D., Rathmell, B., Zarevics, P., Cherubini, M., Walton-Bowen, K., et al. (2012). Effects of STX209 (arbaclofen) on neurobehavioral function in children and adults with fragile X syndrome: a randomized, controlled, phase 2 trial. *Sci. Transl. Med.* 4:152ra127. doi: 10.1126/scitranslmed.3004214

Betancur, C., Sakurai, T., and Buxbaum, J. D. (2009). The emerging role of synaptic cell-adhesion pathways in the pathogenesis of autism spectrum disorders. *Trends Neurosci.* 32, 402–412. doi: 10.1016/j.tins.2009.04.003

Billstedt, E., Gillberg, I. C., and Gillberg, C. (2005). Autism after adolescence: population-based 13- to 22-year follow-up study of 120 individuals with autism diagnosed in childhood. *J. Autism Dev. Disord.* 35, 351–360. doi: 10.1007/s10803-005-3302-5

Blasi, F., Bacchelli, E., Pesaresi, G., Carone, S., Bailey, A. J., Maestrini, E., et al. (2006). Absence of coding mutations in the X-linked genes neuroligin 3 and neuroligin 4 in individuals with autism from the IMGSAC collection. *Am. J. Med. Genet. B Neuropsychiatr. Genet.* 141B, 220–221. doi: 10.1002/ajmg.b.30287

Blatt, G. J., Fitzgerald, C. M., Guptill, J. T., Booker, A. B., Kemper, T. L., and Bauman, M. L. (2001). Density and distribution of hippocampal neurotransmitter receptors in autism: an autoradiographic study. *J. Autism Dev. Disord.* 31, 537–543. doi: 10.1023/A:1013238809666

Boccuto, L., Lauri, M., Sarasua, S. M., Skinner, C. D., Buccella, D., Dwivedi, A., et al. (2013). Prevalence of SHANK3 variants in patients with different subtypes of autism spectrum disorders. *Eur. J. Hum. Genet.* 21, 310–316. doi: 10.1038/ejhg.2012.175

Bolton, P. F., Dennis, N. R., Browne, C. E., Thomas, N. S., Veltman, M. W., Thompson, R. J., et al. (2001). The phenotypic manifestations of interstitial duplications of proximal 15q with special reference to the autistic spectrum disorders. *Am. J. Med. Genet.* 105, 675–685. doi: 10.1002/ajmg.1551

Bozdagi, O., Sakurai, T., Papapetrou, D., Wang, X., Dickstein, D. L., Takahashi, N., et al. (2010). Haploinsufficiency of the autism-associated Shank3 gene leads to deficits in synaptic function, social interaction, and social communication. *Mol. Autism* 1:15. doi: 10.1186/2040-2392-1-15

Bremer, A., Giacobini, M., Eriksson, M., Gustavsson, P., Nordin, V., Fernell, E., et al. (2011). Copy number variation characteristics in subpopulations of patients with autism spectrum disorders. *Am. J. Med. Genet. B Neuropsychiatr. Genet.* 156, 115–124. doi: 10.1002/ajmg.b.31142

Carlsson, M. L. (1998). Hypothesis: is infantile autism a hypoglutamatergic disorder? Relevance of glutamate–serotonin interactions for pharmacotherapy. *J. Neural. Transm.* 105, 525–535. doi: 10.1007/s007020050076

Chen, Y. W., Lin, H. C., Ng, M. C., Hsiao, Y. H., Wang, C. C., Gean, P. W., et al. (2014). Activation of mGluR2/3 underlies the effects of N-acetylcystein on amygdala-associated autism-like phenotypes in a valproate-induced rat model of autism. *Front. Behav. Neurosci.* 8:219. doi: 10.3389/fnbeh.2014.00219

Chez, M. G., Burton, Q., Dowling, T., Chang, M., Khanna, P., and Kramer, C. (2007). Memantine as adjunctive therapy in children diagnosed with autistic spectrum disorders: an observation of initial clinical response and maintenance tolerability. *J. Child Neurol.* 22, 574–579. doi: 10.1177/0883073807302611

Chubykin, A. A., Atasoy, D., Etherton, M. R., Brose, N., Kavalali, E. T., Gibson, J. R., et al. (2007). Activity-dependent validation of excitatory versus inhibitory synapses by neuroligin-1 versus neuroligin-2. *Neuron* 54, 919–931. doi: 10.1016/j.neuron.2007.05.029

Corradi, A., Fadda, M., Piton, A., Patry, L., Marte, A., Rossi, P., et al. (2014). SYN2 is an autism predisposing gene: loss-of-function mutations alter synaptic vesicle cycling and axon outgrowth. *Hum. Mol. Genet.* 23, 90–103. doi: 10.1093/hmg/ddt401

de Anda, F. C., Rosario, A. L., Durak, O., Tran, T., Gräff, J., Meletis, K., et al. (2012). Autism spectrum disorder susceptibility gene TAOK2 affects basal dendrite formation in the neocortex. *Nat. Neurosci.* 15, 1022–1031. doi: 10.1038/nn.3141

Dean, C., and Dresbach, T. (2006). Neuroligins and neurexins: linking cell adhesion, synapse formation and cognitive function. *Trends Neurosci.* 29, 21–29. doi: 10.1016/j.tins.2005.11.003

Depienne, C., Moreno-De-Luca, D., Heron, D., Bouteiller, D., Gennetier, A., Delorme, R., et al. (2009). Screening for genomic rearrangements and methylation abnormalities of the 15q11-q13 region in autism spectrum disorders. *Biol. Psychiatry* 66, 349–359. doi: 10.1016/j.biopsych.2009.01.025

Dhar, S. U., del Gaudio, D., German, J. R., Peters, S. U., Ou, Z., Bader, P. I., et al. (2010). 22q13.3 deletion syndrome: clinical and molecular analysis using array CGH. *Am. J. Med. Genet. A* 152A, 573–581. doi: 10.1002/ajmg.a.33253

Dolen, G., Osterweil, E., Rao, B. S., Smith, G. B., Auerbach, B. D., Chattarji, S., et al. (2007). Correction of fragile X syndrome in mice. *Neuron* 56, 955–962. doi: 10.1016/j.neuron.2007.12.001

Durand, C. M., Betancur, C., Boeckers, T. M., Bockmann, J., Chaste, P., Fauchereau, F., et al. (2007). Mutations in the gene encoding the synaptic scaffolding protein SHANK3 are associated with autism spectrum disorders. *Nat. Genet.* 39, 25–27. doi: 10.1038/ng1933

Elsabbagh, M., Divan, G., Koh, Y. J., Kim, Y. S., Kauchali, S., Marcín, C., et al. (2012). Global prevalence of autism and other pervasive developmental disorders. *Autism Res.* 5, 160–179. doi: 10.1002/aur.239

Erickson, C. A., Veenstra-Vanderweele, J. M., Melmed, R. D., McCracken, J. T., Ginsberg, L. D., Sikich, L., et al. (2014). STX209 (arbaclofen) for autism spectrum disorders: an 8-week open-label study. *J. Autism Dev. Disord.* 44, 958–964. doi: 10.1007/s10803-013-1963-z

Etherton, M. R., Blaiss, C. A., Powell, C. M., and Südhof, T. C. (2009). Mouse neurexin-1alpha deletion causes correlated electrophysiological and behavioral changes consistent with cognitive impairments. *Proc. Natl. Acad. Sci. U.S.A.* 106, 17998–18003. doi: 10.1073/pnas.0910297106

Etherton, M., Földy, C., Sharma, M., Tabuchi, K., Liu, X., Shamloo, M., et al. (2011a). Autism-linked neuroligin-3 R451C mutation differentially alters hippocampal and cortical synaptic function. *Proc. Natl. Acad. Sci. U.S.A.* 108, 13764–13769. doi: 10.1073/pnas.1111093108

Etherton, M. R., Tabuchi, K., Sharma, M., Ko, J., and Südhof, T. C. (2011b). An autism-associated point mutation in the neuroligin cytoplasmic tail selectively impairs AMPA receptor-mediated synaptic transmission in hippocampus. *EMBO J.* 30, 2908–2919. doi: 10.1038/emboj.2011.182

Fassio, A., Patry, L., Congia, S., Onofri, F., Piton, A., Gauthier, J., et al. (2011). SYN1 loss-of-function mutations in autism and partial epilepsy cause impaired synaptic function. *Hum. Mol. Genet.* 20, 2297–2307. doi: 10.1093/hmg/ddr122

Fatemi, S. H., Folsom, T. D., Reutiman, T. J., and Thuras, P. D. (2009). Expression of GABA(B) receptors is altered in brains of subjects with autism. *Cerebellum* 8, 64–69. doi: 10.1007/s12311-008-0075-3

Fatemi, S. H., Halt, A. R., Stary, J. M., Kanodia, R., Schulz, S. C., and Realmuto, G. R. (2002). Glutamic acid decarboxylase 65 and 67 kDa proteins are reduced in autistic parietal and cerebellar cortices. *Biol. Psychiatry* 52, 805–810. doi: 10.1016/S0006-3223(02)01430-0

Feyder, M., Karlsson, R. M., Mathur, P., Lyman, M., Bock, R., Momenan, R., et al. (2010). Association of mouse Dlg4 (PSD-95) gene deletion and human DLG4 gene variation with phenotypes relevant to autism spectrum disorders and Williams' syndrome. *Am. J. Psychiatry* 167, 1508–1517. doi: 10.1176/appi.ajp.2010.10040484

Földy, C., Malenka, R. C., and Südhof, T. C. (2013). Autism-associated neuroligin-3 mutations commonly disrupt tonic endocannabinoid signaling. *Neuron* 78, 498–509. doi: 10.1016/j.neuron.2013.02.036

Fornasiero, E. F., Raimondi, A., Guarnieri, F. C., Orlando, M., Fesce, R., Benfenati, F., et al. (2012). Synapsins contribute to the dynamic spatial organization of synaptic vesicles in an activity-dependent manner. *J. Neurosci.* 32, 12214–12227. doi: 10.1523/JNEUROSCI.1554-12.2012

Friedman, A., and Luiselli, J. K. (2008). Excessive daytime sleep: behavioral assessment and intervention in a child with autism. *Behav. Modif.* 32, 548–555. doi: 10.1177/0145445507312187

Gauthier, J., Bonnel, A., St-Onge, J., Karemera, L., Laurent, S., Mottron, L., et al. (2005). NLGN3/NLGN4 gene mutations are not responsible for autism in the Quebec population. *Am. J. Med. Genet. B Neuropsychiatr. Genet.* 132B, 74–75. doi: 10.1002/ajmg.b.30066

Gauthier, J., Siddiqui, T. J., Huashan, P., Yokomaku, D., Hamdan, F. F., Champagne, N., et al. (2011). Truncating mutations in NRXN2 and NRXN1 in autism spectrum disorders and schizophrenia. *Hum. Genet.* 130, 563–573. doi: 10.1007/s00439-011-0975-z

Gauthier, J., Spiegelman, D., Piton, A., Lafrenière, R. G., Laurent, S., St-Onge, J., et al. (2009). Novel de novo SHANK3 mutation in autistic patients. *Am. J. Med. Genet. B Neuropsychiatr. Genet.* 150B, 421–424. doi: 10.1002/ajmg.b.30822

Glessner, J. T., Wang, K., Cai, G., Korvatska, O., Kim, C. E., Wood, S., et al. (2009). Autism genome-wide copy number variation reveals ubiquitin and neuronal genes. *Nature* 459, 569–573. doi: 10.1038/nature07953

Greco, B., Managò, F., Tucci, V., Kao, H. T., Valtorta, F., and Benfenati, F. (2013). Autism-related behavioral abnormalities in synapsin knockout mice. *Behav. Brain Res.* 251, 65–74. doi: 10.1016/j.bbr.2012.12.015

Gregor, A., Albrecht, B., Bader, I., Bijlsma, E. K., Ekici, A. B., Engels, H., et al. (2011). Expanding the clinical spectrum associated with defects in CNTNAP2 and NRXN1. *BMC Med. Genet.* 12:106. doi: 10.1186/1471-2350-12-106

Grosskreutz, Y., Betz, H., and Kneussel, M. (2003). Rescue of molybdenum cofactor biosynthesis in gephyrin-deficient mice by a Cnx1 transgene. *Biochem. Biophys. Res. Commun.* 301, 450–455. doi: 10.1016/S0006-291X(02)03062-0

Guilmatre, A., Dubourg, C., Mosca, A. L., Legallic, S., Goldenberg, A., Drouin-Garraud, V., et al. (2009). Recurrent rearrangements in synaptic and neurodevelopmental genes and shared biologic pathways in schizophrenia, autism, and mental retardation. *Arch. Gen. Psychiatry* 66, 947–956. doi: 10.1001/archgenpsychiatry.2009.80

Guilmatre, A., Huguet, G., Delorme, R., and Bourgeron, T. (2013). The emerging role of SHANK genes in neuropsychiatric disorders. *Dev. Neurobiol.* 74, 113–122. doi: 10.1002/dneu.22128

Guo, H., Xun, G., Peng, Y., Xiang, X., Xiong, Z., Zhang, L., et al. (2012). Disruption of Contactin 4 in two subjects with autism in Chinese population. *Gene* 505, 201–205. doi: 10.1016/j.gene.2012.06.051

Harada, M., Taki, M. M., Nose, A., Kubo, H., Mori, K., Nishitani, H., et al. (2011). Non-invasive evaluation of the GABAergic/glutamatergic system in autistic patients observed by MEGA-editing proton MR spectroscopy using a clinical 3 tesla instrument. *J. Autism Dev. Disord.* 41, 447–454. doi: 10.1007/s10803-010-1065-0

Henderson, C., Wijetunge, L., Kinoshita, M. N., Shumway, M., Hammond, R. S., Postma, F. R., et al. (2012). Reversal of disease-related pathologies in the fragile X mouse model by selective activation of GABAB receptors with arbaclofen. *Sci. Transl. Med.* 4:152ra128. doi: 10.1126/scitranslmed.3004218

Howlin, P., Goode, S., Hutton, J., and Rutter, M. (2004). Adult outcome for children with autism. *J. Child Psychol. Psychiatry* 45, 212–229. doi: 10.1111/j.1469-7610.2004.00215.x

Hung, A. Y., Futai, K., Sala, C., Valtschanoff, J. G., Ryu, J., Woodworth, M. A., et al. (2008). Smaller dendritic spines, weaker synaptic transmission, but enhanced spatial learning in mice lacking Shank1. *J. Neurosci.* 28, 1697–1708. doi: 10.1523/JNEUROSCI.3032-07.2008

International Schizophrenia Consortium. (2008). Rare chromosomal deletions and duplications increase risk of schizophrenia. *Nature* 455, 237–241. doi: 10.1038/nature07239

Jamain, S., Betancur, C., Quach, H., Philippe, A., Fellous, M., Giros, B., et al. (2002). Linkage and association of the glutamate receptor 6 gene with autism. *Mol. Psychiatry* 7, 302–310. doi: 10.1038/sj.mp.4000979

Jamain, S., Quach, H., Betancur, C., Råstam, M., Colineaux, C., Gillberg, I. C., et al. (2003). Mutations of the X-linked genes encoding neuroligins NLGN3 and NLGN4 are associated with autism. *Nat. Genet.* 34, 27–29. doi: 10.1038/ng1136

Jamain, S., Radyushkin, K., Hammerschmidt, K., Granon, S., Boretius, S., Varoqueaux, F., et al. (2008). Reduced social interaction and ultrasonic communication in a mouse model of monogenic heritable autism. *Proc. Natl. Acad. Sci. U.S.A.* 105, 1710–1715. doi: 10.1073/pnas.0711555105

Kanner, L. (1943). Autistic disturbance of affective contact. *Nerv. Child* 2, 217–250.

Kelleher, R. J. III, Geigenmüller, U., Hovhannisyan, H., Trautman, E., Pinard, R., Rathmell, B., et al. (2012). High-throughput sequencing of mGluR signaling pathway genes reveals enrichment of rare variants in autism. *PLoS ONE* 7:e35003. doi: 10.1371/journal.pone.0035003

Kim, H. G., Kishikawa, S., Higgins, A. W., Seong, I. S., Donovan, D. J., Shen, Y., et al. (2008). Disruption of neurexin 1 associated with autism spectrum disorder. *Am. J. Hum. Genet.* 82, 199–207. doi: 10.1016/j.ajhg.2007.09.011

King, B. H., Wright, D. M., Handen, B. L., Sikich, L., Zimmerman, A. W., McMahon, W., et al. (2001). Double-blind, placebo-controlled study of amantadine hydrochloride in the treatment of children with autistic disorder. *J. Am. Acad. Child Adolesc. Psychiatry* 40, 658–665. doi: 10.1097/00004583-200106000-00010

King, M., and Bearman, P. (2009). Diagnostic change and the increased prevalence of autism. *Int. J. Epidemiol.* 38, 1224–1234. doi: 10.1093/ije/dyp261

Kneussel, M., Brandstätter, J. H., Laube, B., Stahl, S., Müller, U., and Betz, H. (1999). Loss of postsynaptic GABA(A) receptor clustering in gephyrin-deficient mice. *J. Neurosci.* 19, 9289–9297.

Kwasnicka-Crawford, D. A., Roberts, W., and Scherer, S. W. (2007). Characterization of an autism-associated segmental maternal heterodisomy of the chromosome 15q11-13 region. *J. Autism Dev. Disord.* 37, 694–702. doi: 10.1007/s10803-006-0225-8

Lai, M. C., Lombardo, M. V., and Baron-Cohen, S. (2014). Autism. *Lancet* 383, 896–910. doi: 10.1016/S0140-6736(13)61539-1

Laumonnier, F., Bonnet-Brilhault, F., Gomot, M., Blanc, R., David, A., Moizard, M. P., et al. (2004). X-linked mental retardation and autism are associated with a mutation in the NLGN4 gene, a member of the neuroligin family. *Am. J. Hum. Genet.* 74, 552–557. doi: 10.1086/382137

Leblond, C. S., Heinrich, J., Delorme, R., Proepper, C., Betancur, C., Huguet, G., et al. (2012). Genetic and functional analyses of SHANK2 mutations suggest a multiple hit model of autism spectrum disorders. *PLoS Genet.* 8:e1002521. doi: 10.1371/journal.pgen.1002521

Levy, D., Ronemus, M., Yamrom, B., Lee, Y. H., Leotta, A., Kendall, J., et al. (2011). Rare de novo and transmitted copy-number variation in autistic spectrum disorders. *Neuron* 70, 886–897. doi: 10.1016/j.neuron.2011.05.015

Li, X., Zou, H., and Brown, W. T. (2012). Genes associated with autism spectrum disorder. *Brain Res. Bull.* 88, 543–552. doi: 10.1016/j.brainresbull.2012.05.017

Lim, S., Naisbitt, S., Yoon, J., Hwang, J. I., Suh, P. G., Sheng, M., et al. (1999). Characterization of the Shank family of synaptic proteins. Multiple genes, alternative splicing, and differential expression in brain and development. *J. Biol. Chem.* 274, 29510–29518. doi: 10.1074/jbc.274.41.29510

Lintas, C., and Persico, A. M. (2009). Autistic phenotypes and genetic testing: state-of-the-art for the clinical geneticist. *J. Med. Genet.* 46, 1–8. doi: 10.1136/jmg.2008.060871

Lionel, A. C., Crosbie, J., Barbosa, N., Goodale, T., Thiruvahindrapuram, B., Rickaby, J., et al. (2011). Rare copy number variation discovery and cross-disorder comparisons identify risk genes for ADHD. *Sci. Transl. Med.* 3:95ra75. doi: 10.1126/scitranslmed.3002464

Lionel, A. C., Vaags, A. K., Sato, D., Gazzellone, M. J., Mitchell, E. B., Chen, H. Y., et al. (2013). Rare exonic deletions implicate the synaptic organizer Gephyrin (GPHN) in risk for autism, schizophrenia and seizures. *Hum. Mol. Genet.* 22, 2055–2066. doi: 10.1093/hmg/ddt056

Liu, Y., Du, Y., Liu, W., Yang, C., Liu, Y., Wang, H., et al. (2013). Lack of association between NLGN3, NLGN4, SHANK2 and SHANK3 gene variants and autism spectrum disorder in a Chinese population. *PLoS ONE* 8:e56639. doi: 10.1371/journal.pone.0056639

Lotter, V. (1966). Epidemiology of autistic conditions in young children. *Soc. Psychiatry Psychiatr. Epidemiol.* 1, 124–135.

Lugo, J. N., Smith, G. D., Arbuckle, E. P., White, J., Holley, A. J., Floruta, C. M., et al. (2014). Deletion of PTEN produces autism-like behavioral deficits and alterations in synaptic proteins. *Front. Mol. Neurosci.* 7:27. doi: 10.3389/fnmol.2014.00027

Marshall, C. R., Noor, A., Vincent, J. B., Lionel, A. C., Feuk, L., Skaug, J., et al. (2008). Structural variation of chromosomes in autism spectrum disorder. *Am. J. Hum. Genet.* 82, 477–488. doi: 10.1016/j.ajhg.2007.12.009

Martin, E. R., Menold, M. M., Wolpert, C. M., Bass, M. P., Donnelly, S. L., Ravan, S. A., et al. (2000). Analysis of linkage disequilibrium in gamma-aminobutyric acid receptor subunit genes in autistic disorder. *Am. J. Med. Genet.* 96, 43–48. doi: 10.1002/(SICI)1096-8628(20000207)96:1<43::AID-AJMG9>3.0.CO;2-3

Meguro-Horike, M., Yasui, D. H., Powell, W., Schroeder, D. I., Oshimura, M., Lasalle, J. M., et al. (2011). Neuron-specific impairment of inter-chromosomal pairing and transcription in a novel model of human 15q-duplication syndrome. *Hum. Mol. Genet.* 20, 3798–3810. doi: 10.1093/hmg/ddr298

Mendez, M. A., Horder, J., Myers, J., Coghlan, S., Stokes, P., Erritzoe, D., et al. (2013). The brain GABA-benzodiazepine receptor alpha-5 subtype in autism spectrum disorder: a pilot [(11)C]Ro15-4513 positron emission tomography study. *Neuropharmacology* 68, 195–201. doi: 10.1016/j.neuropharm.2012.04.008

Missler, M., Zhang, W., Rohlmann, A., Kattenstroth, G., Hammer, R. E., Gottmann, K., et al. (2003). Alpha-neurexins couple Ca^{2+} channels to synaptic vesicle exocytosis. *Nature* 423, 939–948. doi: 10.1038/nature01755

Moessner, R., Marshall, C. R., Sutcliffe, J. S., Skaug, J., Pinto, D., Vincent, J., et al. (2007). Contribution of SHANK3 mutations to autism spectrum disorder. *Am. J. Hum. Genet.* 81, 1289–1297. doi: 10.1086/522590

Mori, T., Mori, K., Fujii, E., Toda, Y., Miyazaki, M., Harada, M., et al. (2012). Evaluation of the GABAergic nervous system in autistic brain: (123)I-iomazenil SPECT study. *Brain Dev.* 34, 648–654. doi: 10.1016/j.braindev.2011.10.007

Morrow, E. M., Yoo, S. Y., Flavell, S. W., Kim, T. K., Lin, Y., Hill, R. S., et al. (2008). Identifying autism loci and genes by tracing recent shared ancestry. *Science* 321, 218–223. doi: 10.1126/science.1157657

Murdoch, J. D., and State, M. W. (2013). Recent developments in the genetics of autism spectrum disorders. *Curr. Opin. Genet. Dev.* 23, 310–315. doi: 10.1016/j.gde.2013.02.003

Nakatani, J., Tamada, K., Hatanaka, F., Ise, S., Ohta, H., Inoue, K., et al. (2009). Abnormal behavior in a chromosome-engineered mouse model for human 15q11-13 duplication seen in autism. *Cell* 137, 1235–1246. doi: 10.1016/j.cell.2009.04.024

Novarino, G., El-Fishawy, P., Kayserili, H., Meguid, N. A., Scott, E. M., Schroth, J., et al. (2012). Mutations in BCKD-kinase lead to a potentially treatable form of autism with epilepsy. *Science* 338, 394–397. doi: 10.1126/science.1224631

O'Roak, B. J., Vives, L., Girirajan, S., Karakoc, E., Krumm, N., Coe, B. P., et al. (2012). Sporadic autism exomes reveal a highly interconnected protein network of de novo mutations. *Nature* 485, 246–250. doi: 10.1038/nature10989

Oblak, A., Gibbs, T. T., and Blatt, G. J. (2009). Decreased GABAA receptors and benzodiazepine binding sites in the anterior cingulate cortex in autism. *Autism Res.* 2, 205–219. doi: 10.1002/aur.88

Oblak, A., Gibbs, T. T., and Blatt, G. J. (2013). Reduced serotonin receptor subtypes in a limbic and a neocortical region in autism. *Autism Res.* 6, 571–583. doi: 10.1002/aur.1317

Oblak, A. L., Gibbs, T. T., and Blatt, G. J. (2011). Reduced GABAA receptors and benzodiazepine binding sites in the posterior cingulate cortex and fusiform gyrus in autism. *Brain Res.* 1380, 218–228. doi: 10.1016/j.brainres.2010.09.021

Peça, J., Feliciano, C., Ting, J. T., Wang, W., Wells, M. F., Venkatraman, T. N., et al. (2011). Shank3 mutant mice display autistic-like behaviours and striatal dysfunction. *Nature* 472, 437–442. doi: 10.1038/nature09965

Peñagarikano, O., Abrahams, B. S., Herman, E. I., Winden, K. D., Gdalyahu, A., Dong, H., et al. (2011). Absence of CNTNAP2 leads to epilepsy, neuronal migration abnormalities, and core autism-related deficits. *Cell* 147, 235–246. doi: 10.1016/j.cell.2011.08.040

Phelan, M. C. (2008). Deletion 22q13.3 syndrome. *Orphanet J. Rare Dis.* 3:14. doi: 10.1186/1750-1172-3-14

Pinto, D. A., Pagnamenta, T., Klei, L., Anney, R., Merico, D., Regan, R., et al. (2010). Functional impact of global rare copy number variation in autism spectrum disorders. *Nature* 466, 368–372. doi: 10.1038/nature09146

Posey, D. J., Kem, D. L., Swiezy, N. B., Sweeten, T. L., Wiegand, R. E., and McDougle, C. J. (2004). A pilot study of D-cycloserine in subjects with autistic disorder. *Am. J. Psychiatry* 161, 2115–2117. doi: 10.1176/appi.ajp.161.11.2115

Poulopoulos, A., Aramuni, G., Meyer, G., Soykan, T., Hoon, M., Papadopoulos, T., et al. (2009). Neuroligin 2 drives postsynaptic assembly at perisomatic inhibitory synapses through gephyrin and collybistin. *Neuron* 63, 628–642. doi: 10.1016/j.neuron.2009.08.023

Purcell, A. E., Jeon, O. H., Zimmerman, A. W., Blue, M. E., and Pevsner, J. (2001). Postmortem brain abnormalities of the glutamate neurotransmitter system in autism. *Neurology* 57, 1618–1628. doi: 10.1212/WNL.57.9.1618

Ramanathan, S., Woodroffem, A., Flodman, P. L., Mays, L. Z., Hanouni, M., Modahl, C. B., et al. (2004). A case of autism with an interstitial deletion on 4q leading to hemizygosity for genes encoding for glutamine and glycine neurotransmitter receptor sub-units (AMPA 2, GLRA3, GLRB) and neuropeptide receptors NPY1R, NPY5R. *BMC Med. Genet.* 5:10. doi: 10.1186/1471-2350-5-10

Redies, C., Hertel, N., and Hübner, C. A. (2012). Cadherins and neuropsychiatric disorders. *Brain Res.* 1470, 130–144. doi: 10.1016/j.brainres.2012.06.020

Rice, C. (2012). Prevalence of autism spectrum disorders – Autism and Developmental Disabilities Monitoring Network, 14 sites, United States, 2008. *MMWR Surveill. Summ.* 61, 1–19.

Roohi, J., Montagna, C., Tegay, D. H., Palmer, L. E., DeVincent, C., Pomeroy, J. C., et al. (2009). Disruption of contactin 4 in three subjects with autism spectrum disorder. *J. Med. Genet.* 46, 176–182. doi: 10.1136/jmg.2008.057505

Rosahl, T. W., Spillane, D., Missler, M., Herz, J., Selig, D. K., Wolff, J. R., et al. (1995). Essential functions of synapsins I and II in synaptic vesicle regulation. *Nature* 375, 488–493. doi: 10.1038/375488a0

Sadakata, T., Washida, M., Iwayama, Y., Shoji, S., Sato, Y., Ohkura, T., et al. (2007). Autistic-like phenotypes in Cadps2-knockout mice and aberrant CADPS2 splicing in autistic patients. *J. Clin. Invest.* 117, 931–943. doi: 10.1172/JCI29031

Sampath, S., Bhat, S., Gupta, S., O'Connor, A., West, A. B., Arking, D. E., et al. (2013). Defining the contribution of CNTNAP2 to autism susceptibility. *PLoS ONE* 8:e77906. doi: 10.1371/journal.pone.0077906

Sanders, S. J., Ercan-Sencicek, A. G., Hus, V., Luo, R., Murtha, M. T., Moreno-De-Luca, D., et al. (2011). Multiple recurrent de novo CNVs, including duplications of the 7q11.*23* Williams syndrome region, are strongly associated with autism. *Neuron* 70, 863–885. doi: 10.1016/j.neuron.2011.05.002

Sanz-Clemente, A., Nicoll, R. A., and Roche, K. W. (2013). Diversity in NMDA receptor composition: many regulators, many consequences. *Neuroscientist* 19, 62–75. doi: 10.1177/1073858411435129

Sato, D., Lionel, A. C., Leblond, C. S., Prasad, A., Pinto, D., Walker, S., et al. (2012). SHANK1 deletions in males with autism spectrum disorder. *Am. J. Hum. Genet.* 90, 879–887. doi: 10.1016/j.ajhg.2012.03.017

Saunders, J. A., Tatard-Leitman, V. M., Suh, J., Billingslea, E. N., Roberts, T. P., and Siegel, S. J. (2013). Knockout of NMDA receptors in parvalbumin interneurons recreates autism-like phenotypes. *Autism Res.* 6, 69–77. doi: 10.1002/aur.1264

Schmeisser, M. J., Ey, E., Wegener, S., Bockmann, J., Stempel, A. V., Kuebler, A., et al. (2012). Autistic-like behaviours and hyperactivity in mice lacking ProSAP1/Shank2. *Nature* 486, 256–260. doi: 10.1038/nature11015

Schnell, E., Bensen, A. L., Washburn, E. K., and Westbrook, G. L. (2012). Neuroligin-1 overexpression in newborn granule cells in vivo. *PLoS ONE* 7:e48045. doi: 10.1371/journal.pone.0048045

Sheng, M., and Kim, E. (2000). The Shank family of scaffold proteins. *J. Cell Sci.* 113(Pt 11), 1851–1856.

Silverman, J. L., Turner, S. M., Barkan, C. L., Tolu, S. S., Saxena, R., Hung, A. Y., et al. (2011). Sociability and motor functions in Shank1 mutant mice. *Brain Res.* 1380, 120–137. doi: 10.1016/j.brainres.2010.09.026

Simonoff, E., Pickles, A., Charman, T., Chandler, S., Loucas, T., and Baird, G. (2008). Psychiatric disorders in children with autism spectrum disorders: prevalence, comorbidity, and associated factors in a population-derived sample. *J. Am. Acad. Child Adolesc. Psychiatry* 47, 921–929. doi: 10.1097/CHI.0b013e318179964f

Stein, M. B., Yang, B. Z., Chavira, D. A., Hitchcock, C. A., Sung, S. C., Shipon-Blum, E., et al. (2011). A common genetic variant in the neurexin superfamily member CNTNAP2 is associated with increased risk for selective mutism and social anxiety-related traits. *Biol. Psychiatry* 69, 825–831. doi: 10.1016/j.biopsych.2010.11.008

Strauss, K. A., Puffenberger, E. G., Huentelman, M. J., Gottlieb, S., Dobrin, S. E., Parod, J. M., et al. (2006). Recessive symptomatic focal epilepsy and mutant contactin-associated protein-like 2. *N. Engl. J. Med.* 354, 1370–1377. doi: 10.1056/NEJMoa052773

Sundaram, S. K., Huq, A. M., Wilson, B. J., and Chugani, H. T. (2010). Tourette syndrome is associated with recurrent exonic copy number variants. *Neurology* 74, 1583–1590. doi: 10.1212/WNL.0b013e3181e0f147

Tabuchi, K., Blundell, J., Etherton, M. R., Hammer, R. E., Liu, X., Powell, C. M., et al. (2007). A neuroligin-3 mutation implicated in autism increases inhibitory synaptic transmission in mice. *Science* 318, 71–76. doi: 10.1126/science.1146221

Tabuchi, K., and Sudhof, T. C. (2002). Structure and evolution of neurexin genes: insight into the mechanism of alternative splicing. *Genomics* 79, 849–859. doi: 10.1006/geno.2002.6780

Talebizadeh, Z., Bittel, D. C., Veatch, O. J., Butler, M. G., Takahashi, T. N., and Miles, J. H. (2004). Do known mutations in neuroligin genes (NLGN3 and NLGN4) cause autism? *J. Autism Dev. Disord.* 34, 735–736. doi: 10.1007/s10803-004-5295-x

Tarabeux, J., Kebir, O., Gauthier, J., Hamdan, F. F., Xiong, L., Piton, A., et al. (2011). Rare mutations in N-methyl-D-aspartate glutamate receptors in autism spectrum disorders and schizophrenia. *Transl. Psychiatry* 1:e55. doi: 10.1038/tp.2011.52

Vaags, A. K., Lionel, A. C., Sato, D., Goodenberger, M., Stein, Q. P., Curran, S., et al. (2012). Rare deletions at the neurexin 3 locus in autism spectrum disorder. *Am. J. Hum. Genet.* 90, 133–141. doi: 10.1016/j.ajhg.2011.11.025

Vincent, J. B., Kolozsvari, D., Roberts, W. S., Bolton, P. F., Gurling, H. M., and Scherer, S. W. (2004). Mutation screening of X-chromosomal neuroligin genes: no mutations in 196 autism probands. *Am. J. Med. Genet. B Neuropsychiatr. Genet.* 129B, 82–84. doi: 10.1002/ajmg.b.30069

Waga, C., Okamoto, N., Ondo, Y., Fukumura-Kato, R., Goto, Y., Kohsaka, S., et al. (2011). Novel variants of the SHANK3 gene in Japanese autistic patients with severe delayed speech development. *Psychiatr. Genet.* 21, 208–211. doi: 10.1097/YPG.0b013e328341e069

Walsh, T., McClellan, J. M., McCarthy, S. E., Addington, A. M., Pierce, S. B., Cooper, G. M., et al. (2008). Rare structural variants disrupt multiple genes in neurodevelopmental pathways in schizophrenia. *Science* 320, 539–543. doi: 10.1126/science.1155174

Wang, K., Zhang, H., Ma, D., Bucan, M., Glessner, J. T., Abrahams, B. S., et al. (2009). Common genetic variants on 5p14.1 *associate with autism spectrum disorders. Nature* 459, 528–533. doi: 10.1038/nature07999

Wang, X., McCoy, P. A., Rodriguiz, R. M., Pan, Y., Je, H. S., Roberts, A. C., et al. (2011). Synaptic dysfunction and abnormal behaviors in mice lacking major isoforms of Shank3. *Hum. Mol. Genet.* 20, 3093–3108. doi: 10.1093/hmg/ddr212

Weiss, L. A., Shen, Y., Korn, J. M., Arking, D. E., Miller, D. T., Fossdal, R., et al. (2008). Association between microdeletion and microduplication at 16p11.2 *and autism. N. Engl. J. Med.* 358, 667–675. doi: 10.1056/NEJMoa075974

Wermter, A. K., Kamp-Becker, I., Strauch, K., Schulte-Körne, G., and Remschmidt, H. (2008). No evidence for involvement of genetic variants in the X-linked neuroligin genes NLGN3 and NLGN4X in probands with autism spectrum disorder on high functioning level. *Am. J. Med. Genet. B Neuropsychiatr. Genet.* 147B, 535–537. doi: 10.1002/ajmg.b.30618

Wilson, H. L., Crolla, J. A., Walker, D., Artifoni, L., Dallapiccola, B., Takano, T., et al. (2008). Interstitial 22q13 deletions: genes other than SHANK3 have major effects on cognitive and language development. *Eur. J. Hum. Genet.* 16, 1301–1310. doi: 10.1038/ejhg.2008.107

Wilson, H. L., Wong, A. C., Shaw, S. R., Tse, W. Y., Stapleton, G. A., Phelan, M. C., et al. (2003). Molecular characterisation of the 22q13 deletion syndrome supports the role of haploinsufficiency of SHANK3/PROSAP2 in the major neurological symptoms. *J. Med. Genet.* 40, 575–584. doi: 10.1136/jmg.40.8.575

Wöhr, M., Roullet, F. I., Hung, A. Y., Sheng, M., and Crawley, J. N. (2011). Communication impairments in mice lacking Shank1: reduced levels of ultrasonic vocalizations and scent marking behavior. *PLoS ONE* 6:e20631. doi: 10.1371/journal.pone.0020631

Won, H., Lee, H. R., Gee, H. Y., Mah, W., Kim, J. I., Lee, J., et al. (2012). Autistic-like social behaviour in Shank2-mutant mice improved by restoring NMDA receptor function. *Nature* 486, 261–265. doi: 10.1038/nature11208

Yan, J., Oliveira, G., Coutinho, A., Yang, C., Feng, J., Katz, C., et al. (2005). Analysis of the neuroligin 3 and 4 genes in autism and other neuropsychiatric patients. *Mol. Psychiatry* 10, 329–332. doi: 10.1038/sj.mp.4001629

Yang, M., Bozdagi, O., Scattoni, M. L., Wöhr, M., Roullet, F. I., Katz, A. M., et al. (2012). Reduced excitatory neurotransmission and mild autism-relevant phenotypes in adolescent Shank3 null mutant mice. *J. Neurosci.* 32, 6525–6541. doi: 10.1523/JNEUROSCI.6107-11.2012

Yip, J., Soghomonian, J. J., and Blatt, G. J. (2007). Decreased GAD67 mRNA levels in cerebellar Purkinje cells in autism: pathophysiological implications. *Acta Neuropathol.* 113, 559–568. doi: 10.1007/s00401-006-0176-3

Yoo, H. J., Cho, I. H., Park, M., Yang, S. Y., and Kim, S. A. (2012). Family based association of GRIN2A and GRIN2B with Korean autism spectrum disorders. *Neurosci. Lett.* 512, 89–93. doi: 10.1016/j.neulet.2012.01.061

Yoo, J., Bakes, J., Bradley, C., Collingridge, G. L., and Kaang, B. K. (2014). Shank mutant mice as an animal model of autism. *Philos. Trans. R. Soc. Lond. B Biol. Sci.* 369:20130143. doi: 10.1098/rstb.2013.0143

Zhang, D., Cheng, L., Qian, Y., Alliey-Rodriguez, N., Kelsoe, J. R., Greenwood, T., et al. (2009). Singleton deletions throughout the genome increase risk of bipolar disorder. *Mol. Psychiatry* 14, 376–380. doi: 10.1038/mp.2008.144

Zuko, A., Kleijer, K. T., Oguro-Ando, A., Kas, M. J., van Daalen, E., van der Zwaag, B., et al. (2013). Contactins in the neurobiology of autism. *Eur. J. Pharmacol.* 719, 63–74. doi: 10.1016/j.ejphar.2013.07.016

9

Auditory processing in Fragile X Syndrome

Sarah E. Rotschafer[†] and Khaleel A. Razak*

Graduate Neuroscience Program, Department of Psychology, University of California, Riverside, CA, USA

Correspondence:
Khaleel A. Razak, Graduate Neuroscience Program, Department of Psychology, University of California, 900 University Avenue, Riverside, CA 92521, USA
e-mail: khaleel@ucr.edu

[†]Present address:
Sarah E. Rotschafer, Cramer Lab, Neurobiology and Behavior, School of Biological Sciences, University of California, Irvine, CA, USA

Fragile X syndrome (FXS) is an inherited form of intellectual disability and autism. Among other symptoms, FXS patients demonstrate abnormalities in sensory processing and communication. Clinical, behavioral, and electrophysiological studies consistently show auditory hypersensitivity in humans with FXS. Consistent with observations in humans, the *Fmr1* KO mouse model of FXS also shows evidence of altered auditory processing and communication deficiencies. A well-known and commonly used phenotype in pre-clinical studies of FXS is audiogenic seizures. In addition, increased acoustic startle response is seen in the *Fmr1* KO mice. *In vivo* electrophysiological recordings indicate hyper-excitable responses, broader frequency tuning, and abnormal spectrotemporal processing in primary auditory cortex of *Fmr1* KO mice. Thus, auditory hyper-excitability is a robust, reliable, and translatable biomarker in *Fmr1* KO mice. Abnormal auditory evoked responses have been used as outcome measures to test therapeutics in FXS patients. Given that similarly abnormal responses are present in *Fmr1* KO mice suggests that cellular mechanisms can be addressed. Sensory cortical deficits are relatively more tractable from a mechanistic perspective than more complex social behaviors that are typically studied in autism and FXS. The focus of this review is to bring together clinical, functional, and structural studies in humans with electrophysiological and behavioral studies in mice to make the case that auditory hypersensitivity provides a unique opportunity to integrate molecular, cellular, circuit level studies with behavioral outcomes in the search for therapeutics for FXS and other autism spectrum disorders.

Keywords: autism, fragile X syndrome, auditory responses, cortex, biomarkers, audiogenic seizures, sensory hypersensitivity

INTRODUCTION

Autism spectrum disorder is a growing concern, affecting 0.7–1% of all children born in the United States (Centers for Disease Control and Prevention, 2009). The need for more robust and reliable biomarkers for the symptoms of autism is increasing. Autism is diagnosed through evidence for aberrant social behavior, repetitive behavior, and communication disorder; though evidence of sensory processing anomalies is also present in individuals with autism (Gage et al., 2003a,b; Hitoglou et al., 2010; Marco et al., 2011; Alcántara et al., 2012; O'Connor, 2012; Bhatara et al., 2013). Fragile X syndrome (FXS) is a leading known inherited form of autism, with deficiencies in communication and sensory processing (Largo and Schinzel, 1985; Hanson et al., 1986; Miller et al., 1999; Belser and Sudhalter, 2001; Roberts et al., 2001; Frankland et al., 2004; Price et al., 2007, 2008; Roberts et al., 2007a,b; Barnes et al., 2009). Notably, clinical, behavioral, structural, and functional studies indicate abnormalities in auditory structures and processing in humans with FXS (St. Clair et al., 1987; Rojas et al., 2001; Castren et al., 2003; Van der Molen et al., 2012a,b; Schneider et al., 2013). In 1994, a FXS animal model, the *Fmr1* KO mouse, was created (Bakker et al., 1994). Consistent with the results in FXS patients, *Fmr1* KO mice exhibit a variety of abnormal responses to auditory stimuli, and therefore provide a means of studying the neural correlates and mechanisms underlying auditory processing symptoms of human FXS.

FRAGILE X SYNDROME

Fragile X syndrome is a genetic disorder that affects approximately 1 in 4000 individuals (Hagerman et al., 2009). FXS results from expansion and hyper-methylation of CGG trinucleotide repeats in the promoter region of the *FMR1* gene, which leads to a failure to produce fragile x mental retardation protein (FMRP; Bailey et al., 1998; O'Donnell and Warren, 2002). FMRP inhibits translation of synaptic mRNAs in response to mGluR stimulation, and loss of FMRP typically results in an over-production of associated synaptic proteins (Bear et al., 2004; Bassell and Warren, 2008). Individuals with FXS experience a wide array of symptoms, such as hyper-activity, intellectual impairment, macro-orchidism, hyper-sensitivity to sensory stimulus, and language impairments (Hagerman et al., 1986, 1991; Berry-Kravis et al., 2007; Roberts et al., 2007a; Barnes et al., 2009). Additionally, 10–20% of FXS patients experience seizures (Incorpora et al., 2002; Hagerman and Stafstrom, 2009).

Approximately 15–33% of individuals with FXS meet the three diagnostic criteria for autism, with approximately 5% of autism cases attributed to FXS (Bailey et al., 1998; Cohen et al., 2005). Consistent with autism spectrum disorder, many individuals with FXS display deficits in social behavior, repetitive behavior, and abnormalities in communication. In social interactions, children with FXS often display a "pervasive lack of responsiveness to others" in early childhood, are unwilling to engage in peer play or co-operative play, and generally avoid making eye contact (Hagerman et al., 1986). Also, FXS patients often avoid non-verbal social interactions through a lack of social eye contact, or gaze aversion especially with unfamiliar people or environments (Cohen et al., 1988; Hessl et al., 2006). Individuals diagnosed with FXS may demonstrate a strong preference for routines and a variety of repetitive behaviors, including: rocking, hand-flapping, echolalia, repetitive body movements, and self-injurious behavior (Gillberg et al., 1986; Cohen et al., 1988; Baumgardner et al., 1995; Feinstein and Reiss, 1998; Belser and Sudhalter, 2001; Steinhausen et al., 2002; Baranek et al., 2005).

As with autism, FXS patients show communication abnormalities. Generally, aberrant communication manifests through delays in language development (Fidler et al., 2007; Finestack et al., 2009). Using the Reynell Developmental Language Scales, Roberts et al. (2001) demonstrated delays in communication development in FXS patients manifesting as poor expressive and receptive language skills. Receptive language studies focused on verbal comprehension ability and were assessed through FXS patients' ability to recognize sound and word patterns. Expressive language was gaged through the breadth of patients' vocabulary and patients' ability to verbalize ideas (Roberts et al., 2001). In particular, individuals with FXS experience difficulty articulating words, poor co-articulation, substitutions, and omissions of words, reduction in the number of intelligible syllables produced, difficulty sequencing sounds, and echolalia (Largo and Schinzel, 1985; Hanson et al., 1986; Belser and Sudhalter, 2001; Roberts et al., 2001, 2007a; Barnes et al., 2009). It has been suggested that similar language delays seen in autism may be associated with basic auditory processing abnormalities in early sensory cortical regions (Nieto Del Rincón, 2008; Roberts et al., 2011), but basic auditory processing in humans and mouse models of FXS or autism is incompletely characterized. Taken together, many symptoms of FXS and autism spectrum disorders are similar suggesting that studies of neural alterations in FXS may be broadly applicable.

NEUROANATOMICAL AND BEHAVIORAL ABNORMALITIES IN FXS

A variety of neuroanatomical abnormalities are seen in FXS patients including a larger caudate nucleus and hippocampus and a reduced superior temporal gyrus (STG), amygdala, anterior ventral cerebral gray matter, and anterior mid-inferior cerebral gray matter (Hessl et al., 2004; Gothelf et al., 2008). Diffuser tensor imaging found alterations in the frontal-caudate and parietal sensory-motor white matter tracts in FXS patients, which may alter the speed of neural processing or the magnitude of neuronal responses (Barnea-Goraly et al., 2003). At the cellular level, a common feature found in the FXS brain is a profusion of abnormally long and thin dendritic spines, with a reduction in the number of short, mushroom-shaped spines (Rudelli et al., 1985; Hinton et al., 1991; Irwin et al., 2002).

Many FXS symptoms may be attributed to over-arching arousal modulation problems, which may underlie the tendency in FXS to avoid sensory experience (Belser and Sudhalter, 1995; Cohen, 1995; Baranek, 2002; Baranek et al., 2002). In a test of electrodermal responses to olfactory, auditory, visual, tactile, and vestibular stimuli, children with FXS showed greater peak amplitude, more peaks, and a failure to habituate to stimuli, suggesting a general over-arousal to sensory stimuli (Miller et al., 1999).

Fragile X syndrome patients demonstrate unusual responses to auditory stimuli specifically, as indicated by clinical studies and as measured by pre-pulse inhibition (PPI; Frankland et al., 2004; Hessl et al., 2009; Yuhas et al., 2011). In PPI tests, subjects are typically presented with a less intense (quieter) pre-pulse stimulus followed by a more intense (louder) startle stimulus. The pre-pulse stimulus acts to suppress the response to the startle stimulus, as most often measured using ocular electromyogram recordings (Frankland et al., 2004; Hessl et al., 2009). Reduced PPI has been found in individuals with FXS but not autism, and individuals with FXS and autism (Frankland et al., 2004; Hessl et al., 2009; Yuhas et al., 2011; Schneider et al., 2012). The magnitude of the PPI response in FXS patients was associated with the severity of symptoms (as measured through IQ, attention span, autism, and adaptive behaviors; Frankland et al., 2004), and the number of CGG repeats. Overall, impaired performance on auditory tests is thought to reflect an underlying problem with sensory gating in FXS.

AUDITORY PROCESSING IN FXS ASSESSED USING ELECTRO- OR MAGNETO-ENCEPHALOGRAPHY

To assess sensory-cognitive processing in humans with FXS, various event-related brain potential (ERP) techniques have been employed. ERPs reflect the activity of neuronal populations in response to specific sensory-cognitive processes and can be detected using electro-encephalograms (EEG) and magneto-encephalograms (MEG; Luck, 2005). Auditory ERP sensory responses are comprised of N1and P2 components, as well as families of N2 and P3 components (Luck, 2005). The N1 and P2 components are often studied together and can be elicited by simple and complex auditory stimuli, such as pure tones or musical notes (Naatanen and Picton, 1987). Typically, the N1–P2 complex is found within the 80–200 ms following auditory stimulation (Crowley and Colrain, 2004).

The N1 component may be generated by structures within the frontal and temporal lobes (Hari et al., 1982; Naatanen and Picton, 1987). In particular, three basic components have been identified which give rise to a composite N1. There is also MEG and EEG evidence that the auditory cortex is a prime contributor to the N1 component (Zouridakis et al., 1998; Knoth and Lippe, 2012). N1 itself is modulated by the pitch and intensity of auditory stimuli (Beagley and Knight, 1967; Butler, 1968; Pantev et al., 1988; Alain et al., 1997; Butler and Trainor, 2012), and is sensitive to attention effects (Naatanen and Picton, 1987; Luck, 2005; Naatanen et al., 2011a). Specifically, as the intensity of auditory stimulus is increased, the N1 and P2 amplitude increases (Beagley and Knight, 1967; Picton et al., 1970).

Behavioral auditory hyper-sensitivity may result from abnormally increased cortical responses to sound. In six studies using EEG, the N1 component was enlarged in FXS participants (St. Clair et al., 1987; Rojas et al., 2001; Castren et al., 2003; Van der Molen et al., 2012a,b; Schneider et al., 2013). Moreover, there is a reduction in N1 habituation in FXS individuals when presented with repeating trains of single frequency tones (Castren et al., 2003; Schneider et al., 2013). Importantly, the auditory ERP abnormalities can be used as outcome measures in drug treatment in human studies (Schneider et al., 2013). A study using MEG also revealed enlargement and reduced latency of the N100m (the MEG equivalent of the N1 in EEG; Rojas et al., 2001). The N1 amplitude increase may be related to neuroanatomical abnormalities in FXS patients such as related a decrease in STG size (Reiss et al., 1994) and white matter enlargement localized specifically to the temporal lobe (Hazlett et al., 2012). Additionally, fMRI research shows that the STG, along with the medial frontal gyrus, middle temporal gyrus, cerebellum, and pons display higher levels of activation in FXS patients, consistent with the larger N1 component (Hall et al., 2009).

The source of the P2 component has been broadly localized to the temporal lobe, but the specific structures which generate the P2 are somewhat more diffuse (Hari et al., 1980; Knoth and Lippe, 2012). MEG, EEG, and implanted depth electrode evidence suggest that planum temporale and the auditory association cortex (Area 22) are involved in P2 generation (Godey et al., 2001; Crowley and Colrain, 2004). There is also evidence that auditory input to the mesencephalic reticular activating system contribute to the P2 component (Rif et al., 1991; Crowley and Colrain, 2004). P2 amplitude decreases as attention devoted to a stimulus increases (Crowley and Colrain, 2004). Accordingly, the P2 has been suggested to act as an index of task-devoted attention.

Fragile X syndrome-related N1 enhancement is typically accompanied by P2 enhancement as well (St. Clair et al., 1987; Castren et al., 2003; Van der Molen et al., 2012a,b). Because both components seem to stem from temporal lobe activity, it is possible that the structural anomalies and increased temporal lobe activity that likely drives N1 augmentation also contribute to P2. Additionally, P2 enhancement suggests abnormal activation of the mesencephalic reticular activating system, which may contribute to the hyperactivity seen in FXS. Interestingly, alterations in P2 may drive mismatch negativity (MMN), N2b, and P3a abnormalities (Van der Molen et al., 2012b). Structures linked to P2 generation are also responsible for early auditory processing. As such, malfunction of P2-associated structures may create an incorrect memory trace of the target stimulus, which may impair performance on stimulus detection tasks (Naatanen et al., 2007; Naatanen et al., 2011b).

While the N1 and P2 components are readily modulated by altering the spectral components of auditory stimulation, the N2 and P3 component families are generally more heavily involved in task-related selective attention or novelty detection (Breton et al., 1988; Patel and Azzam, 2005). The N2 family is composed of three main components, the N2a/mismatch negativity, the N2b, and the N2c (Patel and Azzam, 2005). N2 components can be elicited with auditory or visual stimulus, and are often probed with an "oddball" paradigm (Patel and Azzam, 2005). Oddball tasks typically involve presenting repetitive trains of a primary stimulus with deviant stimuli interspersed at unpredictable intervals (Breton et al., 1988). N2a, also called MMN, is a feature unique to auditory attention tasks (Cone-Wesson and Wunderlich, 2003). It is associated with bilateral supratemporal processing and right hemisphere frontal lobe activity and is typically seen during tasks that require participants to attend or ignore deviant stimulus (Naatanen et al., 1978; Luck, 2005; Naatanen et al., 2007). Notably, the MMN is present when subjects passively listen to deviant stimuli and when subjects are asked to provide a response to deviant stimuli (Cone-Wesson and Wunderlich, 2003). As MMN is responsive to changes in frequency and intensity of sound, it likely represents the change in attention associated with comparing a deviant tone to the sensory-memory of the control tone (Cone-Wesson and Wunderlich, 2003; Patel and Azzam, 2005; Knoth and Lippe, 2012). The N2b wave can also be generated through oddball tasks, but it is most prominent during voluntary processing of deviant stimuli or when a stimulus is otherwise selectively attended to (Patel and Azzam, 2005). The N2b has also been shown to be modulated by phonological and semantic changes in language (Sanquist et al., 1980). The N2c wave is most strongly associated with visual attention and stimulus context (Folstein and Van Petten, 2008).

Enlargement of the N2b wave (Van der Molen et al., 2012a,b) and increased N2 latency (St. Clair et al., 1987; Van der Molen et al., 2012a) is seen in FXS patients. Despite a general increase in N2 amplitude, the MMN was reduced in individuals with FXS (Van der Molen et al., 2012b). The most likely cause for MMN attenuation is poor memory trace formation of control stimulus (Naatanen et al., 2007). As mentioned earlier, N1 and P2 components are enhanced in FXS. Because N1 and P2 are generated by structures involved in early auditory processing, their aberrant profile may reflect altered perception of auditory stimulus, and therefore an inaccurate representation of the control stimulus (Naatanen et al., 2007). Without an accurate memory trace to compare against deviant tones, individuals with FXS may be less able to identify unexpected stimuli (Naatanen et al., 2007). Interestingly, in studies where participants were asked to respond to, rather than to passively attend deviant stimuli, FXS patients provided more false positives and were slower to respond, suggesting confusion as to the veracity of a stimulus (Scerif et al., 2012; Van der Molen et al., 2012a).

Though the N2b component is typically seen in response to oddball tasks that require participants to attend deviant stimuli, enhancement of N2b may result from a general hypersensitivity to stimuli. In control subjects, the N2b generated in response to the deviant tone was typically larger than the N2b generated by the standard stimulus (Van der Molen et al., 2012b). In FXS subjects, however, there was little difference in the N2b peak amplitudes generated by the deviant and standard stimuli (Van der Molen et al., 2012b). As the N2b peaks generated in response to both the standard and deviant stimuli in FXS participants had greater amplitudes than those of control participants, N2b enhancement in FXS participants may stem from a general increase in sensitivity to any auditory stimuli. Taken together with the reduction in MMN amplitude, oversensitivity to auditory stimulus may impair the ability of FXS participants to discriminate between standard and deviant tones.

The P3 family is comprised of the P3a and P3b components, which are both elicited by infrequent or unpredictable elements introduced into otherwise predictable trains of stimuli. The P3 component typically occurs 300–500 ms after stimulus presentation and is readily evoked with oddball tasks (Hruby and Marsalek, 2003). The source of the P3 component has been localized to the parietal lobe, though there is evidence of hippocampal and temporoparietal structure involvement (Hruby and Marsalek, 2003). The P3a component occurs at 250–280 ms, and is present when infrequent or unpredictable shifts occur during a train of otherwise predictable stimuli regardless of where the participant is asked to direct his or her attention (Squires et al., 1975; Hruby and Marsalek, 2003). As such, the P3a is often described as a "novelty detector" (Comerchero and Polich, 1999; Hruby and Marsalek, 2003). The P3b is also evoked by oddball tasks, and is observed at 250–500 ms (Polich, 2007). Like the P3a, the P3b component is elicited by improbable events. However, the amplitude of the P3b is dependent upon how improbable a stimulus is, with more improbable stimuli resulting in larger amplitude responses (Sutton et al., 1965; Polich, 2007). The P3b response is thought to be distributed across the prefrontal cortex, anterior insula, cingulate gyrus, medial temporal cortex, and hippocampus (Van der Molen et al., 2012a). To gage the predictability of a given stimulus, the ability to recall variations of that stimulus is necessary. As such, short term memory is required for tasks with unpredictable stimuli (Hruby and Marsalek, 2003).

In individuals with FXS, the amplitude of the P3 component was consistently reduced and the latencies to the components were longer (St. Clair et al., 1987; Van der Molen et al., 2012a,b). St. Clair et al. (1987) found a general reduction in P3 amplitude in individuals with FXS, but did not discriminate between P3a and P3b. Van der Molen et al. (2012b) revealed reduced P3a and P3b components in FXS patients. Though the precise source of P3 generation is uncertain, modulation of P3 amplitude or latencies suggest difficulty identifying or responding to infrequent stimuli in FXS patients (Hruby and Marsalek, 2003). Decreased P3b amplitude specifically, may reflect a failure to identify a stimulus as improbable (Sutton et al., 1965), possibly resulting from improper stimulus representation at lower levels of processing, or from short term memory impairments (Polich, 2007). Altered short term memory function may obstruct a FXS patient's ability to recall a previous stimulus (Polich, 2007). The major auditory ERP abnormalities in humans with FXS are summarized in **Table 1**.

Fmr1 KO MOUSE MODEL OF FXS

The *Fmr1* knockout mouse (*Fmr1* KO) was developed as a preclinical model for studying the mechanisms underlying FXS (Bakker et al., 1994). *Fmr1* KO mice lack FMRP and manifest several FXS-associated symptoms (Bernardet and Crusio, 2006; Moy and Nadler, 2008). *Fmr1* KO mice show evidence of social impairments, as demonstrated by social dominance and social interaction tasks (Spencer et al., 2005). Repetitive behaviors have been demonstrated in *Fmr1* KO mice using marble burying tasks (Crawley, 2004, 2007). Through studying ultrasonic vocalization production, evidence has been found that *Fmr1* KO mice experience communication deficits. As pups, *Fmr1* KO mice produce wriggling calls at a higher frequency than their littermate controls, and as adults male *Fmr1* KO mice produce mating calls at a slower rate than male wild type mice (Rotschafer et al., 2012; Roy et al., 2012).

There is also evidence that *Fmr1* KO mice may replicate the heightened anxiety associated with FXS. Elevated plus mazes are a common test for anxiety in mice, but show variable results in *Fmr1* KO mice. Elevated plus mazes usually have four arms, two of which are enclosed, while two remain open. Reluctance to enter the open arms is suggestive of heightened anxiety, and so fewer entries into open arms can serve as a measure of anxiety (Bilousova et al., 2009). While some studies report *Fmr1* KO mice spend less time in the open arms (Bilousova et al., 2009), others do not (Mineur et al., 2002; Zhao et al., 2005). Open field mazes are used to probe exploratory behavior in *Fmr1* KO mice. Results of open field maze tasks are also mixed, but do consistently show increased locomotor activity in *Fmr1* KO mice (Bakker et al., 1994; Mineur et al., 2002). Increased locomotor activity may be related to hyperactivity (Bakker et al., 1994; Mineur et al., 2002). Variability in elevated plus maze tests results may be an artifact of increased locomotor activity or hyperactivity in FXS. Entering the open arms of the plus maze at control levels may reflect *Fmr1* KO mice moving more vigorously within the maze rather than any anomaly in the anxiety the mouse experiences. The 5-choice serial reaction time task (5CSRTT) specifically tested attentional control while performing an operant task. During the 5CSRTT, mice were presented with an array of five holes in which they may find a food reward. When a light appeared in a hole, mice may select that hole for a reward. The ability of a mouse to accurately choose the illuminated hole measures attention to a task, and the ability of an animal to refrain from choosing a hole prior to predictive stimuli measures inhibitory control. Adult *Fmr1* KO mice did not demonstrate impairments in accuracy or inhibitory control during testing. However, *Fmr1* KO mice were hyperactive in novel environments and provided more responses during rule acquisition. During a rule reversal phase, all holes were illuminated and mice had to probe the unilluminated holes to obtain a reward. *Fmr1* KO mice displayed more errors and a general increase in response rate during the rule reversal phase (Kramvis et al., 2013). These data suggest that hyperactivity in

Table 1 | Summary of auditory processing abnormalities in humans with FXS determined using auditory ERP.

ERP component	Changes in FXS patients	Reference
N1	Enhanced peak amplitudes, reduced hemispheric asymmetry, reduced habituation	Rojas et al. (2001), Castren et al. (2003), Van der Molen et al. (2012a,b), Schneider et al. (2013)
P2	Enhanced peak amplitude	Van der Molen et al. (2012b)
MMN	Reduced peak amplitude	Van der Molen et al. (2012b)
N2	Enhanced peak amplitude, reduced sensitization, longer latencies	Castren et al. (2003), Van der Molen et al. (2012a,b)
P3	Reduced peak amplitude, longer latencies, abnormal waveform shape	Van der Molen et al. (2012a,b), St. Clair et al. (1987)

Fmr1 KO is largely driven by heightened arousal resulting from exposure to novel environments. Because the neural mechanisms of these complex behaviors are incompletely understood, it is difficult to interpret the actions of potential therapeutics at a circuit level.

Fmr1 KO MOUSE AUDITORY BEHAVIOR

Consistent with auditory abnormalities in humans with FXS, *Fmr1* KO mice show abnormal behavior in response to auditory stimulus, as seen in audiogenic seizure, PPI, and auditory startle response (ASR) paradigms. In *Fmr1* KO mice, intense auditory stimuli (>100 dB SPL) induces a period of wild running, clonic – tonic seizing, and can result in the death of the animal (Musumeci et al., 2000; Chen and Toth, 2001; Musumeci et al., 2007; Dansie et al., 2013). Reintroduction of FMRP to *Fmr1* KO mice significantly reduced audiogenic seizure susceptibility (Musumeci et al., 2007).

The stimulus protocol on mouse PPI studies is similar to that in human testing, with an intense startle stimulus proceeded by a less intense pre-pulse stimulus (Frankland et al., 2004; Bray et al., 2011). *Fmr1* KO mice reliably show enhanced PPI response, a phenotype that is robust enough to be routinely used as a behavioral outcome measure for potential treatments (Olmos-Serrano et al., 2011; Levenga et al., 2011). The PPI response in KO mice is different from humans with FXS, but the respective enhancements and deficits in PPI are both attributed to an underlying aberration in sensory gating (Frankland et al., 2004).

Fmr1 KO mice show enhanced ASR (Chen and Toth, 2001; Nielsen et al., 2002; Frankland et al., 2004; Yun et al., 2006). Startle enhancement was readily found in *Fmr1* KO mice after 3 weeks of age (Yun et al., 2006). Interestingly, the degree of ASR magnitude was unaffected by stimulus intensity in *Fmr1* KO mice. When wild type mice are presented low intensity stimulus, they respond with relatively small startle response, and relatively large startle responses when presented with high intensity stimulus (Nielsen et al., 2002). By contrast, the magnitude of the *Fmr1* KO mouse startle response did not change with the intensity of the sound stimulus presented (Nielsen et al., 2002). Failure to modulate behavior in response to the magnitude of sensory input is also indicative sensorimotor gating deficits (Nielsen et al., 2002).

ALTERED *IN VIVO* AUDITORY CORTICAL RESPONSES AND PLASTICITY IN *Fmr1* KO MICE

Despite the consistent findings of abnormal auditory behaviors and ERPs in humans and hypersensitive responses to sounds in mice, few studies have examined the neural correlates of auditory processing deficits in FXS (Strumbos et al., 2010; Kim et al., 2013; Rotschafer and Razak, 2013). *In vivo* cortical electrophysiological recordings in response to sounds show that individual neurons in *Fmr1* KO mice are hyper-responsive (Rotschafer and Razak, 2013). Mice were presented with a series of pure tone and frequency modulated (FM) sweep stimuli while single unit extracellular recordings were taken in the primary auditory cortex. In response to pure tones, *Fmr1* KO mouse neurons produced more spikes, prolonged responses, and broader frequency tuning than their wild-type counterparts. Neurons from *Fmr1* KO mice also showed more temporal variability in their responses than WT neurons (Rotschafer and Razak, 2013). When presented with FM sweeps, KO neurons that responded best to fast and intermediate FM sweep rates were less sharply selective for sweep rates than those of wild type (Rotschafer and Razak, 2013). Though excessive cortical response to sound may be partially driven by increased activity in other brain nuclei, it is consistent with the abnormal PPI and ASR responses seen in *Fmr1* KO mice as well as with the audiogenic seizure characteristic of *Fmr1* KO mice.

Fmr1 KO mice also demonstrate mGluR5-associated anomalies in experience-dependent cortical plasticity during the critical period (Kim et al., 2013). An "early" group of *Fmr1* KO mice (P9–P20) and a "late" group of mice (P20–P30) were raised in a sound attenuated chamber while 16 kHz pips were played. Multiunit responses were then used to map frequency representation in the primary auditory cortex of early group, late group, and wild type control mice. Tonotopy in *Fmr1* KO and wild type mice that were not exposed to pure tone stimulus during development was not significantly different. Wild type mice from the early group; however, did demonstrate expanded cortical representation of 16 kHz that the *Fmr1* KO early group failed to replicate, suggesting that cortical plasticity during the critical period may be impaired in *Fmr1* KO mice (Kim et al., 2013). Moreover, neither the wild type nor *Fmr1* KO mice of the late group displayed expanded frequency representation, limiting the window for these plasticity impairments to the critical period. Injections of the mGluR5 antagonist, MPEP, rescued frequency representations in the *Fmr1* KO mouse auditory cortex, implying that heightened mGluR5 activity may underlie this failure of experience dependent plasticity. These data suggest that impaired early developmental plasticity may underlie the abnormalities found in the adult auditory cortical responses (Rotschafer and Razak, 2013). Such cortical deficits may lead to higher order auditory processing deficits such as those involved in language. The major auditory behavioral and processing abnormalities in the *Fmr1* KO mice are summarized in **Table 2**.

ALTERED CORTICAL EXCITATORY-INHIBITORY BALANCE MAY UNDERLIE ABNORMAL AUDITORY RESPONSES

The enhanced single neuron responses in the auditory cortex is consistent with a general increase in the excitability of neurons lacking FMRP, and subsequently, over-active neuronal networks. These responses may be neural correlates of auditory hypersensitivity in humans with FXS, and thus provide functional probes to investigate the underlying receptive field and molecular mechanisms in the mouse model. The heightened activity may stem from a concurrence of dysfunctional intrinsic excitability and GABA receptors, loss of inhibitory neurons, abnormal dendrite morphology, and excessive mGluR activity (Huber et al., 2002a,b; Huber, 2007). For example, neurons in the *Fmr1* KO mouse somatosensory cortex show weakened inhibitory interneuron activity and more excitable pyramidal neurons (Gibson et al., 2008; Hays et al., 2011; Paluszkiewicz et al., 2011). Monosynaptic GABAergic transmission in the barrel cortex of *Fmr1* KO mice is unaffected, but fast spiking (inhibitory) interneurons experience an approximate

Table 2 | Summary of auditory processing abnormalities in the *Fmr1* KO mice.

Auditory deficit	Study method	Reference
Increased propensity for audiogenic seizures	Behavioral response to loud sounds	Musumeci et al. (2000, 2007), Chen and Toth (2001), Dansie et al. (2013)
Increased acoustic startle response	Behavioral observations	Chen and Toth (2001), Nielsen et al. (2002), Frankland et al. (2004), Yun et al. (2006)
Altered auditory cortical responses to sounds		
Increased and prolonged single neuron responses to pure tones	*In vivo* extracellular electrophysiology	Rotschafer and Razak (2013)
Broader frequency tuning curves		
Reduced spectrotemporal selectivity		
Increased variability in response latency		
Reduced critical period plasticity in auditory cortex	Sound exposure during development and *in vivo* electrophysiological mapping	Kim et al. (2013)
Altered tonotopy and reduced experience dependent plasticity of Kv3.1b channel in auditory brainstem	Sound exposure, immunohistochemistry and electrophysiology	Strumbos et al. (2010)

50% decrease in excitatory drive (Gibson et al., 2008). *Fmr1* KO mouse somatosensory neurons are also hyperexcitable, as characterized by longer, less synchronous UP states (Gibson et al., 2008; Hays et al., 2011). UP states were prolonged in cortical slices that did not express *Fmr1* in glutamatergic neuron, while deletion of *Fmr1* in GABAergic neurons had no effect on UP state duration (Hays et al., 2011). Prolonged UP states are generated by the over activity of mGluR5 receptors on excitatory neurons which lack *Fmr1*, rather than any *Fmr1* deficiency in inhibitory neurons (Hays et al., 2011). There might also be abnormalities at the cortical network level as a result of single neuron changes. For example, young (first two post-natal weeks) *Fmr1* KO mice show increased network synchrony when spontaneous firing was assessed with two-photon Ca^{2+} imaging (Gonçalves et al., 2013). In *Fmr1* KO mice, increased network synchrony was strongly correlated with increased action potential production (Gonçalves et al., 2013).

Consistent with behavioral research demonstrating mGluR antagonists and GABA receptor agonists improve *Fmr1* KO mouse responses to auditory stimuli, evidence of both GABA and glutamate imbalances have been found in *Fmr1* KO mice. The mRNA of the α_1, α_3, α_4, β_1, β_2, γ_1, and γ_2 GABA receptor subunits are down-regulated by 35–50% in *Fmr1* KO mice, with a decline in the actual α_1, β_2, and δ GABA receptor subunits (El Idrissi et al., 2005; D'Hulst et al., 2006, 2009; Adusei et al., 2010). Additionally, a 20% reduction in the number of Parvalbumin positive (PV+) cells was found in the somatosensory cortex of *Fmr1* KO mice (Selby et al., 2007). Underlying alterations in GABA receptor function and excessive excitatory input may result in some changes in auditory behavior seen in *Fmr1* KO mice.

Like FXS patients, *Fmr1* KO mice exhibit abnormal cortical and hippocampal dendritic spine morphology. Dendritic spines on pyramidal cells in the visual and temporal cortex of *Fmr1* KO mice are longer, thinner, and generally display a more immature morphology than wild-type mice, with increased spine density along dendrites (Comery et al., 1997; Irwin et al., 2000, 2002; McKinney et al., 2005). The *Fmr1* KO mouse barrel cortex has been studied more extensively and shows a host of dendritic spine abnormalities. Relatively young mice (P25) barrel cortex did not show dendritic spine abnormalities, but older mice (P73–P76) show fewer short/ mature spines and more long/immature spines (Galvez and Greenough, 2005; Till et al., 2012). Transcranial two-photon imaging revealed that dendritic spines in the barrel cortex of *Fmr1* KO mice also display a higher turnover rate, with more pools of new, transient spines (Pan et al., 2010).

The *Fmr1* KO mouse barrel cortex also demonstrates delayed formation, and abnormal dendrite pruning. In mice, each vibrissa (whisker) is represented by a cortical barrel that has a cell body dense septa and cell-sparse hollow. During development, the number of dendrites at the septa decreases, while the number of dendrites growing to the hollow increases. Pruning of dendrites growing toward the septa results in asymmetrical dendrite distribution in wild type adult animals (Greenough and Chang, 1988). In *Fmr1* KO mice, spiny stellate cells in the barrel cortex have an excessive number of dendrites oriented toward the septa, resulting in less asymmetrical cells (Galvez et al., 2003; Till et al., 2012). Barrel cortex neurons of *Fmr1* KO mice also show excessive dendritic spine production and unusually long spines during the first post-natal week. When dendritic spines were examined at post-natal weeks 2 and 4, a trend toward normalization was discovered. While dendritic spines were still longer in *Fmr1* KO mice, the magnitude of difference from wild type animals had decreased. The number dendritic spines in *Fmr1* KO mice had fallen to numbers comparable to WT animals by the second week (Nimchinsky et al., 2001). Disrupted cell morphology and cytoarchitecture during early development of sensory systems may impair an animal's ability to integrate sensory experiences. Functionally, dendritic spines in the *Fmr1* KO mouse barrel cortex are less sensitive to sensory experience modulation. Sensory deprivation (all whiskers on one side of the facial pad were trimmed) resulted in a reduced the rate of dendritic spine elimination in wild type mice, but was unaltered in *Fmr1* KO mice (Zuo et al., 2005; Pan et al., 2010). Alternatively, dendritic spine formation was enhanced in wild type mice when the whiskers were trimmed in a chessboard pattern, while *Fmr1* KO mice failed to show any difference in spine formation. Failure to form or eliminate dendritic spines in response to changing sensory input suggests that barrel cortex neurons in *Fmr1* KO mice may be improperly tuned to sensory stimuli (Pan et al., 2010). A similar pattern if found in the auditory cortex may explain the reduced developmental plasticity (Kim et al., 2013) and abnormal adult responses (Rotschafer and Razak, 2013).

CONCLUSIONS AND FUTURE STUDIES

Converging lines of evidence describe auditory cortical dysfunction in the *Fmr1* KO mice and in patients with FXS. The common underlying phenotype is "auditory hypersensitivity." The mechanisms underlying sensory hypersensitivity may be relatively more tractable compared to more complex social behaviors typically studied in FXS (and autism). Therefore, we propose that auditory hypersensitivity is a robust, reliable, and translatable biomarker to integrate pre-clinical and clinical investigations at multiple levels of analysis to facilitate drug discovery in FXS. Within this framework, the following future studies will be important to perform:

(1) What are the neural mechanisms of individual neuron hyperexcitability in the primary auditory cortex of the *Fmr1* KO mice? Understanding the intrinsic properties, morphological features, and inhibition/excitation balance in auditory cortical neurons is a necessary step in understanding the mechanisms of auditory hypersensitivity in mice and humans. The availability of mice in which FMRP can be deleted specifically in the cortex, in specific types of neurons and at specific developmental time points will make it possible to identify the loci of hyper-excitability.

(2) Fragile X syndrome is a neurodevelopmental disorder, but the developmental changes in functional neural response selectivity are unclear. The focus has been on transient delays or permanent changes in dendritic spine properties and synaptic or intrinsic properties (reviewed in Meredith et al., 2012). The consequence of these synaptic changes to development of behaviorally relevant neural response properties are not known in FXS. Therefore, it is not clear if the observed auditory hypersensitivity in humans with FXS is due to an altered regulation of developmental processes during a sensitive period that persists into adulthood. The majority of studies using *Fmr1* KO mice focus on the neurological responses and behaviors of relatively young mice, neglecting any long term developmental changes *Fmr1* KO may undergo and failing to describe the long term impact of the dysfunction described early in life. Are the results of FMRP loss during a specific sensitive period in life or whether they may better be attributed to the on-going absence of FMRP? It will be useful to determine if there are specific time developmental windows during which the KO and WT mice cortical responses diverge from each other. As summarized by Meredith et al. (2012), it may be possible to target specific developmental windows for therapeutic approaches. Auditory hypersensitivity will provide translatable physiological and behavioral probes to address this possibility and study underlying mechanisms.

(3) Development of methods to monitor long term auditory processing in awake behaving mice. One such technique may be chronic EEG from the temporal cortex of WT and KO mice. This method will not only provide baseline and sound evoked EEG, but also facilitate a study of neural activity during audiogenic seizure induction. Because audiogenic seizure is a commonly used behavior in testing drugs for FXS, having the additional measure of electrical activity during seizure induction, will provide a rich set of biomarkers to measure drug effects. Moreover, the evoked EEGs will allow a more direct comparison with human auditory ERP studies, facilitating translation efforts.

ACKNOWLEDGMENTS

We thank the members of the Razak lab for important discussions leading to this review. The research on FXS in the Razak lab is funded by FRAXA Research Foundation.

REFERENCES

Adusei, D. C., Pacey, L. K., Chen, D., and Hampson, D. R. (2010). Early developmental alterations in GABAergic protein expression in fragile X knockout mice. *Neuropharmacology* 59, 167–171. doi: 10.1016/j.neuropharm.2010.05.002

Alain, C., Woods, D. L., and Covarrubias, D. (1997). Activation of duration-sensitive auditory cortical fields in humans. *Electroencephalogr. Clin. Neurophysiol.* 104, 531–539. doi: 10.1016/S0168-5597(97)00057-9

Alcántara, J. I., Cope, T. E., Cope, W., and Weisblatt, E. J. (2012). Auditory temporal-envelope processing in high-functioning children with Autism Spectrum Disorder. *Neuropsychologia* 50, 1235–1251. doi: 10.1016/j.neuropsychologia.2012.01.034

Bailey, D. B. Jr., Mesibov, G. B., Hatton, D. D., Clark, R. D., Roberts, J. E., and Mayhew, L., et al. (1998). Autistic behavior in young boys with fragile X syndrome. *J. Autism. Dev. Disord.* 28, 499–508. doi: 10.1023/A:1026048027397

Bakker, C. E., Verheij, C., Willemsen, R., Vanderhelm, R., Oerlemans, F., Vermey, M., et al. (1994). FMR1 knockout mice – a model to study fragile-x mental-retardation. *Cell* 78, 23–33. doi:10.1016/0092-8674(94)90569-X

Baranek, G. T. (2002). Efficacy of sensory and motor interventions for children with autism. *J. Autism. Dev. Disord.* 32, 397–422. doi: 10.1023/A:1020541906063

Baranek, G. T., Chin, Y. H., Hess, L. M., Yankee, J. G., Hatton, D. D., and Hooper, S. R. (2002). Sensory processing correlates of occupational performance in children with fragile X syndrome: preliminary findings. *Am. J. Occup. Ther.* 56, 538–546. doi: 10.5014/ajot.56.5.538

Baranek, G. T., Danko, C. D., Skinner, M. L., Bailey, D. B. Jr., Hatton, D. D., Roberts, J. E., et al. (2005). Video analysis of sensory-motor features in infants with fragile X syndrome at 9-12 months of age. *J. Autism. Dev. Disord.* 35, 645–656. doi: 10.1007/s10803-005-0008-7

Barnea-Goraly, N., Eliez, S., Hedeus, M., Menon, V., White, C. D., Moseley, M., et al. (2003). White matter tract alterations in fragile X syndrome: preliminary evidence from diffusion tensor imaging. *Am. J. Med. Genet. B Neuropsychiatr. Genet.* 118B, 81–88. doi: 10.1002/ajmg.b.10035

Barnes, E., Roberts, J., Long, S. H., Martin, G. E., Berni, M. C., Mandulak, K. C., et al. (2009). Phonological accuracy and intelligibility in connected speech of boys with fragile X syndrome or Down syndrome. *J. Speech Lang. Hear. Res.* 52, 1048–1061. doi: 10.1044/1092-4388(2009/08-0001)

Bassell, G. J., and Warren, S. T. (2008). Fragile X syndrome: loss of local mRNA regulation alters synaptic development and function. *Neuron* 60, 201–214. doi: 10.1016/j.neuron.2008.10.004

Baumgardner, T. L., Reiss, A. L., Freund, L. S., and Abrams, M. T. (1995). Specification of the neurobehavioral phenotype in males with fragile X syndrome. *Pediatrics* 95, 744–752.

Beagley, H. A., and Knight, J. J. (1967). Changes in auditory evoked response with intensity. *J. Laryngol. Otol.* 81, 861–873. doi: 10.1017/S0022215100067815

Bear, M. F., Huber, K. M., and Warren, S. T. (2004). The mGluR theory of fragile X mental retardation. *Trends Neurosci.* 27, 370–377. doi: 10.1016/j.tins.2004.04.009

Belser, R. C., and Sudhalter, V. (1995). Arousal difficulties in males with fragile X syndrome: a preliminary report. *Dev. Brain Dysfunct.* 8, 270–279.

Belser, R. C., and Sudhalter, V. (2001). Conversational characteristics of children with fragile X syndrome: repetitive speech. *Am. J. Ment. Retard.* 106, 28–38. doi: 10.1352/0895-8017(2001)106<0028:CCOCWF>2.0.CO;2

Bernardet, M., and Crusio, W. E. (2006). Fmr1 KO mice as a possible model of autistic features. *Scientificworldjournal* 6, 1164–1176. doi: 10.1100/tsw.2006.220

Berry-Kravis, E., Abrams, L., Coffey, S. M., Hall, D. A., Greco, C., Gane, L. W., et al. (2007). Fragile X-associated tremor/ataxia syndrome: clinical features, genetics, and testing guidelines. *Mov. Disord.* 22, 2018–2030; quiz 2140. doi: 10.1002/mds.21493

Bhatara, A., Babikian, T., Laugeson, E., Tachdjian, R., and Sininger, Y. S. (2013). Impaired timing and frequency discrimination in high-functioning autism spectrum disorders. *J. Autism. Dev. Disord.* 43, 1–17. doi: 10.1007/s10803-013-1778-y

Bilousova, T. V., Dansie, L., Ngo, M., Aye, J., Charles, J. R., Ethell, D. W., et al. (2009). Minocycline promotes dendritic spine maturation and improves behavioural performance in the fragile X mouse model. *J. Med. Genet.* 46, 94–102. doi: 10.1136/jmg.2008.061796

Bray, S., Hirt, M., Jo, B., Hall, S. S., Lightbody, A. A., Walter, E., et al. (2011). Aberrant frontal lobe maturation in adolescents with fragile X syndrome is related to delayed cognitive maturation. *Biol. Psychiatry* 70, 852–858. doi: 10.1016/j.biopsych.2011.05.038

Breton, F., Ritter, W., Simson, R., and Vaughan, H. G. Jr. (1988). The N2 component elicited by stimulus matches and multiple targets. *Biol. Psychol.* 27, 23–44. doi: 10.1016/0301-0511(88)90003-8

Butler, B. E., and Trainor, L. J. (2012). Sequencing the cortical processing of pitch-evoking stimuli using EEG analysis and source estimation. *Front. Psychol.* 3:180. doi: 10.3389/fpsyg.2012.00180

Butler, R. A. (1968). Effect of changes in stimulus frequency and intensity on habituation of the human vertex potential. *J. Acoust. Soc. Am.* 44, 945–950. doi: 10.1121/1.1911233

Castren, M., Paakkonen, A., Tarkka, I. M., Ryynanen, M., and Partanen, J. (2003). Augmentation of auditory N1 in children with fragile X syndrome. *Brain Topogr.* 15, 165–171. doi: 10.1023/A:1022606200636

Centers for Disease Control and Prevention. (2009). Prevalence of autism spectrum disorders. Autism and Developmental Disabilities Monitoring Network, United States 2006. *MMWR Surveill. Summ.* 58, 1–20.

Chen, L., and Toth, M. (2001). Fragile X mice develop sensory hyperreactivity to auditory stimuli. *Neuroscience* 103, 1043–1050. doi: 10.1016/S0306-4522(01)00036-7

Cohen, D., Pichard, N., Tordjman, S., Baumann, C., Burglen, L., Excoffier, E., et al. (2005). Specific genetic disorders and autism: clinical contribution towards their identification. *J. Autism. Dev. Disord.* 35, 103–116. doi: 10.1007/s10803-004-1038-2

Cohen, I. L. (1995). A theoretical analysis of the role of hyperarousal in the learning and behavior of fragile X males. *Ment. Retard. Dev. Disabil. Res. Rev.* 1, 286–291. doi: 10.1002/mrdd.1410010410

Cohen, I. L., Fisch, G. S., Sudhalter, V., Wolf-Schein, E. G., Hanson, D., Hagerman, R., et al. (1988). Social gaze, social avoidance, and repetitive behavior in fragile X males: a controlled study. *Am. J. Ment. Retard.* 92, 436–446.

Comerchero, M. D., and Polich, J. (1999). P3a and P3b from typical auditory and visual stimuli. *Clin. Neurophysiol.* 110, 24–30. doi: 10.1016/S0168-5597(98)00033-1

Comery, T. A., Harris, J. B., Willems, P. J., Oostra, B. A., Irwin, S. A., Weiler, I. J., et al. (1997). Abnormal dendritic spines in fragile X knockout mice: maturation and pruning deficits. *Proc. Natl. Acad. Sci. U.S.A.* 94, 5401–5404. doi: 10.1073/pnas.94.10.5401

Cone-Wesson, B., and Wunderlich, J. (2003). Auditory evoked potentials from the cortex: audiology applications. *Curr. Opin. Otolaryngol. Head. Neck. Surg* 11, 372–377. doi: 10.1097/00020840-200310000-00011

Crawley, J. N. (2004). Designing mouse behavioral tasks relevant to autistic-like behaviors. *Ment. Retard. Dev. Disabil. Res. Rev.* 10, 248–258. doi: 10.1002/mrdd.20039

Crawley, J. N. (2007). Mouse behavioral assays relevant to the symptoms of autism. *Brain Pathol.* 17, 448–459. doi: 10.1111/j.1750-3639.2007.00096.x

Crowley, K. E., and Colrain, I. M (2004). A review of the evidence for P2 being an independent component process: age, sleep and modality. *Clin. Neurophysiol.* 115, 732–744. doi: 10.1016/j.clinph.2003.11.021

D'Hulst, C., De Geest, N., Reeve, S. P., Van Dam, D., De Deyn, P. P., Hassan, B. A., et al. (2006). Decreased expression of the GABAA receptor in fragile X syndrome. *Brain Res.* 1121, 238–245. doi: 10.1016/j.brainres.2006.08.115

D'Hulst, C., Heulens, I., Brouwer, J. R., Willemsen, R., De Geest, N., Reeve, S. P., et al. (2009). Expression of the GABAergic system in animal models for fragile X syndrome and fragile X associated tremor/ataxia syndrome (FXTAS). *Brain Res.* 1253, 176–183. doi: 10.1016/j.brainres.2008.11.075

Dansie, L. E., Phommahaxay, K., Okusanya, A. G., Uwadia, J., Huang, M., Rotschafer, S. E., et al. (2013). Long-lasting effects of minocycline on behavior in young but not adult fragile X mice. *Neuroscience* 246, 186–198. doi: 10.1016/j.neuroscience.2013.04.058

El Idrissi, A., Ding, X. H., Scalia, J., Trenkner, E., Brown, W. T., and Dobkin, C. (2005). Decreased GABA(A) receptor expression in the seizure-prone fragile X mouse. *Neurosci. Lett.* 377, 141–146. doi: 10.1016/j.neulet.2004.11.087

Feinstein, C., and Reiss, A. L. (1998). Autism: the point of view from fragile X studies. *J. Autism. Dev. Disord.* 28, 393–405. doi: 10.1023/A:1026000404855

Fidler, D. J., Philofsky, A., and Hepburn, S. L. (2007). Language phenotypes and intervention planning: bridging research and practice. *Ment. Retard. Dev. Disabil. Res. Rev.* 13, 47–57. doi: 10.1002/mrdd.20132

Finestack, L. H., Richmond, E. K., and Abbeduto, L (2009). Language development in individuals with fragile X syndrome. *Top. Lang. Disord.* 29, 133–148. doi: 10.1097/TLD.0b013e3181a72016

Folstein, J. R., and Van Petten, C. (2008). Influence of cognitive control and mismatch on the N2 component of the ERP: a review. *Psychophysiology* 45, 152–170. doi: 10.1111/j.1469-8986.2007.00602.x

Frankland, P. W., Wang, Y., Rosner, B., Shimizu, T., Balleine, B. W., Dykens, E. M. et al. (2004). Sensorimotor gating abnormalities in young males with fragile X syndrome and Fmr1-knockout mice. *Mol. Psychiatry* 9, 417–425. doi: 10.1038/sj.mp.4001432

Gage, N. M., Siegel, B., Callen, M., and Roberts, T. P. (2003a). Cortical sound processing in children with autism disorder: an MEG investigation. *Neuroreport* 14, 2047–2051. doi: 10.1097/00001756-200311140-00008

Gage, N. M., Siegel, B., and Roberts, T. P. (2003b). Cortical auditory system maturational abnormalities in children with autism disorder: an MEG investigation. *Brain Res. Dev. Brain Res.* 144, 201–219. doi: 10.1016/S0165-3806(03)00172-X

Galvez, R., and Greenough, W. T. (2005). Sequence of abnormal dendritic spine development in primary somatosensory cortex of a mouse model of the fragile X mental retardation syndrome. *Am. J. Med. Genet. A* 135, 155–160. doi: 10.1002/ajmg.a.30709

Galvez, R., Gopal, A. R., and Greenough, W. T. (2003). Somatosensory cortical barrel dendritic abnormalities in a mouse model of the fragile X mental retardation syndrome. *Brain Res.* 971, 83–89. doi: 10.1016/S0006-8993(03)02363-1

Gibson, J. R., Bartley, A. F., Hays, S. A., and Huber, K. M. (2008). Imbalance of neocortical excitation and inhibition and altered up states reflect network hyperexcitability in the mouse model of fragile x syndrome. *J. Neurophysiol.* 100, 2615–2626. doi: 10.1152/jn.90752.2008

Gillberg, C., Persson, E., and Wahlstrom, J. (1986). The autism-fragile-X syndrome (AFRAX): a population-based study of ten boys. *J. Ment. Defic. Res.* 30(Pt 1), 27–39.

Godey, B., Schwartz, D., de Graaf, J. B., Chauvel, P., and Liegeois-Chauvel, C. (2001). Neuromagnetic source localization of auditory evoked fields and intracerebral evoked potentials: a comparison of data in the same patients. *Clin. Neurophysiol.* 112, 1850–1859. doi: 10.1016/S1388-2457(01)00636-8

Gonçalves, J. T., Anstey, J. E., Golshani, P., and Portera-Cailliau, C. (2013). Circuit level defects in the developing neocortex of Fragile X mice. *Nat. Neurosci.* 16, 903–909. doi: 10.1038/nn.3415

Gothelf, D., Furfaro, J. A., Hoeft, F., Eckert, M. A., Hall, S. S., O'Hara, R., et al. (2008). Neuroanatomy of fragile X syndrome is associated with aberrant behavior and the fragile X mental retardation protein (FMRP). *Ann. Neurol.* 63, 40–51. doi: 10.1002/ana.21243

Greenough, W. T., and Chang, F. L. (1988). Dendritic pattern formation involves both oriented regression and oriented growth in the barrels of mouse somatosensory cortex. *Brain Res.* 471, 148–152. doi: 10.1016/0165-3806(88)90160-5

Hagerman, P. J., and Stafstrom, C. E. (2009). Origins of epilepsy in fragile X syndrome. *Epilepsy Curr.* 9, 108–112. doi: 10.1111/j.1535-7511.2009.01309.x

Hagerman, R. J., Berry-Kravis, E., Kaufmann, W. E., Ono, M. Y., Tartaglia, N., Lachiewicz, A., et al. (2009). Advances in the treatment of fragile X syndrome. *Pediatrics* 123, 378–390. doi: 10.1542/peds.2008-0317

Hagerman, R. J., Amiri, K., and Cronister, A. (1991). Fragile X checklist. *Am. J. Med. Genet.* 38, 283–287. doi: 10.1002/ajmg.1320380223

Hagerman, R. J., Jackson, A. W. III, Levitas, A., Rimland, B., and Braden, M. (1986). An analysis of autism in fifty males with the fragile X syndrome. *Am. J. Med. Genet.* 23, 359–374. doi: 10.1002/ajmg.1320230128

Hall, S. S., Walter, E., Sherman, E., Hoeft, F., and Reiss, A. L. (2009). The neural basis of auditory temporal discrimination in girls with fragile X syndrome. *J. Neurodev. Disord.* 1, 91–99. doi: 10.1007/s11689-009-9007-x

Hanson, D. M., Jackson, A. W. III, and Hagerman, R. J. (1986). Speech disturbances (cluttering) in mildly impaired males with the Martin-Bell/fragile X syndrome. *Am. J. Med. Genet.* 23, 195–206. doi: 10.1002/ajmg.1320230114

Hari, R., Aittoniemi, K., Jarvinen, M. L., Katila, T., and Varpula, T. (1980). Auditory evoked transient and sustained magnetic fields of the human brain. Localization of neural generators. *Exp. Brain Res.* 40, 237–240. doi: 10.1007/BF00237543

Hari, R., Kaila, K., Katila, T., Tuomisto, T., and Varpula, T. (1982). Interstimulus interval dependence of the auditory vertex response and its magnetic counterpart: implications for their neural generation. *Electroencephalogr. Clin. Neurophysiol.* 54, 561–569. doi: 10.1016/0013-4694(82)90041-4

Hays, S. A., Huber, K. M., and Gibson, J. R. (2011). Altered neocortical rhythmic activity states in Fmr1 KO mice are due to enhanced mGluR5 signaling and involve changes in excitatory circuitry. *J. Neurosci.* 31, 14223–14234. doi: 10.1523/JNEUROSCI.3157-11.2011

Hazlett, H. C., Poe, M. D., Lightbody, A. A., Styner, M., MacFall, J. R., Reiss, A. L., et al. (2012). Trajectories of early brain volume development in fragile x syndrome and autism. *J. Am. Acad. Child. Adolesc. Psychiatry*, 51, 921–933. doi: 10.1016/j.jaac.2012.07.003

Hessl, D., Rivera, S. M., and Reiss, A. L. (2004). The neuroanatomy and neuroendocrinotogy of fragile X syndrome. *Ment. Retard. Dev. Disabil. Res. Rev.* 10, 17–24. doi: 10.1002/mrdd.20004

Hessl, D., Glaser, B., Dyer-Friedman, J., and Reiss, A. L. (2006). Social behavior and cortisol reactivity in children with fragile X syndrome. *J. Child. Psychol. Psychiatry*, 47, 602–610. doi: 10.1111/j.1469-7610.2005.01556.x

Hessl, D., Berry-Kravis, E., Cordeiro, L., Yuhas, J., Ornitz, E. M., Campbell, A., et al. (2009). Prepulse inhibition in fragile X syndrome: feasibility, reliability, and implications for treatment. *Am. J. Med. Genet. B Neuropsychiatr. Genet.* 150B, 545–553. doi: 10.1002/ajmg.b.30858

Hinton, V. J., Brown, W. T., Wisniewski, K., and Rudelli, R. D. (1991). Analysis of neocortex in three males with the fragile X syndrome. *Am. J. Med. Genet.* 41, 289–294. doi: 10.1002/ajmg.1320410306

Hitoglou, M., Ververi, A., Antoniadis, A., and Zafeiriou, D. I. (2010). Childhood autism and auditory system abnormalities. *Pediatr. Neurol.* 42, 309–314. doi: 10.1016/j.pediatrneurol.2009.10.009

Hruby, T., and Marsalek, P. (2003). Event-related potentials – the P3 wave. *Acta Neurobiol. Exp. (Wars)* 63, 55–63.

Huber, K. (2007). Fragile X syndrome: molecular mechanisms of cognitive dysfunction. *Am. J. Psychiatry* 164, 556. doi: 10.1176/appi.ajp.164.4.556

Huber, K. M., Gallagher, S. M., Warren, S. T., and Bear, M. F. (2002a). Altered synaptic plasticity in a mouse model of fragile X mental retardation. *Proc. Natl. Acad. Sci. U.S.A.* 99, 7746–7750. doi: 10.1073/pnas.122205699

Huber, K. M., Gallagher, S. M., Warren, S. T., and Bear, M. F. (2002b). Altered synaptic plasticity in a mouse model of fragile X mental retardation. *Proc. Natl. Acad. Sci. U.S.A.* 99, 7746–7750. doi: 10.1073/pnas.122205699

Incorpora, G., Sorge, G., Sorge, A., and Pavone, L. (2002). Epilepsy in fragile X syndrome. *Brain Dev.* 24, 766–769. doi: 10.1016/S0387-7604(02)00102-X

Irwin, S. A., Galvez, R., and Greenough, W. T. (2000). Dendritic spine structural anomalies in fragile-X mental retardation syndrome. *Cereb. Cortex* 10, 1038–1044. doi: 10.1093/cercor/10.10.1038

Irwin, S. A., Idupulapati, M., Gilbert, M. E., Harris, J. B., Chakravarti, A. B., Rogers, E. J., et al. (2002). Dendritic spine and dendritic field characteristics of layer V pyramidal neurons in the visual cortex of fragile-X knockout mice. *Am. J. Med. Genet.* 111, 140–146. doi: 10.1002/ajmg.10500

Kim, H., Gibboni, R., Kirkhart, C., and Bao, S. (2013). Impaired critical perios plasticity in primary auditory cortex. *J. Neurosci.* 33, 15686–15692. doi: 10.1523/JNEUROSCI.3246-12.2013

Knoth, I. S., and Lippe, S. (2012). Evernt-related potential alterations in fragile x syndrome. *Front. Hum. Neurosci.* 6:264. doi: 10.3389/fnhum.2012.00264

Kramvis, I., Mansvelder, H. D., Loos, M., and Meredith, R. (2013). Hyperactivity, perseverance, and increased responding during attentional rule acquisition in fragile X mouse model. *Front. Behav. Neurosci.* 7:172. doi: 10.3389/fnbeh.2013.00172.

Largo, R. H., Schinzel, A. (1985). Developmental and behavioural disturbances in 13 boys with fragile X syndrome. *Eur. J. Pediatr.* 143, 269–275. doi: 10.1007/BF00442299

Levenga, J., Hayashi, S., de Vrij, F. M., Koekkoek, S. K., van der Linde, H. C., Nieuwenhuizen, I., et al. (2011). AFQ056, a new mGluR5 antagonist for treatment of fragile X syndrome. *Neurobiol. Dis.* 42, 311–317. doi: 10.1016/j.nbd.2011.01.022

Luck, S. (2005). *An Introduction to the Event-Related Potential Technique. In: An Introduction to the Event-Related Potential Technique.* Cambridge, MA: The MIT Press. 38–48.

Marco, E. J., Hinkley, L. B., Hill, S. S., and Nagarajan, S. S. (2011). Sensory processing in autism: a review of neurophysiologic findings. *Pediatr. Res.* 69, 48R–54R. doi: 10.1203/PDR.0b013e3182130c54

McKinney, B. C., Grossman, A. W., Elisseou, N. M., and Greenough, W. T. (2005). Dendritic spine abnormalities in the occipital cortex of C57BL/6 Fmr1 knockout mice. *Am. J. Med. Genet. B Neuropsychiatr. Genet.* 136B, 98–102. doi: 10.1002/ajmg.b.30183

Meredith, R. M., Dawitz, J., and Kramvis, I. (2012). Sensitive time-windows for susceptibility in neurodevelopmental disorders. *Trends Neurosci.* 35, 335–344. doi: 10.1016/j.tins.2012.03.005

Miller, L. J., McIntosh, D. N., McGrath, J., Shyu, V., Lampe, M., Taylor, A. K., et al. (1999). Electrodermal responses to sensory stimuli in individuals with fragile X syndrome: a preliminary report. *Am. J. Med. Genet.* 83, 268–279. doi: 10.1002/(SICI)1096-8628(19990402)83:4<268::AID-AJMG7>3.0.CO;2-K

Mineur, Y. S., Sluyter, F., de Wit, S., Oostra, B. A., and Crusio, W. E. (2002). Behavioral and neuroanatomical characterization of the Fmr1 knockout mouse. *Hippocampus* 12, 39–46. doi: 10.1002/hipo.10005

Moy, S. S., and Nadler, J. J. (2008). Advances in behavioral genetics: mouse models of autism. *Mol. Psychiatry* 13, 4–26. doi: 10.1038/sj.mp.4002082

Musumeci, S. A., Bosco, P., Calabrese, G., Bakker, C., De Sarro, G. B., Elia, M., et al. (2000). Audiogenic seizures susceptibility in transgenic mice with fragile X syndrome. *Epilepsia* 41, 19–23. doi: 10.1111/j.1528-1157.2000.tb01499.x

Musumeci, S. A., Calabrese, G., Bonaccorso, C. M., D'Antoni, S., Brouwer, J. R., Bakker, C. E., et al. (2007). Audiogenic seizure susceptibility is reduced in fragile X knockout mice after introduction of FMR1 transgenes. *Exp. Neurol.* 203, 233–240. doi: 10.1016/j.expneurol.2006.08.007

Naatanen, R., and Picton, T. (1987). The N1 wave of the human electric and magnetic response to sound: a review and an analysis of the component structure. *Psychophysiology* 24, 375–425. doi: 10.1111/j.1469-8986.1987.tb00311.x

Naatanen, R., Gaillard. A. W., and Mantysalo, S. (1978). Early selective-attention effect on evoked potential reinterpreted. *Acta Psychol. (Amst.)*, 42, 313–329. doi: 10.1016/0001-6918(78)90006-9

Naatanen, R., Kujala, T., and Winkler, I. (2011a). Auditory processing that leads to conscious perception: A unique window to central auditory processing opened by the mismatch negativity and related responses. *Psychophysiology* 48, 4–22. doi: 10.1111/j.1469-8986.2010.01114.x

Naatanen, R., Kujala, T., Kreegipuu, K., Carlson, S., Escera, C., Baldeweg, T., et al. (2011b). The mismatch negativity: an index of cognitive decline in neuropsychiatric and neurological diseases and in ageing. *Brain* 134, 3435–3453. doi: 10.1093/brain/awr064

Naatanen, R., Paavilainen, P., Rinne, T., and Alho, K. (2007). The mismatch negativity (MMN) in basic research of central auditory processing: a review. *Clin. Neurophysiol.* 118, 2544–2590. doi: 10.1016/j.clinph.2007.04.026

Nielsen, D. M., Derber, W. J., McClellan, D. A., and Crnic, L. S. (2002). Alterations in the auditory startle response in Fmr1 targeted mutant mouse models of fragile X syndrome. *Brain Res.* 927, 8–17. doi: 10.1016/S0006-8993(01)03309-1

Nieto Del Rincón, P. L. (2008). Autism: alterations in auditory perception. *Rev. Neurosci.* 19, 61–68. doi: 10.1515/REVNEURO.2008.19.1.61

Nimchinsky, E. A., Oberlander, A. M., and Svoboda, K. (2001). Abnormal development of dendritic spines in FMR1 knock-out mice. *J. Neurosci.* 21, 5139–5146.

O'Connor, K. (2012). Auditory processing in autism spectrum disorder: a review. *Neurosci. Biobehav. Rev.* 36, 836–854. doi: 10.1016/j.neubiorev.2011.11.008

O'Donnell, W. T., and Warren, S. T. (2002). A decade of molecular studies of fragile X syndrome. *Annu. Rev. Neurosci.* 25, 315–338. doi: 10.1146/annurev.neuro.25.112701.142909

Olmos-Serrano, J. L., Corbin, J. G., and Burns, M. P. (2011). The GABA(A) receptor agonist THIP ameliorates specific behavioral deficits in the mouse model of fragile X syndrome. *Dev. Neurosci.* 395–403. doi: 10.1159/000332884

Paluszkiewicz, S. M., Olmos-Serrano, J. L., Corbin, J. G., and Huntsman, M. M. (2011). Impaired inhibitory control of cortical synchronization in fragile X syndrome. *J. Neurophysiol.* 106, 2264–2272. doi: 10.1152/jn.00421.2011

Pan, F., Aldridge, G. M., Greenough, W. T., and Gan, W. B. (2010). Dendritic spine instability and insensitivity to modulation by sensory experience in a mouse model of fragile X syndrome. *Proc. Natl. Acad. Sci. U.S.A.* 107, 17768–17773. doi: 10.1073/pnas.1012496107

Pantev, C., Hoke, M., Lehnertz, K., Lutkenhoner, B., Anogianakis, G., and Wittkowski, W. (1988). Tonotopic organization of the human auditory cortex revealed by transient auditory evoked magnetic fields. *Electroencephalogr. Clin. Neurophysiol.* 69, 160–170. doi: 10.1016/0013-4694(88)90211-8

Patel, S. H., and Azzam, P. N. (2005). Characterization of N200 and P300: selected studies of the event-related potential. *Int. J. Med. Sci.* 2, 147–154. doi: 10.7150/ijms.2.147

Picton, T. W., Goodman, W. S., and Bryce, D. P. (1970). Amplitude of evoked responses to tones of high intensity. *Acta Otolaryngol.* 70, 77–82. doi: 10.3109/00016487009181862

Polich, J. (2007). Updating P300: an integrative theory of P3a and P3b. *Clin. Neurophysiol.* 118, 2128–2148. doi: 10.1016/j.clinph.2007.04.019

Price, J., Roberts, J., Vandergrift, N., and Martin, G. (2007). Language comprehension in boys with fragile X syndrome and boys with Down syndrome. *J. Intellect. Disabil. Res.* 51, 318–326. doi: 10.1111/j.1365-2788.2006.00881.x

Price, J. R., Roberts, J. E., Hennon, E. A., Berni, M. C., Anderson, K. L., and Sideris, J. (2008). Syntactic complexity during conversation of boys with fragile X syndrome and Down syndrome. *J. Speech Lang. Hear. Res.* 51, 3–15. doi: 10.1044/1092-4388(2008/001)

Reiss, A. L., Lee, J., and Freund, L. (1994). Neuroanatomy of fragile X syndrome: the temporal lobe. *Neurology* 44, 1317–1324. doi: 10.1212/WNL.44.7.1317

Rif, J., Hari, R., Hamalainen, M. S., and Sams, M. (1991). Auditory attention affects two different areas in the human supratemporal cortex. *Electroencephalogr. Clin. Neurophysiol.* 79, 464–472. doi: 10.1016/0013-4694(91)90166-2

Roberts, J., Price, J., Barnes, E., Nelson, L., Burchinal, M., Hennon, E. A., et al. (2007a). Receptive vocabulary, expressive vocabulary, and speech production of boys with fragile X syndrome in comparison to boys with down syndrome. *Am. J. Ment. Retard.* 112, 177–193. doi: 10.1352/0895-8017(2007)112[177:RVEVAS]2.0.CO;2

Roberts, J. E., Hennon, E. A., Price, J. R., Dear, E., Anderson, K., and Vandergrift, N. A. (2007b). Expressive language during conversational speech in boys with fragile X syndrome. *Am. J. Ment. Retard.* 112, 1–17. doi: 10.1352/0895-8017(2007)112[1:ELDCSI]2.0.CO;2

Roberts, J. E., Mirrett, P., and Burchinal, M. (2001). Receptive and expressive communication development of young males with fragile X syndrome. *Am. J. Ment. Retard.* 106, 216–230. doi: 10.1352/0895-8017(2001)106<0216:RAECDO>2.0.CO;2

Roberts, T. P., Cannon, K. M., Tavabi, K., Blaskey, L., Khan, S. Y., Monroe, J. F., et al. (2011). Auditory magnetic mismatch field latency: a biomarker for language impairment in autism. *Biol. Psychiatry* 70, 263–269. doi: 10.1016/j.biopsych.2011.01.015

Rojas, D. C., Benkers, T. L., Rogers, S. J., Teale, P. D., Reite, M. L., and Hagerman, R. J. (2001). Auditory evoked magnetic fields in adults with fragile X syndrome. *Neuroreport* 12, 2573–2576. doi: 10.1097/00001756-200108080-00056

Rotschafer, S. E., Trujillo, M. S., Dansie, L. E., Ethell, I. M., and Razak, K. A. (2012). Minocycline treatment reverses ultrasonic vocalization production deficit in a mouse model of Fragile X Syndrome. *Brain Res.* 1439, 7–14. doi: 10.1016/j.brainres.2011.12.041

Rotschafer, S., and Razak, K. (2013). Altered auditory processing in a mouse model of fragile X syndrome. *Brain Res.* 1506, 12–24. doi: 10.1016/j.brainres.2013.02.038

Roy, S., Watkins, N., and Heck, D. (2012). Comprehensive analysis of ultrasonic vocalizations in a mouse model of fragile x syndrome reveals limited, call type specific deficits. *PLoS ONE* 7:e44816. doi: 10.1371/journal.pone.0044816

Rudelli, R. D., Brown, W. T., Wisniewski, K., Jenkins, E. C., Laure-Kamionowska, M., Connell, F., et al. (1985). Adult fragile X syndrome. Clinico-neuropathologic findings. *Acta Neuropathol.* 67, 289–295. doi: 10.1007/BF00687814

Sanquist, T. F., Rohrbaugh, J., Syndulko, K., and Lindsley, D. B. (1980). An event-related potential analysis of coding processes in human memory. *Prog. Brain Res.* 54, 655–660. doi: 10.1016/S0079-6123(08)61686-6

Scerif, G., Longhi, E., Cole, V., Karmiloff-Smith, A., and Cornish, K. (2012). Attention across modalities as a longitudinal predictor of early outcomes: the case of fragile X syndrome. *J. Child Psychol. Psychiatry* 53, 641–650. doi: 10.1111/j.1469-7610.2011.02515.x

Schneider, A., Ballinger, E., Chavez, A., Tassone, F., Hagerman, R. J., and Hessl, D. (2012). Prepulse inhibition in patients with fragile X-associated tremor ataxia syndrome. *Neurobiol. Aging* 33, 1045–1053. doi: 10.1016/j.neurobiolaging.2010.09.002

Schneider, A., Leigh, M. J., Adams, P., Nanakul, R., Chechi, T., Olichney, J., et al. (2013). Electrocortical changes associated with minocycline treatment in fragile X syndrome. *J. Psychopharmacol.* 27, 956–963. doi: 10.1177/0269881113494105

Selby, L., Zhang, C. Z., and Sun, Q. Q. (2007). Major defects in neocortical GABAergic inhibitory circuits in mice lacking the fragile X mental retardation protein. *Neurosci. Lett.* 412, 227–232. doi: 10.1016/j.neulet.2006.11.062

Spencer, C. M., Alekseyenko, O., Serysheva, E., Yuva-Paylor, L. A., and Paylor, R. (2005). Altered anxiety-related and social behaviors in the Fmr1 knockout mouse model of fragile X syndrome. *Genes Brain Behav.* 4, 420–430. doi: 10.1111/j.1601-183X.2005.00123.x

Squires, N. K., Squires, K. C., and Hillyard, S. A. (1975). Two varieties of long-latency positive waves evoked by unpredictable auditory stimuli in man. *Electroencephalogr. Clin. Neurophysiol.* 38, 387–401. doi: 10.1016/0013-4694(75)90263-1

St. Clair, D. M., Blackwood, D. H., Oliver, C. J., and Dickens, P. (1987). P3 abnormality in fragile X syndrome. *Biol. Psychiatry* 22, 303–312. doi: 10.1016/0006-3223(87)90148-X

Steinhausen, H. C., Von Gontard, A., Spohr, H. L., Hauffa, B. P., Eiholzer, U., Backes, M., et al. (2002). Behavioral phenotypes in four mental retardation syndromes: fetal alcohol syndrome, Prader-Willi syndrome, fragile X syndrome, and tuberosis sclerosis. *Am. J. Med. Genet.* 111, 381–387. doi: 10.1002/ajmg.10627

Strumbos, J. G., Brown, M. R., Kronengold, J., Polley, D. B., and Kaczmarek, L. K. (2010). Fragile X mental retardation protein is required for rapid experience-dependent regulation of the potassium channel Kv3.1b. *J. Neurosci.* 30, 10263–10271. doi: 10.1523/JNEUROSCI.1125-10.2010

Sutton, S., Braren, M., Zubin, J., and John, E. R. (1965). Evoked-potential correlates of stimulus uncertainty. *Science* 150, 1187–1188. doi: 10.1126/science.150.3700.1187

Till, S. M., Wijetunge, L. S., Seidel, V. G., Harlow, E., Wright, A. K., Bagni, C., et al. (2012). Altered maturation of the primary somatosensory cortex in a mouse model of fragile X syndrome. *Hum. Mol. Genet.* 21, 2143–2156. doi: 10.1093/hmg/dds030

Van der Molen, M. J., Van der Molen, M. W., Ridderinkhof, K. R., Hamel, B. C., Curfs, L. M., Ramakers, G. J. (2012a). Auditory and visual cortical activity during selective attention in fragile X syndrome: a cascade of processing deficiencies. *Clin. Neurophysiol.* 123, 720–729.. doi: 10.1016/j.clinph.2011.08.023

Van der Molen, M. J., Van der Molen, M. W., Ridderinkhof, K. R., Hamel, B. C., Curfs, L. M., Ramakers, G. J. (2012b). Auditory change detection in fragile X syndrome males: a brain potential study. *Clin. Neurophysiol.* 123, 1309–1318. doi: 10.1016/j.clinph.2011.11.039

Yuhas, J., Cordeiro, L., Tassone, F., Ballinger, E., Schneider, A., Long, J. M., et al. (2011). Brief report: Sensorimotor gating in idiopathic autism and autism associated with fragile X syndrome. *J. Autism. Dev. Disord.* 41, 248–253. doi: 10.1007/s10803-010-1040-9

Yun, S. W., Platholi, J., Flaherty, M. S., Fu, W. M., Kottmann, A. H., and Toth, M. (2006). Fmrp is required for the establishment of the startle response during the critical period of auditory development. *Brain Res.* 1110, 159–165. doi: 10.1016/j.brainres.2006.06.086

Zhao, M. G., Toyoda, H., Ko, S. W., Ding, H. K., Wu, L. J., and Zhuo, M. (2005). Deficits in trace fear memory and long-term potentiation in a mouse model for fragile X syndrome. *J. Neurosci.* 25, 7385–7392. doi: 10.1523/JNEUROSCI.1520-05.2005

Zouridakis, G., Simos, P. G., and Papanicolaou, A. C. (1998). Multiple bilaterally asymmetric cortical sources account for the auditory N1m component. *Brain Topogr.* 10, 183–189. doi: 10.1023/A:1022246825461

Zuo, Y., Yang, G., Kwon, E., and Gan, W. B. (2005). Long-term sensory deprivation prevents dendritic spine loss in primary somatosensory cortex. *Nature* 14, 261–265.doi: 10.1038/nature03715

10

The contribution of inhibitory interneurons to circuit dysfunction in Fragile X Syndrome

Christian A. Cea-Del Rio*[1] *and Molly M. Huntsman*[1,2]

[1] *Department of Pharmaceutical Sciences, Skaggs School of Pharmacy and Pharmaceutical Sciences, University of Colorado, Anschutz Medical Campus, Aurora, CO, USA*

[2] *Department of Pediatrics, School of Medicine, University of Colorado, Anschutz Medical Campus, Aurora, CO, USA*

***Correspondence:**
Molly M. Huntsman, Department of Pharmaceutical Sciences, Skaggs School of Pharmacy and Pharmaceutical Sciences, University of Colorado, Anschutz Medical Campus, 12850 E. Montview Blvd., V20-3121, Mail Stop C238, Aurora, CO 80045, USA e-mail: Molly.Huntsman@UCDenver.edu

Many neurological disorders, including neurodevelopmental disorders, report hypersynchrony of neuronal networks. These alterations in neuronal synchronization suggest a link to the function of inhibitory interneurons. In Fragile X Syndrome (FXS), it has been reported that altered synchronization may underlie hyperexcitability, cognitive dysfunction and provide a link to the increased incidence of epileptic seizures. Therefore, understanding the roles of inhibitory interneurons and how they control neuronal networks is of great importance in studying neurodevelopmental disorders such as FXS. Here, we present a review of how interneuron populations and inhibition are important contributors to the loss of excitatory/inhibitory balance seen in hypersynchronous and hyperexcitable networks from neurodevelopmental disorders, and specifically in FXS.

Keywords: GABA, synchronization, inhibitory neurotransmission, synaptic transmission, interneurons

INTRODUCTION

Fragile X Syndrome (FXS) is one of several disorders associated with autism spectrum disorders (ASDs)—a heterogeneous group of behaviorally identified neurodevelopmental disabilities. The prevalence rate of autism in FXS reportedly ranges from 25% to 52% (Kaufmann et al., 2004; García-Nonell et al., 2008; Hall et al., 2008), often presenting ASD features such as social avoidance (Marco and Skuse, 2006). Also, FXS is the most common inherited cause of intellectual disability with an average IQ of 40 (Merenstein et al., 1996). Because of its association to the X chromosome, FXS has a higher prevalence in males as approximately of 1 in 3600–4000, than females (approximately 1 in 4000–6000) (Coffee et al., 2009). FXS is attributed to the transcriptional silencing of the Fragile X Mental Retardation 1 (*FMR1*) gene and the consequent loss of the gene product of *FMR1*—Fragile X Mental Retardation Protein (FMRP; Penagarikano et al., 2007). In the human condition the silencing of *FMR1* is caused by hypermethylation—this occurs when a trinucleotide (CGG) repeat located in the 5' untranslated region of the gene expands to a length of more than 200 repeats. The loss of this protein is far reaching because FMRP interacts with approximately 4–8% of all synaptic mRNAs and regulates the translation of numerous synaptic proteins and receptor systems (Brown et al., 2001).

The FXS phenotype involves hyperactivity, attention deficits, poor eye contact, shyness, self-talk, anxiety, mood instability, hyperarousal to sensory stimuli, and autism (Hagerman and Hagerman, 2002). Defects underlying neurodevelopmental disorders, including FXS, are widely believed to lie at the level of the synapse (Zoghbi, 2003; Ebert and Greenberg, 2013). In FXS, these profound changes include alterations in both excitatory and inhibitory neurotransmission across multiple brain regions (Huber et al., 2002; Bear et al., 2004; Bureau et al., 2008; Harlow et al., 2010; Olmos-Serrano et al., 2010; Till et al., 2012; Van der Molen et al., 2012; Kim et al., 2013). Although excitatory/inhibitory balance has been a recent subject of study in FXS research, not much is known of how interneuron populations contribute to the phenotype. In this review, we summarize current knowledge of FXS behavioral and cognitive phenotype, the circuitry abnormalities related to them and how interneurons are an important subject of study to understand alterations in neuronal networks.

COGNITION AND BEHAVIORAL PROCESSING IN FXS

Since the *FMR1* gene was first identified and linked to FXS in 1991 (Verkerk et al., 1991), tremendous progress has been made to understand the neurological deficits that contribute to the phenotype. Most of the cognition and behavioral abnormalities have been investigated to try to understand how FMRP is involved in the neurobiological processing of brain areas related to these specific tasks. For instance, lack of FMRP found in the mouse model of FXS leads to cerebellar deficits at both the cellular and behavioral levels and raise the possibility that cerebellar dysfunctions can contribute to motor learning deficits in FXS patients (Koekkoek et al., 2005). Indeed, although premutation carriers of FMRP lead to a different syndrome (FXTAS), they showed an absence of cerebellar inhibition over primary motor cortex and a reduced GABA-mediated intracortical and afferent inhibition compared with healthy individuals (Conde et al., 2013) that could potentially also be present in FXS patients. Moreover, FXS patients display specific emotion recognition deficits for angry and neutral (but not happy or fearful) facial expressions through visual scanning tasks (Shaw and Porter, 2013), that in turn is directly related to formation and function of neuronal circuits attributed to behavioral processes such as fear, emotion recognition and anxiety carried out by the amygdala (Olmos-Serrano and Corbin, 2011; Kim et al., 2014). These socio-emotional deficits are also associated with deficits in neuronal processing of sensory systems. Studies have shown that together with a shift change in development for synaptic formation and plasticity in the amygdala (Kratovac and Corbin, 2013; Vislay et al., 2013), impaired critical plasticity periods for auditory, visual and somatosensory cortex also occurred in FXS (Bureau et al., 2008; Harlow et al., 2010; Till et al., 2012; Van der Molen et al., 2012; Kim et al., 2013). Therefore these studies reveal a role for FMRP in shaping sensory circuits during developmental critical periods when time windows of protein expression are vulnerable to alterations (reviewed in Meredith et al., 2012). Dendritic spine stability, branching and density abnormalities are part of the developmental delay observed in these same brain areas (Cruz-Martín et al., 2010; Pan et al., 2010; Till et al., 2012; Lauterborn et al., 2013) and they depend on the environmental context and experience that they are undergoing. Other characteristics of cortical neuronal networks in FXS are hyperesponsivness and hyperexcitability (Gonçalves et al., 2013; Rotschafer and Razak, 2013), making these circuits highly synchronous which taken together suggest excitatory/inhibitory balance abnormalities of the FXS neuronal circuitry. These state-dependent network defects could explain the intellectual and sensory integration dysfunctions associated with FXS.

EXCITATORY/INHIBITORY BALANCE IN FXS NEURONAL NETWORKS

FXS neuronal networks are hyperexcitable (Gibson et al., 2008; Olmos-Serrano et al., 2010; Gonçalves et al., 2013; Rotschafer and Razak, 2013). This explains why most studies focus on excessive excitatory activity. The majority of research about excitatory drive and synaptic plasticity that describes hyperexcitability in FXS is illustrated in the "mGluR theory" (Huber et al., 2002; Bear et al., 2004). Briefly, the mGluR theory explains that the psychiatric and neurological aspects of FXS are a consequence of exaggerated responses to metabotropic glutamate receptor (mGluR) activation (Huber et al., 2002). One response is mediated by a synaptic plasticity process known as long term depression (LTD; Huber et al., 2002; Bear et al., 2004). Additional studies also reveal that pharmacological intervention of mGluR activation can rescue the FXS phenotype in the *Fmr1* mouse model suggesting a therapeutic role for inhibitors of mGluR activity-specifically type 1 and type 5 receptor activity (Dölen et al., 2007; Michalon et al., 2012; Ronesi et al., 2012). Due to initial early success of 2-methyl-6-(phenylethynyl)pyridine (MPEP), fenobam and 2-chloro-4-((2,5-dimethyl-1-(4-(trifluoromethoxy) phenyl)-1H-imidazol-4-yl)ethynyl)pyridine (CTEP), the use of mGluR5 antagonists remains a primary treatment option for FXS (Porter et al., 2005; Yan et al., 2005; Lindemann et al., 2011). However, additional attempts at specific targeting of these receptors have been problematic. Despite mixed success, the development of the mGluR5 antagonist Mavoglurant (AFQ056) has recently been discontinued (April 2014) due to a failure to show improvement over placebo-controlled trials.

Nevertheless, other synaptic proteins have also been involved in the pathology of the syndrome. For instance, loss of FMRP leads to impairments in NMDA receptor-dependent synaptic plasticity in the dentate gyrus (DG), but not in the cornu ammonis area 1 (CA1) subregion (Bostrom et al., 2013), suggesting that functional expression of proteins could be region or even synapse-specific. Additionally, astroglial cells may potentially contribute to enhanced neuronal excitability observed in the mouse model of FXS due to a reduced uptake of glutamate (Higashimori et al., 2013).

On the other hand, we have to account for the excitatory stream counterpart, inhibition, and how this balances circuit activity. Several components of the GABAergic system are also regulated by FMRP expression (reviewed in Paluszkiewicz et al., 2011a). While there is evidence that $GABA_A$ receptor subunits show enhanced surface expression such as the γ_2 subunit (Liu et al., 2013), most other studies suggest the contrary, showing that mRNA expression of α_1, α_3 and $\alpha_4\beta_1$ and β_2, and γ_1 and γ_2, and δ $GABA_A$ receptor subunits in the hippocampus (D'Hulst et al., 2006) and the δ subunit in neocortex (Gantois et al., 2006) are down regulated in *Fmr1* KO mice. Further evidence shows that FMRP binds δ subunit mRNA, suggesting a direct influence of FMRP on the expression of δ subunits (Gantois et al., 2006). This latter study supports the hypothesis that tonic inhibition, which is partially mediated by δ subunit containing $GABA_A$ receptors, is also down-regulated, contributing to hyperexcitability abnormalities in the neuronal networks of *Fmr1* KO mice (Gantois et al., 2006; Olmos-Serrano et al., 2010; Martin et al., 2014). Thus, GABAergic tonic inhibition has been also taken as a potential candidate for therapeutic treatment in FXS (Olmos-Serrano et al., 2010, 2011; Heulens et al., 2012; Martin et al., 2014).

Despite this information on excitatory/inhibitory balance abnormalities in FXS, an important contributor to the balance has been neglected in these studies: the functional and anatomically diverse population of inhibitory interneurons. Although there is information on how $GABA_A$ receptors are affected by the lack of FMRP, few studies address dysfunction of specific presynaptic inhibitory interneurons in FXS. Here we want to summarize some of these studies and discuss how the specific functional properties of different subclasses of inhibitory interneurons are relevant to the study of FXS.

THE CONTRIBUTION OF INHIBITORY INTERNEURONS TO THE FXS PHENOTYPE

Although often overlooked, the importance of local circuit inhibitory interneurons has rapidly gained attention thanks to a number of studies that have provided essential electrophysiological, anatomical and synaptic insight into the function and role(s) played by this large and heterogeneous cell population (Buzsáki et al., 1992; Gulyás et al., 1993a,b; Buhl et al., 1994; Miles et al., 1996; Gupta et al., 2000; Markram et al., 2004). At the most basic level, interneurons are considered to provide inhibitory control over the excitatory flow of the neuronal network. Their physiological properties and connectivity allow them to control the rhythmic output of large populations of excitatory principal cells as well as other populations of inhibitory interneurons (Cobb et al., 1995; Freund and Katona, 2007; Klausberger and Somogyi, 2008). Interneuronal physiological responses *in vivo* often occur in a time-locked form, discharging in the same temporal window of their preferential oscillatory frequency, suggesting their direct involvement in the synchronization and control of pyramidal cells firing (Klausberger and Somogyi, 2008). Thus, it is possible that interneuron subtypes show a differential participation in the FXS phenotype and likely contribute to specific pathophysiological properties of the neuronal networks where they are involved (**Figure 1**).

As earlier stated, cortical networks in FXS are hyperexcitable and highly synchronous (Gonçalves et al., 2013; Rotschafer and Razak, 2013). This could explain state-dependent network defects related to intellectual disability, increased incidence of seizures and sensory integration dysfunctions associated with FXS (reviewed in Musumeci et al., 1999; Hagerman and Stafstrom, 2009; Hagerman et al., 2009). Based on heterogeneous anatomy and function of inhibitory interneurons it is likely that inhibitory circuits play important roles in this phenotype. For example, both perisomatic and dendritic-targeting interneurons are known to be involved in the hyperexcitability of the network. Perisomatic interneurons mainly control pyramidal cell excitability by regulating Na+-dependent action potential initiation (Freund and Katona, 2007). In contrast, inhibition arriving at dendritic locations likely have little influence over somal action potential generation but strongly affect local dendritic integration and regulates dendritic Ca^{2+}-dependent spike initiation and/or propagation (Miles et al., 1996). From this point of view, while perisomatic interneurons have a role in the synchronization of

Interneuron circuitry	Oscillatory activity preferences	Electrical properties	Potential malfunction in fragile-X
FS 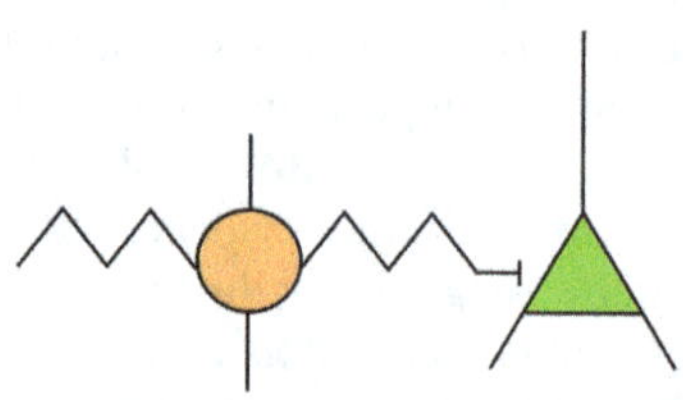	Gamma 40-100Hz	**Firing Pattern:** High, non-accommodating **Action Potential:** Narrow, fast AHP **Input Resistance:** Low	* Receive less excitatory drive * Synchronization of neuronal networks in gamma frequency band * Impact on cognitive or behavioral task depending neuronal area
LTS 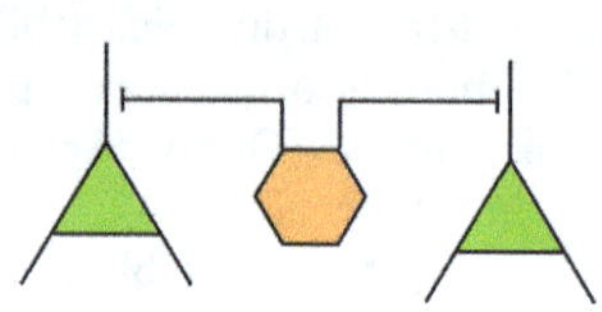	Thetha 4-8Hz	**Firing Pattern:** Moderate, accommodating **Action Potential:** Average, fast AHP followed by slow AHP **Input Resistance:** Large, Ih sag	* Decreased mGluR-mediated synaptic plasticity * Lost capacity of filter ing and/or integration relevant synaptic information * Synchronization of the neuronal network in theta frequency band
NGF 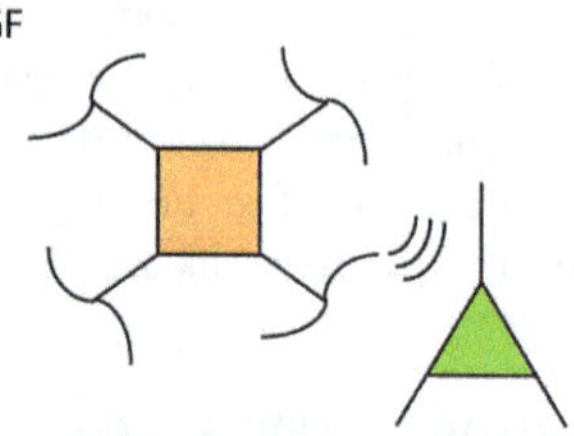	Theta 4-8Hz	**Firing Pattern:** Low, delayed, accommodating **Action Potential:** Average, slow AHP **Input Resistance:** Moderate	* Loss of setting the basal/tonic neuronal activity of the network due to lack of volume transmission * Inability to identify or process relevant information to the network

FIGURE 1 | Comparative table for interneuron populations in FXS. Three different interneuron types (FS: Fast spiking; LTS: Low threshold spiking and NGF: Neurogliaform cells) are compared here regarding their circuitry/connectivity (left panel), oscillatory preferences (left middle panel), electrical properties (right middle panel) and what their failure would represent in FXS (right panel).

network circuits imposing a rhythm, dendritic-targeting cells mainly participate in the propagation of synchronized activity waves throughout the network.

In FXS, EEG recordings show elevated relative theta power and reduced relative upper-alpha power (Van der Molen and Van der Molen, 2013), which can be related to longer UP states seen in the neocortex of *Fmr1* KO mouse model (Gibson et al., 2008; Hays et al., 2011). Indeed, local excitation of fast-spiking (FS) inhibitory interneurons, a perisomatic-targeting interneuron that engage preferably in frequencies between 40–100 Hz (Klausberger et al., 2003), is robustly decreased in neocortex in *Fmr1* KO mice (Selby et al., 2007; Patel et al., 2013), which could explain the decrease in synchrony in gamma frequency (Gibson et al., 2008) of the network (**Figure 1**). However, these inhibitory deficiencies seem to be mediated by polysynaptic responses through local cortical connections instead of monosynaptic or feed-forward responses mediated by thalamic fiber stimulation (Gibson et al., 2008). This is further explained by Patel et al. (2013). When FMRP is conditionally knocked-out in excitatory or inhibitory presynaptic cells, paired recordings reveal that only excitatory responses in inhibitory FS interneurons were decreased by the loss of FMRP (Patel et al., 2013). On the other hand, low threshold spiking (LTS) interneurons, a dendritic-targeting interneuron that contributes to the synchronization of neuronal networks over a wide range of frequencies, including theta and gamma (Szabadics et al., 2001; Blatow et al., 2003), recently have been proposed to control cortical excitability by contributing to the termination of up states in layer II/III (Fanselow and Connors, 2010). Additionally, as opposed to other interneuron subtypes, LTS interneurons respond robustly to metabotropic glutamate receptor (mGluR) activation (Beierlein et al., 2000; Fanselow et al., 2008; Paluszkiewicz et al., 2011b). This robust activation of LTS interneurons is reduced in *Fmr1* KO mice compared to wild type animals (Paluszkiewicz et al., 2011b). The decreased activation of LTS interneurons in *Fmr1* KO mice reduces inhibitory output which in turn alters the synchronization and spike output of excitatory neuronal networks in layer II/III (Paluszkiewicz et al., 2011b). It is also reported that unitary IPSC amplitude mediated by LTS interneurons is increased in somatosensory cortex of *Fmr1* KO mice (Gibson et al., 2008). The fact that this powerful subpopulation of interneurons are tightly coupled by gap junctions (Beierlein et al., 2000; Deans et al., 2001) provides further evidence that the LTS interneuronal microcircuits likely play a key role in hyperexcitable and network synchrony abnormalities in FXS. Moreover, on a network level, LTS interneurons engage in theta frequency activity during mGluR activation (Fanselow et al., 2008; Bostrom et al., 2013) which would explain elevated theta power in EEG from FXS patients (Van der Molen and Van der Molen, 2013).

There is additional evidence that suggest a role for interneurons in FXS with respect to specific activation via neuromodulators. Inhibitory interneurons have differential response to neuromodulators, among them, acetylcholine muscarinic receptors (Cea-del Rio et al., 2010), nicotinic receptors (Bell et al., 2011), serotonin (Chittajallu et al., 2013) and endocannabinoids (eCB; Glickfeld and Scanziani, 2006; Lee et al., 2010). This suggests that alteration of neuromodulatory mechanisms in FXS could differentially affect interneuron cell types. For instance, loss of FMRP broadly affects the eCB signaling system through local 2-arachidonoyl-sn-glycerol (2AG) diminished production (Maccarrone et al., 2010; Zhang and Alger, 2010), possibly because of impaired mGluR5-dependent 2AG formation (Jung et al., 2012). Thus, defects of eCB production will affect inhibitory processes through depolarization suppression of inhibition (DSI; Lee et al., 2010) and slow self-inhibition (SSI; Bacci et al., 2004) mechanisms, suggesting the participation of different set of interneuron cell types in FXS neuronal network abnormalities, including basket cells and LTS cells in the cortex (Bacci et al., 2004; Lee et al., 2010) and basket cells and Schaffer collateral interneurons in the hippocampus (Glickfeld and Scanziani, 2006; Lee et al., 2010). Also, serotonin receptors are affected in the *Fmr1* KO mouse model (Xu et al., 2012b), which can suggest differential regulation of interneuronal cell types such as oriens-laconosum moleculare (O-LM) interneurons of the hippocampus (Chittajallu et al., 2013). Finally, molecular markers such as neuronal nitric oxide synthetase and calbindin are downregulated in FXS (Real et al., 2011; Xu et al., 2012a; Giráldez-Pérez et al., 2013), which suggest that interneurons such as ivy cells, neurogliaform cells (NGF) and bipolar interneuron populations can be diminished in brain circuits of FXS. From these initial studies in the field it is apparent that both monosynaptic and polysynaptic mechanisms of inhibition likely explain some of the neuropathologies observed in FXS. Therefore, more efforts should be addressed to identify specific interneuron populations participating in this syndrome and their roles on network computing and synaptic communication.

Interestingly, inhibitory neurotransmission dysfunction appears to be region selective. As stated above, studies in the cerebral cortex reveal interneuron specific problems. There is a clear lack of excitatory drive to FS interneurons in layer IV (Gibson et al., 2008) and faulty mGluR-dependent activation of LTS interneurons in layer II/III (Paluszkiewicz et al., 2011b). In contrast, inhibitory dysfunction in the amygdala appears to be a "global" loss of inhibitory drive of both phasic (synaptic) and tonic (extrasynaptic) inhibitory neurotransmission onto excitatory principal neurons (Olmos-Serrano et al., 2010; Vislay et al., 2013; Martin et al., 2014). There is also a lack of immunostaining for the synthetic enzyme for GABA and decreased inhibitory connections in the amygdala (Olmos-Serrano et al., 2010). There are biochemical similarities in interneuronal subtypes in the cortex and amygdala, however, there are unique differences to specific spiking properties of specific subtypes such as the parvalbumin-positive interneurons in the amygdala (Woodruff and Sah, 2007a,b). Whether these regional differences are the result of different developmental and migratory patterns of interneuronal populations has yet to be identified. Therefore, further investigation into specific abnormalities in amygdala interneuronal subtypes will need to be explored in future studies in the Fragile-X amygdala.

In summary, while enhanced excitatory neurotransmission leads to hyperexcitable phenotypes, inhibitory interneurons are not just contributing factors but are likely playing a major role in hyperexcitable, hyperresponsiveness and hypersynchronicity of neuronal networks in FXS (Gibson et al., 2008; Hays et al.,

2011; Paluszkiewicz et al., 2011b; Gonçalves et al., 2013; Patel et al., 2013). Principally, somatic and dendritic targeting FS and LTS interneurons seem to be the more relevant cell types in cortical abnormalities (Gibson et al., 2008; Paluszkiewicz et al., 2011b), however we cannot rule out the participation of other cortical interneuron cell types such as chandelier, double bouquet, Martinotti or NGFs. Concurrently, interneurons could operate in a different manner depending on the context in which they are involved, from that point of view it is of high priority to study the role of interneurons in different brain areas than the cortex in order to understand their role in these other neuronal networks. In this regard, studies in the Fragile-X amygdala showed that in conditional KO animals, where FMRP is exclusively expressed in inhibitory interneuron populations, that inhibitory neurotransmission dysfunction is comprised of both presynaptic and postsynaptic components (Vislay et al., 2013); therefore suggesting an important role of interneurons in the development and function of this particular brain region in FXS (Olmos-Serrano et al., 2010; Vislay et al., 2013).

CONCLUDING REMARKS

Since many FXS patients also present with one or more features of ASDs, insights gained from studying the monogenic basis of FXS could pave the way to a greater understanding of the role of inhibitory interneurons in autism. At this point most of the evidence for interneuron participation is indirect in terms of neuromodulatory activation and downstream excitatory network activation, but very promising in terms of the relevance of their contribution. Thus, understanding how interneurons participate in neuronal network abnormalities seen in FXS lends to a greater understanding for neurodevelopmental disorders that fall in the autism spectrum.

ACKNOWLEDGMENTS

This work was supported by the National Institute of Disorders and Stroke (R01NS053719) and a FRAXA research foundation postdoctoral fellowship (CACDR).

REFERENCES

Bacci, A., Huguenard, J. R., and Prince, D. A. (2004). Long-lasting self-inhibition of neocortical interneurons mediated by endocannabinoids. *Nature* 431, 312–316. doi: 10.1038/nature02913

Bear, M. F., Huber, K. M., and Warren, S. T. (2004). The mGluR theory of fragile X mental retardation. *Trends Neurosci.* 27, 370–377. doi: 10.1016/j.tins.2004.04.009

Beierlein, M., Gibson, J. R., and Connors, B. W. (2000). A network of electrically coupled interneurons drives synchronized inhibition in neocortex. *Nat. Neurosci.* 3, 904–910. doi: 10.1038/78809

Bell, K. A., Shim, H., Chen, C. K., and McQuiston, A. R. (2011). Nicotinic excitatory postsynaptic potentials in hippocampal CA1 interneurons are predominantly mediated by nicotinic receptors that contain alpha4 and beta2 subunits. *Neuropharmacology* 61, 1379–1388. doi: 10.1016/j.neuropharm.2011.08.024

Blatow, M., Rozov, A., Katona, I., Hormuzdi, S. G., Meyer, A. H., Whittington, M. A., et al. (2003). A novel network of multipolar bursting interneurons generates theta frequency oscillations in neocortex. *Neuron* 38, 805–817. doi: 10.1016/s0896-6273(03)00300-3

Bostrom, C. A., Majaess, N. M., Morch, K., White, E., Eadie, B. D., and Christie, B. R. (2013). Rescue of NMDAR-Dependent synaptic plasticity in Fmr1 knock-out mice. *Cereb. Cortex* doi: 10.1093/cercor/bht237. [Epub ahead of print].

Brown, V., Jin, P., Ceman, S., Darnell, J. C., O'Donnell, W. T., Tenenbaum, S. A., et al. (2001). Microarray identification of FMRP-associated brain mRNAs and altered mRNA translational profiles in fragile X syndrome. *Cell* 107, 477–487. doi: 10.1016/s0092-8674(01)00568-2

Buhl, E. H., Halasy, K., and Somogyi, P. (1994). Diverse sources of hippocampal unitary inhibitory postsynaptic potentials and the number of synaptic release sites. *Nature* 368, 823–828. doi: 10.1038/368823a0

Bureau, I., Shepherd, G. M., and Svoboda, K. (2008). Circuit and plasticity defects in the developing somatosensory cortex of FMR1 knock-out mice. *J. Neurosci.* 28, 5178–5188. doi: 10.1523/JNEUROSCI.1076-08.2008

Buzsáki, G., Horvath, Z., Urioste, R., Hetke, J., and Wise, K. (1992). High-frequency network oscillation in the hippocampus. *Science* 256, 1025–1027. doi: 10.1126/science.1589772

Cea-del Rio, C. A., Lawrence, J. J., Tricoire, L., Erdelyi, F., Szabo, G., and McBain, C. J. (2010). M3 muscarinic acetylcholine receptor expression confers differential cholinergic modulation to neurochemically distinct hippocampal basket cell subtypes. *J. Neurosci.* 30, 6011–6024. doi: 10.1523/JNEUROSCI.5040-09.2010

Chittajallu, R., Craig, M. T., McFarland, A., Yuan, X., Gerfen, S., Tricoire, L., et al. (2013). Dual origins of functionally distinct O-LM interneurons revealed by differential 5-HT(3A)R expression. *Nat. Neurosci.* 16, 1598–1607. doi: 10.1038/nn.3538

Cobb, S. R., Buhl, E. H., Halasy, K., Paulsen, O., and Somogyi, P. (1995). Synchronization of neuronal activity in hippocampus by individual GABAergic interneurons. *Nature* 378, 75–78. doi: 10.1038/378075a0

Coffee, B., Keith, K., Albizua, I., Malone, T., Mowrey, J., Sherman, S. L., et al. (2009). Incidence of fragile X syndrome by newborn screening for methylated FMR1 DNA. *Am. J. Hum. Genet.* 85, 503–514. doi: 10.1016/j.ajhg.2009.09.007

Conde, V., Palomar, F. J., Lama, M. J., Martinez, R., Carrillo, F., Pintado, E., et al. (2013). Abnormal GABA-mediated and cerebellar inhibition in women with the fragile X premutation. *J. Neurophysiol.* 109, 1315–1322. doi: 10.1152/jn.00730.2012

Cruz-Martín, A., Crespo, M., and Portera-Cailliau, C. (2010). Delayed stabilization of dendritic spines in fragile X mice. *J. Neurosci.* 30, 7793–7803. doi: 10.1523/JNEUROSCI.0577-10.2010

Deans, M. R., Gibson, J. R., Sellitto, C., Connors, B. W., and Paul, D. L. (2001). Synchronous activity of inhibitory networks in neocortex requires electrical synapses containing connexin36. *Neuron* 31, 477–485. doi: 10.1016/s0896-6273(01)00373-7

D'Hulst, C., De Geest, N., Reeve, S. P., Van Dam, D., De Deyn, P. P., Hassan, B. A., et al. (2006). Decreased expression of the GABAA receptor in fragile X syndrome. *Brain Res.* 1121, 238–245. doi: 10.1016/j.brainres.2006.08.115

Dölen, G., Osterweil, E., Rao, B. S., Smith, G. B., Auerbach, B. D., Chattarji, S., et al. (2007). Correction of fragile X syndrome in mice. *Neuron* 56, 955–962. doi: 10.1016/j.neuron.2007.12.001

Ebert, D. H., and Greenberg, M. E. (2013). Activity-dependent neuronal signalling and autism spectrum disorder. *Nature* 493, 327–337. doi: 10.1038/nature11860

Fanselow, E. E., and Connors, B. W. (2010). The roles of somatostatin-expressing (GIN) and fast-spiking inhibitory interneurons in UP-DOWN states of mouse neocortex. *J. Neurophysiol.* 104, 596–606. doi: 10.1152/jn.00206.2010

Fanselow, E. E., Richardson, K. A., and Connors, B. W. (2008). Selective, state-dependent activation of somatostatin-expressing inhibitory interneurons in mouse neocortex. *J. Neurophysiol.* 100, 2640–2652. doi: 10.1152/jn.90691.2008

Freund, T. F., and Katona, I. (2007). Perisomatic inhibition. *Neuron* 56, 33–42. doi: 10.1016/j.neuron.2007.09.012

Gantois, I., Vandesompele, J., Speleman, F., Reyniers, E., D'hooge, R., Severijnen, L. A., et al. (2006). Expression profiling suggests underexpression of the GABA(A) receptor subunit delta in the fragile X knockout mouse model. *Neurobiol. Dis.* 21, 346–357. doi: 10.1016/j.nbd.2005.07.017

García-Nonell, C., Ratera, E. R., Harris, S., Hessl, D., Ono, M. Y., Tartaglia, N., et al. (2008). Secondary medical diagnosis in fragile X syndrome with and without autism spectrum disorder. *Am. J. Med. Genet. A* 146A, 1911–1916. doi: 10.1002/ajmg.a.32290

Gibson, J. R., Bartley, A. F., Hays, S. A., and Huber, K. M. (2008). Imbalance of neocortical excitation and inhibition and altered UP states reflect network hyperexcitability in the mouse model of fragile X syndrome. *J. Neurophysiol.* 100, 2615–2626. doi: 10.1152/jn.90752.2008

Giráldez-Pérez, R. M., Avila, M. N., Feijóo-Cuaresma, M., Heredia, R., De Diego-Otero, Y., Real, M. A., et al. (2013). Males but not females show differences in calbindin immunoreactivity in the dorsal thalamus of the mouse model of fragile X syndrome. *J. Comp. Neurol.* 521, 894–911. doi: 10.1002/cne.23209

Glickfeld, L. L., and Scanziani, M. (2006). Distinct timing in the activity of cannabinoid-sensitive and cannabinoid-insensitive basket cells. *Nat. Neurosci.* 9, 807–815. doi: 10.1038/nn1688

Gonçalves, J. T., Anstey, J. E., Golshani, P., and Portera-Cailliau, C. (2013). Circuit level defects in the developing neocortex of fragile X mice. *Nat. Neurosci.* 16, 903–909. doi: 10.1038/nn.3415

Gulyás, A. I., Miles, R., Hájos, N., and Freund, T. F. (1993a). Precision and variability in postsynaptic target selection of inhibitory cells in the hippocampal CA3 region. *Eur. J. Neurosci.* 5, 1729–1751. doi: 10.1111/j.1460-9568.1993.tb00240.x

Gulyás, A. I., Miles, R., Sík, A., Tóth, K., Tamamaki, N., and Freund, T. F. (1993b). Hippocampal pyramidal cells excite inhibitory neurons through a single release site. *Nature* 366, 683–687. doi: 10.1038/366683a0

Gupta, A., Wang, Y., and Markram, H. (2000). Organizing principles for a diversity of GABAergic interneurons and synapses in the neocortex. *Science* 287, 273–278. doi: 10.1126/science.287.5451.273

Hagerman, R. J., Berry-Kravis, E., Kaufmann, W. E., Ono, M. Y., Tartaglia, N., Lachiewicz, A., et al. (2009). Advances in the treatment of fragile X syndrome. *Pediatrics* 123, 378–390. doi: 10.1542/peds.2008-0317

Hagerman, R. J., and Hagerman, P. J. (2002). The fragile X premutation: into the phenotypic fold. *Curr. Opin. Genet. Dev.* 12, 278–283. doi: 10.1016/s0959-437x(02)00299-x

Hagerman, P. J., and Stafstrom, C. E. (2009). Origins of Epilepsy in fragile X syndrome. *Epilepsy Curr.* 9, 108–112. doi: 10.1111/j.1535-7511.2009.01309.x

Hall, S. S., Lightbody, A. A., and Reiss, A. L. (2008). Compulsive, self-injurious and autistic behavior in children and adolescents with fragile X syndrome. *Am. J. Ment. Retard.* 113, 44–53. doi: 10.1352/0895-8017(2008)113[44:csaabi]2.0.co;2

Harlow, E. G., Till, S. M., Russell, T. A., Wijetunge, L. S., Kind, P., and Contractor, A. (2010). Critical period plasticity is disrupted in the barrel cortex of FMR1 knockout mice. *Neuron* 65, 385–398. doi: 10.1016/j.neuron.2010.01.024

Hays, S. A., Huber, K. M., and Gibson, J. R. (2011). Altered neocortical rhythmic activity states in Fmr1 KO mice are due to enhanced mGluR5 signaling and involve changes in excitatory circuitry. *J. Neurosci.* 31, 14223–14234. doi: 10.1523/JNEUROSCI.3157-11.2011

Heulens, I., D'Hulst, C., Van Dam, D., De Deyn, P. P., and Kooy, R. F. (2012). Pharmacological treatment of fragile X syndrome with GABAergic drugs in a knockout mouse model. *Behav. Brain Res.* 229, 244–249. doi: 10.1016/j.bbr.2012.01.031

Higashimori, H., Morel, L., Huth, J., Lindemann, L., Dulla, C., Taylor, A., et al. (2013). Astroglial FMRP-dependent translational down-regulation of mGluR5 underlies glutamate transporter GLT1 dysregulation in the fragile X mouse. *Hum. Mol. Genet.* 22, 2041–2054. doi: 10.1093/hmg/ddt055

Huber, K. M., Gallagher, S. M., Warren, S. T., and Bear, M. F. (2002). Altered synaptic plasticity in a mouse model of fragile X mental retardation. *Proc. Natl. Acad. Sci. U S A* 99, 7746–7750. doi: 10.1073/pnas.122205699

Jung, K. M., Sepers, M., Henstridge, C. M., Lassalle, O., Neuhofer, D., Martin, H., et al. (2012). Uncoupling of the endocannabinoid signalling complex in a mouse model of fragile X syndrome. *Nat. Commun.* 3:1080. doi: 10.1038/ncomms2045

Kaufmann, W. E., Cortell, R., Kau, A. S., Bukelis, I., Tierney, E., Gray, R. M., et al. (2004). Autism spectrum disorder in fragile X syndrome: communication, social interaction and specific behaviors. *Am. J. Med. Genet. A* 129A, 225–234. doi: 10.1002/ajmg.a.30229

Kim, S. Y., Burris, J., Bassal, F., Koldewyn, K., Chattarji, S., Tassone, F., et al. (2014). Fear-specific amygdala function in children and adolescents on the fragile x spectrum: a dosage response of the FMR1 gene. *Cereb. Cortex* 24, 600–613. doi: 10.1093/cercor/bhs341

Kim, H., Gibboni, R., Kirkhart, C., and Bao, S. (2013). Impaired critical period plasticity in primary auditory cortex of fragile X model mice. *J. Neurosci.* 33, 15686–15692. doi: 10.1523/JNEUROSCI.3246-12.2013

Klausberger, T., Magill, P. J., Márton, L. F., Roberts, J. D., Cobden, P. M., Buzsáki, G., et al. (2003). Brian-state and cell-type-specific firing of hippocampal interneurons in vivo. *Nature* 421, 844–848. doi: 10.1038/nature01374

Klausberger, T., and Somogyi, P. (2008). Neuronal diversity and temporal dynamics: the unity of hippocampal circuit operations. *Science* 321, 53–57. doi: 10.1126/science.1149381

Koekkoek, S. K., Yamaguchi, K., Milojkovic, B. A., Dortland, B. R., Ruigrok, T. J., Maex, R., et al. (2005). Deletion of FMR1 in Purkinje cells enhances parallel fiber LTD, enlarges spines and attenuates cerebellar eyelid conditioning in fragile X syndrome. *Neuron* 47, 339–352. doi: 10.1016/j.neuron.2005.07.005

Kratovac, S., and Corbin, J. G. (2013). Developmental changes in expression of inhibitory neuronal proteins in the fragile X syndrome mouse basolateral amygdala. *Brain Res.* 1537, 69–78. doi: 10.1016/j.brainres.2013.08.052

Lauterborn, J. C., Jafari, M., Babayan, A. H., and Gall, C. M. (2013). Environmental enrichment reveals effects of genotype on hippocampal spine morphologies in the mouse model of fragile X syndrome. *Cereb. Cortex* doi: 10.1093/cercor/bht249. [Epub ahead of print].

Lee, S. H., Foldy, C., and Soltesz, I. (2010). Distinct endocannabinoid control of GABA release at perisomatic and dendritic synapses in the hippocampus. *J. Neurosci.* 30, 7993–8000. doi: 10.1523/JNEUROSCI.6238-09.2010

Lindemann, L., Jaeschke, G., Michalon, A., Vieira, E., Honer, M., Spooren, W., et al. (2011). CTEP: a novel, potent, long-acting and orally bioavailable metabotropic glutamate receptor 5 inhibitor. *J. Pharmacol. Exp. Ther.* 339, 474–486. doi: 10.1124/jpet.111.185660

Liu, B., Li, L., Chen, J., Wang, Z., Li, Z., and Wan, Q. (2013). Regulation of GABAA receptors by fragile X mental retardation protein. *Int. J. Physiol. Pathophysiol. Pharmacol.* 5, 169–176.

Maccarrone, M., Rossi, S., Bari, M., De Chiara, V., Rapino, C., Bernardi, G., et al. (2010). Abnormal mGlu 5 receptor/endocannabinoid coupling in mice lacking FMRP and BC1 RNA. *Neuropsychopharmacology* 35, 1500–1509. doi: 10.1038/npp.2010.19

Marco, E. J., and Skuse, D. H. (2006). Autism-lessons from the X chromosome. *Soc. Cogn. Affect. Neurosci.* 1, 183–193. doi: 10.1093/scan/nsl028

Markram, H., Toledo-Rodriguez, M., Wang, Y., Gupta, A., Silberberg, G., and Wu, C. (2004). Interneurons of the neocortical inhibitory system. *Nat. Rev. Neurosci.* 5, 793–807. doi: 10.1038/nrn1519

Martin, B. S., Corbin, J. G., and Huntsman, M. M. (2014). Deficient tonic GABAergic conductance and synaptic balance in the fragile-X syndrome amygdala. *J. Neurophysiol.* doi: 10.1152/jn.00597.2013. [Epub ahead of print].

Meredith, R. M., Dawitz, J., and Kramvis, I. (2012). Sensitive time-windows for susceptibility in neurodevelopmental disorders. *Trends Neurosci.* 35, 335–344. doi: 10.1016/j.tins.2012.03.005

Merenstein, S. A., Sobesky, W. E., Taylor, A. K., Riddle, J. E., Tran, H. X., and Hagerman, R. J. (1996). Molecular-clinical correlations in males with an expanded FMR1 mutation. *Am. J. Med. Genet.* 64, 388–394. doi: 10.1002/(sici)1096-8628(19960809)64:2<388::aid-ajmg31>3.0.co;2-9

Michalon, A., Sidorov, M., Ballard, T. M., Ozmen, L., Spooren, W., Wettstein, J. G., et al. (2012). Chronic pharmacological mGlu5 inhibition corrects fragile X in adult mice. *Neuron* 74, 49–56. doi: 10.1016/j.neuron.2012.03.009

Miles, R., Tóth, K., Gulyás, A. I., Hájos, N., and Freund, T. F. (1996). Differences between somatic and dendritic inhibition in the hippocampus. *Neuron* 16, 815–823. doi: 10.1016/s0896-6273(00)80101-4

Musumeci, S. A., Hagerman, R. J., Ferri, R., Bosco, P., Dalla Bernardina, B., Tassinari, C. A., et al. (1999). Epilepsy and EEG findings in males with fragile X syndrome. *Epilepsia* 40, 1092–1099. doi: 10.1111/j.1528-1157.1999.tb00824.x

Olmos-Serrano, J. L., and Corbin, J. G. (2011). Amygdala regulation of fear and emotionality in fragile X syndrome. *Dev. Neurosci.* 33, 365–378. doi: 10.1159/000329424

Olmos-Serrano, J. L., Corbin, J. G., and Burns, M. P. (2011). The GABA(A) receptor agonist THIP ameliorates specific behavioral deficits in the mouse model of fragile X syndrome. *Dev. Neurosci.* 33, 395–403. doi: 10.1159/000332884

Olmos-Serrano, J. L., Paluszkiewicz, S. M., Martin, B. S., Kaufmann, W. E., Corbin, J. G., and Huntsman, M. M. (2010). Defective GABAergic neurotransmission and pharmacological rescue of neuronal hyperexcitability in the amygdala in a mouse model of fragile X syndrome. *J. Neurosci.* 30, 9929–9938. doi: 10.1523/JNEUROSCI.1714-10.2010

Paluszkiewicz, S., Martin, B., and Huntsman, M. (2011a). Fragile X syndrome: the GABAergic system and circuit dysfunction. *Dev. Neurosci.* 33, 349–364. doi: 10.1159/000329420

Paluszkiewicz, S. M., Olmos-Serrano, J. L., Corbin, J. G., and Huntsman, M. M. (2011b). Impaired inhibitory control of cortical synchronization in fragile X syndrome. *J. Neurophysiol.* 106, 2264–2272. doi: 10.1152/jn.00421.2011

Pan, F., Aldridge, G. M., Greenough, W. T., and Gan, W. B. (2010). Dendritic spine instability and insensitivity to modulation by sensory experience in a mouse model of fragile X syndrome. *Proc. Natl. Acad. Sci. U S A* 107, 17768–17773. doi: 10.1073/pnas.1012496107

Patel, A. B., Hays, S. A., Bureau, I., Huber, K. M., and Gibson, J. R. (2013). A target cell-specific role for presynaptic Fmr1 in regulating glutamate release onto neocortical fast-spiking inhibitory neurons. *J. Neurosci.* 33, 2593–2604. doi: 10.1523/JNEUROSCI.2447-12.2013

Penagarikano, O., Mulle, J. G., and Warren, S. T. (2007). The pathophysiology of fragile x syndrome. *Annu. Rev. Genomics Hum. Genet.* 8, 109–129. doi: 10.1146/annurev.genom.8.080706.092249

Porter, R. H., Jaeschke, G., Spooren, W., Ballard, T. M., Buttelmann, B., Kolczewski, S., et al. (2005). Fenobam: a clinically validated nonbenzodiazepine anxiolytic is a potent, selective and noncompetitive mGlu5 receptor antagonist with inverse agonist activity. *J. Pharmacol. Exp. Ther.* 315, 711–721. doi: 10.1124/jpet.105.089839

Real, M. A., Simon, M. P., Heredia, R., de Diego, Y., and Guirado, S. (2011). Phenotypic changes in calbindin D28K immunoreactivity in the hippocampus of Fmr1 knockout mice. *J. Comp. Neurol.* 519, 2622–2636. doi: 10.1002/cne.22643

Ronesi, J. A., Collins, K. A., Hays, S. A., Tsai, N. P., Guo, W., Birnbaum, S. G., et al. (2012). Disrupted homer scaffolds mediate abnormal mGluR5 function in a mouse model of fragile X syndrome. *Nat. Neurosci.* 15, 431–440. doi: 10.1038/nn.3033

Rotschafer, S., and Razak, K. (2013). Altered auditory processing in a mouse model of fragile X syndrome. *Brain Res.* 1506, 12–24. doi: 10.1016/j.brainres.2013.02.038

Selby, L., Zhang, C., and Sun, Q. Q. (2007). Major defects in neocortical GABAergic inhibitory circuits in mice lacking the fragile X mental retardation protein. *Neurosci. Lett.* 412, 227–232. doi: 10.1016/j.neulet.2006.11.062

Shaw, T. A., and Porter, M. A. (2013). Emotion recognition and visual-scan paths in fragile X syndrome. *J. Autism. Dev. Disord.* 43, 1119–1139. doi: 10.1007/s10803-012-1654-1

Szabadics, J., Lorincz, A., and Tamas, G. (2001). Beta and gamma frequency synchronization by dendritic gabaergic synapses and gap junctions in a network of cortical interneurons. *J. Neurosci.* 21, 5824–5831.

Till, S. M., Wijetunge, L. S., Seidel, V. G., Harlow, E., Wright, A. K., Bagni, C., et al. (2012). Altered maturation of the primary somatosensory cortex in a mouse model of fragile X syndrome. *Hum. Mol. Genet.* 21, 2143–2156. doi: 10.1093/hmg/dds030

Van der Molen, M. J., and Van der Molen, M. W. (2013). Reduced alpha and exaggerated theta power during the resting-state EEG in fragile X syndrome. *Biol. Psychol.* 92, 216–219. doi: 10.1016/j.biopsycho.2012.11.013

Van der Molen, M. J., Van der Molen, M. W., Ridderinkhof, K. R., Hamel, B. C., Curfs, L. M., and Ramakers, G. J. (2012). Auditory change detection in fragile X syndrome males: a brain potential study. *Clin. Neurophysiol.* 123, 1309–1318. doi: 10.1016/j.clinph.2011.11.039

Verkerk, A., Pieretti, M., Sutcliffe, J. S., Fu, Y. H., Kuhl, D. P., Pizzuti, A., et al. (1991). Identification of a gene (FMR-1) containing a CGG repeat coincident with a breakpoint cluster region exhibiting length variation in fragile X syndrome. *Cell* 65, 905–914. doi: 10.1016/0092-8674(91)90397-h

Vislay, R. L., Martin, B. S., Olmos-Serrano, J. L., Kratovac, S., Nelson, D. L., Corbin, J. G., et al. (2013). Homeostatic responses fail to correct defective amygdala inhibitory circuit maturation in fragile X syndrome. *J. Neurosci.* 33, 7548–7558. doi: 10.1523/JNEUROSCI.2764-12.2013

Woodruff, A. R., and Sah, P. (2007a). Inhibition and synchronization of basal amygdala principal neuron spiking by parvalbumin-positive interneurons. *J. Neurophysiol.* 98, 2956–2961. doi: 10.1152/jn.00739.2007

Woodruff, A. R., and Sah, P. (2007b). Networks of parvalbumin-positive interneurons in the basolateral amygdala. *J. Neurosci.* 27, 553–563. doi: 10.1523/jneurosci.3686-06.2007

Xu, Z. H., Yang, Q., Ma, L., Liu, S. B., Chen, G. S., Wu, Y. M., et al. (2012b). Deficits in LTP induction by 5-HT2A receptor antagonist in a mouse model for fragile X syndrome. *PLoS One* 7:e48741. doi: 10.1371/journal.pone.0048741

Xu, Q., Zhu, Z., Xu, J., Gu, W., and Zhao, Z. (2012a). Depressed nNOS expression during spine transition in the developing hippocampus of FMR1 KO mice. *Braz. J. Med. Biol. Res.* 45, 1234–1239. doi: 10.1590/s0100-879x2012007500158

Yan, Q. J., Rammal, M., Tranfaglia, M., and Bauchwitz, R. P. (2005). Suppression of two major fragile X syndrome mouse model phenotypes by the mGluR5 antagonist MPEP. *Neuropharmacology* 49, 1053–1066. doi: 10.1016/j.neuropharm.2005.06.004

Zhang, L., and Alger, B. E. (2010). Enhanced endocannabinoid signaling elevates neuronal excitability in fragile X syndrome. *J. Neurosci.* 30, 5724–5729. doi: 10.1523/JNEUROSCI.0795-10.2010

Zoghbi, H. Y. (2003). Postnatal neurodevelopmental disorders: meeting at the synapse? *Science* 302, 826–830. doi: 10.1126/science.1089071

11

Late onset deficits in synaptic plasticity in the valproic acid rat model of autism

Henry G. S. Martin[1,2,3] and Olivier J. Manzoni[1,2,3] *

[2] INSERM U901 Pathophysiology of Synaptic Plasticity Group, Marseille, France
[3] Institut de Neurobiologie de la Méditerranée (INMED), Marseille, France
Université de Aix-Marseille, Marseille, France

***Correspondence:**
Olivier J. Manzoni, INSERM and Institut de Neurobiologie de la Méditerranée (INMED), Parc scientifique de Luminy, 163 avenue de Luminy, 13273 Marseille cedex 09, France
e-mail: olivier.manzoni@inserm.fr

Valproic acid (VPA) is a frequently used drug in the treatment of epilepsy, bipolar disorders and migraines; however it is also a potent teratogen. Prenatal exposure increases the risk of childhood malformations and can result in cognitive deficits. In rodents *in utero* exposure to VPA also causes neurodevelopmental abnormalities and is an important model of autism. In early postnatal life VPA exposed rat pups show changes in medial prefrontal cortex (mPFC) physiology and synaptic connectivity. Specifically, principal neurons show decreased excitability but increased local connectivity, coupled with an increase in long-term potentiation (LTP) due to an up-regulation of NMDA receptor (NMDAR) expression. However recent evidence suggests compensatory homeostatic mechanisms lead to normalization of synaptic NMDARs during later postnatal development. Here we have extended study of mPFC synaptic physiology into adulthood to better understand the longitudinal consequences of early developmental abnormalities in VPA exposed rats. Surprisingly in contrast to early postnatal life and adolescence, we find that adult VPA exposed rats show reduced synaptic function. Both NMDAR mediated currents and LTP are lower in adult VPA rats, although spontaneous activity and endocannabinoid dependent long-term depression are normal. We conclude that rather than correcting, synaptic abnormalities persist into adulthood in VPA exposed rats, although a quite different synaptic phenotype is present. This switch from hyper to hypo function in mPFC may be linked to some of the neurodevelopmental defects found in prenatal VPA exposure and autism spectrum disorders in general.

Keywords: valproic acid, prefrontal cortex, synaptic plasticity, autism, age, NMDA receptor

INTRODUCTION

Due to its anti-convulsant action and mood stabilizing properties valproic acid (VPA) is a common treatment for bipolar disorder and childhood epilepsy (McElroy et al., 1989). These stabilizing properties have been attributed to the action of VPA on GABA transaminobutyrate and sodium ion channels, however more recently VPA has been described as a histone deacetylase inhibitor (Göttlicher et al., 2001) leading to renewed interest in VPA for the treatment of a wide range of psychiatric and non-psychiatric diseases (Chateauvieux et al., 2010). Unfortunately VPA is also a potent teratogen and prenatal exposure increases (the risk of congenital malformations and neural tube defects Meador et al., 2008). Specifically VPA exposure *in utero* results in neurodevelopmental delays apparent in poor verbal performance and cognitive impairments (Nadebaum et al., 2011; Meador et al., 2013). Furthermore prenatal VPA exposure is associated with a seven-fold increased risk of developing autism spectrum disorders and is a significant prenatal hazard (Rasalam et al., 2005; Bromley et al., 2008; Christensen et al., 2013).

In utero injection of VPA during neural tube closure in rats and mice results in progeny that model some of the neurodevelopmental changes found in humans. Most prominent is an increase in autistic like behaviors in VPA exposed rodents; notably increased repetitive behaviors, reduced social interaction and hypersensitivity (Schneider and Przewłocki, 2005; Dufour-Rainfray et al., 2010; Gandal et al., 2010; Kim et al., 2011; Mehta et al., 2011). These behaviors have led to the proposal that *in utero* exposure to VPA may represent a useful rodent model of autism and is the basis of the "intense world theory" of autism (Markram et al., 2007).

Changes in local and distant connectivity in the brain have been proposed as a possible cause of autistic behavior (Geschwind and Levitt, 2007). Using the *in utero* VPA exposure model, local changes in principal neuron connectivity and excitability have been found in the rat medial prefrontal cortex (mPFC; Rinaldi et al., 2008a,b). This is perhaps particularly pertinent since the mPFC is linked to autistic behaviors and mPFC abnormalities are found in many neuropsychiatric disorders (Goto et al., 2010). The mPFC synaptic physiology in the VPA exposed rat pups appears to be tuned to a hyper-connected, hyper-excitable state, notable for an increase in NMDA receptor (NMDAR) synaptic expression and an enhancement of long-term potentiation (LTP; Rinaldi et al., 2007, 2008b; Kim et al., 2013). However, recent recordings from older adolescent VPA exposed rats (P30 days) have suggested a normalization of both synaptic physiology and neuronal excitability to naïve levels as pups develop (Walcott et al., 2011). In common with autism spectrum disorders, behavioral deficits are present throughout life in the rat VPA model (Roullet et al., 2013), however a description of adult synaptic physiology is lacking making it unclear if the synaptic compensatory mechanisms found at P30 extend into adulthood.

In this study we have examined synaptic physiology in the mPFC of the prenatally VPA exposed rat from adolescence into adulthood. Surprisingly we find a reversal of the enhanced synaptic NMDAR expression phenotype found in VPA rat pups; such that adult VPA exposed neurons show a deficit in NMDAR mediated currents. Furthermore these adult neurons show a loss of LTP compared to controls, but unaltered long-term depression (LTD).

MATERIALS AND METHODS

ANIMALS

All animals were group housed with 12 h light/dark cycles in compliance with the European Communities Council Directive (86/609/EEC). Time-mated female Wistar rats received a single intra-peritoneal dose of 600 mg/kg VPA (Sigma; prepared as 300 mg/ml saline solution) at gestational day E12 (Schneider and Przewłocki, 2005). Control dams received a single similar volume injection of saline at the same gestational time-point. Adolescent rats were P48 ± 2 days (VPA: 3 males, 1 litter; Saline: 3 males, 1 litter); adult rats were P120 ± 10 days (VPA: 9 males, 2 litters; Saline: 7 males, 2 litters).

SLICE PREPARATION AND ELECTROPHYSIOLOGY

After isoflurane anesthetization and decapitation, brains were sliced (300 μm) in the coronal plane in a sucrose-based solution (in mM: 87 NaCl, 75 sucrose, 25 glucose, 4 KCl, 2.1 $MgCl_2$, 0.5 $CaCl_2$, 18 $NaHCO_3$ and 1.25 NaH_2PO_4). Slices were allowed to recover for 60 min at 32–35°C in artificial cerebrospinal fluid (aCSF; 126 NaCl, 2.5 KCl, 2.4 $MgCl_2$, 1.2 $CaCl_2$, 18 $NaHCO_3$, 1.2 NaH_2PO_4 and 11 glucose; equilibrated with 95% O_2/5% CO_2) before transfer to the recording chamber.

Whole-cell patch-clamp and extra-cellular field recordings were made from layer V/VI pyramidal cells in coronal slices of prelimbic PFC (Lafourcade et al., 2007). For recording, slices were superfused (2 ml/min) with aCSF. All experiments were performed at 32–35°C. The recording aCSF contained picrotoxin (100 μM, Sigma) to block $GABA_A$ receptors. To evoke synaptic currents, 150–200 μs stimuli were delivered at 0.1 Hz through an aCSF-filled glass electrode positioned dorsal-medial to the recording electrode in layer V (**Figure 1A**). Pyramidal neurons were visualized using an infrared microscope (BX-50, Olympus). Patch-clamp experiments were performed with electrodes filled with a cesium methane-sulfonate based solution (in mM; 143 CH_3O_3SCs, 10 NaCl, 1 $MgCl_2$, 1 EGTA, 0.3 $CaCl_2$, 2 Na^{2+}-ATP, 0.3 Na^{+}-GTP, 10 glucose buffered with 10 4-(2-hydroxyethyl)-1-piperazineethanesulfonic acid (HEPES), pH 7.3, osmolarity 290 mOsm). Prior to break-through into the cell, pipette capacitance was compensated and the reference potential of the amplifier was adjusted to zero. Junction potentials were not corrected. Electrode resistance was 3–5 MOhm. If access resistance was greater than 20 MOhm or changed by >20% during the period of recording, the experiment was rejected. During recording holding currents, series resistance and membrane time constant (τ) were monitored. Only monosynaptic excitatory post synaptic currents (EPSCs) were recorded with a latency of <5 ms. In extracellular field experiments, the recording pipette was filled with aCSF. The glutamatergic nature of the field excitatory postsynaptic potential (fEPSP) was confirmed at the end of the experiments using the ionotropic glutamate receptor antagonist 6,7-dinitroquinoxaline-2,3-dione (DNQX, 20 μM; National Institute of Mental Health Chemical Synthesis and Drug Supply Program (NIMH)).

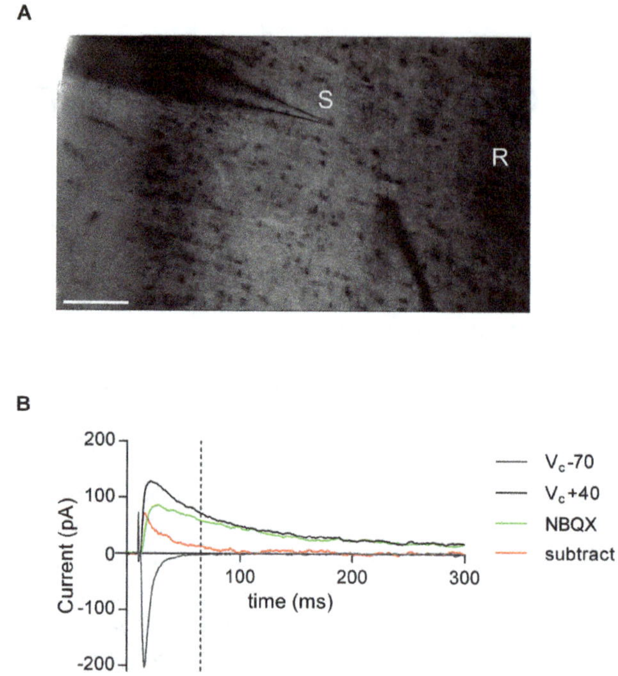

FIGURE 1 | AMPA—NMDA ratio experimental design. (A) Bright-field snapshot of coronal slice detailing prelimbic mPFC division (*x*-axis medial—lateral; *y*-axis dorsal—ventral). Typical positioning of stimulation electrode (S) and patch-clamp recording electrode (R) are indicated (scale bar 100 μm). **(B)** Example traces from AMPA—NMDA ratio calculation. NMDAR mediated current was taken as V_C +40 mV value 50 ms after peak AMPAR mediated current measured at −70 mV (indicated by dashed line). NBQX insensitive current (green) and subtracted current (red) at V_C +40 mV show that AMPAR mediated currents are close to zero at NMDAR current measurement point.

Input-output profiles were recorded for all fEPSP recordings. For time course experiments the stimulation intensity was that necessary give a response 40–60% of the maximal. fEPSPs were recorded at 0.1 Hz. Using the same stimulation intensity as baseline, LTP was induced by a repeated (4 times, 10 s interval) theta burst stimulation (TBS; 4 100 Hz pulses repeated 5 times separated by 200 ms). LTD was likewise induced by a steady 10 Hz stimulation for 10 min.

DATA ACQUISITION AND ANALYSIS

Data was recorded on a MultiClamp700B (Axon Instruments), filtered at 2 kHz, digitized (10 kHz, DigiData 1440A, Axon

Instrument), collected using Clampex 10.2 and analyzed using Clampfit 10.2 (all from Molecular Device, Sunnyvale, USA). Analysis of both area and amplitude of fEPSPs and EPSCs was performed.

The magnitude of LTP and LTD was calculated 25–30 min after tetanus as percentage of baseline responses. To determine the AMPA/NMDA ratio, the AMPAR component amplitude was measured from EPSC at −70 mV. The NMDAR component amplitude was determined 50 ms after the peak AMPAR-evoked EPSC at +40 mV, when the AMPAR component is over (Kasanetz and Manzoni, 2009). In a subset of experiments the AMPAR mediated current was inhibited with the selective antagonist 2,3-dihydroxy-6-nitro-7-sulfamoyl-benzo[f]quinoxaline-2,3-dione (NBQX, 10 μM; NIMH) to confirm the absence of an AMPAR contribution to the measured NMDAR component (**Figure 1B**). Spontaneous EPSCs were analyzed with Axograph X (Axograph). Statistical analysis of data was performed with GraphPad Prism (GraphPad Software Inc., La Jolla, CA) using tests indicated in the main text after Grubbs' outlier subtraction (99% confidence). All values are given as mean ± standard error, n values represent individual animals and statistical significance was set at * $p < 0.05$ and ** $p < 0.01$.

RESULTS

LATE ONSET DEFICITS IN SYNAPTIC CURRENTS ARE FOUND IN THE MEDIAL PREFRONTAL CORTEX (mPFC) OF ADULT VALPROIC ACID (VPA) EXPOSED RATS

Recently it has been reported that mPFC hyper-function found in juvenile rats exposed to the teratogen VPA is corrected in adolescent rats (Walcott et al., 2011). If such a strong compensatory mechanism exists during pup development, we asked if these modifications persist into adulthood. We focused on glutamatergic synapses of principal neurons in layer V/VI of the prelimbic region of the mPFC. These output neurons not only show a full range of synaptic plasticity throughout development into adulthood, but are also implicated in mPFC linked synaptopathologies (Lafourcade et al., 2011; Iafrati et al., 2013; Kasanetz et al., 2013).

We first verified, as reported by Walcott et al. (2011) that synaptic gain function is normalized in adolescent VPA exposed rats by recording evoked synaptic AMPAR and NMDAR currents and using the ratio of the two events as a measure of their modification. Neurons from adolescent rats exposed either to VPA or saline *in utero* reliably showed evoked EPSCs when voltage-clamped at both −70 mV (negative deflections) and +40 mV (positive defections, **Figure 2A**). In the mPFC, at −70 mV fast inward EPSCs are principally AMPAR mediated, whereas at +40 mV a mixed AMPAR and NMDAR outward current is detected. Thus we calculated an index for the ratio AMPAR to NMDAR mediated currents (AMPA-NMDA ratio) by dividing the maximal amplitude of the response at −70 mV (AMPA), by the +40 response amplitude at a predetermined time point after the fast AMPAR event had decayed to zero (NMDA). In agreement with Walcott et al. (2011) we find that this measure is broadly the same in both saline and VPA exposed neurons in adolescent rats (**Figure 2B**).

Given this compensatory rebalancing of synaptic function in adolescent rats, we asked if a similar effect is found in adult rats

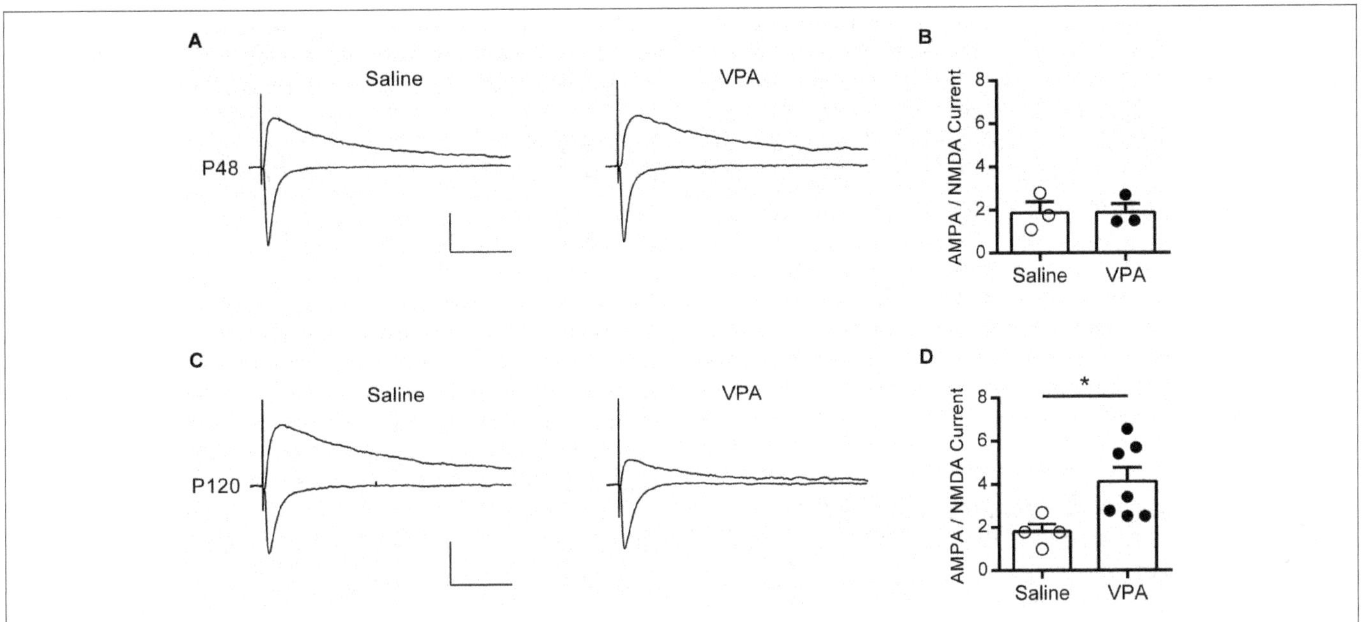

FIGURE 2 | AMPA–NMDA ratio is increased in adult but not adolescent VPA mPFC neurons. (A) Example EPSCs recorded from visually identified pyramidal neurons in layer V/VI mPFC from adolescent rats (P45–P49). Negative traces represent inward evoked currents from neurons patch-clamped at −70 mV, positive traces represent outward evoked currents from neurons patch-clamped at +40 mV. Scale bar 50 ms, 100 pA. **(B)** Average AMPA/NMDA ratio from adolescent rats exposed to saline or VPA *in utero*. **(C)** Similar evoked example EPSC traces from visually identified deep layer pyramidal neurons from adult rats (P110–P130). **(D)** Average AMPA/NMDA ratio from adult rats exposed to saline or VPA *in utero*. Data points represent AMPA/NMDA ratio from individual animals. Data shown as mean ± s.e.m.; * $p < 0.05$.

exposed to VPA *in utero*. At P120 strong EPSCs could be evoked from deep layer mPFC neurons clamped at −70 mV in both saline and VPA treated rats, however responses recorded at +40 mV were notably reduced in VPA neurons (**Figure 2C**). Repeating the same measure used in the adolescent rats, we calculated the AMPA-NMDA in our adult animals (**Figure 2D**). Surprisingly we found that in rats exposed to VPA *in utero* there was a significant increase in the AMPA-NMDA ratio compared to saline controls ($p = 0.024$; Mann-Whitney U-test). Notably saline treated adult rats had an AMPA-NMDA ratio similar to the value calculated for adolescents, whereas VPA treated rats had an elevated AMPA-NMDA ratio compared to both of these groups. Therefore in contrast to the reported reduction in AMPA-NMDA ratio found in mPFC of juvenile VPA exposed rats (Rinaldi et al., 2007, 2008a), we find an increase in this index in adulthood.

Anecdotally the increase in AMPA-NMDA ratio found in adult VPA neurons appeared to be due to a change in NMDAR mediated currents; however a change in this index can be linked to a number of other synaptic parameters. Therefore we further characterized some of the basic properties of these synapses. Taking a systematic approach, we first measured field EPSPs (fEPSP) from layer V/VI neurons to build input-output profiles in saline and VPA neurons. fEPSPs evoked by electrical stimulation in the same layer showed a similar profile in response to increasing stimulation intensity (**Figure 3A**). Furthermore input-output curves from saline and VPA exposed neurons were nearly identical. Therefore these synapses do not show and gross changes in excitability.

To further characterize these synapses, we measured quantal events by recording spontaneous EPSCs (sEPSC). Both saline control and VPA neurons showed robust sEPSCs in adulthood (**Figure 3B**). We used the cumulative distribution of the amplitude of events to gauge any differences between the two groups (**Figure 3C**). However both the distribution and the mean amplitude of spontaneous events were broadly the same in VPA exposed and saline control neurons. At resting membrane potential (−70 mV) these events are principally AMPAR mediated, therefore as previously reported in adolescent animals (Walcott et al., 2011), VPA exposure does not appear to strongly effect AMPAR currents. Likewise, we compared the frequency of sEPSC by comparing the cumulative distribution of the interval between events (**Figure 3D**). Both saline and VPA exposed neurons had a similar distribution and average interval between events. Therefore both presynaptic release and postsynaptic AMPAR are similar in control and VPA exposed neurons in the mPFC.

ADULT VALPROIC ACID (VPA) MEDIAL PREFRONTAL CORTEX (mPFC) NEURONS HAVE DEFICITS IN LONG-TERM POTENTIATION (LTP), BUT NOT LONG-TERM DEPRESSION (LTD)

In juvenile rats exposed to VPA, a decrease in AMPA-NMDA ratio was linked to increased LTP in the mPFC (Rinaldi et al., 2007). Since in adult VPA exposed rats we observe the opposite phenomenon, we asked if adult VPA rats might instead show reduced LTP. We recorded fEPSPs in layer V/VI and challenged slices with a short TBS LTP protocol; this induces a postsynaptic NMDAR dependent form of LTP (Iafrati et al., 2013). In saline controls a robust potentiation of fEPSPs was observed that was stable over the period of recording. In contrast in recordings from VPA exposed neurons, fEPSPs were smaller than saline controls (**Figure 4A**). Taking the fEPSP strength pre- and post-TBS we compared LTP in saline and VPA treated rats (**Figure 4B**). In control slices TBS induced a significant LTP ($p = 0.012$; Paired t-test), whereas in VPA slices there we did not detect a significant potentiation ($p = 0.177$; Paired t-test). Converting the post-TBS fEPSP to a percent LTP, we plotted the cumulative distribution of the percent LTP in individual experiments. The distribution of VPA exposed neurons is left shifted compared to saline controls, indicating a reduction in LTP (**Figure 4C**). Therefore in contrast to juvenile VPA exposed neurons in the mPFC, adult neurons show a reduction in NMDAR mediated LTP.

To confirm this reduction in LTP is a specific phenomenon linked to our observed changes in AMPA-NMDA ratio, we tested another form of activity dependent plasticity that is independent of NMDARs in the mPFC. Endocannabinoid-dependent long-term depression (eCB-LTD) induced by steady 10 Hz stimulation, engages an mGluR5 mediated mechanism that requires retrograde 2-AG signaling to presynaptic cannabinoid receptor type 1 (CB1) receptors (Lafourcade et al., 2007, 2011). Recording fEPSPs from mPFC deep layers, we induced eCB-LTD in saline and VPA *in utero* treated adult rats. Both groups showed an initial strong depression in fEPSP in response to 10 Hz stimulation that stabilized at approximately 80% of the baseline response (**Figure 5A**). Again we compared the response pre- and post-eCB-LTD (**Figure 5B**). In both saline controls and VPA exposed neurons we saw a significant depression of fEPSP (Saline: $p = 0.042$; VPA: $p = 0.005$; Paired t-test). Converting fEPSPs to percent LTD we compared the amount of depression in the two groups. Unlike LTP, the distribution and strength of LTD was similar between control and VPA neurons (**Figure 5C**). Therefore eCB-LTD is unaffected in adult rats exposed to VPA *in utero*.

DISCUSSION

In this study we have traced changes in mPFC synaptic physiology in the VPA rat from adolescence to adulthood. Juvenile rats exposed *in utero* to the teratogen VPA have a hyper-connected mPFC with enhanced NMDAR function (Rinaldi et al., 2007, 2008b). However recent evidence suggests that this phenotype is normalized as pups reach puberty (Walcott et al., 2011). Given the late maturation of the PFC, we wished to extend this synaptic description into adulthood to better understand the developmental consequences of VPA exposure. Surprisingly in contrast to VPA rat pups and adolescents, we found evidence of synaptic hypo-function during adulthood.

Compared to controls, VPA neurons in the mPFC show a reduced and delayed increase in AMPA-NMDA ratio over early postnatal development (Rinaldi et al., 2007; Walcott et al., 2011). However by the time rats reach early adolescence (P30) this parameter is similar in both VPA and saline controls. In concord we find that at puberty (P40–P50) that the AMPA-NMDA ratio is not significantly different between control and VPA rats in the mPFC. However, when we extended measurement of the AMPA-NMDA ratio into young adulthood (P110–P130) we found a significant increase of this index in VPA rats, but not controls.

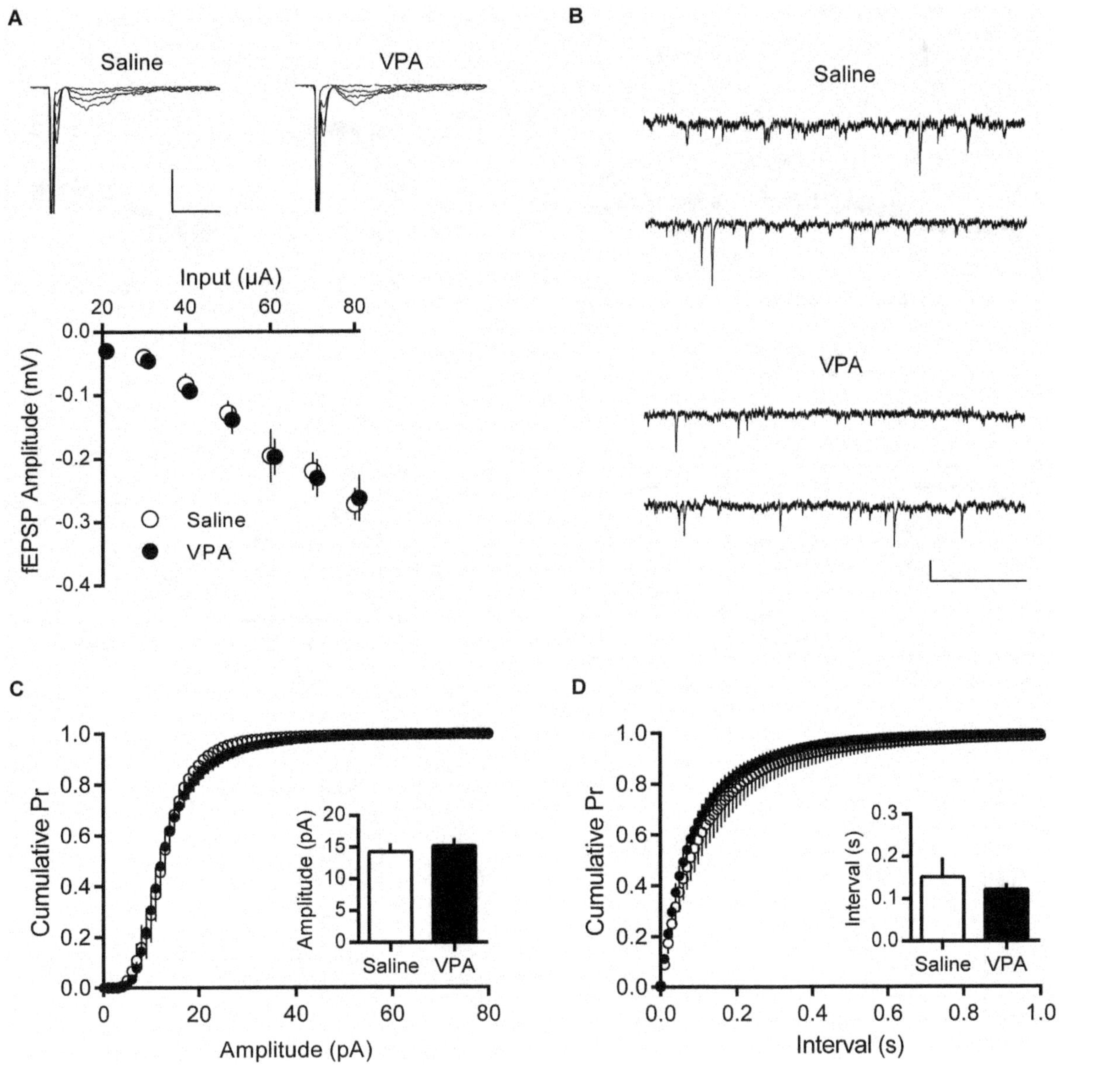

FIGURE 3 | Basal synaptic activity is normal in adult VPA neurons. (A) Input—Output relationships derived from evoked fEPSPs in deep layer mPFC. Sample fEPSP traces from saline and VPA treated rats showing fEPSP change in response to 10 pA stimulation steps (top). Scale bar 10 ms, 0.5 mV. Average fEPSP amplitude from saline and VPA neurons (bottom). **(B)** Spontaneous EPSCs from pyramidal neurons patch-clamped at −70 mV. Scale bar 0.5 s, 10 pA. **(C)** Cumulative probability plot of individual spontaneous EPSCs from adult saline and VPA neurons. Average amplitude EPSC from individual animals (insert; Saline, $n = 5$; VPA, $n = 7$). **(D)** Cumulative probability plot of intervals between spontaneous EPSC events from saline and VPA neurons. Average recorded interval between spontaneous events from individual neurons (insert). Data shown as mean ± s.e.m.

The AMPA-NMDA ratio is a strong measure of synaptic state, particularly the relative number of AMPARs and NMDARs in the post-synapse (Watt et al., 2000), however other synaptic variables may also be involved. Therefore to better interpret the unexpected increase in AMPA-NMDA ratio in adult VPA rats, we measured quantal mPFC activity. Focusing on AMPAR mediated events we recorded spontaneous EPSCs in layer V/VI neurons. We found that neither the average amplitude nor distribution of spontaneous events was different in VPA and saline controls, indicating that synaptic AMPAR are unchanged in these rats. Likewise we failed to observe any change in frequency of spontaneous events. Superficially this is inconsistent with the local hyper-connectivity reported in the mPFC of juvenile VPA rats (Rinaldi et al., 2008b). However our measurements of spontaneous activity do not distinguish between local and distant connections, thus a relative reduction in distant connectivity could account for this inconsistency (Geschwind and Levitt, 2007; Rinaldi et al., 2008b).

The simplest interpretation of our AMPA-NMDA ratio in light of unchanged spontaneous activity is that NMDAR currents are reduced in adult rats exposed to VPA *in utero*. In the young VPA

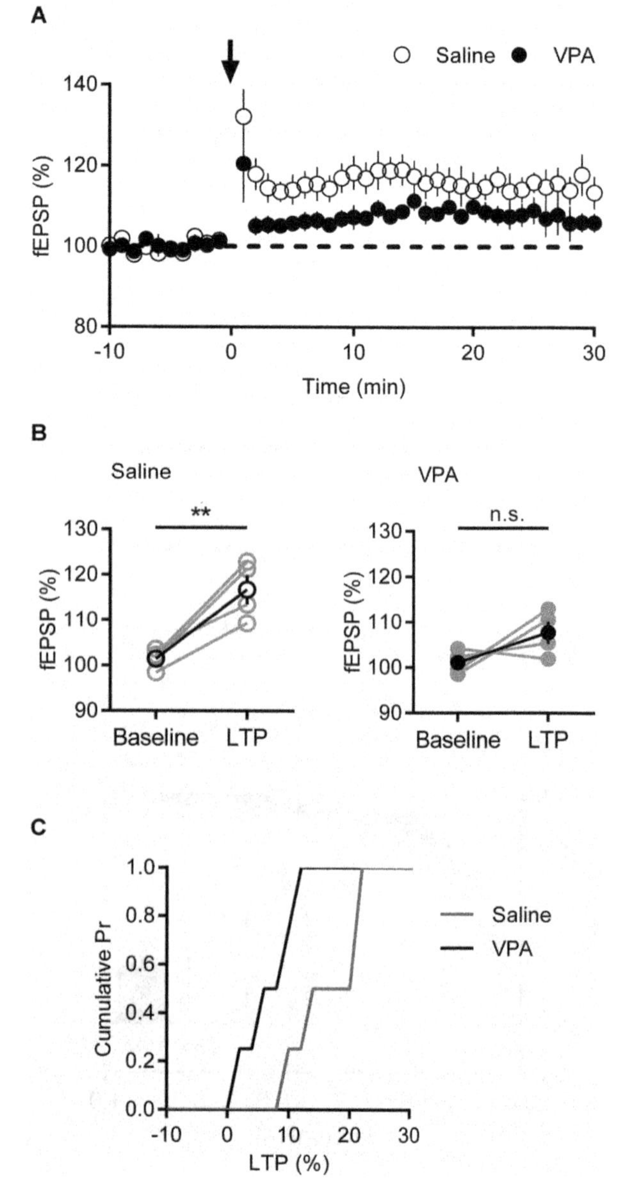

FIGURE 4 | Deficits in LTP are present in VPA exposed mPFC neurons. **(A)** Time course of normalized fEPSP responses from layer V/VI adult rats treated with saline or VPA *in utero*. Theta burst LTP stimulation is indicated by arrow. **(B)** Change in normalized fEPSP pre- (Baseline) and post- (LTP; 25 min after TBS) theta burst stimulation LTP. Darker points represent the mean fEPSP. **(C)** Cumulative probability plot of percent LTP from individual experiments. Data shown as mean ± s.e.m.; ** $p < 0.01$.

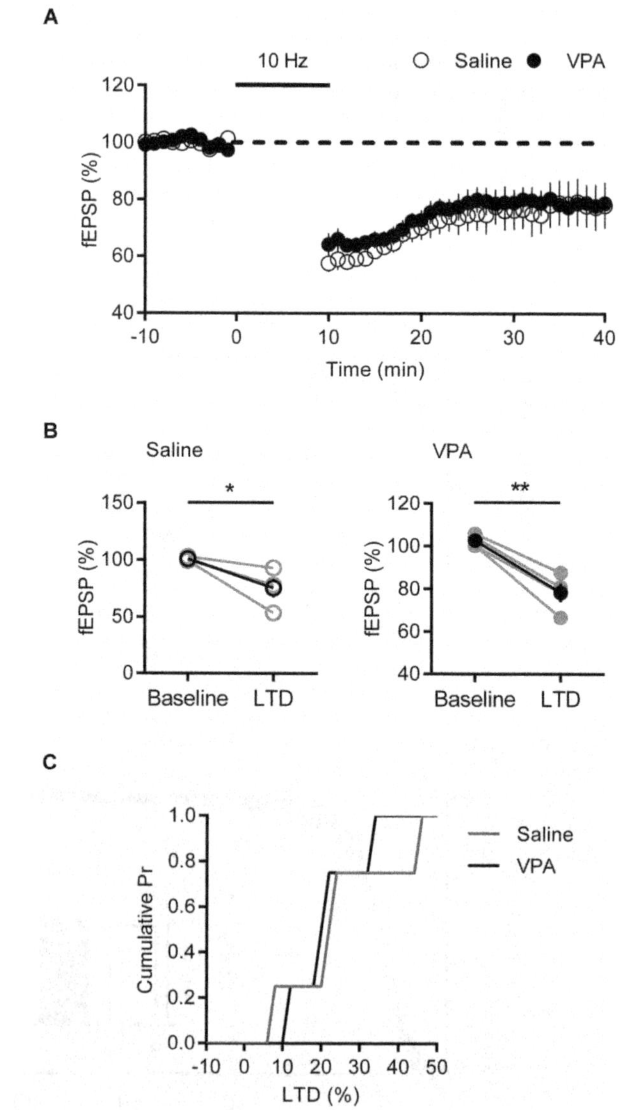

FIGURE 5 | LTD is normal in VPA exposed mPFC neurons. **(A)** Time course of normalized fEPSP responses from layer V/VI adult rats treated with saline or VPA *in utero*. 10 Hz eCB-LTD stimulation is indicated by bar. **(B)** Change in normalized fEPSP pre- (Baseline) and post- (LTD; 25 min after 10 Hz stimulation) eCB-LTD. Darker points represent the mean fEPSP. **(C)** Cumulative probability plot of percent LTD from individual experiments. Data shown as mean ± s.e.m.; * $p < 0.05$, ** $p < 0.01$.

rat, Rinaldi et al. (2007) directly linked a decrease in AMPA-NMDA ratio to an increase in expression of GluN2a and GluN2b and a subsequent increase in LTP. Our increase in AMPA-NMDA ratio in the adult VPA rat was suggestive that the opposite phenomenon might occur in these older animals. Indeed, when we challenged deep layer mPFC neurons with TBS LTP protocol there was a measurable loss in potentiation with VPA exposure compared to saline controls. A similar NMDAR linked loss of LTP is found in a number of mouse genetic models of autism (Ebert and Greenberg, 2013; Jiang and Ehlers, 2013), suggesting the adult VPA rat shares similarities with these mice. We found no change in mGluR5 mediated eCB-LTD in these synapses, demonstrating that this deficit in LTP is not a general loss of synaptic gain function.

Fragile X syndrome (FXS) is a genetic disorder with a complex endophenotype that often includes autism linked behaviors (Cornish et al., 2008). Similar to our findings in VPA rats, FXS mice show a reduction in NMDAR expression in the mPFC and a loss of LTP (Zhao et al., 2005; Meredith et al., 2007; Krueger et al., 2011). Likewise in young FXS mice (2–3 weeks) mGluR5 mediated LTD is unaffected (Desai et al., 2006; Meredith et al., 2007), although in adult mice a deficit in coupling between mGluR5 activation and retrograde signaling appears to be responsible for a loss in eCB-LTD (Jung et al., 2012). Similar to the VPA rat, age and development linked deficits in synaptic physiology appear to be present in the FXS mouse, although differences in early postnatal life suggest these two models of autism are not directly comparable (Desai et al., 2006; Rinaldi et al., 2007).

The surprising finding in this study is that rats prenatally exposed to VPA pass from an enhanced LTP phenotype in early life to a LTP deficit phenotype in adulthood. Immediately before puberty and during adolescence NMDAR mPFC physiology appears similar to saline control suggesting that VPA neurons transition through a normal period between a hyper to hypo synaptic function. It has been proposed that homeostatic compensatory mechanisms may be responsible for the initial normalization of mPFC neuronal function in VPA rats (Walcott et al., 2011). How these compensatory synaptic scaling mechanisms work is unclear, however our results suggest that the action of normalizing hyper function in early life may subsequently lead to the loss of LTP in adulthood. Such a rebound effect may be due to the engagement of feedback loops that act over extended periods of development. It is also noteworthy that in our recordings we average across layer V/VI neuronal responses. This is significant since layer V principal neurons appear to belong to one of two subtypes with differing intrinsic properties and output projects (Dembrow et al., 2010; Lee et al., 2014). Regardless our results strongly argue for the importance of longitudinal studies when investigating early changes in synaptic physiology.

Prenatally treated VPA rats show behavioral deficits that share similarities with core autistic behaviors, in common with a small percentage of children that develop autism due to an exposure to VPA during pregnancy (Roullet et al., 2013). A validation of our observations would be to link autism associated behaviors in the VPA rat at specific ages with deficits in mPFC plasticity. Consistent with a delay in normalizing synaptic currents in early postnatal development, VPA rats and mice show a latency in nest-seeking behavior and bedding odor discrimination compared to control pups (Schneider and Przewłocki, 2005; Roullet et al., 2013), although these behaviors are not mPFC dependent. Deficits in social interaction are more clearly linked to abnormalities in mPFC function and these are consistently reported in the VPA rat (Roullet et al., 2013). However, from the earliest time points (pre-weaning, (Roullet et al., 2010)), into adolescence and adulthood social deficits are found in VPA exposed rats (Schneider and Przewłocki, 2005; Dufour-Rainfray et al., 2010; Kim et al., 2011). Therefore a direct link to social behavior and age dependent changes in NMDAR mediated LTP does not appear to be present. This of course does not exclude the importance of increased synaptic NMDAR and LTP in the formation of a locally hyper-connected state in the VPA rat pup (Rinaldi et al., 2008a,b). Other longitudinal tests of mPFC linked behaviors have not yet been reported in the VPA rat, although an adulthood deficit in radial maze learning is present (Narita et al., 2010). Ultimately a systematic test of mPFC dependent behaviors from adolescence to adulthood will be necessary to identify the specific late-onset behavioral deficits which our findings allude to.

ACKNOWLEDGMENTS

This work was supported by INSERM and ANR "RescueMemo". We thank members from the Manzoni and Chavis laboratories for discussions, the National Institute of Mental Health's Chemical Synthesis and Drug Supply Program (Rockville, MD, USA) for providing DNQX, and Dr. R. Nardou and Dr. D. Ferrari from Neurochlore (www.neurochlore.fr) for providing the VPA-treated rats.

REFERENCES

Bromley, R. L., Mawer, G., Clayton-Smith, J., and Baker, G. A. (2008). Autism spectrum disorders following in utero exposure to antiepileptic drugs. *Neurology* 71, 1923–1924. doi: 10.1212/01.wnl.0000339399.64213.1a

Chateauvieux, S., Morceau, F., Dicato, M., and Diederich, M. (2010). Molecular and therapeutic potential and toxicity of valproic acid. *J. Biomed. Biotechnol.* 2010, 1–18. doi: 10.1155/2010/479364

Christensen, J., Grønborg, T. K., Sørensen, M. J., Schendel, D., Parner, E. T., Pedersen, L. H., et al. (2013). Prenatal valproate exposure and risk of autism spectrum disorders and childhood autism. *JAMA* 309, 1696–1703. doi: 10.1001/jama.2013.2270

Cornish, K., Turk, J., and Hagerman, R. (2008). The fragile X continuum: new advances and perspectives. *J. Intellect. Disabil. Res.* 52, 469–482. doi: 10.1111/j.1365-2788.2008.01056.x

Dembrow, N. C., Chitwood, R. A., and Johnston, D. (2010). Projection-specific neuromodulation of medial prefrontal cortex neurons. *J. Neurosci.* 30, 16922–16937. doi: 10.1523/jneurosci.3644-10.2010

Desai, N. S., Casimiro, T. M., Gruber, S. M., and Vanderklish, P. W. (2006). Early postnatal plasticity in neocortex of Fmr1 knockout mice. *J. Neurophysiol.* 96, 1734–1745. doi: 10.1152/jn.00221.2006

Dufour-Rainfray, D., Vourc'h, P., Le Guisquet, A.-M., Garreau, L., Ternant, D., Bodard, S., et al. (2010). Behavior and serotonergic disorders in rats exposed prenatally to valproate: a model for autism. *Neurosci. Lett.* 470, 55–59. doi: 10.1016/j.neulet.2009.12.054

Ebert, D. H., and Greenberg, M. E. (2013). Activity-dependent neuronal signalling and autism spectrum disorder. *Nature* 493, 327–337. doi: 10.1038/nature11860

Gandal, M. J., Edgar, J. C., Ehrlichman, R. S., Mehta, M., Roberts, T. P. L., and Siegel, S. J. (2010). Validating γ oscillations and delayed auditory responses as translational biomarkers of autism. *Biol. Psychiatry* 68, 1100–1106. doi: 10.1016/j.biopsych.2010.09.031

Geschwind, D. H., and Levitt, P. (2007). Autism spectrum disorders: developmental disconnection syndromes. *Curr. Opin. Neurobiol.* 17, 103–111. doi: 10.1016/j.conb.2007.01.009

Goto, Y., Yang, C. R., and Otani, S. (2010). Functional and dysfunctional synaptic plasticity in prefrontal cortex: roles in psychiatric disorders. *Biol. Psychiatry* 67, 199–207. doi: 10.1016/j.biopsych.2009.08.026

Göttlicher, M., Minucci, S., Zhu, P., Krämer, O. H., Schimpf, A., Giavara, S., et al. (2001). Valproic acid defines a novel class of HDAC inhibitors inducing differentiation of transformed cells. *EMBO J.* 20, 6969–6978. doi: 10.1093/emboj/20.24.6969

Iafrati, J., Orejarena, M. J., Lassalle, O., Bouamrane, L., and Chavis, P. (2013). Reelin, an extracellular matrix protein linked to early onset psychiatric diseases, drives postnatal development of the prefrontal cortex via GluN2B-NMDARs and the mTOR pathway. *Mol. Psychiatry*. doi: 10.1038/mp.2013.148. [Epub ahead of print].

Jiang, Y., and Ehlers, M. D. (2013). Modeling autism by SHANK gene mutations in mice. *Neuron* 78, 8–27. doi: 10.1016/j.neuron.2013.03.016

Jung, K.-M., Sepers, M., Henstridge, C. M., Lassalle, O., Neuhofer, D., Martin, H., et al. (2012). Uncoupling of the endocannabinoid signalling complex in a mouse model of fragile X syndrome. *Nat. Commun.* 3, 1080. doi: 10.1038/ncomms2045

Kasanetz, F., and Manzoni, O. J. (2009). Maturation of excitatory synaptic transmission of the rat nucleus accumbens from juvenile to adult. *J. Neurophysiol.* 101, 2516–2527. doi: 10.1152/jn.91039.2008

Kasanetz, F., Lafourcade, M., Deroche-Gamonet, V., Revest, J.-M., Berson, N., Balado, E., et al. (2013). Prefrontal synaptic markers of cocaine addiction-like behavior in rats. *Mol. Psychiatry* 18, 729–737. doi: 10.1038/mp.2012.59

Kim, K. C., Kim, P., Go, H. S., Choi, C. S., Yang, S.-I., Cheong, J. H., et al. (2011). The critical period of valproate exposure to induce autistic symptoms in Sprague–Dawley rats. *Toxicol. Lett.* 201, 137–142. doi: 10.1016/j.toxlet.2010.12.018

Kim, K. C., Lee, D.-K., Go, H. S., Kim, P., Choi, C. S., Kim, J.-W., et al. (2013). Pax6-dependent cortical glutamatergic neuronal differentiation regulates autism-like behavior in prenatally valproic acid-exposed rat offspring. *Mol. Neurobiol.* doi: 10.1007/s12035-013-8535-2. [Epub ahead of print].

Krueger, D. D., Osterweil, E. K., Chen, S. P., Tye, L. D., and Bear, M. F. (2011). Cognitive dysfunction and prefrontal synaptic abnormalities in a mouse model of fragile X syndrome. *Proc. Natl. Acad. Sci. U S A* 108, 2587–2592. doi: 10.1073/pnas.1013855108

Lafourcade, M., Elezgarai, I., Mato, S., Bakiri, Y., Grandes, P., and Manzoni, O. J. (2007). Molecular components and functions of the endocannabinoid system in mouse prefrontal cortex. *PLoS One* 2:e709. doi: 10.1371/journal.pone.0000709

Lafourcade, M., Larrieu, T., Mato, S., Duffaud, A., Sepers, M., Matias, I., et al. (2011). Nutritional omega-3 deficiency abolishes endocannabinoid-mediated neuronal functions. *Nat. Neurosci.* 14, 345–350. doi: 10.1038/nn.2736

Lee, A. T., Gee, S. M., Vogt, D., Patel, T., Rubenstein, J. L., and Sohal, V. S. (2014). Pyramidal neurons in prefrontal cortex receive subtype-specific forms of excitation and inhibition. *Neuron* 81, 61–68. doi: 10.1016/j.neuron.2013.10.031

Markram, H., Rinaldi, T., and Markram, K. (2007). The intense world syndrome–an alternative hypothesis for autism. *Front. Neurosci.* 15:6. doi: 10.3389/neuro.01.1.1.006.2007

McElroy, S. L., Keck, P. E. Jr., Pope, H. G. Jr., and Hudson, J. I. (1989). Valproate in psychiatric disorders: literature review and clinical guidelines. *J. Clin. Psychiatry* 50, 23–29.

Meador, K. J., Baker, G. A., Browning, N., Cohen, M. J., Bromley, R. L., Clayton-Smith, J., et al. (2013). Fetal antiepileptic drug exposure and cognitive outcomes at age 6 years (NEAD study): a prospective observational study. *Lancet Neurol.* 12, 244–252. doi: 10.1016/s1474-4422(12)70323-x

Meador, K., Reynolds, M. W., Crean, S., Fahrbach, K., and Probst, C. (2008). Pregnancy outcomes in women with epilepsy: a systematic review and meta-analysis of published pregnancy registries and cohorts. *Epilepsy Res.* 81, 1–13. doi: 10.1016/j.eplepsyres.2008.04.022

Mehta, M. V., Gandal, M. J., and Siegel, S. J. (2011). mGluR5-antagonist mediated reversal of elevated stereotyped, repetitive behaviors in the VPA model of autism. *PLoS One* 6:e26077. doi: 10.1371/journal.pone.0026077

Meredith, R. M., Holmgren, C. D., Weidum, M., Burnashev, N., and Mansvelder, H. D. (2007). Increased threshold for spike-timing-dependent plasticity is caused by unreliable calcium signaling in mice lacking fragile X gene FMR1. *Neuron* 54, 627–638. doi: 10.1016/j.neuron.2007.04.028

Nadebaum, C., Anderson, V., Vajda, F., Reutens, D., Barton, S., and Wood, A. (2011). The Australian brain and cognition and antiepileptic drugs study: IQ in school-aged children exposed to sodium valproate and polytherapy. *J. Int. Neuropsychol. Soc.* 17, 133–142. doi: 10.1017/s1355617710001359

Narita, M., Oyabu, A., Imura, Y., Kamada, N., Yokoyama, T., Tano, K., et al. (2010). Nonexploratory movement and behavioral alterations in a thalidomide or valproic acid-induced autism model rat. *Neurosci. Res.* 66, 2–6. doi: 10.1016/j.neures.2009.09.001

Rasalam, A. D., Hailey, H., Williams, J. H. G., Moore, S. J., Turnpenny, P. D., Lloyd, D. J., et al. (2005). Characteristics of fetal anticonvulsant syndrome associated autistic disorder. *Dev. Med. Child Neurol.* 47, 551–555. doi: 10.1017/s0012162205001076

Rinaldi, T., Kulangara, K., Antoniello, K., and Markram, H. (2007). Elevated NMDA receptor levels and enhanced postsynaptic long-term potentiation induced by prenatal exposure to valproic acid. *Proc. Natl. Acad. Sci. U S A* 104, 13501–13506. doi: 10.1073/pnas.0704391104

Rinaldi, T., Perrodin, C., and Markram, H. (2008a). Hyper-connectivity and hyper-plasticity in the medial prefrontal cortex in the valproic acid animal model of autism. *Front. Neural Circuits* 2:4. doi: 10.3389/neuro.04.004.2008

Rinaldi, T., Silberberg, G., and Markram, H. (2008b). Hyperconnectivity of local neocortical microcircuitry induced by prenatal exposure to valproic acid. *Cereb. Cortex* 18, 763–770. doi: 10.1093/cercor/bhm117

Roullet, F. I., Lai, J. K. Y., and Foster, J. A. (2013). In utero exposure to valproic acid and autism—A current review of clinical and animal studies. *Neurotoxicol. Teratol.* 36, 47–56. doi: 10.1016/j.ntt.2013.01.004

Roullet, F. I., Wollaston, L., deCatanzaro, D., and Foster, J. A. (2010). Behavioral and molecular changes in the mouse in response to prenatal exposure to the anti-epileptic drug valproic acid. *Neuroscience* 170, 514–522. doi: 10.1016/j.neuroscience.2010.06.069

Schneider, T., and Przewłocki, R. (2005). Behavioral alterations in rats prenatally exposed to valproic acid: animal model of autism. *Neuropsychopharmacology* 30, 80–89. doi: 10.1038/sj.npp.1300518

Walcott, E. C., Higgins, E. A., and Desai, N. S. (2011). Synaptic and intrinsic balancing during postnatal development in rat pups exposed to valproic acid in utero. *J. Neurosci.* 31, 13097–13109. doi: 10.1523/jneurosci.1341-11.2011

Watt, A. J., van Rossum, M. C. W., MacLeod, K. M., Nelson, S. B., and Turrigiano, G. G. (2000). Activity coregulates quantal AMPA and NMDA currents at neocortical synapses. *Neuron* 26, 659–670. doi: 10.1016/s0896-6273(00)81202-7

Zhao, M.-G., Toyoda, H., Ko, S. W., Ding, H.-K., Wu, L.-J., and Zhuo, M. (2005). Deficits in trace fear memory and long-term potentiation in a mouse model for fragile X syndrome. *J. Neurosci.* 25, 7385–7392. doi: 10.1523/jneurosci.1520-05.2005

12

5-HT$_7$ receptors as modulators of neuronal excitability, synaptic transmission and plasticity: Physiological role and possible implications in autism spectrum disorders

***Lucia Ciranna*[1]* *and Maria Vincenza Catania*[2,3]**

[1] *Department of Biomedical Sciences, University of Catania, Catania, Italy*
[2] *Institute of Neurological Sciences, the National Research Council of Italy (CNR), Catania, Italy*
[3] *Laboratory of Neurobiology, IRCCS Oasi Maria SS, Troina, Italy*

Correspondence:
Lucia Ciranna, Department of Biomedical Sciences, University of Catania, 6, Viale Andrea Doria, Catania 95125, Italy
e-mail: ciranna@unict.it

Serotonin type 7 receptors (5-HT$_7$) are expressed in several brain areas, regulate brain development, synaptic transmission and plasticity, and therefore are involved in various brain functions such as learning and memory. A number of studies suggest that 5-HT$_7$ receptors could be potential pharmacotherapeutic target for cognitive disorders. Several abnormalities of serotonergic system have been described in patients with autism spectrum disorder (ASD), including abnormal activity of 5-HT transporter, altered blood and brain 5-HT levels, reduced 5-HT synthesis and altered expression of 5-HT receptors in the brain. A specific role for 5-HT$_7$ receptors in ASD has not yet been demonstrated but some evidence implicates their possible involvement. We have recently shown that 5-HT$_7$ receptor activation rescues hippocampal synaptic plasticity in a mouse model of Fragile X Syndrome, a monogenic cause of autism. Several other studies have shown that 5-HT$_7$ receptors modulate behavioral flexibility, exploratory behavior, mood disorders and epilepsy, which include core and co-morbid symptoms of ASD. These findings further suggest an involvement of 5-HT$_7$ receptors in ASD. Here, we review the physiological roles of 5-HT$_7$ receptors and their implications in Fragile X Syndrome and other ASD.

Keywords: serotonin, 5-HT$_7$ receptor, synaptic function, autism spectrum disorders, Fragile X Syndrome

INTRODUCTION

The monoamine serotonin (5-HT) is widely distributed in the central nervous system (CNS), where it functions as neurotransmitter and neuro-hormone to control mood, circadian rhythm, nociception, hormone secretion, feeding and sexual behavior (Hannon and Hoyer, 2008; Nichols and Nichols, 2008). 5-HT and its receptors are also present in peripheral tissues where they influence several functions including intestinal motility (Foxx-Orenstein et al., 1996), immune/inflammatory response (Ahern, 2011), modulation of nociception (Cervantes-Duran et al., 2013). Seven families of 5-HT receptors have been identified to date in mammals, 5-HT$_1$ through 5-HT$_7$, each including distinct receptor subtypes. 5-HT$_3$ receptors are ligand-gated ion channels mediating fast depolarization (Sugita et al., 1992). All the other 5-HT receptors are G protein-coupled metabotropic receptors: 5-HT$_1$ and 5-HT$_5$ receptors inhibit adenylate cyclase, 5-HT$_4$, 5-HT$_6$ and 5-HT$_7$ receptors instead stimulate adenylate cyclase, whereas the 5-HT$_2$ receptor family is positively linked to phospholipase C (Hannon and Hoyer, 2008; Millan et al., 2008; Pytliak et al., 2011).

5-HT$_7$ receptors were the last to be cloned in 1993 by different independent laboratories (Lovenberg et al., 1993; Monsma et al., 1993; Ruat et al., 1993) and their role was initially poorly understood. In the last decade, evidence has emerged that 5-HT$_7$ receptors play an important role in the control of body temperature, sleep/wake cycle, nociception, learning and memory (**Table 1**). 5-HT$_7$ receptors are also involved in mood disorders, epilepsy and pain and are starting to be considered as possible targets for these disorders.

The structural, pharmacological and functional features of 5-HT$_7$ receptors have been extensively illustrated in recent reviews (Matthys et al., 2011; Gellynck et al., 2013); thus, we will only briefly outline these receptor properties in the first part of the present work. A core part of our review is dedicated to the physiological functions regulated by 5-HT$_7$ receptors and particularly to 5-HT$_7$ receptor-mediated effects on cognition and mood regulation, two higher brain functions that are strictly related and mutually influence each other. Higher brain functions depend on the activity of brain neuronal networks, which are profoundly affected by changes in neuronal excitability and synaptic efficacy. For this reason, we will describe the effects of 5-HT$_7$ receptor activation on intrinsic neuronal excitability, synaptic transmission and synaptic plasticity, and will discuss the possible functional consequences of these 5-HT$_7$ receptor-mediated effects.

Table 1 | *In vivo* effects of pharmacological activation, pharmacological blockade or genetic ablation of 5-HT$_7$ receptors.

	***In vivo* effects of 5-HT$_7$ receptor manipulation**	**References**
Learning	Genetic ablation of 5-HT$_7$ receptors: impairment of fear-related learning and object location memory	Roberts et al. (2004a) and Sarkisyan and Hedlund (2009)
	Pharmacological activation of 5-HT$_7$ receptors:	
	– improvement of contextual learning	Eriksson et al. (2008, 2012)
	– improvement of instrumental learning	Perez-Garcia and Meneses (2005)
	– improvement of novelty detection	Freret et al. (2014)
	Pharmacological blockade of 5-HT$_7$ receptors: impairment of novelty detection	Ballaz et al. (2007a)
	Pharmacological blockade of 5-HT$_7$ receptors: improvement of long-term memory	Gasbarri et al. (2008)
Behavioral flexibility	Pharmacological blockade of 5-HT$_7$ receptors: improved behavioral flexibility	Nikiforuk (2012) and Nikiforuk and Popik (2013)
Exploratory activity	Pharmacological activation of 5-HT$_7$ receptors:	
	– reduced ambulatory activity	Clissold et al. (2013)
	– enhanced ambulatory activity	Adriani et al. (2012) and Ruocco et al. (2013)
Sleep/wake cycle	Genetic ablation of 5-HT$_7$ receptors: reduced REM sleep	Hedlund et al. (2005)
	Pharmacological blockade of 5-HT$_7$ receptors: reduced REM sleep	Hagan et al. (2000), Thomas et al. (2003), Bonaventure et al. (2007) and Monti et al. (2012)
	Pharmacological activation of 5-HT$_7$ receptors:	
	– reduced REM sleep	Monti et al. (2008, 2014)
	– phase-advance shift of circadian rhythm	Adriani et al. (2012)
Thermoregulation	Pharmacological activation of 5-HT$_7$ receptors: hypothermia	Hagan et al. (2000), Guscott et al. (2003) and Hedlund et al. (2003, 2010)
Nociception	Pharmacological activation of 5-HT$_7$ receptors: central antinociceptive and peripheral pro-nociceptive effects	Yanarates et al. (2010) and Viguier et al. (2012, 2013)
Mood	Genetic ablation of 5-HT$_7$ receptors: antidepressant effects	Hedlund et al. (2005) and Guscott et al. (2005)
	Pharmacological blockade of 5-HT$_7$ receptors: antidepressant effects	Hedlund et al. (2005), Wesolowska et al. (2006a) and Mnie-Filali et al. (2011)
	Non-selective 5-HT$_7$ receptor antagonists (atypical antipsychotics) behave as antidepressant in humans	Abbas et al. (2009), Guilloux et al. (2013) and Woo et al. (2013)
	Genetic ablation of 5-HT$_7$ receptors: no alteration of anxiety	Roberts et al. (2004a) and Guscott et al. (2005)
	Pharmacological blockade of 5-HT$_7$ receptors: anxiolytic effects	Wesolowska et al. (2006a,b)
Epilepsy	Pharmacological blockade of 5-HT$_7$ receptors: antiepileptic effects against:	
	– audiogenic seizures	Bourson et al. (1997)
	– absence epilepsy	Graf et al. (2004)
	– pilocarpine-induced seizures	Yang et al. (2012)
	Pharmacological activation of 5-HT$_7$ receptors: antiepileptic effect against picrotoxin-induced seizures	Pericic and Svob Strac (2007)
	Genetic ablation of 5-HT$_7$ receptors: reduced sensitivity to electrically- and chemically-induced seizures	Witkin et al. (2007)

In the last part, we will review the current literature showing an impairment of the brain serotonin system in autism spectrum disorders (ASD) and its involvement in their pathophysiology. A possible malfunction of 5-HT$_7$ receptors in ASD has not yet been investigated. In this respect, we will highlight a number of reports indicating that 5-HT$_7$ receptors regulate many physiological functions that are altered in ASD. In addition, we will provide indication from different research groups and from our laboratories that pharmacological manipulation of 5-HT$_7$ receptors might be considered as a therapeutic strategy in ASD.

CHARACTERIZATION OF 5-HT$_7$ RECEPTORS

LOCALIZATION, STRUCTURE AND PHARMACOLOGICAL PROFILE

5-HT$_7$ receptors are highly expressed in the thalamus, hypothalamus and hippocampus of mice and rats; significant amounts were detected in cerebral cortex, amygdala, striatum, cerebellum and spinal cord (Belenky and Pickard, 2001; Neumaier et al., 2001; Bickmeyer et al., 2002; Geurts et al., 2002; Muneoka and Takigawa, 2003; Doly et al., 2005; reviewed by Hedlund and Sutcliffe, 2004).

In the human brain, 5-HT$_7$ receptor mRNA was detected in many CNS areas, with highest expression levels in thalamus, hypothalamus, amygdala and hippocampus (Hagan et al., 2000). Autoradiographic studies confirmed that 5-HT_7 receptor levels in human brain are in good correlation with those found in rodents, with high density in thalamus, dorsal raphe, hippocampus (Martin-Cora and Pazos, 2004; Varnäs et al., 2004) and hypothalamus (Varnäs et al., 2004). Unlike in rodents, in the human brain 5-HT_7 receptor binding sites were also found at high levels in caudate nucleus, putamen and substantia nigra (Martin-Cora and Pazos, 2004).

In the rodent brain, the immunoreactivity for 5-HT_7 receptors was high in several regions at birth and then decreased progressively during postnatal development (Muneoka and Takigawa, 2003; García-Alcocer et al., 2006; Kobe et al., 2012). However, in spite of the reported age-related reduction in their brain expression levels, 5-HT_7 receptors exert important functions also in the adult (see Section Physiological Functions Regulated by 5-HT_7 Receptors). This conclusion is supported by several data: first of all, 5-HT_7 receptors have been detected in the brain of adult animals (Neumaier et al., 2001; Geurts et al., 2002; Muneoka and Takigawa, 2003). In the human brain, the presence of 5-HT_7 receptors was confirmed by post-mortem studies on adult subjects (age range 22–73 years; Martin-Cora and Pazos, 2004; Varnäs et al., 2004). Moreover, systemic administration of 5-HT_7 receptor agonists affected body temperature (Naumenko et al., 2011) and circadian rhythms (Adriani et al., 2012; Monti et al., 2014; Romano et al., 2014) in adult animals and improved learning in young adults (Eriksson et al., 2008; Freret et al., 2014). All these data indicate that 5-HT_7 receptor-mediated effects are still present at adult age and exert an important control on various physiological functions.

5-HT_7 receptors display the typical structure of G protein-coupled receptors (GPCRs) with seven transmembrane domains and were initially characterized for their ability to stimulate adenylate cyclase (Bard et al., 1993; Lovenberg et al., 1993; Ruat et al., 1993; Shen et al., 1993).

Among all 5-HT receptor subtypes, 5-HT_7 receptors display the highest affinity (in the low nanomolar range) for the natural agonist serotonin (Ruat et al., 1993). Other high affinity agonists for 5-HT_7 receptors are 5-carboxamidotryptamine (5-CT) and 8-hydroxy-N,N-dipropyl-aminotetralin (8-OH-DPAT), both also showing high affinity for 5-HT_{1A} receptors (Bard et al., 1993; Lovenberg et al., 1993; Ruat et al., 1993). Selective agonists for 5-HT_7 receptors were lacking until recently (Di Pilato et al., 2014). The first compound described as a 5-HT_7 receptor agonist was AS-19, a partial agonist with high affinity but moderate selectivity for 5-HT_7 receptors (Brenchat et al., 2009). The most selective 5-HT_7 receptor agonists described to date are the compounds E-55888 and E-57431 (not commercially available), produced by Esteve pharmaceutical company (Brenchat et al., 2009, 2012). Another high-affinity and selective 5-HT_7 receptor agonist is LP-211 (indicated as compound 25 in the first publication Leopoldo et al., 2008), that shows excellent brain permeation properties (Hedlund et al., 2010). *In vivo* administration of LP-211 induced hypothermia in wild-type but not in 5-HT_7 KO mice (Hedlund et al., 2010) and shifted the sleep-wake cycle (Adriani et al., 2012), two typical 5-HT_7 receptor-mediated effects. Other analogs of LP-211 with improved selectivity and pharmacokinetic properties have been synthesized (Leopoldo, personal communication) and are currently under investigation in our laboratories as possible novel 5-HT_7 receptor agonists.

Concerning antagonists, several antidepressant and antipsychotic drugs showed high affinity for 5-HT_7 receptors and behaved as antagonists on a cyclic adenosine monophosphate (cAMP) formation assay (Shen et al., 1993; Roth et al., 1994; see Section Mood Disorders). Selective and high-affinity antagonists of 5-HT_7 receptors are also available, among which the compound SB-269970 is to date considered the most reliable (Hagan et al., 2000; Guscott et al., 2003; Hedlund et al., 2003).

COUPLING TO INTRACELLULAR TRANSDUCTION MECHANISMS

5-HT_7 receptors display interesting transduction properties, being able to couple to G_s and G_{12} GTP-binding proteins, which activate divergent signaling pathways (reviewed by Woehler and Ponimaskin, 2009; Matthys et al., 2011; Gellynck et al., 2013).

Since their discovery, 5-HT_7 receptors were found to be coupled to G_s and induce adenylate cyclase activation, cAMP formation and activation of protein kinase A (PKA; Bard et al., 1993; Lovenberg et al., 1993; Ruat et al., 1993).

Downstream to cAMP formation, 5-HT_7 receptors can activate the extracellular signal-regulated kinase (ERK), as shown in transfected cells expressing 5-HT_7 receptors (Lin et al., 2003; Norum et al., 2003) and in native rat hippocampal neurons (Errico et al., 2001; Lin et al., 2003). 5-HT_7 receptor-induced activation of ERK was mediated either by PKA (Norum et al., 2003) or by a cAMP-dependent, PKA-independent pathway involving exchange proteins directly activated by cAMP (Epacs) (Lin et al., 2003). In line with this result, cAMP-dependent but PKA-independent 5-HT_7 receptor-mediated effects have been described (Chapin and Andrade, 2001; Bonsi et al., 2007).

5-HT_7 receptors can activate additional intracellular biochemical cascades, among which the kinase Akt (also known as protein kinase B; Hoffman and Mitchell, 2011; Johnson-Farley et al., 2005).

As mentioned above, 5-HT_7 receptors can also couple to G_{12} (Kvachnina et al., 2005), a heterotrimeric G protein that modulates the activity of "small" monomeric GTPases (Hall, 1998), such as members of the Rho family Rho, Rac and Cdc42. Through the G12-dependent activation of RhoA and Cdc42 5-HT_7 receptor activation regulates gene transcription and neuronal morphology (Kvachnina et al., 2005).

The mechanisms regulating 5-HT_7 receptor coupling to G_s or G_{12} are not clear. Recent evidence suggests that agonist-induced dynamic palmitoylation of 5-HT_7 receptors affects its G_s-mediated constitutive activity with no effect on G_{12}-mediated activity (Kvachnina et al., 2009; Gorinski and Ponimaskin, 2013). This result implies that pathways inducing palmitoylation of 5-HT_7 receptors might modify their constitutive activity and switch their intracellular coupling, ultimately changing their final effect.

Another interesting finding is that the expression of G_s remains constant during development, whereas the expression level of G_{12} is higher at early post natal age and parallels the expression level of 5-HT_7 receptors; consistently, 5-HT_7 receptor-mediated effects on synapse formation and function were observed in the hippocampus of juvenile but not adult mice, indicating a crucial role of the 5-HT_7/G_{12} pathway in the development of brain synaptic circuitry (Kobe et al., 2012).

A particular feature of 5-HT_7 receptors, similar to other GPCRs, is the ability to form receptor complexes, either homo- or heterodimers, in which monomers reciprocally modulate receptor trafficking, ligand binding affinity and coupling to intracellular signaling cascades (Renner et al., 2012; Teitler and Klein, 2012). For example, it has been suggested that a 5-HT_{1A}/5-HT_7 heterodimer interaction plays a modulatory role in the control of body temperature (Matthys et al., 2011). This is a further element of complexity in 5-HT receptor-mediated signal transduction mechanisms.

5-HT_7 RECEPTORS REGULATE SYNAPSE DEVELOPMENT

5-HT plays a crucial role in shaping brain structure and circuits during development through modulation of neural cell proliferation, migration and differentiation, as well as neurite outgrowth, axonal guidance and synaptogenesis (Gaspar et al., 2003). Accordingly, early changes in 5-HT brain levels during development affect the functional organization of brain networks and may underlie the pathogenesis of neurodevelopmental disorders including autism (reviewed by Lesch and Waider, 2012). While the role of some 5-HT receptors during brain development has been ascertained (Sodhi and Sanders-Bush, 2004), the involvement of 5-HT_7 receptors has only recently emerged. As mentioned above, the group of Ponimaskin demonstrated that in mouse hippocampal neurons 5-HT_7 receptor activation stimulated the small GTP-ases RhoA and Cdc42 and enhanced neurite elongation, dendritic spine density, the number of synaptic contacts and the amount of AMPA receptors expressed at synapses, leading to increased synaptic efficacy (Kvachnina et al., 2005; Kobe et al., 2012). In line with these results, it was recently shown that the 5-HT_7 receptor agonists 8-OH-DPAT and LP-211 stimulated neurite outgrowth in primary cultures of mouse and rat striatal and cortical neurons by activation of the cyclin-dependent protein kinase 5 (Cdk5), a kinase playing an important role in microtubule assembly and cytoarchitecture rearrangements (Speranza et al., 2013).

MODULATION OF NEURONAL EXCITABILITY BY 5-HT_7 RECEPTORS

5-HT_7 RECEPTOR ACTIVATION EXERTS DEPOLARIZING EFFECTS

Brain 5-HT_7 receptors modulate neuronal networks by playing a crucial role in brain wiring during development. However, as mentioned before, 5-HT_7 receptor-mediated effects are not restricted to a defined developmental window, as a large number of studies show that 5-HT_7 receptors modulate neuronal excitability, synaptic transmission and synaptic plasticity both during development and adult life. 5-HT_7 receptors control neuronal intrinsic excitability by modulating non-synaptic membrane ion currents which directly affect neuronal firing. 5-HT_7 receptor agonists exerted slow depolarizing effects and increased neuronal firing in several brain areas (**Figure 1**), among which the anterodorsal nucleus of the rat thalamus (Chapin and Andrade, 2001), rat globus pallidus (Chen et al., 2008), mouse hippocampal CA1 region (Bickmeyer et al., 2002) and mouse trigeminal nucleus caudalis (Yang et al., 2014). Activation of 5-HT_7 receptors enhanced the firing rate of rat CA1 pyramidal neurons (Tokarski et al., 2003), CA3 pyramidal neurons (Gill et al., 2002), striatal cholinergic interneurons (Bonsi et al., 2007), prefrontal cortex pyramidal neurons (Zhang, 2003; Béïque et al., 2004a) and nucleus accumbens (NAc) neurons (Ishihara et al., 2013). In a spinal cord slice preparation, 5-HT application induced a locomotor-like rhythmic firing activity of motoneurons in wild type but not in 5-HT_7 KO mice, indicating that the excitability of spinal motoneurons was enhanced by 5-HT_7 receptors (Liu et al., 2009).

In many of the studies above cited, 5-HT_7 receptor-induced depolarization was mediated by inhibition of a post-spike AHP or by enhancement of a hyperpolarization-activated inward cation current (Ih).

5-HT_7 RECEPTOR ACTIVATION INHIBITS POST-SPIKE AFTERHYPERPOLARIZATION (AHP)

Action potentials are followed by a negative shift in membrane potential named afterhyperpolarization (AHP), which is mediated by a Ca^{2+}-dependent K^+ current triggered by Ca^{2+} influx. The subsequent efflux of K^+ ions hyperpolarizes the membrane during a few seconds reducing neuronal firing rate, a phenomenon called "spike frequency adaptation" (Sah, 1996). Activation of 5-HT_7 receptors inhibited a slow AHP (sAHP) in thalamic neurons (Goaillard and Vincent, 2002), in CA3 pyramidal neurons (Bacon and Beck, 2000; Gill et al., 2002) and in CA1 pyramidal neurons (Tokarski et al., 2003; **Figure 1**). Likewise, in rat trigeminal motoneurones 5-HT_7 receptor activation reduced a Ca^{2+}-dependent K^+ current responsible for a medium-duration afterhyperpolarization (mAHP), another type of AHP with a time-course faster than the sAHP and with similar inhibitory effects on neuronal excitability (Inoue et al., 2002). Modulation of the AHP by 5-HT_7 receptors was mediated by activation of the cAMP/PKA pathway (Goaillard and Vincent, 2002; Inoue et al., 2002).

Modulation of the AHP has profound effects on neuronal firing. By inhibiting post-spike mAHP and sAHP, 5-HT_7 receptor activation enhances neuronal firing rate and reduces spike frequency adaptation. In addition, 5-HT_7 receptor-mediated modulation of sAHP is likely to involve broader functional consequences, as intrinsic excitability and synaptic inputs mutually influence each other. In fact, Ca^{2+} influx through N-methyl-D-aspartate (NMDA) channels can also activate the sAHP (Lancaster et al., 2001), which implies that synaptic activation also modulates the AHP. Changes in AHP amplitude have been observed following activation of NMDA and kainate receptors (Cherubini et al., 1990) and group I metabotropic glutamate receptors (mGluRs; Ireland and Abraham, 2002).

The AHP in turn reduces NMDA-mediated synaptic transmission: it has been proposed that activation of AHP, by hyperpolarizing the membrane, would favor Mg^{2+} blockade of NMDA channels and reduce NMDA-mediated transmission and plasticity (Wu et al., 2004; Fernández de Sevilla et al., 2007). Vice-versa, conditions reducing the AHP lead to depolarization and removal of Mg^{2+} blockade, thus are likely to enhance NMDA-mediated long term plasticity and

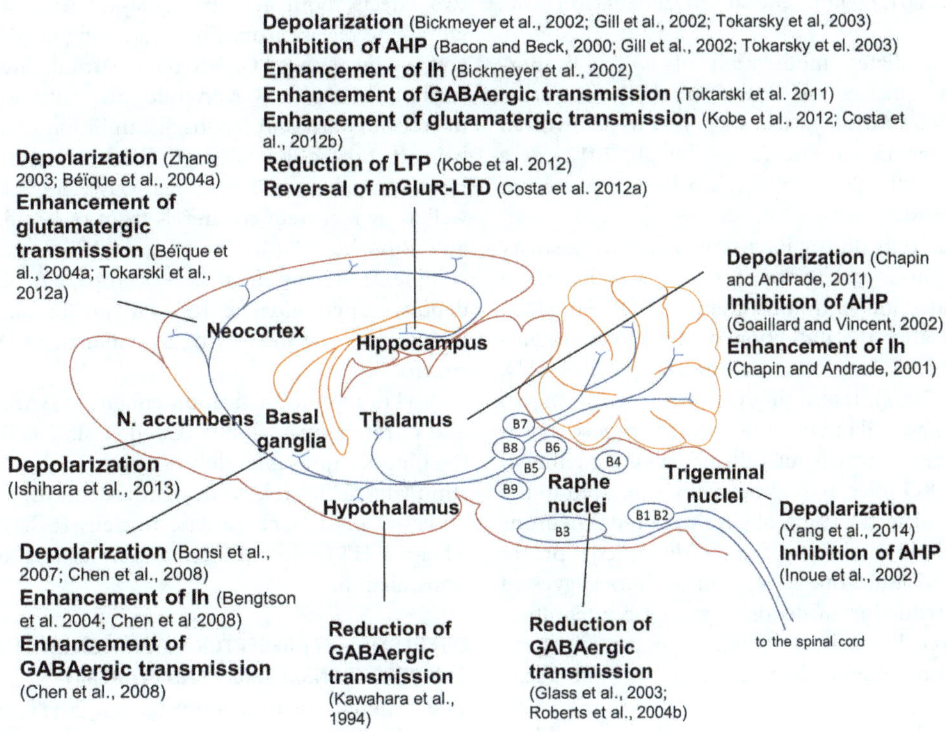

FIGURE 1 | Effects of 5-HT$_7$ receptor activation on neuronal excitability, synaptic transmission and synaptic plasticity in the rodent brain. Activation of 5-HT$_7$ receptors induced depolarization in several brain regions; in many cases, depolarization was mediated by inhibition of a post-spike afterhyperpolarization (AHP) and/or enhancement of a hyperpolatization-activated cation current (Ih; see explanations in the text). Activation of 5-HT$_7$ receptors modulated glutamate-mediated synaptic transmission and plasticity in frontal cortex and hippocampus. 5-HT$_7$ receptors differently modulated GABAergic synaptic transmission in distinct brain areas; notably, activation of 5-HT$_7$ receptors in raphe nuclei inhibited GABAergic interneurons, enhancing the activity of serotonergic raphe neurons and 5-HT release in target structures. Most of the results illustrated here were obtained in the rat, with the following exceptions: mouse (Bickmeyer et al., 2002; Costa et al., 2012a; Yang et al., 2014), hamster (Glass et al., 2003) and guinea pig (Roberts et al., 2004b).

learning. Consistent with this hypothesis, it was shown that the amplitude of AHP in hippocampal neurons was decreased after learning (Disterhoft et al., 1996; Moyer et al., 1996; Oh et al., 2009) and age-related learning deficits are accompanied by increased AHP (Disterhoft et al., 1996; Tombaugh et al., 2005).

Since 5-HT$_7$ receptor activation is able to inhibit post-spike AHP in many brain regions, as described above, the subsequent depolarization might favor NMDA receptor-mediated synaptic plasticity and ultimately enhance learning. As a matter of fact, several studies indicate that 5-HT$_7$ receptor activation exerts pro-cognitive effects (see Section Learning and Memory).

5-HT$_7$ RECEPTOR ACTIVATION ENHANCES A HYPERPOLARIZATION-ACTIVATED CATION CURRENT (I_h)

Another non-synaptic ion current modulated by 5-HT$_7$ receptors is a hyperpolarization-activated cation current (I_h). I_h is carried by Na^+ and K^+ ions and is activated by hyperpolarization beyond −60 mV, thus is already active at resting membrane potential. The voltage-dependence of I_h activation is modulated by cAMP, with increases in cAMP levels facilitating I_h activation (Chen et al., 2001). The physiological consequences of I_h activation are very complex, as it differently affects membrane excitability and synaptic responsiveness. Concerning membrane excitability, I_h shifts the value of resting membrane potential towards depolarization. With respect to synaptic responsiveness, I_h instead exerts a membrane-shunting effect that reduces the amplitude and duration of excitatory post-synaptic potentials. Thus, an enhancement of I_h, although producing a depolarizing shift in membrane potential, ultimately decreases synaptic responsiveness, as it reduces neuronal ability to elicit action potentials in response to synaptic inputs. I_h also reduces the temporal summation of synaptic signals. Notably, the channels responsible for I_h (hyperpolarization-activated cyclic nucleotide-gated non-specific cation channels, HCN) are maximally expressed in distal dendrites, where integration of synaptic signals mostly occurs (Magee, 1998, 1999); reviewed by Mozzachiodi and Byrne (2010).

It was shown that 5-HT$_7$ receptor activation enhanced I_h in dorsal root ganglion neurons (Cardenas et al., 1999), in mouse hippocampus (Bickmeyer et al., 2002), in the anterodorsal thalamic nucleus (Chapin and Andrade, 2001) and in rat globus pallidus (Bengtson et al., 2004; Chen et al., 2008; **Figure 1**). In most cases, 5-HT$_7$ receptor-mediated enhancement of I_h was mediated by an increase in cAMP levels (Cardenas et al., 1999;

Chapin and Andrade, 2001; Bickmeyer et al., 2002; Bengtson et al., 2004).

Neurotransmitter-mediated modulation of I_h has important functional consequences on neuronal rhythmic firing (McCormick and Pape, 1990). I_h is also suggested to be involved in epilepsy, since either an increase (Surges et al., 2012) or a decrease (Jung et al., 2007, 2011) of I_h have been reported in different types of epilepsy.

Changes in I_h also occur during long-term synaptic plasticity (reviewed by Mozzachiodi and Byrne, 2010). I_h was increased during NMDA-mediated long term potentiation (LTP; Fan et al., 2005) and decreased after the induction of metabotropic glutamate receptor-mediated long term depression (mGluR-LTD; Brager and Johnston, 2007). Interestingly, it was recently shown that hippocampal I_h is altered in Fmr1KO mice, the mouse model of Fragile X syndrome, in which mGluR-mediated signaling is deregulated. In Fmr1 KO mice, I_h is abnormally enhanced in the apical dendrites but not in the soma of CA1 pyramidal neurons and NMDA-mediated modulation of I_h is disrupted (Brager et al., 2012; Brager and Johnston, 2014). The authors suggested that the subsequent reduction in dendritic synaptic integration together with enhanced intrinsic excitability may participate to epilepsy, a typical feature of Fmr1KO mice as well as of Fragile X patients.

In summary, modulation of I_h by 5-HT_7 receptors is likely to have important consequences on neuronal firing and synaptic responsiveness and might account for the effects exerted by 5-HT_7 receptor activation on synaptic transmission and on epilepsy (see below).

MODULATORY ROLE OF 5-HT_7 RECEPTORS ON SYNAPTIC TRANSMISSION AND PLASTICITY

EFFECTS OF 5-HT_7 RECEPTOR ACTIVATION ON GABAERGIC SYNAPTIC TRANSMISSION

5-HT_7 receptors differently modulate the activity of GABAergic inhibitory interneurons in distinct brain areas (**Figure 1**). An early study showed that 5-HT_7 receptor activation reduced $GABA_A$ receptor-activated current in cultured rat SCN neurons acting through a post-synaptic cAMP-mediated mechanism (Kawahara et al., 1994). Also in raphe nuclei 5-HT_7 receptor activation reduced GABAergic transmission. In raphe nuclei, GABAergic interneurons exert a negative control on the activity of serotonergic neurons, inhibiting 5-HT release from raphe efferent fibers. When a 5-HT_7 receptor antagonist was applied in raphe nuclei, 5-HT efflux onto target structures was reduced (Glass et al., 2003; Roberts et al., 2004b). Thus, activation of 5-HT_7 receptors in raphe nuclei reduces GABA-mediated inhibition of raphe serotonergic neurons and consequently enhances 5-HT release in target structures.

In the hippocampus, 5-HT_7 receptor activation was instead shown to stimulate the activity of GABAergic interneurons. Application of a 5-HT_7 receptor agonist enhanced the frequency of GABA-mediated spontaneous inhibitory post-synaptic currents (sIPSCs) recorded from rat CA1 pyramidal neurons, indicating an increased GABA release from interneurons (Tokarski et al., 2011). The authors suggest that 5-HT_7 receptors exerted two effects, both at a pre-synaptic level: an enhancement of glutamate release from fibers targeting GABAergic interneurons and an increase of GABA release from interneuron terminals. In the CA1 region, GABAergic interneurons represent a system of feed-forward and feedback inhibition of pyramidal neurons, being activated by afferent fibers (among which the raphe-hippocampal serotonergic pathway), by Schaffer collaterals as well as by recurrent collaterals from pyramidal neurons (Freund and Buzsaki, 1996). Therefore, 5-HT_7 receptors exert a very complex modulation of hippocampal circuits, as they directly depolarize pyramidal neurons (Tokarski et al., 2003) and simultaneously regulate their firing by enhancing GABAergic inhibitory control.

5-HT_7 receptor activation enhanced GABAergic transmission also in rat globus pallidus (Chen et al., 2008). To summarize, in the hippocampus and globus pallidus 5-HT_7 receptor activation stimulates GABA release from interneurons, differing from results observed in suprachiasmatic nucleus (SCN) and dorsal raphe, where 5-HT_7 receptor activation instead reduces GABAergic transmission.

EFFECTS OF 5-HT_7 RECEPTOR ACTIVATION ON GLUTAMATE-MEDIATED SYNAPTIC TRANSMISSION AND PLASTICITY

Two different reports indicate that 5-HT_7 receptor activation can stimulate glutamate release from glutamatergic terminals. In rat frontal cortex, glutamate-mediated synaptic transmission was enhanced by activation of 5-HT_7 receptors (Béïque et al., 2004b) and decreased by the 5-HT_7 receptor antagonist SB-269970 (Tokarski et al., 2012a; **Figure 1**). In both studies, 5-HT_7 receptor-mediated effect was exerted at a pre-synaptic level on glutamatergic terminals.

In the hippocampus, 5-HT_7 receptors modulate glutamate-mediated transmission acting at a post-synaptic level. Field recordings of excitatory post-synaptic potentials (EPSPs) from rat hippocampal slices have shown that serotonin inhibits the perforant path input to the CA1 region, an effect partially mediated by 5-HT_7 receptors and exerted at a post-synaptic level (Otmakhova et al., 2005). The authors suggest that 5-HT_7 receptor-mediated reduction of EPSP amplitude might be due to an enhancement of the hyperpolarization-activated current I_h, similar to what observed in several brain regions (see above).

The other main input to CA1 pyramidal neurons is represented by Schaffer collaterals from CA3 pyramidal neurons. We have studied the effects of serotonin on glutamatergic transmission in the CA3-CA1 synapse in mouse and rat hippocampal slices and showed that activation of post-synaptic 5-HT_7 receptors enhances the amplitude of the AMPA receptor-mediated component of the excitatory post synaptic current ($EPSC_{AMPA}$), which is responsible for basal glutamatergic transmission (Costa et al., 2012b). In the same study, we observed instead that 5-HT_{1A} receptors inhibit AMPA-mediated CA3-CA1 synaptic transmission. These data provide a physiological substrate to the previous observation that 5-HT_7 receptor activation exerts a pro-cognitive action and is able to counteract 5-HT_{1A}-mediated impairment of learning (Eriksson et al., 2008).

In the last few years, evidence has emerged that 5-HT$_7$ receptors can also modulate long-term synaptic plasticity (**Figure 1**). As already mentioned, in mice hippocampal neurons activation of 5-HT$_7$ receptors enhanced basal synaptic transmission by increasing the number of AMPA receptors at synapses but also modulates glutamate-mediated long-term synaptic plasticity, reducing the amount of LTP in the CA3-CA1 synapse (Kobe et al., 2012). The authors suggested that 5-HT$_7$ receptor-mediated enhancement of basal glutamatergic transmission might have prevented further potentiation, thus reducing LTP (Kobe et al., 2012). In contrast with this report, mice lacking 5-HT$_7$ receptors (5-HT$_7$ KO) display decreased LTP in the CA3-CA1 hippocampal synapse (Roberts et al., 2004a), suggesting that 5-HT$_7$ receptors are necessary for LTP. LTP is induced by activation of NMDA receptors and 5-HT$_7$ receptors were shown to exert different short- and long-term effects on NMDA-mediated currents in hippocampal neurons. In particular, acute activation of 5-HT$_7$ receptors enhanced the amplitude of NMDA-mediated currents, whereas a long-term activation of 5-HT$_7$ receptors reduced the cell membrane expression of NMDA receptors through an indirect mechanism involving platelet-derived growth factor (PDGF), an endogenous neurotrophin that protects against NMDA-induced excitotoxicity (Vasefi et al., 2013). This dual action of 5-HT$_7$ receptors, namely a short-term enhancement and a long-term inhibition of NMDA receptors, might also explain different 5-HT$_7$ receptor-mediated effects on LTP.

Another form of long-term depression, mGluR-LTD, is induced by activation of group I mGluRs and is mainly expressed through removal of AMPA receptors from synaptic membrane surface by endocytosis (Luscher and Huber, 2010). We have shown that 5-HT$_7$ receptor activation prevented mGluR-induced endocytosis of AMPA receptors and reversed mGluR-LTD in the CA3-CA1 synapse in mouse hippocampal slices (Costa et al., 2012a). Interestingly, we found that 5-HT$_7$ receptor activation reversed mGluR-mediated endocytosis of AMPA receptors and mGluR-LTD also in Fmr1 KO mice, a mouse model of Fragile X Syndrome, the most common form of inherited intellectual disability associated with epilepsy and autism. Our result that 5-HT$_7$ receptor activation can correct abnormal mGluR-mediated synaptic plasticity in the mouse model of Fragile X Syndrome might suggest new strategies for the therapy of this disorder (see below).

PHYSIOLOGICAL FUNCTIONS REGULATED BY 5-HT$_7$ RECEPTORS

5-HT$_7$ receptors control several body functions including the sleep-wake cycle, body temperature and nociception, and strongly influence mood and learning, two higher brain functions that are strictly related (**Table 1**). Most of the functions regulated by 5-HT$_7$ receptors have been studied using the 5-HT$_7$ receptor knock-out (5-HT$_7$ KO) mice that were generated and characterized by the research group of Dr. Hedlund (Roberts et al., 2004a; Sarkisyan and Hedlund, 2009) and later in other laboratories (Guscott et al., 2005; Witkin et al., 2007).

SLEEP/WAKE CYCLE

Consistent with their abundant expression in the hypothalamus (see Section Localization, Structure and Pharmacological Profile), 5-HT$_7$ receptors play an important role in the regulation of circadian rhythm and sleep (Monti and Jantos, 2014). In the SCN, which is the main regulator of circadian rhythm, 5-HT$_7$ receptors are abundantly expressed (Belenky and Pickard, 2001) and regulate glutamatergic input from the retina (Smith et al., 2001) and serotonergic input from raphe nuclei (Glass et al., 2003).

The role of 5-HT$_7$ receptors in sleep has emerged from studies using both pharmacological and genetic approaches. 5-HT$_7$ KO mice displayed a reduced duration of REM sleep, whereas time spent during wake or non-REM sleep was not different from wild-type mice (Hedlund et al., 2005). Consistently, *in vivo* administration of a 5-HT$_7$ receptor antagonist to wild-type animals reduced the duration of REM sleep (Hagan et al., 2000; Thomas et al., 2003; Bonaventure et al., 2007; Monti et al., 2012). However, in contradiction with these results, systemic administration of a 5-HT$_7$ receptor agonist also enhanced the wake period and reduced the duration of REM sleep (Monti et al., 2008, 2014), together with inducing a phase-shift in the sleep-wake cycle (Adriani et al., 2012). As a possible explanation, it has been proposes that 5-HT$_7$ receptors do not behave according to the classical model of two-state on-off (activation/blockade) ligand-receptor interaction (Monti and Jantos, 2014). In addition, 5-HT$_7$ receptors differently modulate distinct brain areas (dorsal raphe, locus coeruleus, basal forebrain) involved in sleep control (Monti et al., 2012; Monti and Jantos, 2014) and their precise role in each area should be further investigated.

BODY TEMPERATURE

5-HT$_7$ receptors exert a well-established role in thermoregulation (for extensive review on this topic, see Hedlund and Sutcliffe, 2004; Matthys et al., 2011). Administration of 5-HT$_7$ receptor agonists induced hypothermia in wild type guinea pigs and mice (Hagan et al., 2000; Guscott et al., 2003; Hedlund et al., 2003, 2010) but not in 5-HT$_7$ KO mice (Guscott et al., 2003; Hedlund et al., 2003).

Two other 5-HT receptors are involved on thermoregulation, namely 5-HT$_{1A}$ and 5-HT$_3$ receptors, both also inducing hypothermic effects (Hedlund et al., 2004; Naumenko et al., 2011). It has been proposed that 5-HT$_7$ receptors, possessing the highest affinity for 5-HT, are activated by low doses of 5-HT and are responsible for the fine-tuning of body temperature. On the other hand, higher agonist concentrations activate 5-HT$_{1A}$ receptors, which might play a role as a defense against hyperthermia (Hedlund et al., 2004).

NOCICEPTION

Immunohistochemical studies provide evidence for localization of 5-HT$_7$ receptors in the superficial laminae of the dorsal horn and in small and medium sized dorsal root ganglion cells, which is consistent with a role of 5-HT$_7$ receptors in nociception (Doly et al., 2005).

The role of 5-HT$_7$ receptors in the control of pain transmission is multifaceted and has been described in details in recent reviews (Matthys et al., 2011; Viguier et al., 2013). Overall, 5-HT$_7$ receptor agonists induce pro-nociceptive effects on peripheral 5-HT$_7$ receptors and antinociceptive effects on central 5-HT$_7$ receptors (Yanarates et al., 2010; Viguier et al., 2012), with a different outcome depending on preexisting conditions (health vs. neuropathic pain; Viguier et al., 2013).

LEARNING AND MEMORY

In the last decade, an important role of 5-HT$_7$ receptors on learning and memory has emerged (Roberts and Hedlund, 2012; Meneses, 2013). As pointed out in the previous paragraphs, 5-HT$_7$ receptors are expressed at high levels in the hippocampus, one of the brain regions most crucially involved in learning, and modulate hippocampal synaptic transmission and plasticity. Behavioral studies performed on mice lacking 5-HT$_7$ receptors (Roberts et al., 2004a; Sarkisyan and Hedlund, 2009) and on wild-type animals (Manuel-Apolinar and Meneses, 2004; Perez-Garcia and Meneses, 2005; Eriksson et al., 2008, 2012) show that 5-HT$_7$ receptor activation exerts a pro-cognitive action on different types of memory.

5-HT$_7$ KO mice showed no memory impairment in operant food conditioning tests (involving a hippocampus-independent type of memory) and Barnes maze (involving hippocampus-dependent spatial learning) but displayed a memory deficit in the fear conditioning test, which involves hippocampus-dependent contextual learning with emotional aspects. These results indicate that the lack of 5-HT$_7$ receptors did not affect hippocampus-independent memory and among different types of hippocampus-dependent learning, only one with a strong emotional component (fear conditioning) was selectively impaired in 5-HT$_7$ KO mice. The specific contextual learning impairment of 5-HT$_7$ KO mice was accompanied by a decrease of LTP in the CA1 region of the hippocampus (Roberts et al., 2004a).

Further studies from the same laboratory indicated that 5-HT$_7$ KO mice displayed normal recognition of novel objects (Sarkisyan and Hedlund, 2009), a type of visual episodic memory that depends on brain cortex and is believed to correspond to human declarative episodic memory. 5-HT$_7$ KO mice instead showed a selective impairment in the recognition of a novel location, particularly in allocentric spatial memory (a hippocampus-dependent type of memory concerning the location of objects independent from the observer), without any defect in egocentric memory (a striatum-dependent type of memory concerning the position of objects with respect to the observer). The same result was observed in wild-type mice following pharmacological blockade of 5-HT$_7$ receptors (Sarkisyan and Hedlund, 2009).

Behavioral studies on wild-type animals confirmed that activation of 5-HT$_7$ receptors exerts a pro-cognitive effect on hippocampus-dependent contextual learning and revealed that other types of memory are also modulated by 5-HT$_7$ receptors. In mice submitted to the passive avoidance test (involving contextual learning), *in vivo* activation of 5-HT$_7$ receptors was able to exert pro-cognitive effects and counteract a learning impairment induced by 5-HT$_{1A}$ receptor activation (Eriksson et al., 2008, 2012).

5-HT$_7$ receptor stimulation enhanced memory formation in adult rats trained to a learning task involving both conditioning (Pavlonian) and instrumental learning modes: in this experimental protocol, a food reward was delivered with a short delay following a light signal (conditioned learning) but was delivered immediately if the rat pressed a lever (instrumental learning). When the 5-HT$_7$ receptor agonist AS-19 was injected subcutaneously to animals immediately after training, the latency of responses was reduced, indicating enhanced memory performance. AS-19 administration was also able to reverse a memory impairment induced by scopolamine (an anticholinergic agent) or dizocilpine (an NMDA antagonist), suggesting that 5-HT$_7$ receptor activation might exert a pro-cognitive effect by modulating cholinergic and glutamatergic transmission (Perez-Garcia and Meneses, 2005).

Concerning hippocampus-independent memory, different from results on 5-HT$_7$ KO mice (Sarkisyan and Hedlund, 2009), in wild-type mice novel object recognition was enhanced by administration of the 5-HT$_7$ receptor agonist 5-CT and impaired by administration of the 5-HT$_7$ receptor antagonist SB-269970 (Freret et al., 2014), consistent with previous data showing that administration of SB-269970 impaired novel object recognition in wild-type rats (Ballaz et al., 2007a). These data show that 5-HT$_7$ receptor activation exert a pro-cognitive effect also on cortex-dependent memory corresponding to human episodic memory.

To summarize, studies on wild-type animals using 5-HT$_7$ receptor agonists and antagonists have shown that 5-HT$_7$ receptor activation enhances many different types of memory, including some (operant conditioning, novel object recognition) that were not impaired in 5-HT$_7$ KO mice.

5-HT$_7$ receptor-mediated pro-cognitive effects were observed in behavioral tests performed on adult animals, reinforcing the conclusion that 5-HT$_7$ receptors are functional in the adult hippocampus and exert life-long effects on learning and memory.

In one study, blockade rather than activation of 5-HT$_7$ receptors exerted a pro-cognitive effect: *in vivo* administration of the 5-HT$_7$ receptor antagonist SB-269970 to rats submitted to the radial arm maze enhanced long-term reference memory without affecting short-term working memory (Gasbarri et al., 2008).

Heterogeneous results are not surprising considering that different models have been used (either rats or mice; wild-type or 5-HT$_7$ KO animals) and different types of memory were tested, involving different brain areas and distinct circuits. Furthermore, considering that learning and memory are strictly related to stress, 5-HT$_7$ receptor-mediated effects on learning might also be influenced by 5-HT$_7$ receptor-mediated effects on mood (see below).

INVOLVEMENT OF 5-HT$_7$ RECEPTORS IN PATHOLOGY

MOOD DISORDERS

Since the first pharmacological characterization of 5-HT$_7$ receptors, it was evident that several antipsychotics and antidepressants bind these receptors with high affinity (Monsma et al., 1993; Roth et al., 1994). In line with these early results, several studies have later shown that 5-HT$_7$ receptors play a role in mood regulation and thus are potential targets for the therapy of anxiety and depression (Hedlund, 2009; Sarkisyan et al., 2010).

Mice lacking 5-HT$_7$ receptors displayed reduced levels of depression when submitted to forced swimming and tail suspension tests (Guscott et al., 2005; Hedlund et al., 2005). Consistently, pharmacological blockade of 5-HT$_7$ receptors exerted antidepressant effects in wild-type mice and rats submitted to the same stress protocols (Hedlund et al., 2005; Wesolowska et al., 2006a; Mnie-Filali et al., 2011). In addition, 5-HT$_7$ receptor blockade was found to potentiate the effect of other antidepressant drugs: synergistic antidepressant effects were observed when a low and ineffective dose of SB-269970 was administered in combination with a low and ineffective dose of citalopram, a selective serotonin reuptake inhibitor (SSRI; Sarkisyan et al., 2010). In the same study, a synergistic interaction, although to a lesser extent, was also observed between SB-269970 and reuptake inhibitors of norepinephrine (but not dopamine).

With respect to anxiety, 5-HT$_7$ KO mice did not show any alteration in anxiety-related behavior, evaluated by light-dark transfer test (Roberts et al., 2004a) and elevated plus maze (Guscott et al., 2005). On the other side, in wild-type rodents tested in different anxiety protocols (Vogel conflict drinking test; elevated plus maze; four-plate test; open field), administration of the 5-HT$_7$ receptor antagonist SB-269970 induced anxiolytic effects (Wesolowska et al., 2006a,b).

Interestingly, anxiolytic and antidepressant effects were observed also when SB-269970 was administered by local intra-hippocampal injection, indicating the involvement of 5-HT$_7$ receptors located in the hippocampus (Wesolowska et al., 2006a).

It was recently found that second-generation antipsychotic drugs, named atypical antipsychotics, also behave as antagonists of 5-HT$_7$ receptors. Among these substances, the D2/D3 receptor antagonist amisulpride is a high-affinity competitive antagonist of 5-HT$_7$ receptors. Interestingly, the antidepressant effect of amisulpride was absent in 5-HT$_7$ KO mice, indicating that it was mediated exclusively by inhibition of 5-HT$_7$ receptors (Abbas et al., 2009). Lurasidone, another atypical antipsychotic behaving as an antagonist at dopamine D2, 5-HT$_2$, and 5-HT$_7$ receptors (Ishibashi et al., 2010), was shown to exert significant antidepressant effects in patients with bipolar 1 disorder (Woo et al., 2013). Another atypical antipsychotic is vortioxetine, also named Lu AA21004, a multimodal compound that behaves as an antagonist at 5-HT$_3$ and 5-HT$_7$ receptors, a partial agonist at 5-HT$_{1B}$, a full agonist at 5-HT$_{1A}$ receptors and an inhibitor of the serotonin transporter (Guilloux et al., 2013). Vortioxetine proved effective as antidepressant in several clinical studies and was recently approved by the U.S. Food and Drug Administration (FDA) for the treatment of major depressive disorder (Citrome, 2014), confirming that an enhancement of serotonergic transmission associated with 5-HT$_7$ receptor antagonism exerts synergistic antidepressant effects.

These data together indicate that 5-HT$_7$ receptors regulate the balance between anxiety and depression. Mood regulation has crucial consequences on cognition, as stress can improve or impair learning depending on the duration and intensity of stressful conditions. Acute stress enhances learning, particularly when experienced in the same context of learning acquisition (Joëls et al., 2006; Bangasser and Shors, 2010). As underlined above, 5-HT$_7$ receptor activation improves fear-related learning, in which an acute stressor is presented during the paradigms of fear conditioning and passive avoidance (Roberts et al., 2004a; Eriksson et al., 2008). Therefore, an enhancement of anxiety levels by 5-HT$_7$ receptor activation during a stress condition might contribute to 5-HT$_7$ receptor-mediated improvement of stress-related learning.

EPILEPSY

In view of the depolarizing effects exerted by 5-HT$_7$ receptors (see above), their activation is likely to enhance seizure sensitivity. In line with this, a pharmacological study using different mixed antagonists suggested that blockade of 5-HT$_7$ receptors may protect against audiogenic seizures in DBA/2J mice (Bourson et al., 1997). Pharmacological blockade using selective 5-HT$_7$ receptor antagonists decreased cortical epileptic activity in a rat genetic model of absence epilepsy (Graf et al., 2004) and in a pilocarpine-induced rat model of temporal lobe epilepsy (Yang et al., 2012).

In contrast, 5-HT$_7$ receptor activation was instead suggested to exert anticonvulsant effects in other experimental models of epilepsy. Systemic administration of the 5-HT$_7$ receptor agonist 5-CT reduced picrotoxin-induced seizures in mice, an effect abolished by a selective 5-HT$_7$ receptor antagonist (Pericic and Svob Strac, 2007). Consistently, mice lacking 5-HT$_7$ receptors display enhanced sensitivity to electrically and chemically-induced seizures (Witkin et al., 2007).

Thus, 5-HT$_7$ receptor-mediated effects on epilepsy are heterogeneous and apparently controversial, probably due to differences in the models used. Systemic administration of 5-HT$_7$ receptor ligands exerts a complex modulation of the brain serotonin system because, besides directly acting on 5-HT$_7$ receptors on target cells, they also modulate the activity of GABAergic interneurons. As pointed out in the previous paragraphs, in raphe nuclei 5-HT$_7$ receptor activation inhibits GABAergic interneurons targeting serotonergic neurons and subsequently enhance 5-HT release in other brain areas. In the hippocampus, GABAergic interneurons are instead stimulated by 5-HT$_7$ receptor activation. Therefore, the understanding of systemic effects exerted by 5-HT$_7$ receptor ligands is complicated by 5-HT$_7$ receptor-mediated modulation of GABAergic interneurons in distinct brain areas.

Concerning systemic administration of 5-HT$_7$ receptor agonists, it should also be considered that 5-HT$_7$ receptors undergo desensitization following prolonged activation (Shimizu et al., 1998). Desensitization of 5-HT$_7$ receptors was also observed after antagonist treatment (Tokarski et al., 2012b). Thus, systemic treatments of animals should be carefully designed to minimize 5-HT$_7$ receptor desensitization; in this respect, a preferential use of agonists with a short half-life, such as LP-211 and related compounds (Hedlund et al., 2010) might be considered preferentially.

THE SEROTONIN HYPOTHESIS OF AUTISM

A large body of evidence has led to the serotonin hypothesis of autism, which points out a deficiency in the brain serotonin system as a causal mechanism in ASD (Whitaker-Azmitia, 2005; Harrington et al., 2013). Early experimental data (Schain and Freedman, 1961), later confirmed by many research groups (Anderson et al., 1990; Piven et al., 1991; McBride et al., 1998; Mulder et al., 2004), have documented an increase of serotonin levels in blood platelets (hyperserotonemia) in one third of autistic patients. Conversely, a decreased uptake of tryptophan (the precursor of 5-HT) and a reduced 5-HT synthesis were detected in the brain of autistic children by positron emission tomography (PET) using the radioligand tracer alpha-methyl-tryptophan (Chugani et al., 1997, 1999; Chandana et al., 2005). These studies have evidenced that global brain 5-HT synthesis was reduced in autistic patients in an age-dependent manner, with local differences in cortical regions. The localization of 5-HT defect was related to the severity of language problems, as children with the most severe language delay displayed the lowest amount of tryptophan uptake in the left cortex. Overall, in very young autistic children (2–5 years old) the rate of 5-HT synthesis in frontal, temporal and parietal cortex was significantly lower with respect to healthy children of the same age and was gradually increased only later in development (5–14 years old). The authors suggested that a high brain serotonin synthesis normally occurring during early childhood is disrupted in autism (Chugani et al., 1999).

A lack of 5-HT during early stages of development is likely to disrupt the wiring architecture of the brain. Consistently, post mortem observation of brains from young autistic patients showed an abnormal morphology of serotonergic fibers directed to the amygdala and temporal cortex and an increased density of the serotonin transporter (named either 5-HTT or SERT) on these fibers (Azmitia et al., 2011).

The 5-HTT is responsible for 5-HT uptake in CNS serotonergic nerve terminals, reducing the amount of 5-HT in the synaptic cleft. The 5-HTT is also located on blood platelets and up-regulation of 5-HTT activity participates to their increased uptake of serotonin, leading to hyperserotonemia (Marazziti et al., 2000). The gene coding for the 5-HTT, named SLC6A4, exists in various alleles related to different degrees of 5-HTT expression and/or activity. Polymorphism of the SLC6A4 gene has been correlated with autism, although results from different groups are heterogeneous with respect to the polymorphic sites involved and the type of allele associated with autism (Devlin et al., 2005; Cho et al., 2007; Coutinho et al., 2007; Wassink et al., 2007; Cross et al., 2008); however, others did not find any significant association (Ramoz et al., 2006). A SLC6A4 variant coding for an overactive form of 5-HTT has been identified in families of autistic patients (Sutcliffe et al., 2005). Mutant mice expressing this high functioning 5-HTT variant show hyperserotonemia, hypersensitivity of 5-HT receptors (as a result of reduced serotonergic transmission) and autistic behavior (Veenstra-VanderWeele et al., 2012).

Alterations in brain 5-HT receptor density were found in autistic patients. A reduction of 5-HT_{2A} binding sites in the cingulate, frontal, and temporal cortex was detected in adults with Asperger syndrome by single photon emission computed tomography (SPECT; Murphy et al., 2006), although a later PET study found contrasting results (Girgis et al., 2011). A reduced density of 5-HT_{1A} and 5-HT_2 receptors in posterior cingulate cortex and fusiform cortex, brain regions involved in social and emotional behaviors, was observed in post-mortem brain tissue from young adults diagnosed with autism other than Asperger syndrome (Oblak et al., 2013).

To summarize, a large number of clinical studies indicate abnormal synthesis and increased uptake of 5-HT, morphological alteration of serotonergic fibers and reduced expression of 5-HT receptors in the brain of ASD patients. Consistently, neonatal mice depleted of forebrain serotonin by neurotoxin injection at birth (Boylan et al., 2007) and mice genetically depleted of serotonin (Kane et al., 2012) show a delay in development and typical autistic features, and have been proposed as animal models of ASD. Other animal models of ASD were instead generated by manipulations inducing pre-natal hyperserotonemia and postnatal loss of brain 5-HT, such as fetal exposure to sodium valproate (Dufour-Rainfray et al., 2011) or to 5-methoxytryptamine (5-MT), a non-selective agonist of all metabotropic 5-HT receptor types (McNamara et al., 2008). According to a developmental theory of autism, prenatal hyperserotonemia causes increased 5-HT levels in the fetal brain, as the immature blood-brain barrier is permeable to 5-HT; this in turn would cause a loss of serotonergic fibers as a negative feedback mechanism (Whitaker-Azmitia, 2005; McNamara et al., 2008). Thus, prenatal hyperserotonemia would ultimately reduce the function of the brain serotonin system and lead to consequences similar to post-natal serotonin depletion.

Animal studies have confirmed the involvement of 5-HT in ASD and provided some indication about the 5-HT-dependent mechanisms disrupted in ASD. In 5-HTT knockout animals, the lack of 5-HTT during early development altered the connectivity between raphe nuclei and prefrontal cortex (Witteveen et al., 2013), as well as cortical cell density and layer thickness (Altamura et al., 2007; Witteveen et al., 2013). Also neonatal 5-HT depletion in mouse forebrain caused a disruption in neocortical architecture, namely an increase of cortical thickness (Boylan et al., 2007) resembling the increased cortical volume observed in autistic patients (Carper and Courchesne, 2005).

In a hyperserotonemia rat model of autism, a reduced number of oxytocin neurons was detected in the hypothalamic paraventricular nucleus (PVN; McNamara et al., 2008). The PVN projects oxytocin-containing fibers to the NAc, where presynaptic oxytocin receptors stimulate 5-HT release from serotonergic nerve terminals arising from dorsal raphe. Thus, a reduced activity of this pathway might have important implication in the pathophysiology of autistic behavior. As a matter of fact, a recent study shows that 5-HT and oxytocin cooperate in the NAc and their combined activity is crucially involved in social reward, a mechanism disrupted in autism (Dölen et al., 2013).

5-HT_7 RECEPTORS AS A POSSIBLE NOVEL THERAPEUTIC TARGET IN AUTISM SPECTRUM DISORDERS

Little is known about a possible malfunction of 5-HT_7 receptors in ASD. A single base polymorphism was detected in the gene coding for the 5-HT_7 receptor, giving rise to two different alleles; however, analysis of transmission disequilibrium in autistic patients did not evidence any correlation of either allele to autism (Lassig et al., 1999). The expression level of 5-HT$_7$ receptors in the brain of autistic patients has not been specifically investigated and no information is presently available about the functional properties of 5-HT$_7$ receptors in animal models of autism.

Although a dysfunction of 5-HT$_7$ receptors has not been causally linked to ASD, we propose that 5-HT$_7$ receptor ligands might be considered as valuable pharmacological tools in ASD. This suggestion is mainly based on our findings but is also supported by other studies addressing the role of 5-HT$_7$ receptors in behavioral flexibility and repetitive behavior, as discussed below. We have shown that 5-HT$_7$ receptor activation reverses mGluR-LTD in Fmr1KO mice (Costa et al., 2012a), a model of Fragile X Syndrome also considered as an animal model of autism (Bernardet and Crusio, 2006; Pietropaolo et al., 2011). This result might open new perspectives for therapy if pharmacological activation of 5-HT$_7$ receptors, besides correcting the most prominent synaptic defect in the mouse model of FXS, is also able to rescue the symptoms of FXS such as learning deficits, epilepsy and autistic behavior.

A typical feature of ASD is a reduced behavioral flexibility, i.e., a reduced ability to replace a previously acquired rule with a new one, in adaptation to a new environmental context. Behavioral flexibility depends on brain circuits involving pre-frontal cortex (Floresco et al., 2009; Wolfensteller and Ruge, 2012; Logue and Gould, 2014) and can be evaluated in animals as well as in humans using an attentional set-shifting task (Birrell and Brown, 2000; Colacicco et al., 2002). In this test, rodents are trained to discriminate between different stimuli (odor, surface texture, digging medium) as a cue to obtain a reward. After a training period, the rules are changed and animals must learn that a previously relevant cue has become irrelevant and vice-versa. Using attentional set-shifting protocols, recent studies have shown an involvement of 5-HT$_7$ receptors in behavioral flexibility, especially in conditions of stress (Nikiforuk, 2012; Nikiforuk and Popik, 2013). Rats exposed to restraint stress showed reduced behavioral flexibility; administration of amisulpride, an atypical antipsychotic drug and a 5-HT$_7$ receptor antagonist, reversed the restraint-induced cognitive inflexibility and also improved attention in unstressed animals. Administration of the 5-HT$_7$ receptor agonist AS-19 abolished the pro-cognitive effect of amisulpride. The same authors have shown that behavioral inflexibility induced by another protocol (ketamine administration) was reduced by amisulpride and by the 5-HT$_7$ receptor antagonist SB-269970 (Nikiforuk et al., 2013). These results suggest that a lack of behavioral flexibility is associated with increased activation of 5-HT$_7$ receptors. In this respect, antagonists rather than agonist of 5-HT$_7$ receptors might be beneficial to correct the reduced behavioral flexibility observed in ASD. However, further studies are necessary to test the effects of 5-HT$_7$ receptor agonists and antagonist on cognitive flexibility in different pathological conditions. In particular, it would be useful to study the relation between altered synaptic plasticity and behavioral flexibility in different models of intellectual disability and autism. For example, the Fmr1 KO mouse model of Fragile X Syndrome exhibit an abnormally enhanced mGluR-LTD (Huber et al., 2002) and show autistic features and reduced behavioral flexibility (Casten et al., 2011). On the other side, mGluR-LTD is abnormally reduced in other mouse models of syndromic and non syndromic forms of autism, which also show reduced behavioral flexibility. We are currently studying if systemic administration of a 5-HT$_7$ receptor agonist can rescue learning deficits and altered behavior in Fmr1 KO mice. Our hypothesis is that 5-HT$_7$ receptor activation, although reducing behavioral flexibility in wild-type animals (Nikiforuk, 2012; Nikiforuk and Popik, 2013), might restore behavior and thus be beneficial in Fragile X syndrome, a condition in which mGluR-LTD is exaggerated.

Repetitive and stereotypic behavior is considered a core symptom of ASD. A behavioral study has shown that the stereotypical behavior of marble burying, an experimental protocol used to evaluate anxiety and obsessive-compulsive behavior, was reduced in 5-HT$_7$ KO mice and in wild-type mice following pharmacological blockade of 5-HT$_7$ receptors (Hedlund and Sutcliffe, 2007). The authors suggest that this result might also be due to the anxiolytic effect of 5-HT$_7$ receptor blockade (Hedlund, 2009).

Co-morbid symptoms of ASD, observed only in a fraction of patients, include sleep disorders, anxiety, depression, epilepsy, attention deficit and hyperactivity disorder (Spooren et al., 2012). As pointed out in the previous paragraphs, 5-HT$_7$ receptors are crucially involved in the regulation of the sleep/wake cycle, exert either pro- or anti-convulsant effects in different models of epilepsy and play an important role in mood control (reviewed by Bagdy et al., 2007; Matthys et al., 2011). Since 5-HT$_7$ receptor inactivation or blockade exert anxiolytic effects (see above), 5-HT$_7$ receptor activation is likely to enhance the level of anxiety, thus might be expected to reduce hyperactivity. In line with this hypothesis, in highly active rats showing explorative behavior and low levels of anxiety, the expression level of 5-HT$_7$ receptors in the thalamus and in the hippocampus was significantly lower than in low-activity rats (Ballaz et al., 2007b). Accordingly, another study shows that microinjections of the 5-HT$_7$ receptor agonist AS-19 into the NAc decreased ambulatory activity in the rat (Clissold et al., 2013).

Other publications instead show that systemic administration of the 5-HT$_7$ receptor agonist LP-211 enhanced locomotion in wild-type mice (Adriani et al., 2012) and exerted anxiolytic effects, enhancing the exploratory attitude, in a rat model of hyperactivity and attention deficit (Ruocco et al., 2013). Therefore, it would be interesting to further investigate the role of 5-HT$_7$ receptors on different types of anxiety-related behaviors.

CONCLUDING REMARKS

Central 5-HT$_7$ receptors modulate neuronal excitability and synaptic function and are important physiological modulators of learning and mood. Based on these properties, 5-HT$_7$ receptors have been proposed as a pharmacological target in cognitive impairment, depression and epilepsy.

Core and co-morbid symptoms of ASD involve a disruption of several functions, some of which are physiologically regulated by 5-HT$_7$ receptors. In light of this, it would be interesting to investigate the role of 5-HT$_7$ receptors on different features disrupted in ASD. Cognitive functions are likely to be enhanced by

5-HT$_7$ receptor agonists; on the other side, behavioral flexibility, hyperactivity and epilepsy might benefit from blockade of 5-HT$_7$ receptors. In many cases, predictions of a possible outcome by pharmacological manipulation of 5-HT$_7$ receptors are complicated by heterogeneous data present in literature and a direct investigation would be necessary.

ACKNOWLEDGMENTS

We wish to thank Dr. Derek Bowie (McGill University, Montreal, QC, Canada) for critical reading of the manuscript. The present work was financed by FRAXA Research Foundation (call 2013) and Telethon Foundation (grant GGP13145). Part of images from Motifolio drawing toolkit[1] were utilized in the figure preparation.

REFERENCES

Abbas, A. I., Hedlund, P. B., Huang, X. P., Tran, T. B., Meltzer, H. Y., and Roth, B. L. (2009). Amisulpride is a potent 5-HT$_7$ antagonist: relevance for antidepressant actions in vivo. *Psychopharmacology (Berl)* 205, 119–128. doi: 10.1007/s00213-009-1521-8

Adriani, W., Travaglini, D., Lacivita, E., Saso, L., Leopoldo, M., and Laviola, G. (2012). Modulatory effects of two novel agonists for serotonin receptor 7 on emotion, motivation and circadian rhythm profiles in mice. *Neuropharmacology* 62, 833–842. doi: 10.1016/j.neuropharm.2011.09.012

Ahern, G. P. (2011). 5-HT and the immune system. *Curr. Opin. Pharmacol.* 11, 29–33. doi: 10.1016/j.coph.2011.02.004

Altamura, C., Dell'Acqua, M. L., Moessner, R., Murphy, D. L., Lesch, K. P., and Persico, A. M. (2007). Altered neocortical cell density and layer thickness in serotonin transporter knockout mice: a quantitation study. *Cereb. Cortex* 17, 1394–1401. doi: 10.1093/cercor/bhl051

Anderson, G. M., Horne, W. C., Chatterjee, D., and Cohen, D. J. (1990). The hyperserotonemia of autism. *Ann. N Y Acad. Sci.* 600, 331–340; discussion 341–332. doi: 10.1111/j.1749-6632.1990.tb16893.x

Azmitia, E. C., Singh, J. S., and Whitaker-Azmitia, P. M. (2011). Increased serotonin axons (immunoreactive to 5-HT transporter) in postmortem brains from young autism donors. *Neuropharmacology* 60, 1347–1354. doi: 10.1016/j.neuropharm.2011.02.002

Bacon, W. L., and Beck, S. G. (2000). 5-Hydroxytryptamine$_7$ receptor activation decreases slow afterhyperpolarization amplitude in CA3 hippocampal pyramidal cells. *J. Pharmacol. Exp. Ther.* 294, 672–679.

Bagdy, G., Kecskemeti, V., Riba, P., and Jakus, R. (2007). Serotonin and epilepsy. *J. Neurochem.* 100, 857–873. doi: 10.1111/j.1471-4159.2006.04277.x

Ballaz, S. J., Akil, H., and Watson, S. J. (2007a). The 5-HT$_7$ receptor: role in novel object discrimination and relation to novelty-seeking behavior. *Neuroscience* 149, 192–202. doi: 10.1016/j.neuroscience.2007.07.043

Ballaz, S. J., Akil, H., and Watson, S. J. (2007b). Analysis of 5-HT$_6$ and 5-HT$_7$ receptor gene expression in rats showing differences in novelty-seeking behavior. *Neuroscience* 147, 428–438. doi: 10.1016/j.neuroscience.2007.04.024

Bangasser, D. A., and Shors, T. J. (2010). Critical brain circuits at the intersection between stress and learning. *Neurosci. Biobehav. Rev.* 34, 1223–1233. doi: 10.1016/j.neubiorev.2010.02.002

Bard, J. A., Zgombick, J., Adham, N., Vaysse, P., Branchek, T. A., and Weinshank, R. L. (1993). Cloning of a novel human serotonin receptor (5-HT$_7$) positively linked to adenylate cyclase. *J. Biol. Chem.* 268, 23422–23426.

Béïque, J. C., Campbell, B., Perring, P., Hamblin, M. W., Walker, P., Mladenovic, L., et al. (2004a). Serotonergic regulation of membrane potential in developing rat prefrontal cortex: coordinated expression of 5-hydroxytryptamine (5-HT)1A, 5-HT$_{2A}$ and 5-HT$_7$ receptors. *J. Neurosci.* 24, 4807–4817. doi: 10.1523/JNEUROSCI.5113-03.2004

Béïque, J. C., Chapin-Penick, E. M., Mladenovic, L., and Andrade, R. (2004b). Serotonergic facilitation of synaptic activity in the developing rat prefrontal cortex. *J. Physiol.* 556, 739–754. doi: 10.1113/jphysiol.2003.051284

Belenky, M. A., and Pickard, G. E. (2001). Subcellular distribution of 5-HT(1B) and 5-HT$_7$ receptors in the mouse suprachiasmatic nucleus. *J. Comp. Neurol.* 432, 371–388. doi: 10.1002/cne.1109

[1]www.motifolio.com

Bengtson, C. P., Lee, D. J., and Osborne, P. B. (2004). Opposing electrophysiological actions of 5-HT on noncholinergic and cholinergic neurons in the rat ventral pallidum in vitro. *J. Neurophysiol.* 92, 433–443. doi: 10.1152/jn.00543.2003

Bernardet, M., and Crusio, W. E. (2006). Fmr1 KO mice as a possible model of autistic features. *ScientificWorldJournal* 6, 1164–1176. doi: 10.1100/tsw.2006.220

Bickmeyer, U., Heine, M., Manzke, T., and Richter, D. W. (2002). Differential modulation of I(h) by 5-HT receptors in mouse CA1 hippocampal neurons. *Eur. J. Neurosci.* 16, 209–218. doi: 10.1046/j.1460-9568.2002.02072.x

Birrell, J. M., and Brown, V. J. (2000). Medial frontal cortex mediates perceptual attentional set shifting in the rat. *J. Neurosci.* 20, 4320–4324.

Bonaventure, P., Kelly, L., Aluisio, L., Shelton, J., Lord, B., Galici, R., et al. (2007). Selective blockade of 5-hydroxytryptamine (5-HT)$_7$ receptors enhances 5-HT transmission, antidepressant-like behavior and rapid eye movement sleep suppression induced by citalopram in rodents. *J. Pharmacol. Exp. Ther.* 321, 690–698. doi: 10.1124/jpet.107.119404

Bonsi, P., Cuomo, D., Ding, J., Sciamanna, G., Ulrich, S., Tscherter, A., et al. (2007). Endogenous serotonin excites striatal cholinergic interneurons via the activation of 5-HT2C, 5-HT$_6$ and 5-HT$_7$ serotonin receptors: implications for extrapyramidal side effects of serotonin reuptake inhibitors. *Neuropsychopharmacology* 32, 1840–1854. doi: 10.1038/sj.npp.1301294

Bourson, A., Kapps, V., Zwingelstein, C., Rudler, A., Boess, F. G., and Sleight, A. J. (1997). Correlation between 5-HT$_7$ receptor affinity and protection against sound-induced seizures in DBA/2J mice. *Naunyn Schmiedebergs Arch. Pharmacol.* 356, 820–826. doi: 10.1007/PL00005123

Boylan, C. B., Blue, M. E., and Hohmann, C. F. (2007). Modeling early cortical serotonergic deficits in autism. *Behav. Brain Res.* 176, 94–108. doi: 10.1016/j.bbr.2006.08.026

Brager, D. H., Akhavan, A. R., and Johnston, D. (2012). Impaired dendritic expression and plasticity of h-channels in the fmr1(-/y) mouse model of fragile X syndrome. *Cell Rep.* 1, 225–233. doi: 10.1016/j.celrep.2012.02.002

Brager, D. H., and Johnston, D. (2007). Plasticity of intrinsic excitability during long-term depression is mediated through mGluR-dependent changes in I_h in hippocampal CA1 pyramidal neurons. *J. Neurosci.* 27, 13926–13937. doi: 10.1523/JNEUROSCI.3520-07.2007

Brager, D. H., and Johnston, D. (2014). Channelopathies and dendritic dysfunction in fragile X syndrome. *Brain Res. Bull.* 103, 11–17. doi: 10.1016/j.brainresbull.2014.01.002

Brenchat, A., Rocasalbas, M., Zamanillo, D., Hamon, M., Vela, J. M., and Romero, L. (2012). Assessment of 5-HT$_7$ receptor agonists selectivity using nociceptive and thermoregulation tests in knockout versus wild-type mice. *Adv. Pharmacol. Sci.* 2012:312041. doi: 10.1155/2012/312041

Brenchat, A., Romero, L., Garcia, M., Pujol, M., Burgueno, J., Torrens, A., et al. (2009). 5-HT$_7$ receptor activation inhibits mechanical hypersensitivity secondary to capsaicin sensitization in mice. *Pain* 141, 239–247. doi: 10.1016/j.pain.2008.11.009

Cardenas, C. G., Mar, L. P., Vysokanov, A. V., Arnold, P. B., Cardenas, L. M., Surmeier, D. J., et al. (1999). Serotonergic modulation of hyperpolarization-activated current in acutely isolated rat dorsal root ganglion neurons. *J. Physiol.* 518(Pt. 2), 507–523. doi: 10.1111/j.1469-7793.1999.0507p.x

Carper, R. A., and Courchesne, E. (2005). Localized enlargement of the frontal cortex in early autism. *Biol. Psychiatry* 57, 126–133. doi: 10.1016/j.biopsych.2004.11.005

Casten, K. S., Gray, A. C., and Burwell, R. D. (2011). Discrimination learning and attentional set formation in a mouse model of fragile X. *Behav. Neurosci.* 125, 473–479. doi: 10.1037/a0023561

Cervantes-Duran, C., Rocha-Gonzalez, H. I., and Granados-Soto, V. (2013). Peripheral and spinal 5-HT receptors participate in the pronociceptive and antinociceptive effects of fluoxetine in rats. *Neuroscience* 252, 396–409. doi: 10.1016/j.neuroscience.2013.08.022

Chandana, S. R., Behen, M. E., Juhasz, C., Muzik, O., Rothermel, R. D., Mangner, T. J., et al. (2005). Significance of abnormalities in developmental trajectory and asymmetry of cortical serotonin synthesis in autism. *Int. J. Dev. Neurosci.* 23, 171–182. doi: 10.1016/j.ijdevneu.2004.08.002

Chapin, E. M., and Andrade, R. (2001). A 5-HT$_7$ receptor-mediated depolarization in the anterodorsal thalamus. II. Involvement of the hyperpolarization-activated current I(h). *J. Pharmacol. Exp. Ther.* 297, 403–409.

Chen, S., Wang, J., and Siegelbaum, S. A. (2001). Properties of hyperpolarization-activated pacemaker current defined by coassembly of HCN1 and HCN2 subunits and basal modulation by cyclic nucleotide. *J. Gen. Physiol.* 117, 491–504. doi: 10.1085/jgp.117.5.491

Chen, L., Yung, K. K., Chan, Y. S., and Yung, W. H. (2008). 5-HT excites globus pallidus neurons by multiple receptor mechanisms. *Neuroscience* 151, 439–451. doi: 10.1016/j.neuroscience.2007.11.003

Cherubini, E., Rovira, C., Ben-Ari, Y., and Nistri, A. (1990). Effects of kainate on the excitability of rat hippocampal neurones. *Epilepsy Res.* 5, 18–27. doi: 10.1016/0920-1211(90)90062-Z

Cho, I. H., Yoo, H. J., Park, M., Lee, Y. S., and Kim, S. A. (2007). Family-based association study of 5-HTTLPR and the 5-HT$_{2A}$ receptor gene polymorphisms with autism spectrum disorder in Korean trios. *Brain Res.* 1139, 34–41. doi: 10.1016/j.brainres.2007.01.002

Chugani, D. C., Muzik, O., Behen, M., Rothermel, R., Janisse, J. J., Lee, J., et al. (1999). Developmental changes in brain serotonin synthesis capacity in autistic and nonautistic children. *Ann. Neurol.* 45, 287–295. doi: 10.1002/1531-8249(199903)45:3<287::AID-ANA3>3.0.CO;2-9

Chugani, D. C., Muzik, O., Rothermel, R., Behen, M., Chakraborty, P., Mangner, T., et al. (1997). Altered serotonin synthesis in the dentatothalamocortical pathway in autistic boys. *Ann. Neurol.* 42, 666–669. doi: 10.1002/ana.410420420

Citrome, L. (2014). Vortioxetine for major depressive disorder: a systematic review of the efficacy and safety profile for this newly approved antidepressant—what is the number needed to treat, number needed to harm and likelihood to be helped or harmed? *Int. J. Clin. Pract.* 68, 60–82. doi: 10.1111/ijcp.12350

Clissold, K. A., Choi, E., and Pratt, W. E. (2013). Serotonin 1A, 1B, and 7 receptors of the rat medial nucleus accumbens differentially regulate feeding, water intake and locomotor activity. *Pharmacol. Biochem. Behav.* 112, 96–103. doi: 10.1016/j.pbb.2013.10.002

Colacicco, G., Welzl, H., Lipp, H. P., and Wurbel, H. (2002). Attentional set-shifting in mice: modification of a rat paradigm and evidence for strain-dependent variation. *Behav. Brain Res.* 132, 95–102. doi: 10.1016/S0166-4328(01)00391-6

Costa, L., Spatuzza, M., D'Antoni, S., Bonaccorso, C. M., Trovato, C., Musumeci, S. A., et al. (2012a). Activation of 5-HT$_7$ serotonin receptors reverses metabotropic glutamate receptor-mediated synaptic plasticity in wild-type and Fmr1 knockout mice, a model of fragile X syndrome. *Biol. Psychiatry* 72, 924–933. doi: 10.1016/j.biopsych.2012.06.008

Costa, L., Trovato, C., Musumeci, S. A., Catania, M. V., and Ciranna, L. (2012b). 5-HT1A and 5-HT$_7$ receptors differently modulate AMPA receptor-mediated hippocampal synaptic transmission. *Hippocampus* 22, 790–801. doi: 10.1002/hipo.20940

Coutinho, A. M., Sousa, I., Martins, M., Correia, C., Morgadinho, T., Bento, C., et al. (2007). Evidence for epistasis between SLC6A4 and ITGB3 in autism etiology and in the determination of platelet serotonin levels. *Hum. Genet.* 121, 243–256. doi: 10.1007/s00439-006-0301-3

Cross, S., Kim, S. J., Weiss, L. A., Delahanty, R. J., Sutcliffe, J. S., Leventhal, B. L., et al. (2008). Molecular genetics of the platelet serotonin system in first-degree relatives of patients with autism. *Neuropsychopharmacology* 33, 353–360. doi: 10.1038/sj.npp.1301406

Devlin, B., Cook, E. H. Jr., Coon, H., Dawson, G., Grigorenko, E. L., McMahon, W., et al. (2005). Autism and the serotonin transporter: the long and short of it. *Mol. Psychiatry* 10, 1110–1116. doi: 10.1038/sj.mp.4001724

Di Pilato, P., Niso, M., Adriani, W., Romano, E., Travaglini, D., Berardi, F., et al. (2014). Selective agonists for serotonin 7 (5-HT$_7$) receptor and their applications in preclinical models: an overview. *Rev. Neurosci.* 25, 401–415. doi: 10.1515/revneuro-2014-0009

Disterhoft, J. F., Thompson, L. T., Moyer, J. R. Jr., and Mogul, D. J. (1996). Calcium-dependent afterhyperpolarization and learning in young and aging hippocampus. *Life Sci.* 59, 413–420. doi: 10.1016/0024-3205(96)00320-7

Dölen, G., Darvishzadeh, A., Huang, K. W., and Malenka, R. C. (2013). Social reward requires coordinated activity of nucleus accumbens oxytocin and serotonin. *Nature* 501, 179–184. doi: 10.1038/nature12518

Doly, S., Fischer, J., Brisorgueil, M. J., Verge, D., and Conrath, M. (2005). Pre- and postsynaptic localization of the 5-HT$_7$ receptor in rat dorsal spinal cord: immunocytochemical evidence. *J. Comp. Neurol.* 490, 256–269. doi: 10.1002/cne.20667

Dufour-Rainfray, D., Vourc'h, P., Tourlet, S., Guilloteau, D., Chalon, S., and Andres, C. R. (2011). Fetal exposure to teratogens: evidence of genes involved in autism. *Neurosci. Biobehav. Rev.* 35, 1254–1265. doi: 10.1016/j.neubiorev.2010.12.013

Eriksson, T. M., Golkar, A., Ekstrom, J. C., Svenningsson, P., and Ogren, S. O. (2008). 5-HT$_7$ receptor stimulation by 8-OH-DPAT counteracts the impairing effect of 5-HT$_{1A}$ receptor stimulation on contextual learning in mice. *Eur. J. Pharmacol.* 596, 107–110. doi: 10.1016/j.ejphar.2008.08.026

Eriksson, T. M., Holst, S., Stan, T. L., Hager, T., Sjogren, B., Ogren, S. O., et al. (2012). 5-HT$_{1A}$ and 5-HT$_7$ receptor crosstalk in the regulation of emotional memory: implications for effects of selective serotonin reuptake inhibitors. *Neuropharmacology* 63, 1150–1160. doi: 10.1016/j.neuropharm.2012.06.061

Errico, M., Crozier, R. A., Plummer, M. R., and Cowen, D. S. (2001). 5-HT$_7$ receptors activate the mitogen activated protein kinase extracellular signal related kinase in cultured rat hippocampal neurons. *Neuroscience* 102, 361–367. doi: 10.1016/S0306-4522(00)00460-7

Fan, Y., Fricker, D., Brager, D. H., Chen, X., Lu, H. C., Chitwood, R. A., et al. (2005). Activity-dependent decrease of excitability in rat hippocampal neurons through increases in I_h. *Nat. Neurosci.* 8, 1542–1551. doi: 10.1038/nn1568

Fernández de Sevilla, D., Fuenzalida, M., Porto Pazos, A. B., and Buño, W. (2007). Selective shunting of the NMDA EPSP component by the slow afterhyperpolarization in rat CA1 pyramidal neurons. *J. Neurophysiol.* 97, 3242–3255. doi: 10.1152/jn.00422.2006

Floresco, S. B., Zhang, Y., and Enomoto, T. (2009). Neural circuits subserving behavioral flexibility and their relevance to schizophrenia. *Behav. Brain Res.* 204, 396–409. doi: 10.1016/j.bbr.2008.12.001

Foxx-Orenstein, A. E., Kuemmerle, J. F., and Grider, J. R. (1996). Distinct 5-HT receptors mediate the peristaltic reflex induced by mucosal stimuli in human and guinea pig intestine. *Gastroenterology* 111, 1281–1290. doi: 10.1053/gast.1996.v111.pm8898642

Freret, T., Paizanis, E., Beaudet, G., Gusmao-Montaigne, A., Nee, G., Dauphin, F., et al. (2014). Modulation of 5-HT$_7$ receptor: effect on object recognition performances in mice. *Psychopharmacology (Berl)* 231, 393–400. doi: 10.1007/s00213-013-3247-x

Freund, T. F., and Buzsaki, G. (1996). Interneurons of the hippocampus. *Hippocampus* 6, 347–470. doi: 10.1002/(SICI)1098-1063(1996)6:4<347::AID-HIPO1>3.0.CO;2-I

García-Alcocer, G., Segura, L. C., Garcia Pena, M., Martinez-Torres, A., and Miledi, R. (2006). Ontogenetic distribution of 5-HT2C, 5-HT5A and 5-HT$_7$ receptors in the rat hippocampus. *Gene Expr.* 13, 53–57. doi: 10.3727/000000006783991935

Gasbarri, A., Cifariello, A., Pompili, A., and Meneses, A. (2008). Effect of 5-HT$_7$ antagonist SB-269970 in the modulation of working and reference memory in the rat. *Behav. Brain Res.* 195, 164–170. doi: 10.1016/j.bbr.2007.12.020

Gaspar, P., Cases, O., and Maroteaux, L. (2003). The developmental role of serotonin: news from mouse molecular genetics. *Nat. Rev. Neurosci.* 4, 1002–1012. doi: 10.1038/nrn1256

Gellynck, E., Heyninck, K., Andressen, K. W., Haegeman, G., Levy, F. O., Vanhoenacker, P., et al. (2013). The serotonin 5-HT$_7$ receptors: two decades of research. *Exp. Brain Res.* 230, 555–568. doi: 10.1007/s00221-013-3694-y

Geurts, F. J., De Schutter, E., and Timmermans, J. P. (2002). Localization of 5-HT$_{2A}$, 5-HT3, 5-HT5A and 5-HT$_7$ receptor-like immunoreactivity in the rat cerebellum. *J. Chem. Neuroanat.* 24, 65–74. doi: 10.1016/S0891-0618(02)00020-0

Gill, C. H., Soffin, E. M., Hagan, J. J., and Davies, C. H. (2002). 5-HT$_7$ receptors modulate synchronized network activity in rat hippocampus. *Neuropharmacology* 42, 82–92. doi: 10.1016/S0028-3908(01)00149-6

Girgis, R. R., Slifstein, M., Xu, X., Frankle, W. G., Anagnostou, E., Wasserman, S., et al. (2011). The 5-HT$_{2A}$ receptor and serotonin transporter in Asperger's disorder: a PET study with [^{11}C]MDL 100907 and [^{11}C]DASB. *Psychiatry Res.* 194, 230–234. doi: 10.1016/j.pscychresns.2011.04.007

Glass, J. D., Grossman, G. H., Farnbauch, L., and DiNardo, L. (2003). Midbrain raphe modulation of nonphotic circadian clock resetting and 5-HT release in the mammalian suprachiasmatic nucleus. *J. Neurosci.* 23, 7451–7460.

Goaillard, J. M., and Vincent, P. (2002). Serotonin suppresses the slow afterhyperpolarization in rat intralaminar and midline thalamic neurones by activating 5-HT$_7$ receptors. *J. Physiol.* 541, 453–465. doi: 10.1113/jphysiol.2001.013896

Gorinski, N., and Ponimaskin, E. (2013). Palmitoylation of serotonin receptors. *Biochem. Soc. Trans.* 41, 89–94. doi: 10.1042/BST20120235

Graf, M., Jakus, R., Kantor, S., Levay, G., and Bagdy, G. (2004). Selective 5-HT$_{1A}$ and 5-HT$_7$ antagonists decrease epileptic activity in the WAG/Rij rat model of absence epilepsy. *Neurosci. Lett.* 359, 45–48. doi: 10.1016/j.neulet.2004.01.072

Guilloux, J. P., Mendez-David, I., Pehrson, A., Guiard, B. P., Reperant, C., Orvoen, S., et al. (2013). Antidepressant and anxiolytic potential of the multimodal antidepressant vortioxetine (Lu AA21004) assessed by behavioural and neurogenesis outcomes in mice. *Neuropharmacology* 73, 147–159. doi: 10.1016/j.neuropharm.2013.05.014

Guscott, M., Bristow, L. J., Hadingham, K., Rosahl, T. W., Beer, M. S., Stanton, J. A., et al. (2005). Genetic knockout and pharmacological blockade studies of the 5-HT$_7$ receptor suggest therapeutic potential in depression. *Neuropharmacology* 48, 492–502. doi: 10.1016/j.neuropharm.2004.11.015

Guscott, M. R., Egan, E., Cook, G. P., Stanton, J. A., Beer, M. S., Rosahl, T. W., et al. (2003). The hypothermic effect of 5-CT in mice is mediated through the 5-HT$_7$ receptor. *Neuropharmacology* 44, 1031–1037. doi: 10.1016/S0028-3908(03)00117-5

Hagan, J. J., Price, G. W., Jeffrey, P., Deeks, N. J., Stean, T., Piper, D., et al. (2000). Characterization of SB-269970-A, a selective 5-HT$_7$ receptor antagonist. *Br. J. Pharmacol.* 130, 539–548.

Hall, A. (1998). G proteins and small GTPases: distant relatives keep in touch. *Science* 280, 2074–2075. doi: 10.1126/science.280.5372.2074

Hannon, J., and Hoyer, D. (2008). Molecular biology of 5-HT receptors. *Behav. Brain Res.* 195, 198–213. doi: 10.1016/j.bbr.2008.03.020

Harrington, R. A., Lee, L. C., Crum, R. M., Zimmerman, A. W., and Hertz-Picciotto, I. (2013). Serotonin hypothesis of autism: implications for selective serotonin reuptake inhibitor use during pregnancy. *Autism Res.* 6, 149–168. doi: 10.1002/aur.1288

Hedlund, P. B. (2009). The 5-HT$_7$ receptor and disorders of the nervous system: an overview. *Psychopharmacology (Berl)* 206, 345–354. doi: 10.1007/s00213-009-1626-0

Hedlund, P. B., Danielson, P. E., Thomas, E. A., Slanina, K., Carson, M. J., and Sutcliffe, J. G. (2003). No hypothermic response to serotonin in 5-HT$_7$ receptor knockout mice. *Proc. Natl. Acad. Sci. U S A* 100, 1375–1380. doi: 10.1073/pnas.0337340100

Hedlund, P. B., Huitron-Resendiz, S., Henriksen, S. J., and Sutcliffe, J. G. (2005). 5-HT$_7$ receptor inhibition and inactivation induce antidepressantlike behavior and sleep pattern. *Biol. Psychiatry* 58, 831–837. doi: 10.1016/j.biopsych.2005.05.012

Hedlund, P. B., Kelly, L., Mazur, C., Lovenberg, T., Sutcliffe, J. G., and Bonaventure, P. (2004). 8-OH-DPAT acts on both 5-HT$_{1A}$ and 5-HT$_7$ receptors to induce hypothermia in rodents. *Eur. J. Pharmacol.* 487, 125–132. doi: 10.1016/j.ejphar.2004.01.031

Hedlund, P. B., Leopoldo, M., Caccia, S., Sarkisyan, G., Fracasso, C., Martelli, G., et al. (2010). LP-211 is a brain penetrant selective agonist for the serotonin 5-HT$_7$ receptor. *Neurosci. Lett.* 481, 12–16. doi: 10.1016/j.neulet.2010.06.036

Hedlund, P. B., and Sutcliffe, J. G. (2004). Functional, molecular and pharmacological advances in 5-HT$_7$ receptor research. *Trends Pharmacol. Sci.* 25, 481–486. doi: 10.1016/j.tips.2004.07.002

Hedlund, P. B., and Sutcliffe, J. G. (2007). The 5-HT$_7$ receptor influences stereotypic behavior in a model of obsessive-compulsive disorder. *Neurosci. Lett.* 414, 247–251. doi: 10.1016/j.neulet.2006.12.054

Hoffman, M. S., and Mitchell, G. S. (2011). Spinal 5-HT$_7$ receptor activation induces long-lasting phrenic motor facilitation. *J. Physiol.* 589, 1397–1407. doi: 10.1113/jphysiol.2010.201657

Huber, K. M., Gallagher, S. M., Warren, S. T., and Bear, M. F. (2002). Altered synaptic plasticity in a mouse model of fragile X mental retardation. *Proc. Natl. Acad. Sci. U S A* 99, 7746–7750. doi: 10.1073/pnas.122205699

Inoue, T., Itoh, S., Wakisaka, S., Ogawa, S., Saito, M., and Morimoto, T. (2002). Involvement of 5-HT$_7$ receptors in serotonergic effects on spike afterpotentials in presumed jaw-closing motoneurons of rats. *Brain Res.* 954, 202–211. doi: 10.1016/S0006-8993(02)03286-9

Ireland, D. R., and Abraham, W. C. (2002). Group I mGluRs increase excitability of hippocampal CA1 pyramidal neurons by a PLC-independent mechanism. *J. Neurophysiol.* 88, 107–116. doi: 10.1152/jn.00679.2001

Ishibashi, T., Horisawa, T., Tokuda, K., Ishiyama, T., Ogasa, M., Tagashira, R., et al. (2010). Pharmacological profile of lurasidone, a novel antipsychotic agent with potent 5-hydroxytryptamine 7 (5-HT$_7$) and 5-HT$_{1A}$ receptor activity. *J. Pharmacol. Exp. Ther.* 334, 171–181. doi: 10.1124/jpet.110.167346

Ishihara, K., Takahashi, N., Komoto, N., Yoshikawa, C., Fukumoto, S., Ide, S., et al. (2013). Serotonergic modulation of neuronal activity in the nucleus accumbens following repeated methamphetamine administration in rats. *J. Pharmacol. Sci.* 123, 140–146. doi: 10.1254/jphs.13100FP

Joëls, M., Pu, Z., Wiegert, O., Oitzl, M. S., and Krugers, H. J. (2006). Learning under stress: how does it work? *Trends Cogn. Sci.* 10, 152–158. doi: 10.1016/j.tics.2006.02.002

Johnson-Farley, N. N., Kertesy, S. B., Dubyak, G. R., and Cowen, D. S. (2005). Enhanced activation of Akt and extracellular-regulated kinase pathways by simultaneous occupancy of Gq-coupled 5-HT$_{2A}$ receptors and Gs-coupled 5-HT$_{7A}$ receptors in PC12 cells. *J. Neurochem.* 92, 72–82. doi: 10.1111/j.1471-4159.2004.02832.x

Jung, S., Jones, T. D., Lugo, J. N. Jr., Sheerin, A. H., Miller, J. W., D'Ambrosio, R., et al. (2007). Progressive dendritic HCN channelopathy during epileptogenesis in the rat pilocarpine model of epilepsy. *J. Neurosci.* 27, 13012–13021. doi: 10.1523/JNEUROSCI.3605-07.2007

Jung, S., Warner, L. N., Pitsch, J., Becker, A. J., and Poolos, N. P. (2011). Rapid loss of dendritic HCN channel expression in hippocampal pyramidal neurons following status epilepticus. *J. Neurosci.* 31, 14291–14295. doi: 10.1523/JNEUROSCI.1148-11.2011

Kane, M. J., Angoa-Perez, M., Briggs, D. I., Sykes, C. E., Francescutti, D. M., Rosenberg, D. R., et al. (2012). Mice genetically depleted of brain serotonin display social impairments, communication deficits and repetitive behaviors: possible relevance to autism. *PLoS One* 7:e48975. doi: 10.1371/journal.pone.0048975

Kawahara, F., Saito, H., and Katsuki, H. (1994). Inhibition by 5-HT$_7$ receptor stimulation of GABAA receptor-activated current in cultured rat suprachiasmatic neurones. *J. Physiol.* 478(Pt. 1), 67–73.

Kobe, F., Guseva, D., Jensen, T. P., Wirth, A., Renner, U., Hess, D., et al. (2012). 5-HT$_7$R/G12 signaling regulates neuronal morphology and function in an age-dependent manner. *J. Neurosci.* 32, 2915–2930. doi: 10.1523/JNEUROSCI.2765-11.2012

Kvachnina, E., Dumuis, A., Wlodarczyk, J., Renner, U., Cochet, M., Richter, D. W., et al. (2009). Constitutive Gs-mediated, but not G12-mediated, activity of the 5-hydroxytryptamine 5-HT$_{7a}$ receptor is modulated by the palmitoylation of its C-terminal domain. *Biochim. Biophys. Acta* 1793, 1646–1655. doi: 10.1016/j.bbamcr.2009.08.008

Kvachnina, E., Liu, G., Dityatev, A., Renner, U., Dumuis, A., Richter, D. W., et al. (2005). 5-HT$_7$ receptor is coupled to G alpha subunits of heterotrimeric G12-protein to regulate gene transcription and neuronal morphology. *J. Neurosci.* 25, 7821–7830. doi: 10.1523/JNEUROSCI.1790-05.2005

Lancaster, B., Hu, H., Ramakers, G. M., and Storm, J. F. (2001). Interaction between synaptic excitation and slow afterhyperpolarization current in rat hippocampal pyramidal cells. *J. Physiol.* 536, 809–823. doi: 10.1111/j.1469-7793.2001.00809.x

Lassig, J. P., Vachirasomtoon, K., Hartzell, K., Leventhal, M., Courchesne, E., Courchesne, R., et al. (1999). Physical mapping of the serotonin 5-HT$_7$ receptor gene (HTR7) to chromosome 10 and pseudogene (HTR7P) to chromosome 12 and testing of linkage disequilibrium between HTR7 and autistic disorder. *Am. J. Med. Genet.* 88, 472–475. doi: 10.1002/(SICI)1096-8628(19991015)88:5<472::AID-AJMG7>3.0.CO;2-G

Leopoldo, M., Lacivita, E., De Giorgio, P., Fracasso, C., Guzzetti, S., Caccia, S., et al. (2008). Structural modifications of N-(1,2,3,4-tetrahydronaphthalen-1-yl)-4-aryl-1-piperazinehexanamides: influence on lipophilicity and 5-HT$_7$ receptor activity. Part III. *J. Med. Chem.* 51, 5813–5822. doi: 10.1021/jm800615e

Lesch, K. P., and Waider, J. (2012). Serotonin in the modulation of neural plasticity and networks: implications for neurodevelopmental disorders. *Neuron* 76, 175–191. doi: 10.1016/j.neuron.2012.09.013

Lin, S. L., Johnson-Farley, N. N., Lubinsky, D. R., and Cowen, D. S. (2003). Coupling of neuronal 5-HT$_7$ receptors to activation of extracellular-regulated kinase through a protein kinase A-independent pathway that can utilize Epac. *J. Neurochem.* 87, 1076–1085. doi: 10.1046/j.1471-4159.2003.02076.x

Liu, J., Akay, T., Hedlund, P. B., Pearson, K. G., and Jordan, L. M. (2009). Spinal 5-HT$_7$ receptors are critical for alternating activity during locomotion: in vitro neonatal and in vivo adult studies using 5-HT$_7$ receptor knockout mice. *J. Neurophysiol.* 102, 337–348. doi: 10.1152/jn.91239.2008

Logue, S. F., and Gould, T. J. (2014). The neural and genetic basis of executive function: attention, cognitive flexibility and response inhibition. *Pharmacol. Biochem. Behav.* 123C, 45–54. doi: 10.1016/j.pbb.2013.08.007

Lovenberg, T. W., Baron, B. M., de Lecea, L., Miller, J. D., Prosser, R. A., Rea, M. A., et al. (1993). A novel adenylyl cyclase-activating serotonin receptor (5-HT$_7$) implicated in the regulation of mammalian circadian rhythms. *Neuron* 11, 449–458. doi: 10.1016/0896-6273(93)90149-L

Luscher, C., and Huber, K. M. (2010). Group 1 mGluR-dependent synaptic long-term depression: mechanisms and implications for circuitry and disease. *Neuron* 65, 445–459. doi: 10.1016/j.neuron.2010.01.016

Magee, J. C. (1998). Dendritic hyperpolarization-activated currents modify the integrative properties of hippocampal CA1 pyramidal neurons. *J. Neurosci.* 18, 7613–7624.

Magee, J. C. (1999). Dendritic Ih normalizes temporal summation in hippocampal CA1 neurons. *Nat. Neurosci.* 2, 848. doi: 10.1038/12229

Manuel-Apolinar, L., and Meneses, A. (2004). 8-OH-DPAT facilitated memory consolidation and increased hippocampal and cortical cAMP production. *Behav. Brain Res.* 148, 179–184. doi: 10.1016/S0166-4328(03)00186-4

Marazziti, D., Muratori, F., Cesari, A., Masala, I., Baroni, S., Giannaccini, G., et al. (2000). Increased density of the platelet serotonin transporter in autism. *Pharmacopsychiatry* 33, 165–168. doi: 10.1055/s-2000-7588

Martin-Cora, F. J., and Pazos, A. (2004). Autoradiographic distribution of 5-HT_7 receptors in the human brain using [3H]mesulergine: comparison to other mammalian species. *Br. J. Pharmacol.* 141, 92–104. doi: 10.1038/sj.bjp.07 05576

Matthys, A., Haegeman, G., Van Craenenbroeck, K., and Vanhoenacker, P. (2011). Role of the 5-HT_7 receptor in the central nervous system: from current status to future perspectives. *Mol. Neurobiol.* 43, 228–253. doi: 10.1007/s12035-011-8175-3

McBride, P. A., Anderson, G. M., Hertzig, M. E., Snow, M. E., Thompson, S. M., Khait, V. D., et al. (1998). Effects of diagnosis, race and puberty on platelet serotonin levels in autism and mental retardation. *J. Am. Acad. Child Adolesc. Psychiatry* 37, 767–776. doi: 10.1097/00004583-199807000-00017

McCormick, D. A., and Pape, H. C. (1990). Properties of a hyperpolarization-activated cation current and its role in rhythmic oscillation in thalamic relay neurones. *J. Physiol.* 431, 291–318.

McNamara, I. M., Borella, A. W., Bialowas, L. A., and Whitaker-Azmitia, P. M. (2008). Further studies in the developmental hyperserotonemia model (DHS) of autism: social, behavioral and peptide changes. *Brain Res.* 1189, 203–214. doi: 10.1016/j.brainres.2007.10.063

Meneses, A. (2013). 5-HT systems: emergent targets for memory formation and memory alterations. *Rev. Neurosci.* 24, 629–664. doi: 10.1515/revneuro-2013-0026

Millan, M. J., Marin, P., Bockaert, J., and la Cour, C. M. (2008). Signaling at G-protein-coupled serotonin receptors: recent advances and future research directions. *Trends Pharmacol. Sci.* 29, 454–464. doi: 10.1016/j.tips.2008.06.007

Mnie-Filali, O., Faure, C., Lambas-Senas, L., El Mansari, M., Belblidia, H., Gondard, E., et al. (2011). Pharmacological blockade of 5-HT_7 receptors as a putative fast acting antidepressant strategy. *Neuropsychopharmacology* 36, 1275–1288. doi: 10.1038/npp.2011.13

Monsma, F. J. Jr., Shen, Y., Ward, R. P., Hamblin, M. W., and Sibley, D. R. (1993). Cloning and expression of a novel serotonin receptor with high affinity for tricyclic psychotropic drugs. *Mol. Pharmacol.* 43, 320–327.

Monti, J. M., and Jantos, H. (2014). The role of serotonin 5-HT_7 receptor in regulating sleep and wakefulness. *Rev. Neurosci.* 25, 429–437. doi: 10.1515/revneuro-2014-0016

Monti, J. M., Leopoldo, M., and Jantos, H. (2008). The serotonin 5-HT_7 receptor agonist LP-44 microinjected into the dorsal raphe nucleus suppresses REM sleep in the rat. *Behav. Brain Res.* 191, 184–189. doi: 10.1016/j.bbr.2008.03.025

Monti, J. M., Leopoldo, M., and Jantos, H. (2014). Systemic administration and local microinjection into the central nervous system of the 5-HT_7 receptor agonist LP-211 modify the sleep-wake cycle in the rat. *Behav. Brain Res.* 259, 321–329. doi: 10.1016/j.bbr.2013.11.030

Monti, J. M., Leopoldo, M., Jantos, H., and Lagos, P. (2012). Microinjection of the 5-HT_7 receptor antagonist SB-269970 into the rat brainstem and basal forebrain: site-dependent effects on REM sleep. *Pharmacol. Biochem. Behav.* 102, 373–380. doi: 10.1016/j.pbb.2012.05.012

Moyer, J. R. Jr., Thompson, L. T., and Disterhoft, J. F. (1996). Trace eyeblink conditioning increases CA1 excitability in a transient and learning-specific manner. *J. Neurosci.* 16, 5536–5546.

Mozzachiodi, R., and Byrne, J. H. (2010). More than synaptic plasticity: role of nonsynaptic plasticity in learning and memory. *Trends Neurosci.* 33, 17–26. doi: 10.1016/j.tins.2009.10.001.

Mulder, E. J., Anderson, G. M., Kema, I. P., de Bildt, A., van Lang, N. D., den Boer, J. A., et al. (2004). Platelet serotonin levels in pervasive developmental disorders and mental retardation: diagnostic group differences, within-group distribution and behavioral correlates. *J. Am. Acad. Child Adolesc. Psychiatry* 43, 491–499. doi: 10.1097/00004583-200404000-00016

Muneoka, K. T., and Takigawa, M. (2003). 5-Hydroxytryptamine7 (5-HT_7) receptor immunoreactivity-positive 'stigmoid body'-like structure in developing rat brains. *Int. J. Dev. Neurosci.* 21, 133–143. doi: 10.1016/S0736-5748(03)00029-7

Murphy, D. G., Daly, E., Schmitz, N., Toal, F., Murphy, K., Curran, S., et al. (2006). Cortical serotonin 5-HT_{2A} receptor binding and social communication in adults with Asperger's syndrome: an in vivo SPECT study. *Am. J. Psychiatry* 163, 934–936. doi: 10.1176/appi.ajp.163.5.934

Naumenko, V. S., Kondaurova, E. M., and Popova, N. K. (2011). On the role of brain 5-HT_7 receptor in the mechanism of hypothermia: comparison with hypothermia mediated via 5-HT_{1A} and 5-HT3 receptor. *Neuropharmacology* 61, 1360–1365. doi: 10.1016/j.neuropharm.2011.08.022

Neumaier, J. F., Sexton, T. J., Yracheta, J., Diaz, A. M., and Brownfield, M. (2001). Localization of 5-HT_7 receptors in rat brain by immunocytochemistry, in situ hybridization and agonist stimulated cFos expression. *J. Chem. Neuroanat.* 21, 63–73. doi: 10.1016/S0891-0618(00)00092-2

Nichols, D. E., and Nichols, C. D. (2008). Serotonin receptors. *Chem. Rev.* 108, 1614–1641. doi: 10.1021/cr078224o

Nikiforuk, A. (2012). Selective blockade of 5-HT_7 receptors facilitates attentional set-shifting in stressed and control rats. *Behav. Brain Res.* 226, 118–123. doi: 10. 1016/j.bbr.2011.09.006

Nikiforuk, A., Kos, T., Fijal, K., Holuj, M., Rafa, D., and Popik, P. (2013). Effects of the selective 5-HT_7 receptor antagonist SB-269970 and amisulpride on ketamine-induced schizophrenia-like deficits in rats. *PLoS One* 8:e66695. doi: 10.1371/journal.pone.0066695

Nikiforuk, A., and Popik, P. (2013). Amisulpride promotes cognitive flexibility in rats: the role of 5-HT_7 receptors. *Behav. Brain Res.* 248, 136–140. doi: 10.1016/j. bbr.2013.04.008

Norum, J. H., Hart, K., and Levy, F. O. (2003). Ras-dependent ERK activation by the human G(s)-coupled serotonin receptors 5-HT4(b) and 5-HT_7(a). *J. Biol. Chem.* 278, 3098–3104. doi: 10.1074/jbc.M206237200

Oblak, A., Gibbs, T. T., and Blatt, G. J. (2013). Reduced serotonin receptor subtypes in a limbic and a neocortical region in autism. *Autism Res.* 6, 571–583. doi: 10. 1002/aur.1317

Oh, M. M., McKay, B. M., Power, J. M., and Disterhoft, J. F. (2009). Learning-related postburst afterhyperpolarization reduction in CA1 pyramidal neurons is mediated by protein kinase A. *Proc. Natl. Acad. Sci. U S A* 106, 1620–1625. doi: 10.1073/pnas.0807708106

Otmakhova, N. A., Lewey, J., Asrican, B., and Lisman, J. E. (2005). Inhibition of perforant path input to the CA1 region by serotonin and noradrenaline. *J. Neurophysiol.* 94, 1413–1422. doi: 10.1152/jn.00217.2005

Perez-Garcia, G. S., and Meneses, A. (2005). Effects of the potential 5-HT_7 receptor agonist AS 19 in an autoshaping learning task. *Behav. Brain Res.* 163, 136–140. doi: 10.1016/j.bbr.2005.04.014

Pericic, D., and Svob Strac, D. (2007). The role of 5-HT_7 receptors in the control of seizures. *Brain Res.* 1141, 48–55. doi: 10.1016/j.brainres.2007.01.019

Pietropaolo, S., Guilleminot, A., Martin, B., D'Amato, F. R., and Crusio, W. E. (2011). Genetic-background modulation of core and variable autistic-like symptoms in Fmr1 knock-out mice. *PLoS One* 6:e17073. doi: 10.1371/journal. pone.0017073

Piven, J., Tsai, G. C., Nehme, E., Coyle, J. T., Chase, G. A., and Folstein, S. E. (1991). Platelet serotonin, a possible marker for familial autism. *J. Autism Dev. Disord.* 21, 51–59. doi: 10.1007/BF02206997

Pytliak, M., Vargova, V., Mechirova, V., and Felsoci, M. (2011). Serotonin receptors—from molecular biology to clinical applications. *Physiol. Res.* 60, 15–25.

Ramoz, N., Reichert, J. G., Corwin, T. E., Smith, C. J., Silverman, J. M., Hollander, E., et al. (2006). Lack of evidence for association of the serotonin transporter gene SLC6A4 with autism. *Biol. Psychiatry* 60, 186–191. doi: 10.1016/j.biopsych. 2006.01.009

Renner, U., Zeug, A., Woehler, A., Niebert, M., Dityatev, A., Dityateva, G., et al. (2012). Heterodimerization of serotonin receptors 5-HT_{1A} and 5-HT_7 differentially regulates receptor signalling and trafficking. *J. Cell Sci.* 125, 2486–2499. doi: 10.1242/jcs.101337

Roberts, A. J., and Hedlund, P. B. (2012). The 5-HT_7 receptor in learning and memory. *Hippocampus* 22, 762–771. doi: 10.1002/hipo.20938

Roberts, A. J., Krucker, T., Levy, C. L., Slanina, K. A., Sutcliffe, J. G., and Hedlund, P. B. (2004a). Mice lacking 5-HT receptors show specific impairments in contextual learning. *Eur. J. Neurosci.* 19, 1913–1922. doi: 10.1111/j.1460-9568.2004.03288.x

Roberts, C., Thomas, D. R., Bate, S. T., and Kew, J. N. (2004b). GABAergic modulation of 5-HT$_7$ receptor-mediated effects on 5-HT efflux in the guinea-pig dorsal raphe nucleus. *Neuropharmacology* 46, 935–941. doi: 10.1016/j.neuropharm.2004.01.010

Romano, E., Ruocco, L. A., Nativio, P., Lacivita, E., Ajmone-Cat, M. A., Boatto, G., et al. (2014). Modulatory effects following subchronic stimulation of brain 5-HT$_7$-R system in mice and rats. *Rev. Neurosci.* 25, 383–400. doi: 10.1515/revneuro-2014-0007

Roth, B. L., Craigo, S. C., Choudhary, M. S., Uluer, A., and Monsma, F. J. Jr. (1994). Binding of typical and atypical antipsychotic agents to 5-hydroxytryptamine-6 and 5-hydroxytryptamine-7 receptors. *J. Pharmacol. Exp. Ther.* 268, 1403–1410.

Ruat, M., Traiffort, E., Leurs, R., Tardivel-Lacombe, J., Diaz, J., Arrang, J. M., et al. (1993). Molecular cloning, characterization and localization of a high-affinity serotonin receptor (5-HT$_7$) activating cAMP formation. *Proc. Natl. Acad. Sci. U S A* 90, 8547–8551. doi: 10.1073/pnas.90.18.8547

Ruocco, L. A., Romano, E., Treno, C., Lacivita, E., Claudio, A., Gironi-Carnevale, U. A., et al. (2013). Emotional and risk seeking behavior after prepuberal subchronic or adult acute stimulation of 5-HT$_7$-Rs in naples high excitability rats. *Synapse* 68, 159–167. doi: 10.1002/syn.21724

Sah, P. (1996). Ca(2+)-activated K+ currents in neurones: types, physiological roles and modulation. *Trends Neurosci.* 19, 150–154. doi: 10.1016/S0166-2236(96)80026-9

Sarkisyan, G., and Hedlund, P. B. (2009). The 5-HT$_7$ receptor is involved in allocentric spatial memory information processing. *Behav. Brain Res.* 202, 26–31. doi: 10.1016/j.bbr.2009.03.011

Sarkisyan, G., Roberts, A. J., and Hedlund, P. B. (2010). The 5-HT$_7$ receptor as a mediator and modulator of antidepressant-like behavior. *Behav. Brain Res.* 209, 99–108. doi: 10.1016/j.bbr.2010.01.022

Schain, R. J., and Freedman, D. X. (1961). Studies on 5-hydroxyindole metabolism in autistic and other mentally retarded children. *J. Pediatr.* 58, 315–320.

Shen, Y., Monsma, F. J. Jr., Metcalf, M. A., Jose, P. A., Hamblin, M. W., and Sibley, D. R. (1993). Molecular cloning and expression of a 5-hydroxytryptamine7 serotonin receptor subtype. *J. Biol. Chem.* 268, 18200–18204.

Shimizu, M., Nishida, A., Zensho, H., Miyata, M., and Yamawaki, S. (1998). Agonist-induced desensitization of adenylyl cyclase activity mediated by 5-hydroxytryptamine7 receptors in rat frontocortical astrocytes. *Brain Res.* 784, 57–62.

Smith, B. N., Sollars, P. J., Dudek, F. E., and Pickard, G. E. (2001). Serotonergic modulation of retinal input to the mouse suprachiasmatic nucleus mediated by 5-HT1B and 5-HT7 receptors. *J. Biol. Rhythms* 16, 25–38. doi: 10.1177/074873040101600104

Sodhi, M. S., and Sanders-Bush, E. (2004). Serotonin and brain development. *Int. Rev. Neurobiol.* 59, 111–174. doi: 10.1016/S0074-7742(04)59006-2

Speranza, L., Chambery, A., Di Domenico, M., Crispino, M., Severino, V., Volpicelli, F., et al. (2013). The serotonin receptor 7 promotes neurite outgrowth via ERK and Cdk5 signaling pathways. *Neuropharmacology* 67, 155–167. doi: 10.1016/j.neuropharm.2012.10.026

Spooren, W., Lindemann, L., Ghosh, A., and Santarelli, L. (2012). Synapse dysfunction in autism: a molecular medicine approach to drug discovery in neurodevelopmental disorders. *Trends Pharmacol. Sci.* 33, 669–684. doi: 10.1016/j.tips.2012.09.004

Sugita, S., Shen, K. Z., and North, R. A. (1992). 5-hydroxytryptamine is a fast excitatory transmitter at 5-HT3 receptors in rat amygdala. *Neuron* 8, 199–203. doi: 10.1016/0896-6273(92)90121-S

Surges, R., Kukley, M., Brewster, A., Ruschenschmidt, C., Schramm, J., Baram, T. Z., et al. (2012). Hyperpolarization-activated cation current Ih of dentate gyrus granule cells is upregulated in human and rat temporal lobe epilepsy. *Biochem. Biophys. Res. Commun.* 420, 156–160. doi: 10.1016/j.bbrc.2012.02.133

Sutcliffe, J. S., Delahanty, R. J., Prasad, H. C., McCauley, J. L., Han, Q., Jiang, L., et al. (2005). Allelic heterogeneity at the serotonin transporter locus (SLC6A4) confers susceptibility to autism and rigid-compulsive behaviors. *Am. J. Hum. Genet.* 77, 265–279. doi: 10.1086/432648

Teitler, M., and Klein, M. T. (2012). A new approach for studying GPCR dimers: drug-induced inactivation and reactivation to reveal GPCR dimer function in vitro, in primary culture and in vivo. *Pharmacol. Ther.* 133, 205–217. doi: 10.1016/j.pharmthera.2011.10.007

Thomas, D. R., Melotto, S., Massagrande, M., Gribble, A. D., Jeffrey, P., Stevens, A. J., et al. (2003). SB-656104-A, a novel selective 5-HT$_7$ receptor antagonist, modulates REM sleep in rats. *Br. J. Pharmacol.* 139, 705–714. doi: 10.1038/sj.bjp.0705290

Tokarski, K., Kusek, M., and Hess, G. (2011). 5-HT$_7$ receptors modulate GABAergic transmission in rat hippocampal CA1 area. *J. Physiol. Pharmacol.* 62, 535–540.

Tokarski, K., Kusek, M., and Hess, G. (2012a). Repeated blockade of 5-HT$_7$ receptors depresses glutamatergic transmission in the rat frontal cortex. *J. Physiol. Pharmacol.* 63, 173–177.

Tokarski, K., Zahorodna, A., Bobula, B., and Hess, G. (2003). 5-HT$_7$ receptors increase the excitability of rat hippocampal CA1 pyramidal neurons. *Brain Res.* 993, 230–234. doi: 10.1016/j.brainres.2003.09.015

Tokarski, K., Zelek-Molik, A., Duszynska, B., Satala, G., Bobula, B., Kusek, M., et al. (2012b). Acute and repeated treatment with the 5-HT$_7$ receptor antagonist SB 269970 induces functional desensitization of 5-HT$_7$ receptors in rat hippocampus. *Pharmacol. Rep.* 64, 256–265. doi: 10.1016/S1734-1140(12)70763-6

Tombaugh, G. C., Rowe, W. B., and Rose, G. M. (2005). The slow afterhyperpolarization in hippocampal CA1 neurons covaries with spatial learning ability in aged Fisher 344 rats. *J. Neurosci.* 25, 2609–2616. doi: 10.1523/JNEUROSCI.5023-04.2005

Varnäs, K., Thomas, D. R., Tupala, E., Tiihonen, J., and Hall, H. (2004). Distribution of 5-HT$_7$ receptors in the human brain: a preliminary autoradiographic study using [3H]SB-269970. *Neurosci. Lett.* 367, 313–316. doi: 10.1016/j.neulet.2004.06.025

Vasefi, M. S., Kruk, J. S., Heikkila, J. J., and Beazely, M. A. (2013). 5-Hydroxytryptamine type 7 receptor neuroprotection against NMDA-induced excitotoxicity is PDGFβ receptor dependent. *J. Neurochem.* 125, 26–36. doi: 10.1111/jnc.12157

Veenstra-VanderWeele, J., Muller, C. L., Iwamoto, H., Sauer, J. E., Owens, W. A., Shah, C. R., et al. (2012). Autism gene variant causes hyperserotonemia, serotonin receptor hypersensitivity, social impairment and repetitive behavior. *Proc. Natl. Acad. Sci. U S A* 109, 5469–5474. doi: 10.1073/pnas.1112345109

Viguier, F., Michot, B., Hamon, M., and Bourgoin, S. (2013). Multiple roles of serotonin in pain control mechanisms–implications of 5-HT$_7$. and other 5-HT receptor types. *Eur. J. Pharmacol.* 716, 8–16. doi: 10.1016/j.ejphar.2013.01.074

Viguier, F., Michot, B., Kayser, V., Bernard, J. F., Vela, J. M., Hamon, M., et al. (2012). GABA, but not opioids, mediates the anti-hyperalgesic effects of 5-HT$_7$ receptor activation in rats suffering from neuropathic pain. *Neuropharmacology* 63, 1093–1106. doi: 10.1016/j.neuropharm.2012.07.023

Wassink, T. H., Hazlett, H. C., Epping, E. A., Arndt, S., Dager, S. R., Schellenberg, G. D., et al. (2007). Cerebral cortical gray matter overgrowth and functional variation of the serotonin transporter gene in autism. *Arch. Gen. Psychiatry* 64, 709–717. doi: 10.1001/archpsyc.64.6.709

Wesolowska, A., Nikiforuk, A., and Stachowicz, K. (2006a). Potential anxiolytic and antidepressant effects of the selective 5-HT$_7$ receptor antagonist SB 269970 after intrahippocampal administration to rats. *Eur. J. Pharmacol.* 553, 185–190. doi: 10.1016/j.ejphar.2006.09.064

Wesolowska, A., Nikiforuk, A., Stachowicz, K., and Tatarczynska, E. (2006b). Effect of the selective 5-HT$_7$ receptor antagonist SB 269970 in animal models of anxiety and depression. *Neuropharmacology* 51, 578–586. doi: 10.1016/j.neuropharm.2006.04.017

Whitaker-Azmitia, P. M. (2005). Behavioral and cellular consequences of increasing serotonergic activity during brain development: a role in autism? *Int. J. Dev. Neurosci.* 23, 75–83. doi: 10.1016/j.ijdevneu.2004.07.022

Witkin, J. M., Baez, M., Yu, J., Barton, M. E., and Shannon, H. E. (2007). Constitutive deletion of the serotonin-7 (5-HT$_7$) receptor decreases electrical and chemical seizure thresholds. *Epilepsy Res.* 75, 39–45. doi: 10.1016/j.eplepsyres.2007.03.017

Witteveen, J. S., Middelman, A., van Hulten, J. A., Martens, G. J., Homberg, J. R., and Kolk, S. M. (2013). Lack of serotonin reuptake during brain development alters rostral raphe-prefrontal network formation. *Front. Cell. Neurosci.* 7:143. doi: 10.3389/fncel.2013.00143

Woehler, A., and Ponimaskin, E. G. (2009). G protein–mediated signaling: same receptor, multiple effectors. *Curr. Mol. Pharmacol.* 2, 237–248. doi: 10.2174/1874467210902030237

Wolfensteller, U., and Ruge, H. (2012). Frontostriatal mechanisms in instruction-based learning as a hallmark of flexible goal-directed behavior. *Front. Psychol.* 3:192. doi: 10.3389/fpsyg.2012.00192

Woo, Y. S., Wang, H. R., and Bahk, W. M. (2013). Lurasidone as a potential therapy for bipolar disorder. *Neuropsychiatr. Dis. Treat.* 9, 1521–1529. doi: 10.2147/NDT.S51910

Wu, W. W., Chan, C. S., and Disterhoft, J. F. (2004). Slow afterhyperpolarization governs the development of NMDA receptor-dependent afterdepolarization in CA1 pyramidal neurons during synaptic stimulation. *J. Neurophysiol.* 92, 2346–2356. doi: 10.1152/jn.00977.2003

Yanarates, O., Dogrul, A., Yildirim, V., Sahin, A., Sizlan, A., Seyrek, M., et al. (2010). Spinal 5-HT_7 receptors play an important role in the antinociceptive and antihyperalgesic effects of tramadol and its metabolite, O-Desmethyltramadol, via activation of descending serotonergic pathways. *Anesthesiology* 112, 696–710. doi: 10.1097/ALN.0b013e3181cd7920

Yang, E. J., Han, S. K., and Park, S. J. (2014). Functional expression of 5-HT_7 receptor on the substantia gelatinosa neurons of the trigeminal subnucleus caudalis in mice. *Brain Res.* 1543, 73–82. doi: 10.1016/j.brainres.2013.10.041

Yang, Z., Liu, X., Yin, Y., Sun, S., and Deng, X. (2012). Involvement of 5-HT_7 receptors in the pathogenesis of temporal lobe epilepsy. *Eur. J. Pharmacol.* 685, 52–58. doi: 10.1016/j.ejphar.2012.04.011

Zhang, Z. W. (2003). Serotonin induces tonic firing in layer V pyramidal neurons of rat prefrontal cortex during postnatal development. *J. Neurosci.* 23, 3373–3384.

13

Genetic aspects of autism spectrum disorders: Insights from animal models

Swati Banerjee*, Maeveen Riordan and Manzoor A. Bhat*

Department of Physiology, Center for Biomedical Neuroscience, School of Medicine, University of Texas Health Science Center, San Antonio, TX, USA

Correspondence:
Swati Banerjee and Manzoor A. Bhat, Department of Physiology, Center for Biomedical Neuroscience, School of Medicine, University of Texas Health Science Center, 7703 Floyd Curl Drive, San Antonio, TX 78229-3900, USA
e-mail: banerjees@uthscsa.edu; bhatm@uthscsa.edu

Autism spectrum disorders (ASDs) are a complex neurodevelopmental disorder that display a triad of core behavioral deficits including restricted interests, often accompanied by repetitive behavior, deficits in language and communication, and an inability to engage in reciprocal social interactions. ASD is among the most heritable disorders but is not a simple disorder with a singular pathology and has a rather complex etiology. It is interesting to note that perturbations in synaptic growth, development, and stability underlie a variety of neuropsychiatric disorders, including ASD, schizophrenia, epilepsy, and intellectual disability. Biological characterization of an increasing repertoire of synaptic mutants in various model organisms indicates synaptic dysfunction as causal in the pathophysiology of ASD. Our understanding of the genes and genetic pathways that contribute toward the formation, stabilization, and maintenance of functional synapses coupled with an in-depth phenotypic analysis of the cellular and behavioral characteristics is therefore essential to unraveling the pathogenesis of these disorders. In this review, we discuss the genetic aspects of ASD emphasizing on the well conserved set of genes and genetic pathways implicated in this disorder, many of which contribute to synapse assembly and maintenance across species. We also review how fundamental research using animal models is providing key insights into the various facets of human ASD.

Keywords: autism spectrum disorder, synapse, animal models, genetics, epigenetics, environment, cell adhesion molecules, scaffolding proteins

INTRODUCTION

Autism spectrum disorders (ASDs) are a complex set of heterogeneous neurodevelopmental disorders categorized by a triad of key behavioral anomalies. Characteristic behavioral abnormalities consist of restricted interests accompanied by repetitive behavior, deficits in language and communication, and the inability to engage in reciprocal social interactions (Abrahams and Geschwind, 2008; Betancur et al., 2009; Levitt and Campbell, 2009; Peca et al., 2011b; Zoghbi and Bear, 2012). Autism is not a singular disease entity. The disorder encompasses a spectrum of wide ranging phenotypic manifestations which span from debilitating impairments to mild behavioral and personality traits. Therefore, autism is rightfully referred to as "autism spectrum disorders" (Persico and Bourgeron, 2006).

Autism spectrum disorder appears to be involved in early brain development. Obvious signs and symptoms show early onset within the first 3 years of life and persist into adulthood. According to the recent reports from the Center for Disease Control, an estimated 1 in 88 children has been identified with ASD. Interestingly, these disorders show a gender bias where males are affected almost five times more than females (http://www.cdc.gov/Features/CountingAutism/). ASD is among the most heritable disorders evidenced by family and twin studies with a concordance rate of 70–90% for monozygotic twins (Folstein and Rutter, 1977; Steffenburg et al., 1989; Bailey et al., 1995; Folstein and Rosen-Sheidley, 2001). Nevertheless, heritability in this case is more complex due to the differences in manifestations of its core symptoms, gradual changes over time, and differing degrees of response to interventions (Abrahams and Geschwind, 2008; Levitt and Campbell, 2009). 10–25% of ASD cases seem to have an underlying genetic disorder such as fragile X syndrome, tuberous sclerosis (TSC), and Rett syndrome (Betancur et al., 2009).

Recent studies have highlighted numerous potential risk factors that may contribute to ASD. These risk factors range from genetic, to epigenetic, to environmental factors. Detection of copy number variations (CNV), point mutations, and identification of rare variants in synaptic cell adhesion proteins and pathways are some of the ways researchers are providing insight into the pathophysiology of ASD (Sebat et al., 2007; Malhotra and Sebat, 2012; Zoghbi and Bear, 2012). It is worthwhile to note that the genes and the genetic pathways implicated in ASD, and the identification of any causal rare variants are accessible to modeling in experimental systems. Research findings both from studying human genetics and animal models of ASD suggest that disruption of synapse formation and stabilization processes is a key underlying feature in ASD etiology. Dysfunctions in the assembly or structure of transmembrane and scaffolding proteins needed for building and maintaining synapses, and disruption in cellular signaling pathways controlling synaptogenesis are major contributing factors in ASD.

A large portion of this review will emphasize the well-conserved sets of genes and genetic pathways implicated in ASD, many of which contribute to synapse assembly and maintenance across different species. Given the complexity and heterogeneity of this disorder, it has proved challenging to unravel the underlying causes of ASD from human clinical population alone. Nevertheless, numerous animal models have been utilized that have enormously contributed toward understanding specific aspects that constitute the spectrum of these disorders.

HISTORICAL OVERVIEW OF AUTISM SPECTRUM DISORDERS

Leo Kanner, a psychiatrist, initially described autism well over half a century ago (Kanner, 1943, 1968, 1971). Studies on the relationship between autism and abnormal electroencephalogram were among the first to suggest autism as a disorder of brain function (Creak and Pampiglione, 1969). Despite these ground-breaking observations on autism, early identification of autism was marred by lack of adequate diagnostic criteria. It was not until the introduction of the concept of "autism triad" that highlighted the now well-established characteristics of impairment in social interaction, language and communication did Autism become a recognizable disorder. Since then the clinical conceptualizations of ASD have consistently evolved together with a steady rise in the number of ASD cases. Our current understanding of ASD is that of a complex neurological disorder that continues to challenge our ability to identify the underlying causal mechanisms.

MANY FACETS OF AUTISM SPECTRUM DISORDERS

GENETICS – COPY NUMBER VARIATION

Copy number variation is among the most widespread of structural variations in the human genome, and is increasingly being implicated as a major contributor to the pathophysiology of complex neurodevelopmental disorders (Sebat et al., 2007, 2009; Christian et al., 2008; Kumar et al., 2008; Marshall et al., 2008; Weiss et al., 2008; Bucan et al., 2009; Glessner et al., 2009; Merikangas et al., 2009; Luo et al., 2012; Malhotra and Sebat, 2012). CNVs largely comprise of duplications and deletions and can be *de novo* or familial. *De novo* CNVs are more prevalent in causing sporadic genomic disorders (McCarroll et al., 2008). The duplication or deletion events disrupt gene structure, expression, and function and are a common cause of developmental delay. Several studies suggest important role of CNVs in disease etiology, susceptibility, and inheritance (Beckmann et al., 2007; Estivill and Armengol, 2007). Large-scale genome-wide association studies are credited for detection of CNVs in rare cases of ASD (Ma et al., 2009a). Duplications and microdeletions in many loci are associated with ASD. Several studies identified duplication CNVs within 15q13 (Christian et al., 2008; Miller et al., 2009) and microdeletions at many loci in 16p11.2 (Sebat et al., 2007; Marshall et al., 2008; Weiss et al., 2008; Levy et al., 2011; Sanders et al., 2011), Williams syndrome locus 7q11.23, DiGeorge syndrome locus 22q11.2, 1q21.1, and Prader–Willi and Angelman syndromes at 15q11-13 (Glessner et al., 2009; Sanders et al., 2011).

Interestingly, genes associated with CNVs in ASD are involved in regulating synaptogenesis. Some of the genes include *NEUROLIGIN 4* (*NLGN4*; Jamain et al., 2003; Laumonnier et al., 2004), *SHANK3* (Durand et al., 2007; Moessner et al., 2007; Gauthier et al., 2009), *TBX1*, *PCDH10*, and *NHE9* (Morrow et al., 2008). Recent findings further reiterate a correlation between synapse formation and autism (Glessner et al., 2009; Mitne-Neto et al., 2011). In addition to these genes, some of the other genes recognized as risk factors in ASD include *NEUREXIN 1* (*NRXN1*; Kim et al., 2008; Bucan et al., 2009), *SHANK2* (Berkel et al., 2010), CNTN4 (Fernandez et al., 2004), *CNTNAP2* (Bakkaloglu et al., 2008; Penagarikano et al., 2011), *DPYD* and *DPP6* (Marshall et al., 2008); NLG1 (Glessner et al., 2009) and SYNGAP1, DLGAP2 (Pinto et al., 2010). A detailed list of genes, their potential functions and genetic pathways linked to ASD are summarized in **Table 1**.

EPIGENETICS

Epigenetic mechanisms underlie several human neurodevelopmental disorders. Genomic imprinting, epimutations, DNA methylation, and histone modifications are all examples of epigenetic mechanisms linked to the development of certain disorders. These mechanisms involve modifications of nucleotides or chromosomes without altering the genetic sequence (Zoghbi, 2003; Egger et al., 2004). Thus causing modifications in gene expression that may increase the likelihood of developing a particular disease. Epigenetic mechanisms are believed to function at the interface between genetic and environmental factors (Jiang et al., 2004; Qiu, 2006). Studies linking these two factors are gaining importance for understanding the etiologies of complex disorders and could play a role in the development of ASD.

While epigenetic mechanisms are implicated in the development of many disorders, they are also an intrinsic phenomenon for normal brain development. Genomic imprinting is an example of an epigenetic mechanism that occurs normally throughout life. This is when one of the two parental alleles for an imprinted gene becomes inactive due to DNA methylation resulting in monoallelic gene expression. This phenomenon occurs quite frequently in humans but was also discovered in fungi, plants, and other animals (Martienssen and Colot, 2001; Jiang and Kohler, 2012). Using genome-wide scans, several areas on chromosomes known as, hot spots for genomic imprinting, were located on loci 7q and 15q (Reik and Walter, 2001; Luedi et al., 2007). Interestingly, these loci are highly affected in individuals with ASD (International Molecular Genetic Study of Autism Consortium, 2001; Lamb et al., 2005). Several studies have linked duplication or deletion events on the active chromosome to ASD (Cook et al., 1997; Schroer et al., 1998; Koochek et al., 2006). Individuals with Angelman syndrome (Mabb et al., 2011; Huang et al., 2012) and Prader–Willi syndrome (Miyake et al., 2012) show a defect in the active allele that leads to loss of gene expression. Such correlations provide compelling evidence for the role of genetic and epigenetic mechanisms in the etiology of ASD.

Additionally, DNA methylation is an important basic step in epigenetic gene control. Methyl-CpG binding proteins bind to the methylated DNA regions to control gene expression. Mutations in methyl-CpG binding protein 2 (MeCP2) cause Rett syndrome which shows characteristic autistic-like behavior in addition to seizures, ataxia, and stereotypic hand movements (Amir et al., 1999). More recently, MeCP2 was shown to regulate several genes involved in synaptic plasticity, neuronal cell proliferation and neuronal transcription factors including: brain-derived neurotrophic

Table 1 | Conserved genes implicated in ASD.

Gene	Protein description	Nature of abnormality	Reference
NRXN1	Transmembrane	Mutation, CNVs	Feng et al. (2006)
NRXN2	Transmembrane	Mutation	Arstikaitis et al. (2011)
NRXN3	Transmembrane	Mutation	Vaags et al. (2012)
NLGN1	Transmembrane	Genetic association	Glessner et al. (2009)
NLGN3	Transmembrane	Mutation	Jamain et al. (2003)
NLGN4	Transmembrane	Mutation, CNVs	Jamain et al. (2003)
CNTN3	Ig-CAM	Mutation, CNVs	Morrow et al. (2008)
CNTN 4	Ig-CAM	Mutation	Roohi et al. (2009)
CNTNAP2	Transmembrane	Mutation, genetic association	Arking et al. (2008)
NrCAM	Ig-CAM	Genetic association	Marui et al. (2009)
CDH9/10	Transmembrane	Genetic association	Bucan et al. (2009)
CDH18	Transmembrane	Chromosomal abnormality	Marshall et al. (2008)
PCDH9	Transmembrane	Mutation	Marshall et al. (2008)
PCDH10	Transmembrane	Mutation	Morrow et al. (2008)
PCDH19	Transmembrane	Mutation	Dibbens et al. (2008)
SHANK1	Scaffolding	Mutation	Sato et al. (2012)
SHANK2	Scaffolding	Mutation	Berkel et al. (2010)
SHANK3	Scaffolding	Mutation	Durand et al. (2007)
DLG4 (disk large homolog 4)	Scaffolding	SNPs	Feyder et al. (2010)
HOMER1	Scaffolding	Mutation	Kelleher et al. (2012)
cAMP-GEF (guanine exchange factor)	Cytoskeletal	Mutation	Bacchelli et al. (2003)
RELN (Reelin)	Secreted	Genetic association	Persico et al. (2001)
EN2 (Engrailed 2)	Transcription factor	Genetic association	Gharani et al. (2004)

factor (BDNF), distal-less homeobox 5 (DlX5), and insulin-like growth factor binding protein 3 (IGF3; Chen et al., 2003; Martinowich et al., 2003; reviewed in Miyake et al., 2012). Thus, epigenetic misregulation of synaptic genes could potentially contribute to ASD (Beaudet, 2007). Yet another set of studies suggest that extrinsic factors like the environment can alter epigenetic make up leading to defective neuronal functions (Jessberger et al., 2007; Ma et al., 2009b).

ENVIRONMENT AND OTHER FACTORS

Environmental contributions and other modulating factors are emerging as potential risk factors for ASD. Heavy metals, parental age, immunological proteins, environmental pesticides and insecticides, and food contaminants are thought to act as modulators of ASD (Durkin et al., 2008). These factors could contribute toward an increase in the prevalence of ASD but may not be sufficient to cause ASD. Nonetheless, a major challenge is to identify environmental factors relevant to ASD that could influence susceptibility, severity, and intervention outcomes. Heritable genetic vulnerabilities can magnify the adverse effects triggered by environmental factors. If both genes and environment converge, a resulting dysfunction of neurotransmitters and signaling pathways could take place at key developmental time points (Pessah et al., 2008). The toxicological literature point toward several environmental chemicals of concern to human health that can either directly or indirectly affect signaling pathways impaired in ASD.

Prenatal exposure to certain pesticides and insecticides are known to inhibit acetylcholine (ACh) and γ-aminobutyric acid (GABA; Shelton et al., 2012). Studies show these neurotransmitter systems are altered in a subset of autistic individuals. Similarly, environmentally induced alterations in calcium signaling pathways caused by organic pollutants, impact a broad range of neurotransmitter systems like the cholinergic, GABAergic, and dopaminergic systems (Pessah et al., 2008; Corrales and Herbert, 2011). In addition to disruptions in important neuronal signaling pathways, pesticides can cause oxidative stress, neuroinflammation, and mitochondrial dysfunction, all contributors to neuronal cell-death and dysfunction (Herbert, 2010; Shelton et al., 2012). Furthermore, cytokine-mediated influences and immune-related proteins are also listed as modulating factors for ASD (Ashwood et al., 2011; Onore et al., 2012). Families with ASD often show clustering of autoimmune disorders (Croen et al., 2005; Currenti, 2010). Several reports indicate the presence of serum antibody reactivity against human cortical and cerebellar regions of the brain in autistic patients (Silva et al., 2004). This process is thought to begin *in utero* and is associated with placental transfer of maternal autoantibodies to neuronal proteins potentially leading to neuronal dysfunction.

ANIMAL MODELS OF AUTISM SPECTRUM DISORDERS

Autism spectrum disorder is a complex disorder with no singular pathology and because of this a collective and collaborative approach is the key to understanding its etiology and design of rational interventions. Studies in animals are aimed at modeling the core phenotypes associated with ASD, including communication and social impairments, restricted interests, and repetitive behaviors in an attempt to uncover the mechanisms that underscore the entire spectrum of the disorder. In this section, we will uncover the wide range of both invertebrate and vertebrate model systems utilized by researchers that have collectively made significant contributions toward understanding the mechanisms that underlie ASD (summarized in **Table 3**).

NON-HUMAN PRIMATES

One of the animal models largely believed to help bridge the gap between humans and lower vertebrate systems is the non-human primate (NHP) model. NHP model is relevant for understanding ASD due to its high degree of correspondence to human behavior and their striking homology in the anatomy of neural circuits that mediate social behavior (for review, see Ongur and Price, 2000; Watson and Platt, 2012). Some of the behavioral correlates that NHPs have with human behavioral deficits seen in ASD include repetitive behaviors (Lutz et al., 2003; Alarcon et al., 2008), social communication (Ghazanfar and Santos, 2004), and their ability to follow other's gazes, a tendency that is compromised in Autism. For example, ablation studies in NHPs especially of the superior temporal sulcus region reveal difficulties in responding to social cues like eye gaze (Campbell et al., 1990). The lesion model involving the amygdala in NHPs is used to study alterations in socio-emotional behaviors (Amaral et al., 2003). Some papers speculate on the involvement of mirror neurons in the development of ASD (Oberman et al., 2005). In early childhood development, mirror neurons may play a key role in mimicking behaviors, actions, and language. A failure in the development or proper organization of mirror neurons might be linked to some of the behavioral phenotypes associated with ASD (Williams et al., 2001). NHP, like humans, possess mirror neurons and their use as a model system could provide some insight into the involvement of mirror neurons in ASD. NHP models are also used to investigate immunological factors in the etiology of ASD. Autoantibodies present in children with ASD have prompted investigators to analyze the affects of maternal IgG antibodies on the fetal brain during gestation. Injections of IgG antibodies from human mothers who had multiple children with ASD to pregnant rhesus monkeys resulted in abnormal stereotyped behaviors in offspring, and increased activity of offspring compared to controls (Martin et al., 2008). Although use of NHP model has the capability of contributing to some of the more behavioral aspects of ASD research, the absence of genetic knockouts in NHPs modeling ASD together with the careful considerations of ethical implications of NHP research tend to pose limitations that can be better addressed using rodents and invertebrate model systems.

RODENTS

Mouse models recapitulating symptoms of ASD through selective manipulations of genes and neural circuitry is a much more amenable model system compared to NHP models. Currently, there is a sizeable number of autism mouse models available made possible due to generation of specific gene knockouts; mutations in these genes are thought to contribute to ASD together with the emergence of CNVs and high-end genome-wide sequencing studies. Mouse models of human disorders have limitations in recapitulating the entire phenotypic spectrum (Arguello and Gogos, 2006). The validity of mouse models of human disorders are based on three criteria: (i) construct validity as provided by knock outs that carry a mutation in a gene that is affected in the human disorder (Peca et al., 2011a), (ii) face validity as reflected in animals that bear many of the core and ancillary physical or behavioral resemblances to the human disorder (Crawley, 2004), and (iii) predictive validity, which by far, is the most challenging to accomplish and indicates a similar response in the mouse model to an intervention that is known to be effective in human patients with that disorder.

Some of the mouse models representing syndromic forms of ASD include mice modeling Phelan–McDermid syndrome (SHANK3; Bangash et al., 2011; Peca et al., 2011a), Rett syndrome (MeCP2; Shahbazian et al., 2002; Moretti et al., 2006), fragile X syndrome (FMR1; Ronesi et al., 2012), Timothy syndrome (TS; CACNA1C; Bader et al., 2011), and others (see also **Table 2**). Neuroligin 3 knock out mice serve as a model for non-syndromic

Table 2 | Genetic syndromes with ASD-related phenotypes.

Syndrome	Chromosome	Genes	Reference
Angelman	15q11	Ube3A	Nurmi et al. (2001)
Phelan–McDermid	22q13	Shank3	Durand et al. (2007)
Rett	Xq28	MeCP2	Amir et al. (1999)
Tuberous sclerosis	9q34	TSC1	Baker et al. (1998), Smalley (1998)
	16p13	TSC2	
Timothy	16p13	CACNA1C	Splawski et al. (2004)
Fragile X	Xq27	FMR1	Rogers et al. (2001)
Cortical dysplasia-focal epilepsy syndrome	7q35	CNTNAP2	Arking et al. (2008)
Smith–Lemli–Opitz	11q13	DHCR7	Tierney et al. (2001)

Table 3 | Phenotypic analyses and relevant animal models of ASD.

Phenotype	Animal models								
	Non-human primate	Mouse	Rat	Prairie vole	Songbird	Zebrafish	*Drosophila*	*Aplysia*	*C. elegans*
Genetic analyses		+	+			+	+	+	+
Molecular analyses		+	+		+	+	+	+	+
Hyperactivity and repetitive behavior	+	+	+						
Social communication	+	+	+	+	+				
Cognition		+	+						
Impaired vocalization		+			+				

autism (Baudouin et al., 2012). Other examples of mouse models to study characteristics of ASD include Purkinje-specific knock out of TSC1 (Tsai et al., 2012), chromosome-engineered mouse model for human 15q11-13 (Nakatani et al., 2009), model for 16p11.2 lesion found in autism (Horev et al., 2011), 22q11.2 mice lacking PTEN (Zhou et al., 2009), CNTNAP2 (Penagarikano et al., 2011), SHANK2 (Won et al., 2012), and SCN1A (Han et al., 2012). The impressive array of mouse models displaying behaviors that are reflective of the human behavioral and cognitive ASD symptoms is highly informative. On the other hand, the behavioral phenotypes between mouse models with ablation of the same gene show variations based on either their genetic backgrounds (Crabbe et al., 1999), or how individual laboratories conduct their behavioral assays further underscoring the impact of the genetic background or the local environment on the displayed phenotypes. In any case, a complete understanding of the similarities and differences in the behavioral phenotypes across the ASD mouse models will provide key insights into the underlying neural circuitry behind these behaviors.

Other emerging rodent models of ASD include rat and prairie vole (McGraw and Young, 2010). Rats that are injected with valproic acid (VPA) serve as an environmentally triggered model of autism and this method has emerged as a new way to study ASD in rats (Rodier et al., 1997). VPA injected to gestational mothers before neural tube closure causes autistic-like phenotypes in offspring such as a reduction in the number of cerebellar Purkinje cells and disruption in inhibitory circuits (Gogolla et al., 2009). Furthermore, these animals show similar behavioral phenotypes

Table 4 | Receptors, transporters, and channel proteins in ASD.

Gene	Gene name	Genetic abnormality	Reference
AGTR2	Angiotensin II receptor, type 2	Mutation	Vervoort et al. (2002)
ADRB2	Adrenergic β-2 receptor	Genetic association	Cheslack-Postava et al. (2007)
AVPR1A	Arginine vasopressin receptor 1A	Mutation, genetic association	Yirmiya et al. (2006)
DRD3	Dopamine receptor D3	Genetic association	de Krom et al. (2009)
ESRRB	Estrogen-related receptor β	Genetic association	Wang et al. (2009)
GABRB3	GABA A receptor, β3	Genetic association	Cook et al. (1998)
GABR4/GABRB1	GABA A receptor, α4/β1	Genetic association	Ma et al. (2005)
GRIP1	Glutamate receptor interacting protein	Mutation, genetic association	Mejias et al. (2011)
GRIK2	Glutamate receptor, kainate 2	Genetic association	Jamain et al. (2002)
GRIN2A	Glutamate receptor, ionotropic, *N*-methyl D-aspartate 2A	Mutation	Barnby et al. (2005)
GRIN2B	Glutamate recepto14r, ionotropic, *N*-methyl D-aspartate 2B	Mutation	O'Roak et al. (2011)
GRID1	Glutamate receptor, δ1	Mutation	Glessner et al. (2009)
GRID2	Glutamate receptor, δ2	Mutation	Schaaf et al. (2011)
GRM5	Glutamate receptor metabotropic 5	Mutation	Iossifov et al. (2012)
OXTR	Oxytocin receptor	Genetic association	Wu et al. (2005)
SL6A4	Solute carrier family 6 (serotonin transporter)	Genetic association	Sutcliffe et al. (2005)
SLC25A13	Solute carrier family 25 (aspartate-glutamate carrier)	Genetic association	Ramoz et al. (2004)
CACNA1C	Calcium channel, α1B subunit	Mutation	Splawski et al. (2004)
SCN1A/SCN2A	Sodium channel, α subunit	Mutation	Weiss et al. (2003)
KCNJ10	Potassium channel subfamily	Genetic association	Sicca et al. (2011)

associated with autism including lower sensitivity to pain and higher sensitivity to non-painful stimuli, repetitive behaviors, hyperactivity, and decreased number of social behaviors. They also show delayed mental impairments and lower body weight (Schneider and Przewlocki, 2005; Favre et al., 2013). Prairie voles also generated interest in the area of ASD because of their ability to form lasting social bonds and their nurturing behavior. Impaired social behaviors and deficits in various aspects of social cognition are some of the signature of ASD in humans. Thus, development of genetic, molecular, and genomic tools in prairie vole will likely be useful in basic and translational research that may be relevant to ASD (McGraw and Young, 2010).

ZEBRAFISH

Zebrafish are widely used as a model for studying vertebrate development and although not as popular as the mouse model for studying ASD, zebrafish are being used to dissect the genetic basis of autism due to a multitude of genetic techniques available. These include lineage tracing using fluorescent tracers or labeling cells with lipophilic dyes, loss of function analyses using chemicals, transposable elements, and gain of function assays such as those involving microinjection of synthetic mRNA. In addition, morpholino technology is widely used as an efficient reverse genetic approach to understand gene function (Tropepe and Sive, 2003). Furthermore, fast oogenesis and embryogenesis, and high fecundity allows for rapid experimental assays in this model. Transparency and external development of embryos allows for the study of growth and development of cells and tissues in live embryos (Tropepe and Sive, 2003). Additionally, zebrafish are an excellent model for use in carrying out genetic screens to identify new genes of interest and are useful in designing genetic screens to uncover specific enhancers or suppressors of particular phenotype (Dooley and Zon, 2000). These screens identified several candidate genes, such as Reelin and MET that confers susceptibility to human ASD in zebrafish (Rice and Curran, 2001). The presence of structurally and functionally homologous regions in zebrafish brain, which are perturbed in human autistic patients, is another avenue that zebrafish researchers are taking advantage of to study brain development and neuronal connections. Although zebrafish is an excellent model to study some of the genetic aspects of ASD, the behavioral phenotypes associated with ASD are difficult to recapitulate (Tropepe and Sive, 2003). Thus, other model systems might be useful in studying some of the behavioral phenotypes associated with ASD.

SONGBIRDS

Songbirds can be used both as a molecular and a behavioral model for understanding the etiology of ASD. Songbirds are socially sophisticated and display characteristically human traits like monogamy and cultural inheritance while demonstrating the ability to learn vocalizations (Clayton et al., 2009). Vocal learning is an important element of language. Impairments in vocal and language learning are some of the core deficits in autism. Thus, understanding vocal learning through songbirds has emerged as an important model to study some aspects of ASD.

Speech in humans and bird songs display striking parallels in that both seem to have a critical developmental time window for learning, a homologous underlying neural circuitry involving a loop between the cerebral cortex, basal ganglia, and thalamus, and a role for social influences in the learning of vocalizations (Panaitof, 2012). Studies from songbird indicate that CNTNAP2, which is implicated in human ASD and is enriched in human language related neural circuits (Alarcon et al., 2008), might play a role in vocal communication in songbirds as well (Panaitof et al., 2010). Similar to developing human brain where CNTNAP2 shows a gradient distribution in frontal cortical areas, Cntnap2 expression is either enhanced or reduced in key song control nuclei in songbird brain. In the absence of an animal model that can address language deficits, songbird model may prove useful for further exploration of the cellular and molecular mechanisms underlying the homologous neural circuitry that underscore language development in humans. Recently, using microarray and *in situ* hybridization analyses, large databases have been compiled that reveal expression patterns of certain genes in specific regions of the brain (Warren et al., 2010). Expansion on the molecular aspects of these observations has further increased the validity of behavioral songbird research. While linking behavior and genetics in songbirds is a tall order, it might still provide important clues about neuronal circuitry and language acquisition in the complex and heterogeneous nature of ASD and its behavioral manifestations.

INVERTEBRATE MODELS

Despite being millions of years apart on the evolutionary scale there is a surprising degree of genetic conservation between invertebrates and humans. Invertebrate models have made seminal contributions toward a basic understanding of human neurological disorders that are hard to ignore. One such classic invertebrate model for studying human neurodevelopmental disorders is the fruit fly, *Drosophila*. The fruit fly has proven to be an important model time and again to study various disorders where a single, causative genetic defect has been identified in Rett syndrome (Cukier et al., 2008), fragile X syndrome (Morales et al., 2002), and Angelman syndrome (Wu et al., 2008; see also **Table 2**). *Drosophila* studies have advanced our fundamental understanding of some of these human disease gene functions, which show features of ASD. Recent studies in *Drosophila* have started to unravel some of the key genes, such as Neurexin 1 (Li et al., 2007; Zeng et al., 2007), Neuroligin 1 (Banovic et al., 2010), and Neuroligin 2 (Chen et al., 2012), which are the fly homologs of human NRXNs and NLGNs, respectively, that are implicated in ASD (De Jaco et al., 2005; Sudhof, 2008). With the unmatched power of *Drosophila* genetics and the potential of carrying out large scale screens using the sophisticated genetic tools available, *Drosophila* will undoubtedly continue to provide key mechanistic insights to dissect the genetic basis of ASD and likely facilitate the design of therapeutics. Apart from *Drosophila*, other invertebrate models that are being used to study aspects of ASD are *C. elegans* (Calahorro and Ruiz-Rubio, 2011, 2012) and *Aplysia* (Choi et al., 2011; Ye and Carew, 2011).

A recent study in *Aplysia* showed that trans-synaptic Neurexin–Neuroligin interactions govern synaptic remodeling and regulates signaling required for the storage of long-term memory, including emotional memory, an ability that is affected in ASD patients

(Choi et al., 2011). This study showed that long-term facilitation and associated pre-synaptic growth were compromised when neurexin or neuroligin was depleted from pre- and post-synaptic machineries. In addition, an introduction of R451C mutation of NLGN3 associated with human ASD blocked both intermediate- and long-term facilitation in *Aplysia* (Choi et al., 2011).

Another genetically tractable animal model is the nematode, *C. elegans*, which are utilized to understand the underlying mechanisms and abnormalities in neuronal synaptic communications in complex human neurological disorders like Alzheimer's and ASD (Calahorro and Ruiz-Rubio, 2012). *C. elegans* have orthologs for ASD-related genes such as *NLGNs*, *NRXNs*, and *SHANK*. Recent reports highlight behavioral phenotypes in *C. elegans* reminiscent of ASD following removal of neuroligin homolog, nlg-1 (Hunter et al., 2010; Calahorro and Ruiz-Rubio, 2012) and subsequent functional phenotypic rescue by human NLGN1 (Calahorro and Ruiz-Rubio, 2012). Additionally, trans-synaptic NRX-1 and NLG-1 in *C. elegans* are found to mediate retrograde synaptic inhibition of neurotransmitter release at the neuromuscular junction (Hu et al., 2012) further underscoring the function of these molecules in synaptic modulation.

Thus determining the biological underpinnings of ASD will require a concerted effort involving studies from human clinical populations and several different animal models. This effort will provide complementary and critical insights toward understanding the complex and unknown ASD etiology. Since testing the causality and exploring the molecular and cellular mechanisms of ASD are either severely limited or off limits in human populations, research using various animal models will provide clues to the range of functional deficits that cause the disorder and may even hint at the underlying neural circuits that drive the behavioral deficits.

GENES IMPLICATED IN ASD

With the growing repertoire of synaptic genes implicated in ASD, it is becoming increasingly clear that synaptic dysfunction at multiple levels may underlie ASD. Synapses comprise of pre- and post-synaptic elements (**Figure 1**; see also review by Delorme et al., 2013) like synaptic cell adhesion molecules (CAMs), ion channels, neurotransmitter receptors, scaffolding and cytoskeletal proteins that work harmoniously to provide synaptic structural integrity and functionality (refer **Tables 1** and **4**). Perturbations in synaptic assembly or function are commonly reported in many neuropsychiatric disorders (Blanpied and Ehlers, 2004).

CELL ADHESION MOLECULES

Neuroligins

Neuroligins (NLGNs) are post-synaptic CAMs localized at glutamatergic or GABAergic synapses (Song et al., 1999; Varoqueaux et al., 2004). NLGNs have a large extracellular cholinesterase-like domain, and a small intracellular domain with PDZ-binding motif. There are five NLGNs, which include two X-linked genes (*NlgN3* and *NlgN4X*) and one Y-linked (*NlgN4Y*). The identification of ASD-linked mutations in NLGN3 and NLGN4X was an important finding that implicated these genes in the etiology of ASD (Jamain et al., 2003) and linked ASD to molecules with synaptic function. *In vitro* studies using mutant forms of *NlgN3* and *NlgN4X* showed retention of the mutant proteins in endoplasmic reticulum resulting in reduced cell surface binding to Neurexin (NRXN; Chih et al., 2004; Comoletti et al., 2004; Boucard et al., 2005). Some of the mutations of NLGNs seen in ASD patients were generated in mice and other model systems. For example, *NlgN3* R451C knock-in mice showed challenged social interactions, enhanced inhibitory synaptic transmission, and altered spatial learning abilities (Jamain et al., 2003; Tabuchi et al., 2007; Chadman et al., 2008). This arginine to cysteine point mutation at the analogous position as the human NLGN3 R451C was recently made in *Aplysia* revealing abnormal synaptic facilitation (Choi et al., 2011). *NLGN3* knock out mice showed reduced ultrasound vocalization together and a lack of social novelty preference (Radyushkin et al., 2009). *NlgN4* knock out mice displayed reduced reciprocal social interactions and vocalizations consistent with observations in human ASD patients (Jamain et al., 2008). Studies on *NlgN1* knock out mice showed impaired NMDA receptor signaling, while *NlgN2* knock out mutants revealed reduced inhibitory synaptic transmission (Chubykin et al., 2007). Studies in vertebrate and invertebrates alike have now established that NLGNs are essential for proper synapse maturation, maintenance, and function as opposed to initial synapse formation (Chih et al., 2005; Varoqueaux et al., 2006; Sudhof, 2008; Banovic et al., 2010; Chen et al., 2012).

Recent studies on null mutants of *Drosophila neuroligin 2* (*dnlg2*), which is the fly homolog of human *NlgN3* showed reduced synaptic bouton numbers and synaptic transmission (Chen et al., 2012). Interestingly, *dnlg2* is required both pre- and post-synaptically for proper synapse structure and function. Another study in *C. elegans* reported presence of Neuroligin at both pre- and post-synaptic regions (Feinberg et al., 2008). These studies highlight the exceptions to the traditional role and localization of NLGNs at the post-synaptic terminals as seen at most vertebrate synapses. It also raises interesting questions about how synaptic organization might be fine tuned, and how signaling pathways might regulate the expression of pre- and post-synaptic proteins during synaptic development and function. Thus, studies on NLGNs using various model systems will provide key insights into how these synaptic CAMs are involved in human ASD.

Neurexins

Neurexins (NRXNs) are predominantly presynaptic CAMs (Ichtchenko et al., 1995), although they were also reported to be expressed post-synaptically (Taniguchi et al., 2007). There are three *Nrxn* genes, *Nrxn1*, *Nrxn2*, and *Nrxn3*, each of which encode α- and β-isoforms. The α-Neurexin extracellular domain consists of six LNS domains interspersed by three EGF-like repeats and interacts with various proteins in the synaptic cleft. Mouse knock out mutants of individual Nrxns do not show gross abnormalities in synaptic ultrastructure or in synapse number while triple α-Nrxn knock out mice die prenatally due to respiratory complications. These mice show impaired synaptic transmission, but not synapse formation suggesting that like their Nlgn ligands, α-NRXNs are required for proper synaptic maintenance and function, and not initial synapse formation (Missler et al., 2003).

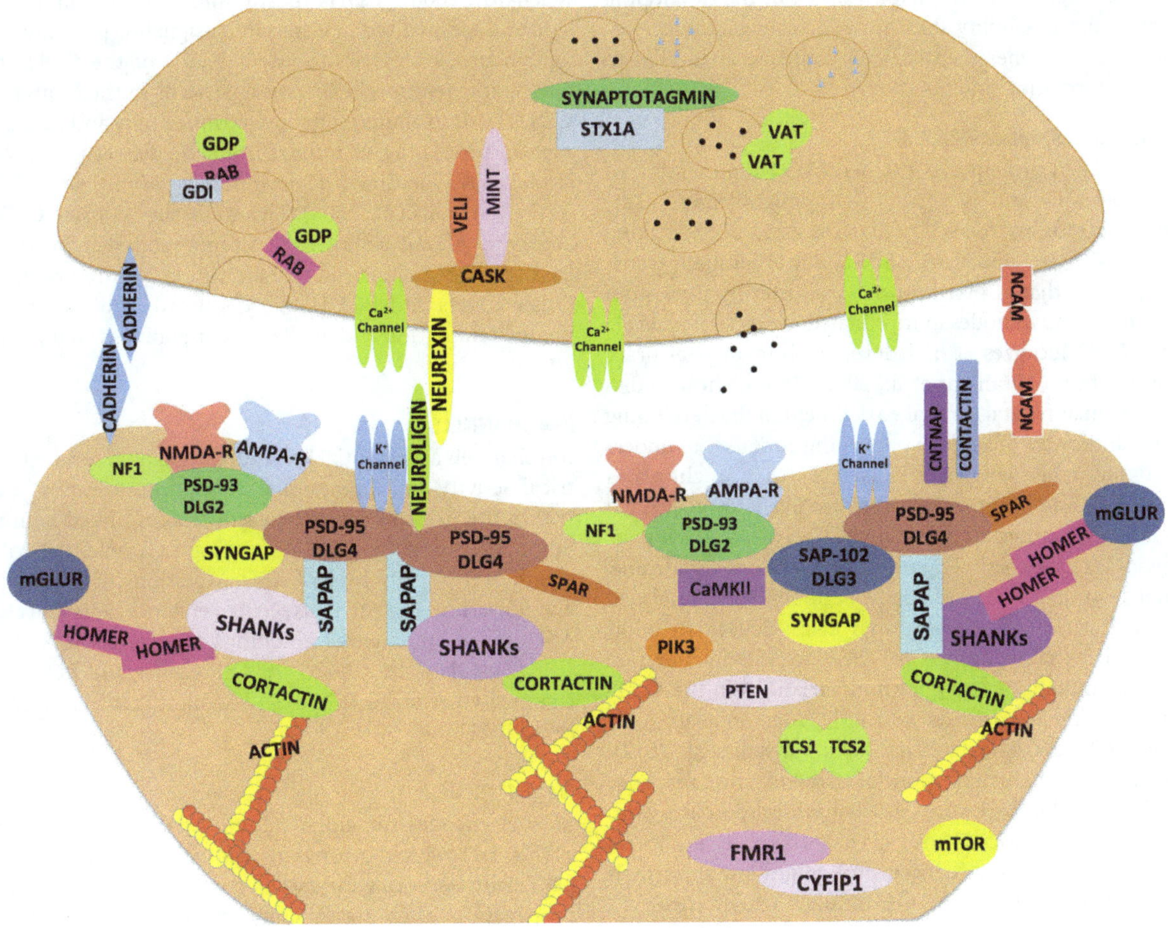

FIGURE 1 | Synaptic proteins implicated in neurodevelopmental and neuropsychiatric disorders. A schematic illustration of an ensemble of pre- and post-synaptic proteins. The majority of these proteins are highly conserved across species, and thought to confer susceptibility to a host of neurodevelopmental and neuropsychiatric disorders including ASD. The cellular machinery of synapses is comprised of transmembrane heterophilic (such as Neurexin and Neuroligin) and homophilic cell-adhesion molecules (such as Cadherins and NCAM), cytoplasmic scaffolding proteins (such as PSD-95, Cask, and Shank) and cytoskeletal proteins (such as Homer and Cortactin) that link transmembrane and membrane-associated protein complexes with the underlying actin cytoskeleton. One of the emerging models in ASD is based on synaptic dysfunction in a molecular pathway that is orchestrated by trans-synaptic Neurexin–Neuroligin-dependent proteins complexes. This molecular assembly aligns the pre- and post-synaptic apparatus facilitating functional activation and modulation of ion channels that are in proximity to the neurotransmitter containing synaptic vesicles on the pre-synaptic side. These protein complexes recruit other proteins both pre- and post-synaptically and help organize functional neural networks. The cytoskeletal scaffolding protein Cask is one such notable protein which binds to the C-terminus of Neurexin. At the post-synaptic density, Neuroligin binds to PSD-95, other molecules such as PSD-93, SAP97, and the SAPAP family of proteins as well as the Shank family of scaffolding proteins help orchestrate the post-synaptic area. Homer and Shank function is thought to stabilize the post-synaptic density and serve as a platform to incorporate the post-synaptic receptors (such as NMDAR, AMPAR, and mGluR) into the machinery. The synaptic dysfunction in ASD may occur at multiple levels whereby failure to organize proper protein–protein interactions at the synapse may compromise neuronal functions (*refer text for more details*).

Pre-synaptic calcium channel function is also disrupted in α-*Nrxn* knock out mice. Interestingly, compared to three NRXNs in mammals, *Drosophila* has a single *neurexin-1* (*dnrx*) gene which like its vertebrate counterparts is pre-synaptic and is required for proper synaptic growth and neurotransmission (Li et al., 2007).

NRXN1 has emerged as a strong candidate in ASD since the identification of overlapping *de novo* deletions in *Nrxn1* in individuals with ASD. Although rare, missense mutations (Feng et al., 2006; Kim et al., 2008) and deletions, and chromosomal aberrations in the *NRXN1* were also found in ASD patients (Marshall et al., 2008; Zahir et al., 2008; Glessner et al., 2009). Interestingly, NRXN1 deletions also confer risk for schizophrenia pointing to an overlap between the two neurodevelopmental disorders (Betancur et al., 2009; Rujescu et al., 2009).

Contactins

The Contactins (CNTNs) are glycosyl phosphatidyl-inositol (GPI) anchored immunoglobulin (Ig) superfamily proteins with diverse functions ranging from myelination (Berglund et al., 1999; Bhat et al., 2001) to synapse formation and plasticity (Betancur et al., 2009). Disruption of *CNTN4* is associated with ASD (Fernandez et al., 2004). Deletion and duplication in *CNTN4* and small deletions near *CNTN3* have been identified in various patients with ASD (Roohi et al., 2009). Since *CNTN3* and *CNTN4* expression and localization overlaps with synaptogenesis in the developing brain, it raises the possibility that mutations or genomic rearrangements in these genes seen in ASD could be attributed to altered synapse formation and function.

Contactin-associated protein like 2

Contactin-associated protein like 2 (CNTNAP2) is a member of Neurexin superfamily and is a locus that is significantly associated with susceptibility for ASD (Alarcon et al., 2008; Arking et al., 2008). *CNTNAP2* encodes CASPR2, a multidomain transmembrane protein that is best known for clustering potassium channels at the juxtaparanodes in myelinated axons (Poliak et al., 2003). CNTNAP2 localizes at high levels in human fetal brain prior to myelination (Abrahams et al., 2007). It also shows a distribution gradient as frontal cortical enrichment in the developing human brain, indicative of a role in patterning circuits that underlie higher cognition and language. Thus, *CNTNAP2* might play a role in the developing brain regions that are likely to be affected in ASD. A recessive frameshift mutation in *CNTNAP2* was identified in individuals with cortical dysplasia focal epilepsy syndrome, a congenital disorder, where majority of individuals displayed characteristic features of ASD (Strauss et al., 2006). In addition, other studies that attribute *CNTNAP2* to ASD include rare single base pair mutations and common variations in the *CNTNAP2* locus identified in patients with ASD (Alarcon et al., 2008; Arking et al., 2008; Bakkaloglu et al., 2008; Falivelli et al., 2012). Recent phenotypic characterization of *Cntnap2* mutant mice revealed deficits in the three core ASD behavioral domains with hyperactivity and epileptic seizures (Penagarikano et al., 2011). These mutant mice also showed neuronal migration abnormalities, a significant reduction in the number of interneurons, and abnormal neuronal network activity before the onset of seizures. Most importantly, treatment with the FDA-approved drug risperidone led to amelioration of the repetitive behaviors in the mutant mice further demonstrating a functional role for CNTNAP2 in neuronal development and opening of new avenues for therapeutic intervention in ASD (Penagarikano et al., 2011).

NrCAM

NrCAM is a CAM that has gene homology to NgCAM and is capable of homophilic cell adhesion as well as heterophilic interactions with other non-NrCAM molecules such as Contactin-1, Contactin-2/TAG1, and Neurofascin (Suter et al., 1995; Volkmer et al., 1996; Pavlou et al., 2002). More recently, association analysis has linked NrCAM to ASD (Sakurai et al., 2006). This study showed over transmission of particular haplotypes of NrCAM that modulate NrCAM expression in the brain, are associated with a specific subset of autism with a severe obsessive–compulsive behavior. Several single nucleotide polymorphisms (SNPs) in the NrCAM gene were also found to be associated with autism (Marui et al., 2009) further underscoring NrCAM as a strong candidate gene in ASD.

Cadherins

Cadherins (CDH) and protocadherins (PCDH) include a large family of CAMs, a number of which are required for synaptic formation and function (Weiner et al., 2005; Arikkath and Reichardt, 2008). CDHs mostly undergo homophilic cell adhesion and are involved in intracellular signaling pathways associated with neuropsychiatric disorders. Many of the CDHs have specific spatio-temporal expression patterns in the brain and loss of CDHs leads to altered functional connectivity and neuronal information processing in human brain (Redies et al., 2012). Recent studies have identified *de novo* translocation deleting *CDH18* in ASD (Marshall et al., 2008). This study also reported CNVs associated with *PCDH9* gene in ASD. Homozygous deletions in *PCDH10* have also been shown in autistic children (Morrow et al., 2008). Other CDHs and PCDHs are disrupted in disorders related to mental retardation and intellectual disabilities (Weiner and Jontes, 2013).

ION CHANNELS

Ion channels are essential for regulating axonal conduction of electrical activity and maintaining the optimum level of excitability within the nervous system. Recent studies linked neuronal excitation alterations with ASD pointing to a potential role for ion channels in the etiology of ASD. Mutations in calcium, sodium, and potassium ion channels seem to enhance neuronal excitability. ASD-linked ion channel mutations involve the *SCN1A* ($Na_V1.1$), *CACNA1C* ($Ca_V1.2$), *KCNMA1* (BK Ca^{2+}), and *KCNJ10* (Kir4.1) channels (Ji et al., 2009; Liao and Soong, 2010; Li et al., 2011; Sicca et al., 2011).

$Na_V1.1$

SCN1A encodes the alpha subunit of the sodium channel type 1 ($Na_V1.1$) which belongs to the voltage-gated sodium channel family necessary for axonal conduction and action potential propagation. These transmembrane proteins possess a large pore-forming alpha subunit and two auxiliary beta subunits. This organization is important for allowing sodium ions to move through the axonal membrane to initiate and propagate action potentials. Recently, *SCN1A* has emerged as the most important gene in epilepsy (Mulley et al., 2005). More that 70% of individuals with epileptic encephalopathy posses a mutation in the region encoding SCN1A causing severe myoclonic epilepsy in infancy, also known as Dravet syndrome (DS; Harkin et al., 2007). This disorder is often accompanied by certain behavioral abnormalities such as hyperactivity, sleep-disorder, anxiety, attention deficit, impaired social interactions, restricted interests, and severe cognitive defects (Weiss et al., 2003; Ramoz et al., 2008; O'Roak et al., 2012). Such behaviors are very similar to those observed in patients with ASD and emerging evidence has linked SCNA1 and ASD (Li et al., 2011). Researchers found that mice with a loss of function mutation for *SCN1A* phenocopy DS and show autistic-like behaviors (Han et al., 2012). It was suggested that the autism-related traits in DS mice might be caused by a decrease in inhibitory neurotransmission in GABAergic interneurons due to SCN1A haploinsufficiency providing further evidence that impaired GABAergic signaling may underlie ASD (Chao et al., 2010).

$Ca_V1.2$

The calcium channels, voltage-dependent, L type, alpha 1C subunit, also known as $Ca_V1.2$ encoded by the gene *CACNA1C* has been implicated in ASD. $Ca_V 1.2$ channels are important in the activation of transcription factors and play a key role in promoting neuronal survival and dendritic arborization (Krey and Dolmetsch, 2007). A mutation in the G406R region of the CACNA1C gene is known to cause TS, a rare genetic disorder that results in malformations of multi-organ systems, neurological and developmental defects, and autism (Liao and Soong, 2010). The mutation in this region causes prolonged inward current and has dramatic effects on calcium channel inactivation (Splawski et al., 2004). The cellular and molecular consequences of this mutation are not yet known. Future studies should address the physiological relationship between calcium channel inactivation and ASD.

Kir4.1 and BKCa

Recent studies have linked potassium channel proteins Kir4.1 and BKCa to ASD. Mutational screens identified several missense mutations in the *KCNJ10* region encoding the potassium ion channel Kir4.1. This ATP sensitive inward rectifier type potassium channel is characterized by having a greater tendency to allow potassium ions to flow into the cell and is suggested to be responsible for the buffering action of glial cells in the brain. Individuals who possess a mutation in the region show symptoms consistent with the DSM-IV-TR criteria for ASD along with seizure and intellectual disability (Sicca et al., 2011). BKCa is a potassium channel known for its large conductance of potassium ions across cell membranes. The gene *KCNMA1* encodes BKCa. which is thought to function as a synaptic regulator of neuronal excitability which seems to be disrupted in patients with ASD (Laumonnier et al., 2006). Disruption of this gene caused a decrease in BKCa channel activity and haploinsufficiency in Autism patients further implicating excessive ion channel activity to ASD (Ji et al., 2009).

SCAFFOLDING PROTEINS

Scaffolding proteins are essential molecules of the synaptic architecture. They are enriched in post-synaptic densities (PSDs) and function in synapse biogenesis by trafficking and anchoring synaptic proteins and clustering of membrane-associated proteins. Most importantly, the scaffolding proteins serve to link post-synaptic receptors with their downstream signaling components and regulate cytoskeletal dynamics (Verpelli et al., 2012).

Shank

Shank protein family is one such synaptic scaffolding family of proteins that includes Shank1, Shank2, and Shank3. They have multiple protein–protein interaction domains and are also known as proline-rich synapse-associated proteins (ProSAPs). Shank proteins are enriched in PSDs and stabilize the PSD-95/SAPAP/Shank/Homer complex (Tu et al., 1999; Sala et al., 2001). Additionally, Shank interacts with NMDA receptors/PSD-95/GKAP complex and actin regulatory protein, Cortactin (Naisbitt et al., 1999; refer **Figure 1**). Strong genetic and molecular evidence has linked *SHANK2* and *SHANK3* to the development of ASD phenotypes.

SHANK2

Mutations in *ProSAP1/Shank2* gene result in an upregulation of glutamate receptors in certain brain regions, an increase in Shank3 at the synapse, and a decrease in dendritic spine morphology and synaptic transmission (Schmeisser et al., 2012). *ProSAP/Shank2* mutants also display behavioral phenotypes that are consistent with those seen in ASD. *Shank2* mutant mice are hyperactive, exhibit repetitive grooming, and have impairments in social and vocal behaviors (Schmeisser et al., 2012). Such phenotypic manifestations are linked to the reduction of NMDAR function that results from the absence of the Shank2 protein (Won et al., 2012). Human studies using microarray analyses have identified several variants in *SHANK2* that are associated with ASD and mental retardation (Berkel et al., 2010).

SHANK3

Shank3 is an important member of Shank family of proteins and interacts with NLGN (Gerrow et al., 2006) to play a key role in spine morphogenesis and synaptic plasticity (Sala et al., 2001). Recent studies on Shank3 using knockout mice suggest its involvement in the regulation of glutamatergic synapse size, shape, and structure (Jiang and Ehlers, 2013). In *Shank3* knockout mice, synaptic ultrastructure is compromised. Overall, shank3 loss leads to a reduction in spine volume, decreased PSD thickness, and loss of dendritic spines (Bozdagi et al., 2010; Peca et al., 2011a; Wang et al., 2011; Jiang and Ehlers, 2013). Furthermore, *Shank3* knockout mice show abnormal social behaviors, communication patterns, repetitive behaviors, and impairments in learning and memory (Bozdagi et al., 2010; Peca et al., 2011a; Wang et al., 2011).

There is growing evidence of the involvement of Shank3 in ASD. Molecular characterization of individuals with 22q13.3 deletion syndrome that display autism behavior identified a deletion disrupting *Shank3* among other genes (Wilson et al., 2003). Haploinsufficiency of *Shank3* has been confirmed to account for 22q13 deletion phenotype of developmental and speech delays (Durand et al., 2007). Other studies that attributed a role of Shank3 in ASD include identification of *de novo* splice site mutation in ASD (Gauthier et al., 2009). More recently, Shank3 mutations identified in patients with ASD show a modification in dendritic spine induction and morphology as well as actin accumulation in spines affecting growth cone motility (Durand et al., 2007). Furthermore, a microdeletion in *Shank1* locus has been discovered using microarray analysis in individuals with ASD (Sato et al., 2012). Recent studies have further uncovered the functional role of Shank3 as *Shank3* duplication in mice leads to hyperactivity and spontaneous seizures much like human subjects who have small duplications in the *SHANK3* locus. These recent studies further underscore the function of Shank3 in neuronal function and possibly in the maintenance of a balance between the excitatory and inhibitory (E/I) synaptic mechanisms (Han et al., 2013).

SynGAP1

SynGAP1 encodes the RAS GTPase-activating protein (GAPs) which is a critical component of the PSD. At the PSD, SynGAP1 regulates synapse development and maintenance of proper synaptic function. It is known to interact with PSD-95 and colocalizes with excitatory NMDA receptor complexes (Chen et al., 1998). SynGAP is shown to play a critical role in the PSD during early postnatal development as SYNGAP1 knockout mice for die during early development (Kim et al., 2003). Furthermore, mice heterozygous for SynGAP1 show impairments in learning and memory consistent with its involvement in NMDA receptor complexes (Komiyama et al., 2002). In humans, sequencing of the *SYNGAP1* locus revealed mutations linked to non-syndromic mental retardation evidencing the importance of SynGAP in synaptic plasticity and learning (Hamdan et al., 2009). SynGap1 was recently implicated ASD because many of its key interacting partners including PSD-95/DLG4, SAP-102/DLG3, PSD-93/DLG2, Neurexins, and Neuroligins have previously been associated with ASD (van de Lagemaat and Grant, 2010). Recent evidence suggests that SynGAP may play a crucial role in controlling the E/I balance in cortical neurons through the regulation on ERK signaling pathways (Wang et al., 2013). This is interesting because the E/I balance seems to be altered in individuals with ASD (Eichler and Meier, 2008; Won et al., 2013). Further characterization of SynGAP as a regulator of synaptic function will provide additional insight into its involvement in ASD.

CYTOSKELETAL PROTEINS

A set of cytoskeletal proteins is also mutated in individuals with ASD. These include factors regulating dynamics of actin cytoskeleton, such as GAPs and guanosine exchange factors (GEFs; Newey et al., 2005). Rare non-synonymous variants in *cAMP-GEFII* are among candidate genes for autism in chromosome 2q (Bacchelli et al., 2003). Mutations in tumor suppressor genes *TSC1* and *TSC2* are also linked to ASD as the mutant proteins are thought to perturb cytoskeletal dynamics and dendritic spine structure in mutant animals (Folstein and Rosen-Sheidley, 2001). More recently, microtubule associated protein, KATNAL2, has emerged as a credible risk factor for ASD (Neale et al., 2012).

Apart from CAMs, scaffolding and cytoskeletal proteins, a host of other receptors, transporters and channel proteins are known to contribute toward the etiology of ASD (summarized in **Table 4**). Discovery of more and more genes and genetic pathways are expanding the genetic landscape of ASD. It is interesting to note that these genes include chromatin modifiers, DNA binding proteins, ion channels, and neurotransmitter receptors (State and Sestan, 2012). Recently, CNVs in new candidate genes within GABAergic signaling and neural development pathways associated with ASD were identified using genome wide SNP array (Griswold et al., 2012). These genes include an allosteric binder of GABA receptor, DB1, the GABA receptor-associated protein, GABARAPL1 and a post-synaptic GABA transporter, SLC6A11. Other genes contributing to the genetics of ASD include glutamate receptors, such as GRID1, GRIK2, and GRIK4, synaptic regulators, such as SLC6A8 and SYN3, and transcription factors, such as Engrailed 2 (EN2; Griswold et al., 2012).

SIGNALING PATHWAYS

Signaling pathways are a complex system of communication within cells that function to organize cellular activities. Signaling pathways and cascades have long been implicated in many disease models. Understanding signaling pathways may play a central role in developing pharmacological or other agents to better treat disease. Currently, disruptions in signaling pathways are being linked to the development of ASD phenotypes. One such pathway connected to ASD is the mammalian target of rapamycin (mTOR) pathway.

mTOR PATHWAY

Mammalian target of rapamycin is a serine/threonine protein kinase involved in the regulation of cell proliferation, cell growth, cell survival, protein synthesis, and transcription. The mTOR signaling cascade plays a very important role in synapse protein synthesis and several studies have linked this pathway to ASD (Hay and Sonenberg, 2004; Hoeffer and Klann, 2010). Many of the signaling components of the mTOR cascade are located at the synapses where they have been shown to regulate dendritic spine morphology and synaptogenesis (Kumar et al., 2005). Mutations in the proteins known to inhibit mTOR signaling including NF1, PTEN, TSC1, and TSC2 are all linked to neurological disease and autistic-like behavioral phenotypes (Williams and Hersh, 1998; Butler et al., 2005; Won et al., 2013). Furthermore, mutations in the downstream targets of the mTOR signaling cascade have been identified in patients with ASD. The mTOR signaling cascade works by the phosphorylation of 4E-BP by mTOR. This causes 4E-BP to dissociate from the eIF4E initiation factor resulting in cap-dependent translation and elongation of mRNA (Laplante and Sabatini, 2009; Wang and Doering, 2013). Genomic sequence analyses of the eIF4E promoter region identified a SNP in autism patients that enhanced the promoter activity of eIF4E (Neves-Pereira et al., 2009). Additionally, 4E-BP knockout mice as well as mice with an overexpression of eIF4E show autistic like behaviors, enhanced translational of Neuroligins, and disruptions in the E/I balance (Gkogkas et al., 2013; Won et al., 2013). Analyses of monogenetic sources of ASD found that approximately 8–10% of all ASD are involved in regulation of the mTOR pathway (Moldin et al., 2006; Kelleher and Bear, 2008; Hoeffer and Klann, 2010). Of those, 1–2% of ASD cases result due to a mutation in the gene encoding PTEN, an upstream member of the mTOR pathway (Hoeffer and Klann, 2010). The other upstream members, TSC1 and TSC2, form a heterodimer complex. Mutations in the genes encoding this complex cause TSC which is defined clinically by the appearance and growth of benign hamartomas throughout the body and brain (Smalley, 1998). TSC patients suffer from mental retardation and epilepsy. Recent studies show that 25–50% of patients with TSC show behaviors that are consistent with ASD behavioral phenotypes (Hoeffer and Klann, 2010). Pharmacological manipulations to identify therapeutic targets that may be enhancers and suppressors of mTOR signaling cascades and mRNA translation are currently being explored to combat some of the phenotypic manifestations associated with ASD (Carson et al., 2012). Further studies into the downstream and upstream targets of the mTOR signaling cascade will provide additional insights into the functional relationship between the mTOR pathway and ASD.

CONCLUDING REMARKS

Current efforts to identify the constellation of genes that confer the characteristic phenotypic manifestations within the autism spectrum have improved our understanding of this complex disorder.

While modeling mutations in experimental animal model systems will highlight the underlying disruptions in conserved signaling pathways, the daunting task will still be to establish ASD-specific phenotypes at the molecular, cellular and neural circuit levels. The staggering number of genes already discovered in ASD holds the promise to translate the knowledge into designing new therapeutic interventions. The very interesting and equally challenging observation from the recent genetic studies has been a high degree of overlap of risk factors for various neurodevelopmental disorders, such as ASD, epilepsy, and schizophrenia. This pattern of overlap provides the feasibility to address which genes and genetic pathways intersect and specify the spatio-temporal sequence of events that occur within the developing human brain. The recent advent of comprehensive maps of spatio-temporal gene expression in the human brain (Kang et al., 2011) will greatly help toward providing a powerful developmentally informed approach to studying disorders such as ASD.

Although concerted efforts from studies of human clinical ASD populations and various ASD-related animal models have provided a better understanding of the genetic, molecular, and circuit level aberrations in ASD, several intriguing, yet significant questions still remain. For instance, how can the compound effects of genetics, epigenetics, and environment be consolidated in understanding ASD pathogenesis? What other events play a role in determining the appearance and trajectory of ASD symptoms? How do the majority of the genetic susceptibility loci in ASD affect synapse assembly, maintenance and functional modulation? Finally, how would the future treatments and interventions be designed and organized to accommodate the ever-changing genetic landscape of ASD?

ACKNOWLEDGMENTS

The work in our laboratory has been generously supported by the grants from the Simons Foundation Autism Research Initiative (SFARI-177037), the National Institutes of Health (GM063074, NS050356), and the University of Texas Health Science Center, San Antonio, TX, USA. We sincerely regret that the work of many authors related to the topic could not be cited here due to space limitations.

REFERENCES

Abrahams, B. S., and Geschwind, D. H. (2008). Advances in autism genetics: on the threshold of a new neurobiology. *Nat. Rev. Genet.* 9, 341–355. doi: 10.1038/nrg2346

Abrahams, B. S., Tentler, D., Perederiy, J. V., Oldham, M. C., Coppola, G., and Geschwind, D. H. (2007). Genome-wide analyses of human perisylvian cerebral cortical patterning. *Proc. Natl. Acad. Sci. U.S.A.* 104, 17849–17854. doi: 10.1073/pnas.0706128104

Alarcon, M., Abrahams, B. S., Stone, J. L., Duvall, J. A., Perederiy, J. V., Bomar, J. M., et al. (2008). Linkage, association, and gene-expression analyses identify CNTNAP2 as an autism-susceptibility gene. *Am. J. Hum. Genet.* 82, 150–159. doi: 10.1016/j.ajhg.2007.09.005

Amaral, D. G., Bauman, M. D., and Schumann, C. M. (2003). The amygdala and autism: implications from non-human primate studies. *Genes Brain Behav.* 2, 295–302. doi: 10.1034/j.1601-183X.2003.00043.x

Amir, R. E., Van Den Veyver, I. B., Wan, M., Tran, C. Q., Francke, U., and Zoghbi, H. Y. (1999). Rett syndrome is caused by mutations in X-linked MECP2, encoding methyl-CpG-binding protein 2. *Nat. Genet.* 23, 185–188. doi: 10.1038/13810

Arguello, P. A., and Gogos, J. A. (2006). Modeling madness in mice: one piece at a time. *Neuron* 52, 179–196. doi: 10.1016/j.neuron.2006.09.023

Arikkath, J., and Reichardt, L. F. (2008). Cadherins and catenins at synapses: roles in synaptogenesis and synaptic plasticity. *Trends Neurosci.* 31, 487–494. doi: 10.1016/j.tins.2008.07.001

Arking, D. E., Cutler, D. J., Brune, C. W., Teslovich, T. M., West, K., Ikeda, M., et al. (2008). A common genetic variant in the neurexin superfamily member CNTNAP2 increases familial risk of autism. *Am. J. Hum. Genet.* 82, 160–164. doi: 10.1016/j.ajhg.2007.09.015

Arstikaitis, P., Gauthier-Campbell, C., Huang, K., El-Husseini, A., and Murphy, T. H. (2011). Proteins that promote filopodia stability, but not number, lead to more axonal-dendritic contacts. *PLoS ONE* 6:e16998. doi: 10.1371/journal.pone.0016998

Ashwood, P., Krakowiak, P., Hertz-Picciotto, I., Hansen, R., Pessah, I., and Van De Water, J. (2011). Elevated plasma cytokines in autism spectrum disorders provide evidence of immune dysfunction and are associated with impaired behavioral outcome. *Brain Behav. Immun.* 25, 40–45. doi: 10.1016/j.bbi.2010.08.003

Bacchelli, E., Blasi, F., Biondolillo, M., Lamb, J. A., Bonora, E., Barnby, G., et al. (2003). Screening of nine candidate genes for autism on chromosome 2q reveals rare nonsynonymous variants in the cAMP-GEFII gene. *Mol. Psychiatry* 8, 916–924. doi: 10.1038/sj.mp.4001340

Bader, P. L., Faizi, M., Kim, L. H., Owen, S. F., Tadross, M. R., Alfa, R. W., et al. (2011). Mouse model of Timothy syndrome recapitulates triad of autistic traits. *Proc. Natl. Acad. Sci. U.S.A.* 108, 15432–15437. doi: 10.1073/pnas.1112667108

Bailey, A., Le Couteur, A., Gottesman, I., Bolton, P., Simonoff, E., Yuzda, E., et al. (1995). Autism as a strongly genetic disorder: evidence from a British twin study. *Psychol. Med.* 25, 63–77. doi: 10.1017/S0033291700028099

Baker, P., Piven, J., and Sato, Y. (1998). Autism and tuberous sclerosis complex: prevalence and clinical features. *J. Autism Dev. Disord.* 28, 279–285. doi: 10.1023/A:1026004501631

Bakkaloglu, B., O'Roak, B. J., Louvi, A., Gupta, A. R., Abelson, J. F., Morgan, T. M., et al. (2008). Molecular cytogenetic analysis and resequencing of contactin associated protein-like 2 in autism spectrum disorders. *Am. J. Hum. Genet.* 82, 165–173. doi: 10.1016/j.ajhg.2007.09.017

Bangash, M. A., Park, J. M., Melnikova, T., Wang, D., Jeon, S. K., Lee, D., et al. (2011). Enhanced polyubiquitination of Shank3 and NMDA receptor in a mouse model of autism. *Cell* 145, 758–772. doi: 10.1016/j.cell.2011.03.052

Banovic, D., Khorramshahi, O., Owald, D., Wichmann, C., Riedt, T., Fouquet, W., et al. (2010). *Drosophila neuroligin* 1 promotes growth and postsynaptic differentiation at glutamatergic neuromuscular junctions. *Neuron* 66, 724–738. doi: 10.1016/j.neuron.2010.05.020

Barnby, G., Abbott, A., Sykes, N., Morris, A., Weeks, D. E., Mott, R., et al. (2005). Candidate-gene screening and association analysis at the autism-susceptibility locus on chromosome 16p: evidence of association at GRIN2A and ABAT. *Am. J. Hum. Genet.* 76, 950–966. doi: 10.1086/430454

Baudouin, S. J., Gaudias, J., Gerharz, S., Hatstatt, L., Zhou, K., Punnakkal, P., et al. (2012). Shared synaptic pathophysiology in syndromic and nonsyndromic rodent models of autism. *Science* 338, 128–132. doi: 10.1126/science.1224159

Beaudet, A. L. (2007). Autism: highly heritable but not inherited. *Nat. Med.* 13, 534–536. doi: 10.1038/nm0507-534

Beckmann, J. S., Estivill, X., and Antonarakis, S. E. (2007). Copy number variants and genetic traits: closer to the resolution of phenotypic to genotypic variability. *Nat. Rev. Genet.* 8, 639–646. doi: 10.1038/nrg2149

Berglund, E. O., Murai, K. K., Fredette, B., Sekerkova, G., Marturano, B., Weber, L., et al. (1999). Ataxia and abnormal cerebellar microorganization in mice with ablated contactin gene expression. *Neuron* 24, 739–750. doi: 10.1016/S0896-6273(00)81126-5

Berkel, S., Marshall, C. R., Weiss, B., Howe, J., Roeth, R., Moog, U., et al. (2010). Mutations in the SHANK2 synaptic scaffolding gene in autism spectrum disorder and mental retardation. *Nat. Genet.* 42, 489–491. doi: 10.1038/ng.589

Betancur, C., Sakurai, T., and Buxbaum, J. D. (2009). The emerging role of synaptic cell-adhesion pathways in the pathogenesis of autism spectrum disorders. *Trends Neurosci.* 32, 402–412. doi: 10.1016/j.tins.2009.04.003

Bhat, M. A., Rios, J. C., Lu, Y., Garcia-Fresco, G. P., Ching, W., St Martin, M., et al. (2001). Axon–glia interactions and the domain organization of myelinated axons requires neurexin IV/Caspr/Paranodin. *Neuron* 30, 369–383. doi: 10.1016/S0896-6273(01)00294-X

Blanpied, T. A., and Ehlers, M. D. (2004). Microanatomy of dendritic spines: emerging principles of synaptic pathology in psychiatric and neurological disease. *Biol. Psychiatry* 55, 1121–1127. doi: 10.1016/j.biopsych.2003.10.006

Boucard, A. A., Chubykin, A. A., Comoletti, D., Taylor, P., and Sudhof, T. C. (2005). A splice code for trans-synaptic cell adhesion mediated by binding of neuroligin 1 to alpha- and beta-neurexins. *Neuron* 48, 229–236. doi: 10.1016/j.neuron.2005.08.026

Bozdagi, O., Sakurai, T., Papapetrou, D., Wang, X., Dickstein, D. L., Takahashi, N., et al. (2010). Haploinsufficiency of the autism-associated Shank3 gene leads to deficits in synaptic function, social interaction, and social communication. *Mol. Autism* 1, 15. doi: 10.1186/2040-2392-1-15

Bucan, M., Abrahams, B. S., Wang, K., Glessner, J. T., Herman, E. I., Sonnenblick, L. I., et al. (2009). Genome-wide analyses of exonic copy number variants in a family-based study point to novel autism susceptibility genes. *PLoS Genet.* 5:e1000536. doi: 10.1371/journal.pgen.1000536

Butler, M. G., Dasouki, M. J., Zhou, X. P., Talebizadeh, Z., Brown, M., Takahashi, T. N., et al. (2005). Subset of individuals with autism spectrum disorders and extreme macrocephaly associated with germline PTEN tumour suppressor gene mutations. *J. Med. Genet.* 42, 318–321. doi: 10.1136/jmg.2004.024646

Calahorro, F., and Ruiz-Rubio, M. (2011). *Caenorhabditis elegans* as an experimental tool for the study of complex neurological diseases: Parkinson's disease, Alzheimer's disease and autism spectrum disorder. *Invert. Neurosci.* 11, 73–83. doi: 10.1007/s10158-011-0126-1

Calahorro, F., and Ruiz-Rubio, M. (2012). Functional phenotypic rescue of Caenorhabditis elegans neuroligin-deficient mutants by the human and rat NLGN1 genes. *PLoS ONE* 7:e39277. doi: 10.1371/journal.pone.0039277

Campbell, R., Heywood, C. A., Cowey, A., Regard, M., and Landis, T. (1990). Sensitivity to eye gaze in prosopagnosic patients and monkeys with superior temporal sulcus ablation. *Neuropsychologia* 28, 1123–1142. doi: 10.1016/0028-3932(90)90050-X

Carson, R. P., Van Nielen, D. L., Winzenburger, P. A., and Ess, K. C. (2012). Neuronal and glia abnormalities in Tsc1-deficient forebrain and partial rescue by rapamycin. *Neurobiol. Dis.* 45, 369–380. doi: 10.1016/j.nbd.2011.08.024

Chadman, K. K., Gong, S., Scattoni, M. L., Boltuck, S. E., Gandhy, S. U., Heintz, N., et al. (2008). Minimal aberrant behavioral phenotypes of neuroligin-3 R451C knockin mice. *Autism Res.* 1, 147–158. doi: 10.1002/aur.22

Chao, H. T., Chen, H., Samaco, R. C., Xue, M., Chahrour, M., Yoo, J., et al. (2010). Dysfunction in GABA signalling mediates autism-like stereotypies and Rett syndrome phenotypes. *Nature* 468, 263–269. doi: 10.1038/nature09582

Chen, H. J., Rojas-Soto, M., Oguni, A., and Kennedy, M. B. (1998). A synaptic Ras-GTPase activating protein (p135 SynGAP) inhibited by CaM kinase II. *Neuron* 20, 895–904. doi: 10.1016/S0896-6273(00)80471-7

Chen, W. G., Chang, Q., Lin, Y., Meissner, A., West, A. E., Griffith, E. C., et al. (2003). Derepression of BDNF transcription involves calcium-dependent phosphorylation of MeCP2. *Science* 302, 885–889. doi: 10.1126/science.1086446

Chen, Y. C., Lin, Y. Q., Banerjee, S., Venken, K., Li, J., Ismat, A., et al. (2012). *Drosophila neuroligin* 2 is required presynaptically and postsynaptically for proper synaptic differentiation and synaptic transmission. *J. Neurosci.* 32, 16018–16030. doi: 10.1523/JNEUROSCI.1685-12.2012

Cheslack-Postava, K., Fallin, M. D., Avramopoulos, D., Connors, S. L., Zimmerman, A. W., Eberhart, C. G., et al. (2007). beta2-Adrenergic receptor gene variants and risk for autism in the AGRE cohort. *Mol. Psychiatry* 12, 283–291. doi: 10.1038/sj.mp.4001940

Chih, B., Afridi, S. K., Clark, L., and Scheiffele, P. (2004). Disorder-associated mutations lead to functional inactivation of neuroligins. *Hum. Mol. Genet.* 13, 1471–1477. doi: 10.1093/hmg/ddh158ddh158

Chih, B., Engelman, H., and Scheiffele, P. (2005). Control of excitatory and inhibitory synapse formation by neuroligins. *Science* 307, 1324–1328. doi: 10.1126/science.1107470

Choi, Y. B., Li, H. L., Kassabov, S. R., Jin, I., Puthanveettil, S. V., Karl, K. A., et al. (2011). Neurexin–neuroligin transsynaptic interaction mediates learning-related synaptic remodeling and long-term facilitation in aplysia. *Neuron* 70, 468–481. doi: 10.1016/j.neuron.2011.03.020

Christian, S. L., Brune, C. W., Sudi, J., Kumar, R. A., Liu, S., Karamohamed, S., et al. (2008). Novel submicroscopic chromosomal abnormalities detected in autism spectrum disorder. *Biol. Psychiatry* 63, 1111–1117. doi: 10.1016/j.biopsych.2008.01.009

Chubykin, A. A., Atasoy, D., Etherton, M. R., Brose, N., Kavalali, E. T., Gibson, J. R., et al. (2007). Activity-dependent validation of excitatory versus inhibitory synapses by neuroligin-1 versus neuroligin-2. *Neuron* 54, 919–931. doi: 10.1016/j.neuron.2007.05.029

Clayton, D. F., Balakrishnan, C. N., and London, S. E. (2009). Integrating genomes, brain and behavior in the study of songbirds. *Curr. Biol.* 19, R865–R873. doi: 10.1016/j.cub.2009.07.006

Comoletti, D., De Jaco, A., Jennings, L. L., Flynn, R. E., Gaietta, G., Tsigelny, I., et al. (2004). The Arg451Cys-neuroligin-3 mutation associated with autism reveals a defect in protein processing. *J. Neurosci.* 24, 4889–4893. doi: 10.1523/JNEUROSCI.0468-04.200424/20/4889

Cook, E. H. Jr., Courchesne, R. Y., Cox, N. J., Lord, C., Gonen, D., Guter, S. J., et al. (1998). Linkage-disequilibrium mapping of autistic disorder, with 15q11-13 markers. *Am. J. Hum. Genet.* 62, 1077–1083. doi: 10.1086/301832

Cook, E. H. Jr., Lindgren, V., Leventhal, B. L., Courchesne, R., Lincoln, A., Shulman, C., et al. (1997). Autism or atypical autism in maternally but not paternally derived proximal 15q duplication. *Am. J. Hum. Genet.* 60, 928–934.

Corrales, M., and Herbert, M. (2011). "Autism and environmental genomics: synergistic systems approaches to autism complexity," in *Autism Spectrum Disorders*, eds D. Amaral, G. Dawson, and D. H. Geschwind (New York: Oxford University Press), 875–892. doi: 10.1093/med/9780195371826.003.0056

Crabbe, J. C., Wahlsten, D., and Dudek, B. C. (1999). Genetics of mouse behavior: interactions with laboratory environment. *Science* 284, 1670–1672. doi: 10.1126/science.284.5420.1670

Crawley, J. N. (2004). Designing mouse behavioral tasks relevant to autistic-like behaviors. *Ment. Retard. Dev. Disabil. Res. Rev.* 10, 248–258. doi: 10.1002/mrdd.20039

Creak, M., and Pampiglione, G. (1969). Clinical and EEG studies on a group of 35 psychotic children. *Dev. Med. Child Neurol.* 11, 218–227. doi: 10.1111/j.1469-8749.1969.tb01420.x

Croen, L. A., Grether, J. K., Yoshida, C. K., Odouli, R., and Van De Water, J. (2005). Maternal autoimmune diseases, asthma and allergies, and childhood autism spectrum disorders: a case–control study. *Arch. Pediatr. Adolesc. Med.* 159, 151–157. doi: 10.1001/archpedi.159.2.151

Cukier, H. N., Perez, A. M., Collins, A. L., Zhou, Z., Zoghbi, H. Y., and Botas, J. (2008). Genetic modifiers of MeCP2 function in *Drosophila*. *PLoS Genet.* 4:e1000179. doi: 10.1371/journal.pgen.1000179

Currenti, S. A. (2010). Understanding and determining the etiology of autism. *Cell. Mol. Neurobiol.* 30, 161–171. doi: 10.1007/s10571-009-9453-8

De Jaco, A., Kovarik, Z., Comoletti, D., Jennings, L. L., Gaietta, G., Ellisman, M. H., et al. (2005). A single mutation near the C-terminus in alpha/beta hydrolase fold protein family causes a defect in protein processing. *Chem. Biol. Interact.* 157–158, 371–372. doi: 10.1016/j.cbi.2005.10.057

de Krom, M., Staal, W. G., Ophoff, R. A., Hendriks, J., Buitelaar, J., Franke, B., et al. (2009). A common variant in DRD3 receptor is associated with autism spectrum disorder. *Biol. Psychiatry* 65, 625–630. doi: 10.1016/j.biopsych.2008.09.035

Delorme, R., Ey, E., Toro, R., Leboyer, M., Gillberg, C., and Bourgeron, T. (2013). Progress toward treatments for synaptic defects in autism. *Nat. Med.* 19, 685–694. doi: 10.1038/nm.3193

Dibbens, L. M., Tarpey, P. S., Hynes, K., Bayly, M. A., Scheffer, I. E., Smith, R., et al. (2008). X-linked protocadherin 19 mutations cause female-limited epilepsy and cognitive impairment. *Nat. Genet.* 40, 776–781. doi: 10.1038/ng.149

Dooley, K., and Zon, L. I. (2000). Zebrafish: a model system for the study of human disease. *Curr. Opin. Genet. Dev.* 10, 252–256. doi: 10.1016/S0959-437X(00)00074-5

Durand, C. M., Betancur, C., Boeckers, T. M., Bockmann, J., Chaste, P., Fauchereau, F., et al. (2007). Mutations in the gene encoding the synaptic scaffolding protein SHANK3 are associated with autism spectrum disorders. *Nat. Genet.* 39, 25–27. doi: 10.1038/ng1933

Durkin, M. S., Maenner, M. J., Newschaffer, C. J., Lee, L. C., Cunniff, C. M., Daniels, J. L., et al. (2008). Advanced parental age and the risk of autism spectrum disorder. *Am. J. Epidemiol.* 168, 1268–1276. doi: 10.1093/aje/kwn250

Egger, G., Liang, G., Aparicio, A., and Jones, P. A. (2004). Epigenetics in human disease and prospects for epigenetic therapy. *Nature* 429, 457–463. doi: 10.1038/nature02625

Eichler, S. A., and Meier, J. C. (2008). E-I balance and human diseases – from molecules to networking. *Front. Mol. Neurosci.* 1:2. doi: 10.3389/neuro.02.002.2008

Estivill, X., and Armengol, L. (2007). Copy number variants and common disorders: filling the gaps and exploring complexity in genome-wide association studies. *PLoS Genet.* 3:1787–1799. doi: 10.1371/journal.pgen.0030190

Falivelli, G., De Jaco, A., Favaloro, F. L., Kim, H., Wilson, J., Dubi, N., et al. (2012). Inherited genetic variants in autism-related CNTNAP2 show perturbed trafficking and ATF6 activation. *Hum. Mol. Genet.* doi: 10.1093/hmg/dds320

Favre, M. R., Barkat, T. R., Lamendola, D., Khazen, G., Markram, H., and Markram, K. (2013). General developmental health in the VPA-rat model of autism. *Front. Behav. Neurosci.* 7:88. doi: 10.3389/fnbeh.2013.00088

Feinberg, E. H., Vanhoven, M. K., Bendesky, A., Wang, G., Fetter, R. D., Shen, K., et al. (2008). GFP Reconstitution Across Synaptic Partners (GRASP) defines cell contacts and synapses in living nervous systems. *Neuron* 57, 353–363. doi: 10.1016/j.neuron.2007.11.030

Feng, J., Schroer, R., Yan, J., Song, W., Yang, C., Bockholt, A., et al. (2006). High frequency of neurexin 1beta signal peptide structural variants in patients with autism. *Neurosci. Lett.* 409, 10–13. doi: 10.1016/j.neulet.2006.08.017

Fernandez, T., Morgan, T., Davis, N., Klin, A., Morris, A., Farhi, A., et al. (2004). Disruption of contactin 4 (CNTN4) results in developmental delay and other features of 3p deletion syndrome. *Am. J. Hum. Genet.* 74, 1286–1293. doi: 10.1086/421474AJHG40899

Feyder, M., Karlsson, R. M., Mathur, P., Lyman, M., Bock, R., Momenan, R., et al. (2010). Association of mouse Dlg4 (PSD-95) gene deletion and human DLG4 gene variation with phenotypes relevant to autism spectrum disorders and Williams' syndrome. *Am. J. Psychiatry* 167, 1508–1517. doi: 10.1176/appi.ajp.2010.10040484

Folstein, S., and Rutter, M. (1977). Genetic influences and infantile autism. *Nature* 265, 726–728. doi: 10.1038/265726a0

Folstein, S. E., and Rosen-Sheidley, B. (2001). Genetics of autism: complex aetiology for a heterogeneous disorder. *Nat. Rev. Genet.* 2, 943–955. doi: 10.1038/351 03559

Gauthier, J., Spiegelman, D., Piton, A., Lafreniere, R. G., Laurent, S., St-Onge, J., et al. (2009). Novel de novo SHANK3 mutation in autistic patients. *Am. J. Med. Genet. B Neuropsychiatr. Genet.* 150B, 421–424. doi: 10.1002/ajmg.b.30822

Gerrow, K., Romorini, S., Nabi, S. M., Colicos, M. A., Sala, C., and El-Husseini, A. (2006). A preformed complex of postsynaptic proteins is involved in excitatory synapse development. *Neuron* 49, 547–562. doi: 10.1016/j.neuron.2006.01.015

Gharani, N., Benayed, R., Mancuso, V., Brzustowicz, L. M., and Millonig, J. H. (2004). Association of the homeobox transcription factor, ENGRAILED 2, 3, with autism spectrum disorder. *Mol. Psychiatry* 9, 474–484. doi: 10.1038/sj.mp.4001498

Ghazanfar, A. A., and Santos, L. R. (2004). Primate brains in the wild: the sensory bases for social interactions. *Nat. Rev. Neurosci.* 5, 603–616. doi: 10.1038/nrn1473

Gkogkas, C. G., Khoutorsky, A., Ran, I., Rampakakis, E., Nevarko, T., Weatherill, D. B., et al. (2013). Autism-related deficits via dysregulated eIF4E-dependent translational control. *Nature* 493, 371–377. doi: 10.1038/nature 11628

Glessner, J. T., Wang, K., Cai, G., Korvatska, O., Kim, C. E., Wood, S., et al. (2009). Autism genome-wide copy number variation reveals ubiquitin and neuronal genes. *Nature* 459, 569–573. doi: 10.1038/nature07953

Gogolla, N., Leblanc, J. J., Quast, K. B., Sudhof, T. C., Fagiolini, M., and Hensch, T. K. (2009). Common circuit defect of excitatory-inhibitory balance in mouse models of autism. *J. Neurodev. Disord.* 1, 172–181. doi: 10.1007/s11689-009-9023-x

Griswold, A. J., Ma, D., Cukier, H. N., Nations, L. D., Schmidt, M. A., Chung, R. H., et al. (2012). Evaluation of copy number variations reveals novel candidate genes in autism spectrum disorder-associated pathways. *Hum. Mol. Genet.* 21, 3513–3523. doi: 10.1093/hmg/dds164

Hamdan, F. F., Gauthier, J., Spiegelman, D., Noreau, A., Yang, Y., Pellerin, S., et al. (2009). Mutations in SYNGAP1 in autosomal nonsyndromic mental retardation. *N. Engl. J. Med.* 360, 599–605. doi: 10.1056/NEJMoa0805392

Han, K., Holder, J. L. Jr., Schaaf, C. P., Lu, H., Chen, H., Kang, H., et al. (2013). SHANK3 overexpression causes manic-like behaviour with unique pharmacogenetic properties. *Nature* 503, 72–77. doi: 10.1038/nature12630

Han, S., Tai, C., Westenbroek, R. E., Yu, F. H., Cheah, C. S., Potter, G. B., et al. (2012). Autistic-like behaviour in Scn1a$^{+/-}$ mice and rescue by enhanced GABA-mediated neurotransmission. *Nature* 489, 385–390. doi: 10.1038/nature11356

Harkin, L. A., Mcmahon, J. M., Iona, X., Dibbens, L., Pelekanos, J. T., Zuberi, S. M., et al. (2007). The spectrum of SCN1A-related infantile epileptic encephalopathies. *Brain* 130, 843–852. doi: 10.1093/brain/awm002

Hay, N., and Sonenberg, N. (2004). Upstream and downstream of mTOR. *Genes Dev.* 18, 1926–1945. doi: 10.1101/gad.1212704

Herbert, M. R. (2010). Contributions of the environment and environmentally vulnerable physiology to autism spectrum disorders. *Curr. Opin. Neurol.* 23, 103–110. doi: 10.1097/WCO.0b013e328336a01f

Hoeffer, C. A., and Klann, E. (2010). mTOR signaling: at the crossroads of plasticity, memory and disease. *Trends Neurosci.* 33, 67–75. doi: 10.1016/j.tins.2009.11.003

Horev, G., Ellegood, J., Lerch, J. P., Son, Y. E., Muthuswamy, L., Vogel, H., et al. (2011). Dosage-dependent phenotypes in models of 16p11.2 lesions found in autism. *Proc. Natl. Acad. Sci. U.S.A.* 108, 17076–17081. doi: 10.1073/pnas.1114042108

Hu, Z., Hom, S., Kudze, T., Tong, X. J., Choi, S., Aramuni, G., et al. (2012). Neurexin and neuroligin mediate retrograde synaptic inhibition in *C. elegans*. *Science* 337, 980–984. doi: 10.1126/science.1224896

Huang, H. S., Allen, J. A., Mabb, A. M., King, I. F., Miriyala, J., Taylor-Blake, B., et al. (2012). Topoisomerase inhibitors unsilence the dormant allele of Ube3a in neurons. *Nature* 481, 185–189. doi: 10.1038/nature10726

Hunter, J. W., Mullen, G. P., Mcmanus, J. R., Heatherly, J. M., Duke, A., and Rand, J. B. (2010). Neuroligin-deficient mutants of *C. elegans* have sensory processing deficits and are hypersensitive to oxidative stress and mercury toxicity. *Dis. Model. Mech.* 3, 366–376. doi: 10.1242/dmm.003442

Ichtchenko, K., Hata, Y., Nguyen, T., Ullrich, B., Missler, M., Moomaw, C., et al. (1995). Neuroligin 1: a splice site-specific ligand for beta-neurexins. *Cell* 81, 435–443. doi: 10.1016/0092-8674(95)90396-8

International Molecular Genetic Study of Autism Consortium. (2001). Further characterization of the autism susceptibility locus AUTS1 on chromosome 7q. *Hum. Mol. Genet.* 10, 973–982. doi: 10.1093/hmg/10.9.973

Iossifov, I., Ronemus, M., Levy, D., Wang, Z., Hakker, I., Rosenbaum, J., et al. (2012). De novo gene disruptions in children on the autistic spectrum. *Neuron* 74, 285–299. doi: 10.1016/j.neuron.2012.04.009

Jamain, S., Betancur, C., Quach, H., Philippe, A., Fellous, M., Giros, B., et al. (2002). Linkage and association of the glutamate receptor 6 gene with autism. *Mol. Psychiatry* 7, 302–310. doi: 10.1038/sj.mp.4000979

Jamain, S., Quach, H., Betancur, C., Rastam, M., Colineaux, C., Gillberg, I. C., et al. (2003). Mutations of the X-linked genes encoding neuroligins NLGN3 and NLGN4 are associated with autism. *Nat. Genet.* 34, 27–29. doi: 10.1038/ng1136ng1136

Jamain, S., Radyushkin, K., Hammerschmidt, K., Granon, S., Boretius, S., Varoqueaux, F., et al. (2008). Reduced social interaction and ultrasonic communication in a mouse model of monogenic heritable autism. *Proc. Natl. Acad. Sci. U.S.A.* 105, 1710–1715. doi: 10.1073/pnas.0711555105

Jessberger, S., Nakashima, K., Clemenson, G. D. Jr., Mejia, E., Mathews, E., Ure, k., et al. (2007). Epigenetic modulation of seizure-induced neurogenesis and cognitive decline. *J. Neurosci.* 27, 5967–5975. doi: 10.1523/JNEUROSCI.0110-07.2007

Ji, L., Chauhan, A., Brown, W. T., and Chauhan, V. (2009). Increased activities of Na^+/K^+-ATPase and Ca^{2+}/Mg^{2+}-ATPase in the frontal cortex and cerebellum of autistic individuals. *Life Sci.* 85, 788–793. doi: 10.1016/j.lfs.2009.10.008

Jiang, H., and Kohler, C. (2012). Evolution, function, and regulation of genomic imprinting in plant seed development. *J. Exp. Bot.* 63, 4713–4722. doi: 10.1093/jxb/ers145

Jiang, Y. H., Bressler, J., and Beaudet, A. L. (2004). Epigenetics and human disease. *Annu. Rev. Genomics Hum. Genet.* 5, 479–510. doi: 10.1146/annurev.genom.5.061903.180014

Jiang, Y. H., and Ehlers, M. D. (2013). Modeling autism by SHANK gene mutations in mice. *Neuron* 78, 8–27. doi: 10.1016/j.neuron.2013.03.016

Kang, H. J., Kawasawa, Y. I., Cheng, F., Zhu, Y., Xu, X., Li, M., et al. (2011). Spatio-temporal transcriptome of the human brain. *Nature* 478, 483–489. doi: 10.1038/nature10523

Kanner, L. (1943). Autistic disturbances of affective contact. *Nervous Child* 2, 34.

Kanner, L. (1968). Autistic disturbances of affective contact. *Acta Paedopsychiatr.* 35, 100–136.

Kanner, L. (1971). Follow-up study of eleven autistic children originally reported in 1943. *J. Autism Child. Schizophr.* 1, 119–145. doi: 10.1007/BF01537953

Kelleher, R. J. III, and Bear, M. F. (2008). The autistic neuron: troubled translation? *Cell* 135, 401–406. doi: 10.1016/j.cell.2008.10.017

Kelleher, R. J. III, Geigenmuller, U., Hovhannisyan, H., Trautman, E., Pinard, R., Rathmell, B., et al. (2012). High-throughput sequencing of mGluR signaling pathway genes reveals enrichment of rare variants in autism. *PLoS ONE* 7:e35003. doi: 10.1371/journal.pone.0035003

Kim, H. G., Kishikawa, S., Higgins, A. W., Seong, I. S., Donovan, D. J., Shen, Y., et al. (2008). Disruption of neurexin 1 associated with autism spectrum disorder. *Am. J. Hum. Genet.* 82, 199–207. doi: 10.1016/j.ajhg.2007.09.011

Kim, J. H., Lee, H. K., Takamiya, K., and Huganir, R. L. (2003). The role of synaptic GTPase-activating protein in neuronal development and synaptic plasticity. *J. Neurosci.* 23, 1119–1124.

Komiyama, N. H., Watabe, A. M., Carlisle, H. J., Porter, K., Charlesworth, P., Monti, J., et al. (2002). SynGAP regulates ERK/MAPK signaling, synaptic plasticity, and learning in the complex with postsynaptic density 95 and NMDA receptor. *J. Neurosci.* 22, 9721–9732.

Koochek, M., Harvard, C., Hildebrand, M. J., Van Allen, M., Wingert, H., Mickelson, E., et al. (2006). 15q duplication associated with autism in a multiplex family with a familial cryptic translocation t(14; 15)(q11.2; q13.3) detected using array-CGH. *Clin. Genet.* 69, 124–134. doi: 10.1111/j.1399-0004.2005.00560.x

Krey, J. F., and Dolmetsch, R. E. (2007). Molecular mechanisms of autism: a possible role for Ca^{2+} signaling. *Curr. Opin. Neurobiol.* 17, 112–119. doi: 10.1016/j.conb.2007.01.010

Kumar, R. A., Karamohamed, S., Sudi, J., Conrad, D. F., Brune, C., Badner, J. A., et al. (2008). Recurrent 16p11.2 microdeletions in autism. *Hum. Mol. Genet.* 17, 628–638. doi: 10.1093/hmg/ddm376

Kumar, V., Zhang, M. X., Swank, M. W., Kunz, J., and Wu, G. Y. (2005). Regulation of dendritic morphogenesis by Ras–PI3K–Akt–mTOR and Ras–MAPK signaling pathways. *J. Neurosci.* 25, 11288–11299. doi: 10.1523/JNEUROSCI.2284-05.2005

Lamb, J. A., Barnby, G., Bonora, E., Sykes, N., Bacchelli, E., Blasi, F., et al. (2005). Analysis of IMGSAC autism susceptibility loci: evidence for sex limited and parent of origin specific effects. *J. Med. Genet.* 42, 132–137. doi: 10.1136/jmg.2004.025668

Laplante, M., and Sabatini, D. M. (2009). mTOR signaling at a glance. *J. Cell Sci.* 122, 3589–3594. doi: 10.1242/jcs.051011

Laumonnier, F., Bonnet-Brilhault, F., Gomot, M., Blanc, R., David, A., Moizard, M. P., et al. (2004). X-linked mental retardation and autism are associated with a mutation in the NLGN4 gene, a member of the neuroligin family. *Am. J. Hum. Genet.* 74, 552–557. doi: 10.1086/382137AJHG40657

Laumonnier, F., Roger, S., Guerin, P., Molinari, F., M'Rad, R., Cahard, D., et al. (2006). Association of a functional deficit of the BKCa channel, a synaptic regulator of neuronal excitability, with autism and mental retardation. *Am. J. Psychiatry* 163, 1622–1629. doi: 10.1176/appi.ajp.163.9.1622

Levitt, P., and Campbell, D. B. (2009). The genetic and neurobiologic compass points toward common signaling dysfunctions in autism spectrum disorders. *J. Clin. Invest.* 119, 747–754. doi: 10.1172/JCI37934

Levy, D., Ronemus, M., Yamrom, B., Lee, Y. H., Leotta, A., Kendall, J., et al. (2011). Rare de novo and transmitted copy-number variation in autistic spectrum disorders. *Neuron* 70, 886–897. doi: 10.1016/j.neuron.2011.05.015

Li, B. M., Liu, X. R., Yi, Y. H., Deng, Y. H., Su, T., Zou, X., et al. (2011). Autism in Dravet syndrome: prevalence, features, and relationship to the clinical characteristics of epilepsy and mental retardation. *Epilepsy Behav.* 21, 291–295. doi: 10.1016/j.yebeh.2011.04.060

Li, J., Ashley, J., Budnik, V., and Bhat, M. A. (2007). Crucial role of *Drosophila neurexin* in proper active zone apposition to postsynaptic densities, synaptic growth, and synaptic transmission. *Neuron* 55, 741–755. doi: 10.1016/j.neuron.2007.08.002

Liao, P., and Soong, T. W. (2010). CaV1.2 channelopathies: from arrhythmias to autism, bipolar disorder, and immunodeficiency. *Pflugers Arch.* 460, 353–359. doi: 10.1007/s00424-009-0753-0

Luedi, P. P., Dietrich, F. S., Weidman, J. R., Bosko, J. M., Jirtle, R. L., and Hartemink, A. J. (2007). Computational and experimental identification of novel human imprinted genes. *Genome Res.* 17, 1723–1730. doi: 10.1101/gr.6584707

Luo, R., Sanders, S. J., Tian, Y., Voineagu, I., Huang, N., Chu, S. H., et al. (2012). Genome-wide transcriptome profiling reveals the functional impact of rare de novo and recurrent CNVs in autism spectrum disorders. *Am. J. Hum. Genet.* 91, 38–55. doi: 10.1016/j.ajhg.2012.05.011

Lutz, C., Well, A., and Novak, M. (2003). Stereotypic and self-injurious behavior in rhesus macaques: a survey and retrospective analysis of environment and early experience. *Am. J. Primatol.* 60, 1–15. doi: 10.1002/ajp.10075

Ma, D., Salyakina, D., Jaworski, J. M., Konidari, I., Whitehead, P. L., Andersen, A. N., et al. (2009a). A genome-wide association study of autism reveals a common novel risk locus at 5p14.1. *Ann. Hum. Genet.* 73, 263–273. doi: 10.1111/j.1469-1809.2009.00523.x

Ma, D. K., Jang, M. H., Guo, J. U., Kitabatake, Y., Chang, M. L., Pow-Anpongkul, N., et al. (2009b). Neuronal activity-induced Gadd45b promotes epigenetic DNA demethylation and adult neurogenesis. *Science* 323, 1074–1077. doi: 10.1126/science.1166859

Ma, D. Q., Whitehead, P. L., Menold, M. M., Martin, E. R., Ashley-Koch, A. E., Mei, H., et al. (2005). Identification of significant association and gene–gene interaction of GABA receptor subunit genes in autism. *Am. J. Hum. Genet.* 77, 377–388. doi: 10.1086/433195

Mabb, A. M., Judson, M. C., Zylka, M. J., and Philpot, B. D. (2011). Angelman syndrome: insights into genomic imprinting and neurodevelopmental phenotypes. *Trends Neurosci.* 34, 293–303. doi: 10.1016/j.tins.2011.04.001

Malhotra, D., and Sebat, J. (2012). CNVs: harbingers of a rare variant revolution in psychiatric genetics. *Cell* 148, 1223–1241. doi: 10.1016/j.cell.2012.02.039

Marshall, C. R., Noor, A., Vincent, J. B., Lionel, A. C., Feuk, L., Skaug, J., et al. (2008). Structural variation of chromosomes in autism spectrum disorder. *Am. J. Hum. Genet.* 82, 477–488. doi: 10.1016/j.ajhg.2007.12.009

Martienssen, R. A., and Colot, V. (2001). DNA methylation and epigenetic inheritance in plants and filamentous fungi. *Science* 293, 1070–1074. doi: 10.1126/science.293.5532.1070

Martin, L. A., Ashwood, P., Braunschweig, D., Cabanlit, M., Van De Water, J., and Amaral, D. G. (2008). Stereotypies and hyperactivity in rhesus monkeys exposed to IgG from mothers of children with autism. *Brain Behav. Immun.* 22, 806–816. doi: 10.1016/j.bbi.2007.12.007

Martinowich, K., Hattori, D., Wu, H., Fouse, S., He, F., Hu, Y., et al. (2003). DNA methylation-related chromatin remodeling in activity-dependent BDNF gene regulation. *Science* 302, 890–893. doi: 10.1126/science.1090842

Marui, T., Funatogawa, I., Koishi, S., Yamamoto, K., Matsumoto, H., Hashimoto, O., et al. (2009). Association of the neuronal cell adhesion molecule (NRCAM) gene variants with autism. *Int. J. Neuropsychopharmacol.* 12, 1–10. doi: 10.1017/S1461145708009127

McCarroll, S. A., Kuruvilla, F. G., Korn, J. M., Cawley, S., Nemesh, J., Wysoker, A., et al. (2008). Integrated detection and population-genetic analysis of SNPs and copy number variation. *Nat. Genet.* 40, 1166–1174. doi: 10.1038/ng.238

McGraw, L. A., and Young, L. J. (2010). The prairie vole: an emerging model organism for understanding the social brain. *Trends Neurosci.* 33, 103–109. doi: 10.1016/j.tins.2009.11.006

Mejias, R., Adamczyk, A., Anggono, V., Niranjan, T., Thomas, G. M., Sharma, K., et al. (2011). Gain-of-function glutamate receptor interacting protein 1 variants alter GluA2 recycling and surface distribution in patients with autism. *Proc. Natl. Acad. Sci. U.S.A.* 108, 4920–4925. doi: 10.1073/pnas.1102233108

Merikangas, A. K., Corvin, A. P., and Gallagher, L. (2009). Copy-number variants in neurodevelopmental disorders: promises and challenges. *Trends Genet.* 25, 536–544. doi: 10.1016/j.tig.2009.10.006

Miller, D. T., Shen, Y., Weiss, L. A., Korn, J., Anselm, I., Bridgemohan, C., et al. (2009). Microdeletion/duplication at 15q13.2q13.3 among individuals with features of autism and other neuropsychiatric disorders. *J. Med. Genet.* 46, 242–248. doi: 10.1136/jmg.2008.059907

Missler, M., Zhang, W., Rohlmann, A., Kattenstroth, G., Hammer, R. E., Gottmann, K., et al. (2003). Alpha-neurexins couple Ca^{2+} channels to synaptic vesicle exocytosis. *Nature* 423, 939–948. doi: 10.1038/nature01755

Mitne-Neto, M., Machado-Costa, M., Marchetto, M. C., Bengtson, M. H., Joazeiro, C. A., Tsuda, H., et al. (2011). Downregulation of VAPB expression in motor neurons derived from induced pluripotent stem cells of ALS8 patients. *Hum. Mol. Genet.* 20, 3642–3652. doi: 10.1093/hmg/ddr284

Miyake, K., Hirasawa, T., Koide, T., and Kubota, T. (2012). Epigenetics in autism and other neurodevelopmental diseases. *Adv. Exp. Med. Biol.* 724, 91–98. doi: 10.1007/978-1-4614-0653-2_7

Moessner, R., Marshall, C. R., Sutcliffe, J. S., Skaug, J., Pinto, D., Vincent, J., et al. (2007). Contribution of SHANK3 mutations to autism spectrum disorder. *Am. J. Hum. Genet.* 81, 1289–1297. doi: 10.1086/522590

Moldin, S. O., Rubenstein, J. L., and Hyman, S. E. (2006). Can autism speak to neuroscience? *J. Neurosci.* 26, 6893–6896. doi: 10.1523/JNEUROSCI.1944-06.2006

Morales, J., Hiesinger, P. R., Schroeder, A. J., Kume, K., Verstreken, P., Jackson, F. R., et al. (2002). Drosophila fragile X protein, DFXR, regulates neuronal morphology and function in the brain. *Neuron* 34, 961–972. doi: 10.1016/S0896-6273(02)00731-6

Moretti, P., Levenson, J. M., Battaglia, F., Atkinson, R., Teague, R., Antalffy, B., et al. (2006). Learning and memory and synaptic plasticity are impaired in a mouse model of Rett syndrome. *J. Neurosci.* 26, 319–327. doi: 10.1523/JNEUROSCI.2623-05.2006

Morrow, E. M., Yoo, S. Y., Flavell, S. W., Kim, T. K., Lin, Y., Hill, R. S., et al. (2008). Identifying autism loci and genes by tracing recent shared ancestry. *Science* 321, 218–223. doi: 10.1126/science.1157657

Mulley, J. C., Scheffer, I. E., Petrou, S., Dibbens, L. M., Berkovic, S. F., and Harkin, L. A. (2005). SCN1A mutations and epilepsy. *Hum. Mutat.* 25, 535–542. doi: 10.1002/humu.20178

Naisbitt, S., Kim, E., Tu, J. C., Xiao, B., Sala, C., Valtschanoff, J., et al. (1999). Shank, a novel family of postsynaptic density proteins that binds to the NMDA receptor/PSD-95/GKAP complex and cortactin. *Neuron* 23, 569–582. doi: 10.1016/S0896-6273(00)80809-0

Nakatani, J., Tamada, K., Hatanaka, F., Ise, S., Ohta, H., Inoue, K., et al. (2009). Abnormal behavior in a chromosome-engineered mouse model for human 15q11-13 duplication seen in autism. *Cell* 137, 1235–1246. doi: 10.1016/j.cell.2009.04.024

Neale, B. M., Kou, Y., Liu, L., Ma'ayan, A., Samocha, K. E., Sabo, A., et al. (2012). Patterns and rates of exonic de novo mutations in autism spectrum disorders. *Nature* 485, 242–245. doi: 10.1038/nature11011

Neves-Pereira, M., Muller, B., Massie, D., Williams, J. H., O'Brien, P. C., Hughes, A., et al. (2009). Deregulation of EIF4E: a novel mechanism for autism. *J. Med. Genet.* 46, 759–765. doi: 10.1136/jmg.2009.066852

Newey, S. E., Velamoor, V., Govek, E. E., and Van Aelst, L. (2005). Rho GTPases, dendritic structure, and mental retardation. *J. Neurobiol.* 64, 58–74. doi: 10.1002/neu.20153

Nurmi, E. L., Bradford, Y., Chen, Y., Hall, J., Arnone, B., Gardiner, M. B., et al. (2001). Linkage disequilibrium at the Angelman syndrome gene UBE3A in autism families. *Genomics* 77, 105–113. doi: 10.1006/geno.2001.6617

Oberman, L. M., Hubbard, E. M., Mccleery, J. P., Altschuler, E. L., Ramachandran, V. S., and Pineda, J. A. (2005). EEG evidence for mirror neuron dysfunction in autism spectrum disorders. *Brain Res. Cogn. Brain Res.* 24, 190–198. doi: 10.1016/j.cogbrainres.2005.01.014

Ongur, D., and Price, J. L. (2000). The organization of networks within the orbital and medial prefrontal cortex of rats, monkeys and humans. *Cereb. Cortex* 10, 206–219. doi: 10.1093/cercor/10.3.206

Onore, C., Careaga, M., and Ashwood, P. (2012). The role of immune dysfunction in the pathophysiology of autism. *Brain Behav. Immun.* 26, 383–392. doi: 10.1016/j.bbi.2011.08.007

O'Roak, B. J., Deriziotis, P., Lee, C., Vives, L., Schwartz, J. J., Girirajan, S., et al. (2011). Exome sequencing in sporadic autism spectrum disorders identifies severe de novo mutations. *Nat. Genet.* 43, 585–589. doi: 10.1038/ng.835

O'Roak, B. J., Vives, L., Girirajan, S., Karakoc, E., Krumm, N., Coe, B. P., et al. (2012). Sporadic autism exomes reveal a highly interconnected protein network of de novo mutations. *Nature* 485, 246–250. doi: 10.1038/nature 10989

Panaitof, S. C. (2012). A songbird animal model for dissecting the genetic bases of autism spectrum disorder. *Dis. Markers* 33, 241–249. doi: 10.3233/DMA-2012–2918

Panaitof, S. C., Abrahams, B. S., Dong, H., Geschwind, D. H., and White, S. A. (2010). Language-related Cntnap2 gene is differentially expressed in sexually dimorphic song nuclei essential for vocal learning in songbirds. *J. Comp. Neurol.* 518, 1995–2018. doi: 10.1002/cne.22318

Pavlou, O., Theodorakis, K., Falk, J., Kutsche, M., Schachner, M., Faivre-Sarrailh, C., et al. (2002). Analysis of interactions of the adhesion molecule TAG-1 and its domains with other immunoglobulin superfamily members. *Mol. Cell. Neurosci.* 20, 367–381. doi: 10.1006/mcne.2002.1105

Peca, J., Feliciano, C., Ting, J. T., Wang, W., Wells, M. F., Venkatraman, T. N., et al. (2011a). Shank3 mutant mice display autistic-like behaviours and striatal dysfunction. *Nature* 472, 437–442. doi: 10.1038/nature09965

Peca, J., Ting, J., and Feng, G. (2011b). SnapShot: autism and the synapse. *Cell* 147, 706–706.e1. doi: 10.1016/j.cell.2011.10.015

Penagarikano, O., Abrahams, B. S., Herman, E. I., Winden, K. D., Gdalyahu, A., Dong, H., et al. (2011). Absence of CNTNAP2 leads to epilepsy, neuronal migration abnormalities, and core autism-related deficits. *Cell* 147, 235–246. doi: 10.1016/j.cell.2011.08.040

Persico, A. M., and Bourgeron, T. (2006). Searching for ways out of the autism maze: genetic, epigenetic and environmental clues. *Trends Neurosci.* 29, 349–358. doi: 10.1016/j.tins.2006.05.010

Persico, A. M., D'Agruma, L., Maiorano, N., Totaro, A., Militerni, R., Bravaccio, C., et al. (2001). Reelin gene alleles and haplotypes as a factor predisposing to autistic disorder. *Mol. Psychiatry* 6, 150–159. doi: 10.1038/sj.mp.4000850

Pessah, I. N., Seegal, R. F., Lein, P. J., Lasalle, J., Yee, B. K., Van De Water, J., et al. (2008). Immunologic and neurodevelopmental susceptibilities of autism. *Neurotoxicology* 29, 532–545. doi: 10.1016/j.neuro.2008.02.006

Pinto, D., Pagnamenta, A. T., Klei, L., Anney, R., Merico, D., Regan, R., et al. (2010). Functional impact of global rare copy number variation in autism spectrum disorders. *Nature* 466, 368–372. doi: 10.1038/nature09146

Poliak, S., Salomon, D., Elhanany, H., Sabanay, H., Kiernan, B., Pevny, L., et al. (2003). Juxtaparanodal clustering of Shaker-like K^+ channels in myelinated axons depends on Caspr2 and TAG-1. *J. Cell Biol.* 162, 1149–1160. doi: 10.1083/jcb.200305018jcb.200305018

Qiu, J. (2006). Epigenetics: unfinished symphony. *Nature* 441, 143–145. doi: 10.1038/441143a

Radyushkin, K., Hammerschmidt, K., Boretius, S., Varoqueaux, F., El-Kordi, A., Ronnenberg, A., et al. (2009). Neuroligin-3-deficient mice: model of a monogenic heritable form of autism with an olfactory deficit. *Genes Brain Behav.* 8, 416–425. doi: 10.1111/j.1601-183X.2009.00487.x

Ramoz, N., Cai, G., Reichert, J. G., Silverman, J. M., and Buxbaum, J. D. (2008). An analysis of candidate autism loci on chromosome 2q24-q33: evidence for association to the STK39 gene. *Am. J. Med. Genet. B Neuropsychiatr. Genet.* 147B, 1152–1158. doi: 10.1002/ajmg.b.30739

Ramoz, N., Reichert, J. G., Smith, C. J., Silverman, J. M., Bespalova, I. N., Davis, K. L., et al. (2004). Linkage and association of the mitochondrial aspartate/glutamate carrier SLC25A12 gene with autism. *Am. J. Psychiatry* 161, 662–669. doi: 10.1176/appi.ajp.161.4.662

Redies, C., Hertel, N., and Hubner, C. A. (2012). Cadherins and neuropsychiatric disorders. *Brain Res.* 1470, 130–144. doi: 10.1016/j.brainres.2012.06.020

Reik, W., and Walter, J. (2001). Genomic imprinting: parental influence on the genome. *Nat. Rev. Genet.* 2, 21–32. doi: 10.1038/35047554

Rice, D. S., and Curran, T. (2001). Role of the reelin signaling pathway in central nervous system development. *Annu. Rev. Neurosci.* 24, 1005–1039. doi: 10.1146/annurev.neuro.24.1.1005

Rodier, P. M., Ingram, J. L., Tisdale, B., and Croog, V. J. (1997). Linking etiologies in humans and animal models: studies of autism. *Reprod. Toxicol.* 11, 417–422. doi: 10.1016/S0890-6238(97)80001-U

Rogers, S. J., Wehner, D. E., and Hagerman, R. (2001). The behavioral phenotype in fragile X: symptoms of autism in very young children with fragile X syndrome, idiopathic autism, and other developmental disorders. *J. Dev. Behav. Pediatr.* 22, 409–417. doi: 10.1097/00004703-200112000-00008

Ronesi, J. A., Collins, K. A., Hays, S. A., Tsai, N. P., Guo, W., Birnbaum, S. G., et al. (2012). Disrupted Homer scaffolds mediate abnormal mGluR5 function in a mouse model of fragile X syndrome. *Nat. Neurosci.* 15, 431–440, S431. doi: 10.1038/nn.3033

Roohi, J., Montagna, C., Tegay, D. H., Palmer, L. E., Devincent, C., Pomeroy, J. C., et al. (2009). Disruption of contactin 4 in three subjects with autism spectrum disorder. *J. Med. Genet.* 46, 176–182. doi: 10.1136/jmg.2008.057505

Rujescu, D., Ingason, A., Cichon, S., Pietilainen, O. P., Barnes, M. R., Toulopoulou, T., et al. (2009). Disruption of the neurexin 1 gene is associated with schizophrenia. *Hum. Mol. Genet.* 18, 988–996. doi: 10.1093/hmg/ddn351

Sakurai, T., Ramoz, N., Reichert, J. G., Corwin, T. E., Kryzak, L., Smith, C. J., et al. (2006). Association analysis of the NrCAM gene in autism and in subsets of families with severe obsessive–compulsive or self-stimulatory behaviors. *Psychiatr. Genet.* 16, 251–257. doi: 10.1097/01.ypg.0000242196.81891.c9

Sala, C., Piech, V., Wilson, N. R., Passafaro, M., Liu, G., and Sheng, M. (2001). Regulation of dendritic spine morphology and synaptic function by Shank and Homer. *Neuron* 31, 115–130. doi: 10.1016/S0896-6273(01)00339-7

Sanders, S. J., Ercan-Sencicek, A. G., Hus, V., Luo, R., Murtha, M. T., Moreno-De-Luca, D., et al. (2011). Multiple recurrent de novo CNVs, including duplications of the 7q11.23 Williams syndrome region, are strongly associated with autism. *Neuron* 70, 863–885. doi: 10.1016/j.neuron.2011.05.002

Sato, D., Lionel, A. C., Leblond, C. S., Prasad, A., Pinto, D., Walker, S., et al. (2012). SHANK1 deletions in males with autism spectrum disorder. *Am. J. Hum. Genet.* 90, 879–887. doi: 10.1016/j.ajhg.2012.03.017

Schaaf, C. P., Sabo, A., Sakai, Y., Crosby, J., Muzny, D., Hawes, A., et al. (2011). Oligogenic heterozygosity in individuals with high-functioning autism spectrum disorders. *Hum. Mol. Genet.* 20, 3366–3375. doi: 10.1093/hmg/ddr243

Schmeisser, M. J., Ey, E., Wegener, S., Bockmann, J., Stempel, A. V., Kuebler, A., et al. (2012). Autistic-like behaviours and hyperactivity in mice lacking ProSAP1/Shank2. *Nature* 486, 256–260. doi: 10.1038/nature11015

Schneider, T., and Przewlocki, R. (2005). Behavioral alterations in rats prenatally exposed to valproic acid: animal model of autism. *Neuropsychopharmacology* 30, 80–89. doi: 10.1038/sj.npp.1300518

Schroer, R. J., Phelan, M. C., Michaelis, R. C., Crawford, E. C., Skinner, S. A., Cuccaro, M., et al. (1998). Autism and maternally derived aberrations of chromosome 15q. *Am. J. Med. Genet.* 76, 327–336. doi: 10.1002/(SICI)1096-8628(19980401)76:4<327::AID-AJMG8>3.0.CO;2-M

Sebat, J., Lakshmi, B., Malhotra, D., Troge, J., Lese-Martin, C., Walsh, T., et al. (2007). Strong association of de novo copy number mutations with autism. *Science* 316, 445–449. doi: 10.1126/science.1138659

Sebat, J., Levy, D. L., and Mccarthy, S. E. (2009). Rare structural variants in schizophrenia: one disorder, multiple mutations; one mutation, multiple disorders. *Trends Genet.* 25, 528–535. doi: 10.1016/j.tig.2009.10.004

Shahbazian, M., Young, J., Yuva-Paylor, L., Spencer, C., Antalffy, B., Noebels, J., et al. (2002). Mice with truncated MeCP2 recapitulate many Rett syndrome features and display hyperacetylation of histone H3. *Neuron* 35, 243–254. doi: 10.1016/S0896-6273(02)00768-7

Shelton, J. F., Hertz-Picciotto, I., and Pessah, I. N. (2012). Tipping the balance of autism risk: potential mechanisms linking pesticides and autism. *Environ. Health Perspect.* 120, 944–951. doi: 10.1289/ehp.1104553

Sicca, F., Imbrici, P., D'Adamo, M. C., Moro, F., Bonatti, F., Brovedani, P., et al. (2011). Autism with seizures and intellectual disability: possible causative role of gain-of-function of the inwardly-rectifying K^+ channel Kir4.1. *Neurobiol. Dis.* 43, 239–247. doi: 10.1016/j.nbd.2011.03.016

Silva, S. C., Correia, C., Fesel, C., Barreto, M., Coutinho, A. M., Marques, C., et al. (2004). Autoantibody repertoires to brain tissue in autism nuclear families. *J. Neuroimmunol.* 152, 176–182. doi: 10.1016/j.jneuroim.2004.03.015

Smalley, S. L. (1998). Autism and tuberous sclerosis. *J. Autism Dev. Disord.* 28, 407–414. doi: 10.1023/A:1026052421693

Song, J. Y., Ichtchenko, K., Sudhof, T. C., and Brose, N. (1999). Neuroligin 1 is a postsynaptic cell-adhesion molecule of excitatory synapses. *Proc. Natl. Acad. Sci. U.S.A.* 96, 1100–1105. doi: 10.1073/pnas.96.3.1100

Splawski, I., Timothy, K. W., Sharpe, L. M., Decher, N., Kumar, P., Bloise, R., et al. (2004). Ca(V)1.2 calcium channel dysfunction causes a multisystem disorder including arrhythmia and autism. *Cell* 119, 19–31. doi: 10.1016/j.cell.2004.09.011

State, M. W., and Sestan, N. (2012). Neuroscience. The emerging biology of autism spectrum disorders. *Science* 337, 1301–1303. doi: 10.1126/science.1224989

Steffenburg, S., Gillberg, C., Hellgren, L., Andersson, L., Gillberg, I. C., Jakobsson, G., et al. (1989). A twin study of autism in Denmark, Finland, Iceland, Norway and Sweden. *J. Child Psychol. Psychiatry* 30, 405–416. doi: 10.1111/j.1469-7610.1989.tb00254.x

Strauss, K. A., Puffenberger, E. G., Huentelman, M. J., Gottlieb, S., Dobrin, S. E., Parod, J. M., et al. (2006). Recessive symptomatic focal epilepsy and mutant contactin-associated protein-like 2. *N. Engl. J. Med.* 354, 1370–1377. doi: 10.1056/NEJMoa052773

Sudhof, T. C. (2008). Neuroligins and neurexins link synaptic function to cognitive disease. *Nature* 455, 903–911. doi: 10.1038/nature07456

Sutcliffe, J. S., Delahanty, R. J., Prasad, H. C., Mccauley, J. L., Han, Q., Jiang, L., et al. (2005). Allelic heterogeneity at the serotonin transporter locus (SLC6A4) confers susceptibility to autism and rigid-compulsive behaviors. *Am. J. Hum. Genet.* 77, 265–279. doi: 10.1086/432648

Suter, D. M., Pollerberg, G. E., Buchstaller, A., Giger, R. J., Dreyer, W. J., and Sonderegger, P. (1995). Binding between the neural cell adhesion molecules axonin-1 and Nr-CAM/Bravo is involved in neuron-glia interaction. *J. Cell Biol.* 131, 1067–1081. doi: 10.1083/jcb.131.4.1067

Tabuchi, K., Blundell, J., Etherton, M. R., Hammer, R. E., Liu, X., Powell, C. M., et al. (2007). A neuroligin-3 mutation implicated in autism increases inhibitory synaptic transmission in mice. *Science* 318, 71–76. doi: 10.1126/science.1146221

Taniguchi, H., Gollan, L., Scholl, F. G., Mahadomrongkul, V., Dobler, E., Limthong, N., et al. (2007). Silencing of neuroligin function by postsynaptic neurexins. *J. Neurosci.* 27, 2815–2824. doi: 10.1523/JNEUROSCI.0032-07.2007

Tierney, E., Nwokoro, N. A., Porter, F. D., Freund, L. S., Ghuman, J. K., and Kelley, R. I. (2001). Behavior phenotype in the RSH/Smith–Lemli–Opitz syndrome. *Am. J. Med. Genet.* 98, 191–200. doi: 10.1002/1096-8628(20010115)98:2<191::AID-AJMG1030>3.0.CO;2-M

Tropepe, V., and Sive, H. L. (2003). Can zebrafish be used as a model to study the neurodevelopmental causes of autism? *Genes Brain Behav.* 2, 268–281. doi: 10.1034/j.1601-183X.2003.00038.x

Tsai, P. T., Hull, C., Chu, Y., Greene-Colozzi, E., Sadowski, A. R., Leech, J. M., et al. (2012). Autistic-like behaviour and cerebellar dysfunction in Purkinje cell Tsc1 mutant mice. *Nature* 488, 647–651. doi: 10.1038/nature11310

Tu, J. C., Xiao, B., Naisbitt, S., Yuan, J. P., Petralia, R. S., Brakeman, P., et al. (1999). Coupling of mGluR/Homer and PSD-95 complexes by the Shank family of postsynaptic density proteins. *Neuron* 23, 583–592. doi: 10.1016/S0896-6273(00)80810-7

Vaags, A. K., Lionel, A. C., Sato, D., Goodenberger, M., Stein, Q. P., Curran, S., et al. (2012). Rare deletions at the neurexin 3 locus in autism spectrum disorder. *Am. J. Hum. Genet.* 90, 133–141. doi: 10.1016/j.ajhg.2011.11.025

van de Lagemaat, L. N., and Grant, S. G. (2010). Genome variation and complexity in the autism spectrum. *Neuron* 67, 8–10. doi: 10.1016/j.neuron.2010.06.026

Varoqueaux, F., Aramuni, G., Rawson, R. L., Mohrmann, R., Missler, M., Gottmann, K., et al. (2006). Neuroligins determine synapse maturation and function. *Neuron* 51, 741–754. doi: 10.1016/j.neuron.2006.09.003

Varoqueaux, F., Jamain, S., and Brose, N. (2004). Neuroligin 2 is exclusively localized to inhibitory synapses. *Eur. J. Cell Biol.* 83, 449–456. doi: 10.1078/0171-9335-00410

Verpelli, C., Schmeisser, M. J., Sala, C., and Boeckers, T. M. (2012). Scaffold proteins at the postsynaptic density. *Adv. Exp. Med. Biol.* 970, 29–61. doi: 10.1007/978-3-7091-0932-8_2

Vervoort, V. S., Beachem, M. A., Edwards, P. S., Ladd, S., Miller, K. E., De Mollerat, X., et al. (2002). AGTR2 mutations in X-linked mental retardation. *Science* 296, 2401–2403. doi: 10.1126/science.1072191

Volkmer, H., Leuschner, R., Zacharias, U., and Rathjen, F. G. (1996). Neurofascin induces neurites by heterophilic interactions with axonal NrCAM while NrCAM requires F11 on the axonal surface to extend neurites. *J. Cell Biol.* 135, 1059–1069. doi: 10.1083/jcb.135.4.1059

Wang, C. C., Held, R. G., and Hall, B. J. (2013). SynGAP regulates protein synthesis and homeostatic synaptic plasticity in developing cortical networks. *PLoS ONE* 8:e83941. doi: 10.1371/journal.pone.0083941

Wang, H., and Doering, L. C. (2013). Reversing autism by targeting downstream mTOR signaling. *Front. Cell. Neurosci.* 7:28. doi: 10.3389/fncel.2013.00028

Wang, K., Zhang, H., Ma, D., Bucan, M., Glessner, J. T., Abrahams, B. S., et al. (2009). Common genetic variants on 5p14.1 associate with autism spectrum disorders. *Nature* 459, 528–533. doi: 10.1038/nature07999

Wang, X., Mccoy, P. A., Rodriguiz, R. M., Pan, Y., Je, H. S., Roberts, A. C., et al. (2011). Synaptic dysfunction and abnormal behaviors in mice lacking major isoforms of Shank3. *Hum. Mol. Genet.* 20, 3093–3108. doi: 10.1093/hmg/ddr212

Warren, W. C., Clayton, D. F., Ellegren, H., Arnold, A. P., Hillier, L. W., Kunstner, A., et al. (2010). The genome of a songbird. *Nature* 464, 757–762. doi: 10.1038/nature08819

Watson, K. K., and Platt, M. L. (2012). Of mice and monkeys: using non-human primate models to bridge mouse- and human-based investigations of autism spectrum disorders. *J. Neurodev. Disord.* 4, 21. doi: 10.1186/1866-1955-4-21

Weiner, J. A., and Jontes, J. D. (2013). Protocadherins, not prototypical: a complex tale of their interactions, expression, and functions. *Front. Mol. Neurosci.* 6:4. doi: 10.3389/fnmol.2013.00004

Weiner, J. A., Wang, X., Tapia, J. C., and Sanes, J. R. (2005). Gamma protocadherins are required for synaptic development in the spinal cord. *Proc. Natl. Acad. Sci. U.S.A.* 102, 8–14. doi: 10.1073/pnas.0407931101

Weiss, L. A., Escayg, A., Kearney, J. A., Trudeau, M., Macdonald, B. T., Mori, M., et al. (2003). Sodium channels SCN1A, SCN2A and SCN3A in familial autism. *Mol. Psychiatry* 8, 186–194. doi: 10.1038/sj.mp.40012414001241

Weiss, L. A., Shen, Y., Korn, J. M., Arking, D. E., Miller, D. T., Fossdal, R., et al. (2008). Association between microdeletion and microduplication at 16p11.2 and autism. *N. Engl. J. Med.* 358, 667–675. doi: 10.1056/NEJMoa075974

Williams, J. H., Whiten, A., Suddendorf, T., and Perrett, D. I. (2001). Imitation, mirror neurons and autism. *Neurosci. Biobehav. Rev.* 25, 287–295. doi: 10.1016/S0149-7634(01)00014-8

Williams, P. G., and Hersh, J. H. (1998). Brief report: the association of neurofibromatosis type 1 and autism. *J. Autism Dev. Disord.* 28, 567–571. doi: 10.1023/A:1026012414193

Wilson, H. L., Wong, A. C., Shaw, S. R., Tse, W. Y., Stapleton, G. A., Phelan, M. C., et al. (2003). Molecular characterisation of the 22q13 deletion syndrome supports the role of haploinsufficiency of SHANK3/PROSAP2 in the major neurological symptoms. *J. Med. Genet.* 40, 575–584. doi: 10.1136/jmg.40.8.575

Won, H., Lee, H. R., Gee, H. Y., Mah, W., Kim, J. I., Lee, J., et al. (2012). Autistic-like social behaviour in Shank2-mutant mice improved by restoring NMDA receptor function. *Nature* 486, 261–265. doi: 10.1038/nature11208

Won, H., Mah, W., and Kim, E. (2013). Autism spectrum disorder causes, mechanisms, and treatments: focus on neuronal synapses. *Front. Mol. Neurosci.* 6:19. doi: 10.3389/fnmol.2013.00019

Wu, S., Jia, M., Ruan, Y., Liu, J., Guo, Y., Shuang, M., et al. (2005). Positive association of the oxytocin receptor gene (OXTR) with autism in the Chinese Han population. *Biol. Psychiatry* 58, 74–77. doi: 10.1016/j.biopsych.2005.03.013

Wu, Y., Bolduc, F. V., Bell, K., Tully, T., Fang, Y., Sehgal, A., et al. (2008). A *Drosophila* model for Angelman syndrome. *Proc. Natl. Acad. Sci. U.S.A.* 105, 12399–12404. doi: 10.1073/pnas.0805291105

Ye, X., and Carew, T. J. (2011). Transsynaptic coordination of presynaptic and postsynaptic modifications underlying enduring synaptic plasticity. *Neuron* 70, 379–381. doi: 10.1016/j.neuron.2011.04.016

Yirmiya, N., Rosenberg, C., Levi, S., Salomon, S., Shulman, C., Nemanov, L., et al. (2006). Association between the arginine vasopressin 1a receptor (AVPR1a) gene and autism in a family-based study: mediation by socialization skills. *Mol. Psychiatry* 11, 488–494. doi: 10.1038/sj.mp.4001812

Zahir, F. R., Baross, A., Delaney, A. D., Eydoux, P., Fernandes, N. D., Pugh, T., et al. (2008). A patient with vertebral, cognitive and behavioural abnormalities and a de novo deletion of NRXN1alpha. *J. Med. Genet.* 45, 239–243. doi: 10.1136/jmg.2007.054437

Zeng, X., Sun, M., Liu, L., Chen, F., Wei, L., and Xie, W. (2007). Neurexin-1 is required for synapse formation and larvae associative learning in *Drosophila*. *FEBS Lett.* 581, 2509–2516. doi: 10.1016/j.febslet.2007.04.068

Zhou, J., Blundell, J., Ogawa, S., Kwon, C. H., Zhang, W., Sinton, C., et al. (2009). Pharmacological inhibition of mTORC1 suppresses anatomical, cellular, and behavioral abnormalities in neural-specific Pten knockout mice. *J. Neurosci.* 29, 1773–1783. doi: 10.1523/JNEUROSCI.5685-08.2009

Zoghbi, H. Y. (2003). Postnatal neurodevelopmental disorders: meeting at the synapse? *Science* 302, 826–830. doi: 10.1126/science.1089071302/5646/826

Zoghbi, H. Y., and Bear, M. F. (2012). Synaptic dysfunction in neurodevelopmental disorders associated with autism and intellectual disabilities. *Cold Spring Harb. Perspect. Biol.* 4, 1–22. doi: 10.1101/cshperspect.a009886

14

Targeted pharmacological treatment of autism spectrum disorders: Fragile X and Rett syndromes

Hansen Wang[1]*, Sandipan Pati[2], Lucas Pozzo-Miller[3]* and Laurie C. Doering[4]*

[1] *Faculty of Medicine, University of Toronto, 1 King's College Circle, Toronto, ON, Canada*
[2] *Department of Neurology, Epilepsy Division, The University of Alabama at Birmingham, Birmingham, AL, USA*
[3] *Department of Neurobiology, Civitan International Research Center, The University of Alabama at Birmingham, Birmingham, AL, USA*
[4] *Faculty of Health Sciences, Department of Pathology and Molecular Medicine, McMaster University, Hamilton, ON, Canada*

***Correspondence:**
Hansen Wang, Faculty of Medicine, University of Toronto, 1 King's College Circle, Toronto, ON M5S 1A8, Canada
e-mail: hansen.wang@utoronto.ca;
Lucas Pozzo-Miller, Department of Neurobiology, Civitan International Research Center, The University of Alabama at Birmingham, Birmingham, AL, 35294 USA
e-mail: lucaspm@uab.edu;
Laurie C. Doering, Faculty of Health Sciences, Department of Pathology and Molecular Medicine, McMaster University, HSC 1R1, 1280 Main Street West, Hamilton, ON L8S 4K1, Canada
e-mail: doering@mcmaster.ca

Autism spectrum disorders (ASDs) are genetically and clinically heterogeneous and lack effective medications to treat their core symptoms. Studies of syndromic ASDs caused by single gene mutations have provided insights into the pathophysiology of autism. Fragile X and Rett syndromes belong to the syndromic ASDs in which preclinical studies have identified rational targets for drug therapies focused on correcting underlying neural dysfunction. These preclinical discoveries are increasingly translating into exciting human clinical trials. Since there are significant molecular and neurobiological overlaps among ASDs, targeted treatments developed for fragile X and Rett syndromes may be helpful for autism of different etiologies. Here, we review the targeted pharmacological treatment of fragile X and Rett syndromes and discuss related issues in both preclinical studies and clinical trials of potential therapies for the diseases.

Keywords: fragile X syndrome, Rett syndrome, autism spectrum disorders, pharmacotherapy, treatment, synaptic deficits, FMRP, MeCP2

INTRODUCTION

Autism spectrum disorders (ASDs) encompass a group of neurodevelopmental disorders which are of different etiologies and characterized by impairments in socialization and communication, abnormalities in language development, restricted interests, and repetitive and stereotyped behaviors (Mefford et al., 2012; Zoghbi and Bear, 2012; Murdoch and State, 2013; Anagnostou et al., 2014b; Lai et al., 2014). These disorders are estimated to affect approximately 1% of the population. The genetic causes of ASDs show a high degree of heterogeneity, with hundreds of ASD-associated genes now identified (Mefford et al., 2012; Huguet et al., 2013; Murdoch and State, 2013; Lai et al., 2014; Ronemus et al., 2014). However, recent studies suggest that these ASD genes may functionally converge into a relatively smaller subset of cellular and biochemical pathways affecting distinct neuronal functions (Auerbach et al., 2011; Zoghbi and Bear, 2012; Ebert and Greenberg, 2013; Doll and Broadie, 2014; Krumm et al., 2014). In a subset of ASDs, such as the syndromic ASD fragile X syndrome, Rett syndrome (RTT) and tuberous sclerosis, mutations of genes have been found to be related to synaptic function, suggesting that abnormal neuronal homeostasis is a risk factor for ASD (Auerbach et al., 2011; Santoro et al., 2012; Zoghbi and Bear, 2012; Ebert and Greenberg, 2013; Banerjee et al., 2014). This subset of ASDs belong to a larger group of neurological conditions called "synaptopathies", which refer to disorders with altered synaptic function and/or morphology as primary neuropathology (Auerbach et al., 2011; Zoghbi and Bear, 2012; Krumm et al., 2014). The functional convergence on particular signaling pathways and the shared synaptopathology of ASDs have raised the hope that similar therapeutic strategies may be effective for different forms of ASDs which are related, but genetically distinct (Zoghbi and Bear, 2012; Delorme et al., 2013; Wang and Doering, 2013).

Fragile X and Rett syndromes are two of the most widely and intensively studied monogenetic ASDs (Santoro et al., 2012; Zoghbi and Bear, 2012; Castro et al., 2013; Chapleau et al., 2013a; Banerjee et al., 2014). Numerous studies have investigated the possibility of treating fragile X and Rett syndromes in their relative animal models. Strategies to alleviate abnormal phenotypes include genetic manipulation, cellular therapy, pharmacological intervention and environmental stimulation (Wang and Doering, 2012; Zoghbi and Bear, 2012; Castro et al., 2013; Chapleau et al., 2013a; Delorme et al., 2013; Ebert and Greenberg, 2013). Most encouraging, some of these fundamental studies have led to the development of drugs that are in clinical trials.

In this review, we summarize the potential therapeutic targets and relative pharmacological interventions in fragile X and Rett syndromes. The challenges in preclinical studies and clinical trials, and the implications of these targeted pharmacological treatments for other ASDs and related neurodevelopmental disorders are also discussed.

TARGETED PHARMACOTHERAPY FOR FRAGILE X SYNDROME

Fragile X syndrome is one of the most common genetic causes of intellectual disability and autism. It is mostly caused by the mutation of the trinucleotide CGG expansion in the 5′-untranslated region of the fragile X mental retardation (*FMR1*) gene, which eventually leads to the absence of its protein product, fragile X mental retardation protein (FMRP) (Garber et al., 2008; Bhakar et al., 2012; Santoro et al., 2012; Hagerman et al., 2014). FMRP is ubiquitous with the most abundance in the central nervous system (Santoro et al., 2012; Wang et al., 2012a; Sidorov et al., 2013) and exists in both neurons and glial cells (Wang et al., 2004; Pacey and Doering, 2007).

FMRP, a RNA binding protein, binds its mRNA targets and regulates the transport and translation of those mRNAs (Bear et al., 2004; Penagarikano et al., 2007; Bhakar et al., 2012; Santoro et al., 2012; Wang et al., 2012a; Sidorov et al., 2013; Abekhoukh and Bardoni, 2014). The mRNA targets of FMRP encode pre- and post-synaptic proteins and some of these proteins are implicated in other ASDs, suggesting a molecular overlap between fragile X syndrome and other neurodevelopmental disorders (Bhakar et al., 2012; Wang et al., 2012a; Sidorov et al., 2013). FMRP normally acts as a translational repressor, especially at synapses. Its absence has profound consequences on neural development and synaptic plasticity. Alterations in synaptic structure and function are believed to underlie the fragile X symptoms. Dysregulated protein synthesis is central to fragile X synaptopathy (Bear et al., 2004; Penagarikano et al., 2007; Bassell and Warren, 2008; Wang et al., 2010a; Bhakar et al., 2012; Santoro et al., 2012; Sidorov et al., 2013).

Over the past two decades, efforts have been made to elucidate the molecular and cellular events that give rise to synaptic dysfunction in fragile X syndrome. Studies in animal models have revealed defects in multiple neurotransmitter systems and relative signaling pathways/molecules that are responsible for fragile X synaptopathy (Wang et al., 2010b; Bhakar et al., 2012; Gross et al., 2012; Santoro et al., 2012; Zoghbi and Bear, 2012; Delorme et al., 2013; Ebert and Greenberg, 2013). Advances in neurobiology of fragile X syndrome have led to the development of therapeutic agents that target the underlying mechanisms of the disease (Summarized in **Figure 1**; **Tables 1, 2**).

TARGETING NEUROTRANSMITTER/NEUROMODULATOR SYSTEMS

Metabotropic glutamate receptors

Metabotropic glutamate receptors (mGluRs) play important roles in synaptic plasticity, learning and memory (Bortolotto et al., 1999; Bear et al., 2004; Wang et al., 2008a; Wang and Zhuo, 2012; Mukherjee and Manahan-Vaughan, 2013). Activation of group 1 mGluRs (mGluR1s and mGluR5s) leads to local translation of pre-existing mRNAs and triggers long-term depression (LTD) (Weiler and Greenough, 1993; Bortolotto et al., 1999; Raymond et al., 2000; Penagarikano et al., 2007; Ronesi and Huber, 2008a; Upreti et al., 2013). FMRP is one of these newly synthesized proteins and serves as a repressor of the translation of other synaptic mRNAs that encode LTD proteins such as activity-regulated cytoskeleton-associated protein (Arc), microtubule associated protein (MAP) 1B and Striatal-enriched protein tyrosine phosphatase (STEP), which mediate a-amino-3-hydroxyl-4-isoxazole propionic acid receptor (AMPAR) internalization and LTD stabilization (Bhakar et al., 2012; Santoro et al., 2012; Wang et al., 2012a; Darnell and Klann, 2013; Sidorov et al., 2013). In fragile X conditions, protein synthesis is elevated and mGluR-LTD in the hippocampus is exaggerated in the absence of FMRP; the enhanced mGluR-LTD is no longer protein synthesis dependent as a result of increased basal protein synthesis. The mGluR theory of fragile X syndrome thus postulates that the core symptoms of the disease result from exaggerated group 1 mGluR mediated signaling including mGluR-LTD (Bear et al., 2004; Garber et al., 2008; Bhakar et al., 2012; Santoro et al., 2012; Sidorov et al., 2013).

The mGluR theory and its therapeutic significance have been validated in both genetic and pharmacological rescue studies (Dölen and Bear, 2008; Hays et al., 2011; Thomas et al., 2011; Gandhi et al., 2014; Michalon et al., 2014; Pop et al., 2014). In *Fmr1* knockout mice, the mGluR5 antagonist 2-methyl-6-(phenylethynyl)-pyridine (MPEP) stabilized hippocampal protein synthesis, increased the density or rescued the morphology of hippocampal dendritic spines, corrected altered brain network function, reduced audiogenic seizures and repetitive and/or perseverative behaviors (marble burying), rescued the deficits in prepulse inhibition of startle response, and improved the maze and motor learning (Yan et al., 2005; de Vrij et al., 2008; Hays et al., 2011; Thomas et al., 2012; Gandhi et al., 2014). Other mGluR5 antagonists tested in fragile X animal models include CTEC, fenobam and AFQ056. Acute treatment with CTEC corrected the elevated hippocampal LTD, protein synthesis, and audiogenic seizures; chronic treatment rescued cognitive deficits, auditory hypersensitivity, aberrant dendritic spine density, overactive extracellular signal regulated kinase (ERK) and mammalian target of rapamycin (mTOR) signaling, and partially corrected macroorchidism in adult fragile X mice (Michalon et al., 2012). Chronic CTEP treatment also corrected learning deficit in the inhibitory avoidance and extinction test, and partially normalized altered local brain activity in these animals (Michalon et al., 2014). Fenobam reversed some synaptic alterations in the cortex (Wang et al., 2014) and corrected deficits in associative motor learning and avoidance behaviors in fragile X mice

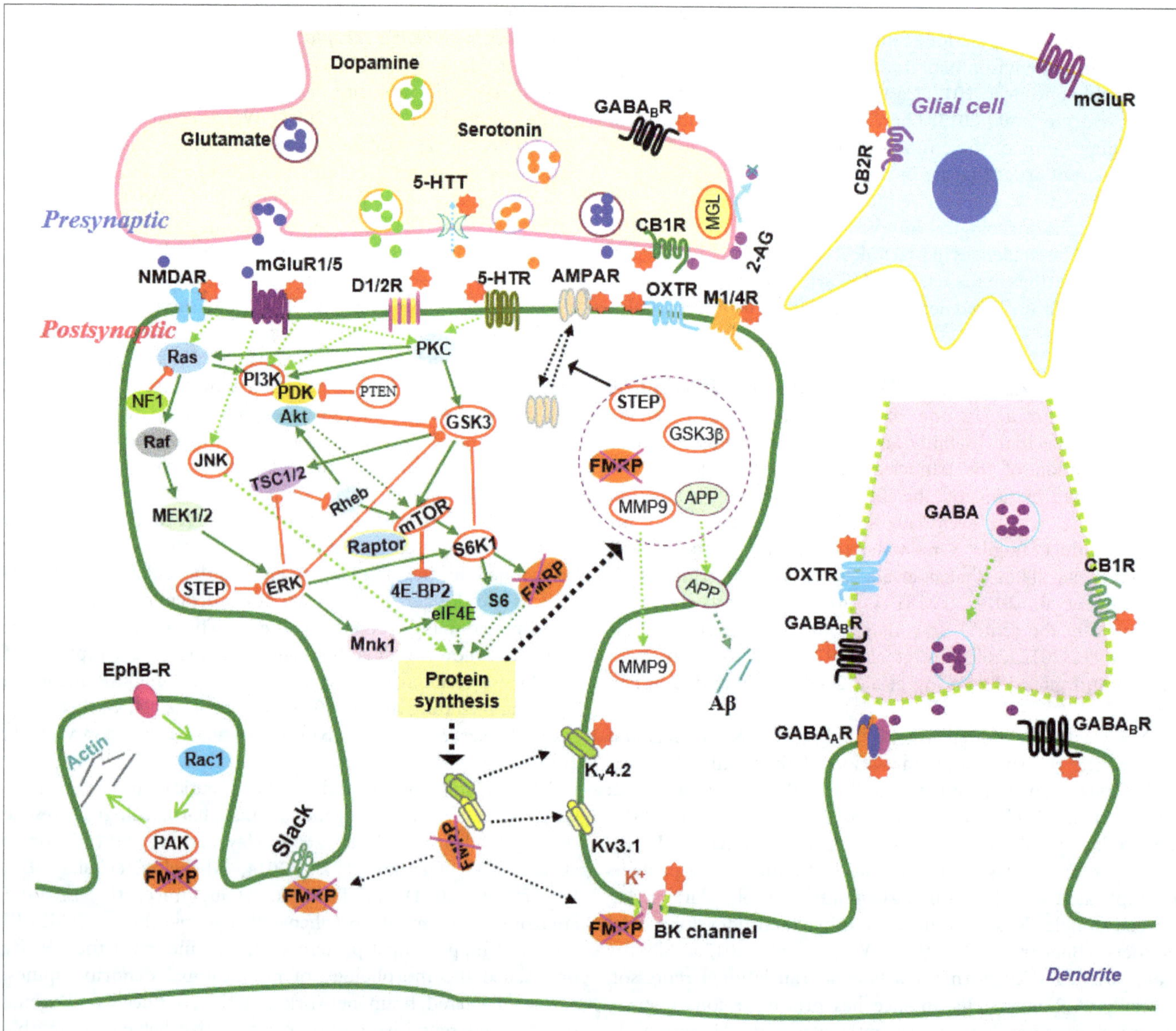

FIGURE 1 | Signaling molecules and pathways in the neurobiology of fragile X syndrome. In signaling pathways, arrows indicate positive (green) or inhibitory (red) consequence on downstream components, but they do not necessarily represent direct interactions. Potential therapeutic targets which have been validated by genetic or pharmacological manipulation are indicated by red stars or highlighted by red circles. Abbreviations: 2-AG, 2-arachidonoyl-sn-glycerol; 4E-BP2, eIF4E-binding protein 2; 5-HT, serotonin; 5-HTR, serotonin receptors; 5-HTT, serotonin transporters; Akt (PKB), protein kinase B; AMPAR, α-amino-3-hydroxyl-4-isoxazole propionic acid receptors; APP, amyloid precursor protein; CB1(2)R, cannabinoid receptor 1(2); EphB-R, EphB receptors; ERK, extracellular signal related kinase; FMRP, fragile X mental retardation protein; GABA, gamma aminobutyric acid; GABA$_{A(B)}$R, GABA$_{A(B)}$ receptors; GSK3, glycogen synthase kinase-3; JNK, c-Jun N-terminal kinase; M1/4R, muscarinic acetylcholine receptor 1/4; MEK, mitogen-activated protein kinase/ERK kinase; MGL, monoacylglycerol lipase; mGluR, metabotropic glutamate receptor; MMP9, matrix metalloproteinase 9; MSK, mitogen and stress-activated protein kinase; mTOR, mammalian target of rapamycin; NF1, neurofibromatosis 1; NMDAR, N-methyl-d-aspartate receptors; OXTR, oxytocin receptor; PAK, p21-activated kinase; PI3K, phosphatidylinositol 3-kinase; PKC, protein kinase C; PP2A, protein phosphatase 2A; PTEN, Phosphatase and tensin homolog; Raptor, regulatory-associated protein of mTOR; RSK, p90 ribosomal S6 kinase; S6K1, p70 ribosomal kinase 1; STEP, striatal-enriched protein tyrosine phosphatase; TSC1/2, tuberous sclerosis complex 1/2.

(Vinueza Veloz et al., 2012). AFQ056 was found to be able to correct aberrant hippocampal dendritic spine morphology (Levenga et al., 2011; Pop et al., 2014), and rescue deficits in prepulse inhibition of acoustic startle response and abnormal social behaviors (Levenga et al., 2011; Gantois et al., 2013) in *Fmr1* knockout mice. Treatment with mGluR1 antagonists (JNJ16259685 or LY367385) decreased repetitive and/or perseverative behaviors (Thomas et al., 2012), and rescued dysregulated synaptic protein synthesis in fragile X mice (Gross et al., 2010; Guo et al., 2012). These preclinical studies have been paving the way for treatments with mGluR antagonists in humans.

Table 1 | Therapeutic targets and relative drugs in preclinical studies of fragile X syndrome.

Targets		Drugs	Action
Neurotransmitter receptors or transporters	mGluR5	MPEP, CTEC, fenobam, AFQ056	Antagonists
	mGluR1	JNJ16259685, LY367385	Antagonists
	$GABA_A$ receptor	THIP, ganaxolone	Agonists
	$GABA_B$ receptor	Baclofen, arbaclofen (STX209)	Agonists
	$5\text{-}HT_7$ receptor	8-OH-DPAT	Agonist
	$5\text{-}HT_{2B}$ receptor	BW723C86	Agonist
	$5\text{-}HT_{2A}$ receptor	αMe-5HT, MDL11939	Antagonists
	5-HTT	Fluoxetine	5-HT reuptake inhibitor
	Dopamine D1 receptor	SKF81297	Agonist
	CB1R	Rimonabant	Antagonist
	CB2R	AM630	Antagonist
	MGL	JZL184	Inhibitor
	M1R	Dicyclomine	Antagonist
	M4R	Tropicamide	Antagonist
	NMDAR	Memantine	Antagonist
Protein kinases or other enzymes	ERK	SL327, U0126, lovastatin	Inhibitors
	JNK	SP600125	Inhibitor
	PI3K	LY294002, TGX-221	Inhibitors
	PTEN	BpV	Inhibitor
	mTOR	Temsirolimus, rapamycin, LY294002, TGX221	Inhibitors
	GSK3	Lithium, SB216763 TDZD-8, YP0.7	Inhibitors
	MMP9	Minocycline	Inhibitor
	PAK	FRAX486	Inhibitor
Ion channels	Kv4 channel	HpTx2	Blocker
	BK channel	BMS-204352	Opener

Table 2 | Drugs in clinical trials of fragile X syndrome.

Drugs	Action	Study designs	Publications
Fenobam	mGluR5 antagonist	Open label pilot study; single dose	Berry-Kravis et al. (2009)
AFQ056	mGluR5 antagonist	Randomized, double-blind, two treatment, two-period crossover study	Jacquemont et al. (2011)
RO4917523	mGluR5 antagonist	Randomized, double-blinded, placebo-controlled study	Discontinued due to negative results†
Ganaxolone	$GABA_A$ receptor agonist	Double-blind, controlled trial	www.clinicaltrials.gov
Acamprosate	GABA receptor agonist	Open-label, uncontrolled trial	Erickson et al. (2010, 2013)
Arbaclofen (STX209)	$GABA_B$ receptor agonist	Randomized, double-blind, placebo-controlled study	Berry-Kravis et al. (2012)
Oxytocin	OXTR agonist	Double-blind, placebo-controlled study	Hall et al. (2012)
CX516	AMPAR positive modulator	Randomized, double-blind, placebo-controlled study	Berry-Kravis et al. (2006)
Memantine	NMDAR antagonist	Open-label study	Erickson et al. (2009)
Lovastatin	ERK inhibitor	Open-label study	Çaku et al. (2014)
Lithium	GSK3 inhibitor	Open-label study	Berry-Kravis et al. (2008)
Minocycline	MMP9 inhibitor	Open-label add-on pilot trial	Paribello et al. (2010)
		Randomized, double-blind, placebo-controlled and crossover trial	Leigh et al. (2013)

† *www.fragilex.org*

Fenobam, the first mGluR antagonist used in patients, showed beneficial effects, such as reduced anxiety and hyperarousal, improved prepulse inhibition of startle, and better accuracy on a continuous performance task, in adults with fragile X syndrome (Berry-Kravis et al., 2009). The pharmacokinetics and side effects of fenobam are currently tested in adult healthy volunteers.[1] AFQ056 also showed improvements in inappropriate speech, stereotypic behavior, and hyperactivity and efficacy in adult patients with fully methylated *FMR1* (Jacquemont et al., 2011). However, the mGluR5 negative allosteric modulator RG7090 (RO4917523) in fragile X was recently discontinued by Roche due to negative phase II clinical study results from fragile X patients.[2] More drugs targeting mGluRs with higher efficacy and better safety need to be developed in the future (Berry-Kravis, 2014; Hagerman et al., 2014).

[1] www.clinicaltrials.gov

[2] www.fragilex.org

GABAergic receptors

The γ-aminobutyric acid (GABA) is the main inhibitory neurotransmitter in brain and signals through $GABA_A$ and $GABA_B$ receptors (Ben-Ari et al., 2012; Gassmann and Bettler, 2012; Sigel and Steinmann, 2012). The deficiencies in GABA receptor expression and GABA receptor-mediated inhibition have been demonstrated in fragile X animal models, linking GABA receptors to fragile X phenotypes and leading to the hypothesis that fragile X syndrome may result from an imbalance between excitation and inhibition, and increasing inhibition may ameliorate some fragile X pathophysiologies, including dysregulated protein synthesis (D'Hulst et al., 2006, 2009; Chang et al., 2008; Pacey et al., 2009; Olmos-Serrano et al., 2010; Paluszkiewicz et al., 2011; He et al., 2014). The potential of GABA receptors as a therapeutic target for fragile X syndrome has been validated in animal models. Treatment with a selective $GABA_A$ receptor agonist THIP (gaboxadol) corrected neuronal hyperexcitability in the amygdala (Olmos-Serrano et al., 2010), and attenuated hyperactivity and deficits in prepulse inhibition of the acoustic startle response of fragile X mice (Olmos-Serrano et al., 2011). Treatment with ganaxolone, a positive allosteric modulator of $GABA_A$ receptors, could prevent audiogenic seizures in *Fmr1* knockout mice (Heulens et al., 2012). The $GABA_B$ receptor agonist baclofen reduced locomotor activity and hyperactivity (Zupan and Toth, 2008), and ameliorated audiogenic seizure susceptibility of *Fmr1* knockout mice (Pacey et al., 2009, 2011). Notably, arbaclofen (STX209), the R-isomer of baclofen, was also able to attenuate audiogenic seizures in fragile X mice (Henderson et al., 2012). In addition, arbaclofen corrected dysregulated protein synthesis in the hippocampus, restored the elevated AMPA receptor internalization and the increased spine density, and thus corrected synaptic abnormalities which are central to fragile X pathophysiologies, suggesting that arbaclofen could be potentially used to treat the core symptoms of fragile X patients (Henderson et al., 2012).

A large clinical trial with ganaxolone is currently ongoing in children and adolescents with fragile X syndrome between 6 to 17 years of age (Wijetunge et al., 2013; Berry-Kravis, 2014; Hagerman et al., 2014).[3] A controlled trial of arbaclofen in 63 fragile X patients between 6 to 40 years of age has revealed significant beneficial treatment effects, such as improvements in socialization and social avoidance scores, particularly in those with more severe social impairments, suggesting that $GABA_B$ receptor agonists have potential to improve social function and behaviors in fragile X patients (Berry-Kravis et al., 2012). However, this clinical trial for arbaclofen failed to fulfill its initial endpoints and had to be terminated by Seaside Therapeutics due to resource limitations.[4] Acamprosate, with agonist properties on both $GABA_A$ and $GABA_B$ receptors, was well tolerated and was found to significantly improve social behavior and reduce inattention/hyperactivity in 12 fragile X children aged 6–17 years in a prospective open-label 10-week trial. Additionally, an increase in brain-derived neurotrophic factor (BDNF) in blood was observed with treatment and might become a useful biomarker for future clinical studies (Erickson et al., 2010, 2013). A double-blind, placebo-controlled study will be needed to further assess the effect of acamprosate. As a whole, it is hopeful that some of the GABA receptor agonists may eventually become clinically applicable.

Serotonin receptors/transporters

The serotonin (5-Hydroxytryptamine, 5-HT) system is involved in various brain functions, including synaptic plasticity, learning and memory (Matthys et al., 2011; Lesch and Waider, 2012; Gellynck et al., 2013). It has been shown that 5-HT7 receptor (agonist 8-OH-DPAT) activation could reverse mGluR-induced AMPA receptor internalization and correct excessive mGluR-LTD in hippocampal neurons of *Fmr1* knockout mice, suggesting that 5-HT receptors may represent a novel therapeutic target for fragile X syndrome (Costa et al., 2012). Interestingly, a recent study has demonstrated that compounds activating 5-HT2B receptors or inhibiting 5-HT2A receptors could enhance phosphoinositide 3-kinase (PI3K) signaling transduction and AMPA GluR1 dependent synaptic plasticity, and restore learning in *Fmr1* knockout mice, further linking 5-HT receptors to fragile X syndrome (Lim et al., 2014).

The alteration of 5-HT and its transporters have been known to associate with autism (Chugani, 2002; Devlin et al., 2005; Prasad et al., 2009; Veenstra-VanderWeele et al., 2012; Harrington et al., 2013). 5-HT transporters are the main target for widely used antidepressant agents including fluoxetine (Wong et al., 2005). Fluoxetine binds to 5-HT transporters and blocks 5-HT uptake from the synaptic cleft into presynaptic vesicles in the central nervous system (Wong et al., 2005; Tavoulari et al., 2009). Studies have suggested that fluoxetine may be beneficial to individuals with autism (Hollander et al., 2005, 2012; Kolevzon et al., 2006). Treatment with fluoxetine has shown some effect in fragile X mice and patients (Hagerman et al., 1999; Uutela et al., 2014). However, fluoxetine has some possible side effects in clinic, such as mood changes, agitation, restlessness, and aggression, and may not be suitable to all individuals with fragile X syndrome and other ASDs (Wernicke, 2004; Kolevzon et al., 2006; Uutela et al., 2014).

Dopamine receptors

Dopamine plays critical roles in synaptic plasticity, cognitive functioning and neuropsychiatic pathologies (Jay, 2003; Seamans and Yang, 2004; Surmeier et al., 2009; Cerovic et al., 2013). Deficits in the dopamine system have been demonstrated in both fragile X animal models and patients (Roberts et al., 2005; Wang et al., 2008b; Weinshenker and Warren, 2008; Fulks et al., 2010; Paul et al., 2013; Rogers et al., 2013). Electrophysiological studies have found that dopaminergic modulation of synaptic transmission and potentiation are impaired in fragile X mice (Wang et al., 2008b; Paul et al., 2013). Biochemical studies have further revealed that dopamine D1 receptor mediated synapse-associated protein synthesis, AMPA GluR1 receptor surface expression and subsequent internalization are defective in these mice (Wang et al., 2008b, 2010a). Application of

[3]www.clinicaltrials.gov
[4]www.clinicaltrials.gov

the D1 receptor agonist and/or D2 receptor antagonist could promote PI3K signaling and AMPA GluR1 receptor delivery, and improve learning behaviors in *Fmr1* knockout mice (Lim et al., 2014). The dopamine D1 receptor agonist also partially rescued the hyperactivity and enhanced motor function of fragile X mice (Wang et al., 2008b). These findings suggest that dopamine receptors could be a potential target for effectively treating cognitive impairment associated with fragile X syndrome.

Cannabinoid receptors

The endocannabinoids N-arachidonoyl ethanolamine and 2-arachidonoyl glycerol (2-AG) activate cannabinoid receptors (CB1R and CB2R), and modulate synaptic plasticity and cognitive function (Chevaleyre et al., 2006; Heifets and Castillo, 2009; Oudin et al., 2011). Alterations in endocannabinoid signaling contribute to cognitive dysfunction associated with fragile X syndrome. Various abnormalities in endocannabinoid signaling, such as CB1R-driven long-term regulation of synaptic strength due to mGluR5 activation, have been observed in several brain areas of *Fmr1* knockout mice (Maccarrone et al., 2010; Zhang and Alger, 2010; Busquets-Garcia et al., 2013). FMRP exerts a regulatory control over the endocannabinoid system at central synapses (Maccarrone et al., 2010). Loss of FMRP affects endocannabinoid signaling, possibly through local 2-AG production (Straiker et al., 2013). In fragile X mice, the linkage between mGluR5 and the 2-AG producing enzyme, diacylglycerol lipase-α (DGL-α), is disrupted and mGluR5-dependent 2-AG formation is compromised, leading to impairment of endocannabinoid-mediated LTD in the ventral striatum and prefrontal cortex (Jung et al., 2012).

Pharmacological enhancement of 2-AG signaling by inhibiting 2-AG-deactivating enzyme monoacylglycerol lipase (MGL) with JZL184, normalized this synaptic defect and corrected behavioral abnormalities (hyperactivity and abnormal anxiety) in fragile X mice (Jung et al., 2012). Interestingly, dampening of endocannabinoid signaling through pharmacological or genetic approaches also benefit these mice. CB1R blockade with rimonabant or genetic reduction of CB1R, normalized cognitive impairment, nociceptive desensitization, susceptibility to audiogenic seizures, overactivated mTOR signaling and altered spine morphology in the male *Fmr1* knockout (*Fmr1*(-/y)) mice, whereas CB2R antagonism with AM630 normalized anxiolytic-like behaviors in those mice (Busquets-Garcia et al., 2013). These studies thus demonstrate that targeting endocannabinoid signaling might provide a new therapeutic strategy for fragile X syndrome. Further investigation is needed to clarify the therapeutic value of this potential target.

Muscarinic acetylcholine receptors

The G-protein coupled muscarinic acetylcholine receptors (mAChRs, subtypes M1–M5) are widely expressed in the central nervous system and mediate the metabotropic actions of acetylcholine (Volpicelli and Levey, 2004; Picciotto et al., 2012). M1 mAChR activation facilitates synaptic plasticity, learning and memory. Activation of M1 mAChRs stimulates synthesis of synaptic proteins including FMRP, and induces protein synthesis dependent LTD similar to group 1 mGluR-LTD (McCoy and McMahon, 2007; Volk et al., 2007). In the absence of FMRP, hippocampal M1 mAChR-dependent LTD is enhanced, indicating overactive mAChR signaling in *Fmr1* knockout mice (Volk et al., 2007). Genetic reduction of M4 mAChRs corrected the analgesic response and partly rescued the acoustic startle response in *Fmr1* knockout mice (Veeraragavan et al., 2012). These studies suggest new therapeutic strategies for using mAChR antagonists in fragile X syndrome.

The subtype selective mAChR modulators, including the M1 receptor antagonist dicyclomine and M4 receptor antagonist tropicamide, have been tested in the fragile X mouse model. The M1 receptor antagonist dicyclomine decreased repetitive and/or perseverative behavior (marble burying) and reduced susceptibility to audiogenic seizures in *Fmr1* knockout mice (Veeraragavan et al., 2011b). Similarly, the M4 receptor antagonist tropicamide also attenuated audiogenic seizure susceptibility in *Fmr1* knockout mice (Veeraragavan et al., 2011a). Noteworthy, treatment with tropicamide reduced repetitive and/or perseverative behaviors, improved performance in the passive avoidance task in both wild-type and fragile X mice, and reduced audiogenic seizures in fragile X mice (Veeraragavan et al., 2011a). These studies indicate that pharmacological inhibition of mAChRs modulates specific behavioral responses and further support these receptors as therapeutic targets for fragile X syndrome.

Oxytocin receptors

Oxytocin acts as a neuromodulator through its receptors in various brain areas and regulates social cognition and behaviors (Neumann, 2008; Meyer-Lindenberg et al., 2011; Neumann and Landgraf, 2012; Knobloch and Grinevich, 2014). It is emerging as a target for treatment of anxiety and depression-related diseases or social dysfunction including autism (Neumann, 2008; Meyer-Lindenberg et al., 2011; Neumann and Landgraf, 2012; Anagnostou et al., 2014a; Preti et al., 2014). The perinatal excitatory-to-inhibitory shift of GABA is mediated by oxytocin receptors. Oxytocin-mediated GABA inhibition during delivery could attenuate autism pathogenesis in rodent offsprings. Application of the oxytocin receptor antagonist SSR126768A in naïve mothers could produce offspring which have the electrophysiological and behavioral autistic-like features (Tyzio et al., 2014). In fragile X mice, oxytocin is reduced in some brain regions and the oxytocin-mediated neuroprotective GABA excitatory-inhibitory shift during delivery is absent (Tyzio et al., 2014). This study thus indicates the importance of the oxytocin system in the pathogenesis of autism and fragile X sydrome.

The clinical actions of oxytocin have been validated in ASD patients, providing preliminary evidence that oxytocin is able to enhance brain function and improve social behaviors in autistic patients (Andari et al., 2010; Domes et al., 2013; Gordon et al., 2013; Anagnostou et al., 2014a; Preti et al., 2014; Scheele et al., 2014; Watanabe et al., 2014). Intranasal administration of oxytocin could ameliorate symptoms of social anxiety in children with fragile X syndrome (Hall et al., 2012).

The double-blind placebo-controlled studies of oxytocin will be needed for further validation of its effect on fragile X patients.

AMPA receptors

The surface expression and synaptic delivery of AMPA receptors (GluR1) is impaired in *Fmr1* knockout mice, altering signal transmission and synaptic plasticity (Nakamoto et al., 2007; Hu et al., 2008; Suvrathan et al., 2010; Wang et al., 2010a). AMPA receptor modulators have been tested in fragile X patients. CX516 is a positive allosteric modulator that potentiates glutamate activation with the final outcome of strengthening synapses (O'Neill et al., 2004; O'Neill and Witkin, 2007). In a double-blind placebo-controlled trial in adult patients with fragile X syndrome, 4-week treatment with CX516 produced no significant improvement in cognitive or behavioral measures (Berry-Kravis et al., 2006). The failure could be due to the potency of CX516 or its dosage which may be inadequate for a therapeutic effect. It is thus unclear whether modulation of AMPA receptors is a feasible therapeutic strategy for treatment of fragile X syndrome.

NMDA receptors

The defects in NMDA receptors observed in the hippocampus, prefrontal cortex and other brain areas of fragile X mice are believed to contribute to fragile X phenotypes (Pilpel et al., 2009; Suvrathan et al., 2010; Krueger et al., 2011; Yun and Trommer, 2011; Eadie et al., 2012; Gocel and Larson, 2012). Memantine is an uncompetitive NMDA receptor antagonist and has been shown to improve language function and social behavior in autistic patients (Erickson and Chambers, 2006; Chez et al., 2007; Niederhofer, 2007). A study in cultured cerebellar granule cells from *Fmr1* knockout mice suggested that memantine may exert therapeutic capacity for fragile X syndrome through a stimulatory effect on dendritic spine maturation and excitatory synapse formation (Wei et al., 2012). Although a pilot study showed that memantine was modestly effective in several patients with fragile X syndrome, a systematic clinical study is needed to further evaluate its effectiveness (Erickson et al., 2009).

TARGETING SIGNALING PATHWAYS DOWNSTREAM OF NEUROTRANSMITTER RECEPTORS

Studies in fragile X animal models have revealed defects in intracellular signaling pathways [Mitogen-activated protein kinases (MAPKs), PI3K, mTOR and glycogen synthase kinase-3 (GSK3)] which could be downstream of neurotransmitter receptors such as glutamate, GABA, endocannabinoid, 5-HT, dopamine or mACh receptors. These signaling pathways may serve as therapeutic targets for fragile X syndrome (**Figure 1**; **Tables 1, 2**).

Mitogen-activated protein kinases

MAPKs are a family of serine/threonine protein kinases, including ERKs, p38 MAPKs, and c-Jun N-terminal kinase (JNK; Wang and Zhuo, 2012). The ERK1/2 pathway, which is activated by the Ras-mitogen-activated protein kinase/ERK kinase (MEK) and eventually leads to gene transcription or mRNA translation, plays critical roles in synaptic plasticity (Kelleher et al., 2004; Thomas and Huganir, 2004; Wiegert and Bading, 2011; Wang and Zhuo, 2012). A number of studies have investigated ERK signaling under basal conditions or upon mGluR-induction using brain tissues from fragile X animal models or patients (Kim et al., 2008; Weng et al., 2008; Wang et al., 2012b; Curia et al., 2013). Although these studies sometimes have presented conflicting results, most of them have shown that the ERK1/2 pathway is altered in fragile X conditions, suggesting that the ERK pathway is likely to have translational implications for fragile X syndrome (Weng et al., 2008; Wang et al., 2012b; Curia et al., 2013). Indeed, treatment with MEK1/2 inhibitor SL327 could prevent audiogenic seizures in *Fmr1* knockout mice (Wang et al., 2012b). Inhibition of ERK1/2 with the MEK1/2-ERK1/2 inhibitor U0126 also reduced elevated protein synthesis in hippocampus of fragile X mice (Osterweil et al., 2010). These findings further support that ERK1/2 pathway and the neurotransmitter systems that stimulate ERK1/2 may represent additional therapeutic targets for fragile X syndrome. Interestingly, statins, drug widely prescribed to treat hypercholesterolemia, have shown potentials for treating fragile X syndrome. Lovastatin corrected the excess protein synthesis and the exaggerated mGluR-LTD in the hippocampal slices of *Fmr1* knockout mice, attenuated hyperexcitability in visual cortex, and reduced audiogenic seizures in those mice (Osterweil et al., 2013). In a recent Phase I clinical trial, lovastatin was found to improve aberrant behaviors (social avoidance/unresponsiveness, stereotypy, hyperactivity and irritability) in majority (12/15) of fragile X patients after 12-weeks of treatment; the effect was significant after 4-week treatment at the lower dose, with further improvement during the 4–12 week treatment (Çaku et al., 2014). Although it was suggested that statins may alter membrane cholesterol and lipid rafts, thus modulating group I mGluRs or/and other neurotransmitter systems to correct fragile X phenotypes, the drugs might also exert the effects through direct inhibition of Ras–ERK activity (Kumari et al., 2013; Osterweil et al., 2013; Wang, 2014).

The JNK pathway is known to regulate mGluR-dependent gene transcription (Wang and Zhuo, 2012). A recent study has shown that JNK is essential for mGluR-dependent expression of FMRP target proteins. In addition, JNK activity is upregulated in synapses of *Fmr1* knockout mice, and inhibition of JNK with SP600125 decreased elevated postsynaptic protein synthesis in these mice, suggesting that JNK could be a key signaling downstream of mGluR in regulating FMRP-dependent protein synthesis and may provide a strategy to restore the deficits in fragile X syndrome (Schmit et al., 2013).

Phosphoinositide 3-kinase

PI3K transduces signals from cell surface receptors to the Akt/mTOR pathway and is essential for dendritic spine development and synaptic plasticity underlying learning and memory (Horwood et al., 2006; Hu et al., 2008; Cuesto et al., 2011). The PI3K catalytic subunit p110beta can be regulated by FMRP. Both p110beta level and PI3K activity are elevated and insensitive to mGluR stimulation in *Fmr1* knockout neurons, suggesting that dysregulated PI3K signaling may underlie synaptic deficits in fragile X syndrome (Gross et al., 2010; Gross and Bassell, 2014). PI3K inhibitor LY294002 corrected dysregulated synaptic protein synthesis, excess AMPA receptor internalization and the increased spine density in *Fmr1* knockout neurons, supporting PI3K as a potential therapeutic target for fragile X syndrome (Gross et al., 2010). Development of specific inhibitors for PI3K subunits may help to translate this strategy to patients since selective inhibition of the p110b-subunit with TGX-221 has been found to rescue excess protein synthesis in synaptoneurosomes from fragile X mice and in patient cells (Gross et al., 2010; Gross and Bassell, 2012, 2014). Conversely, one recent study showed that promoting PI3K signaling by dipotassium bisperoxo (5-hydroxypyridine-2-carboxyl)oxovanadate (BpV), a phosphatase and tensin homolog (PTEN) inhibitor, reversed deficits in both basal turnover and activity-mediated spine stabilization in hippocampal slices, restored defective long-term potentiation (LTP) mechanisms in slices and improved reversal learning in *Fmr1* knockout mice (Boda et al., 2014). Thus, the specific role of PI3K signaling in fragile X syndrome needs to be further investigated due to the complexity of its upstream cell surface receptors and interactions with other signaling pathways.

Mammalian target of rapamycin

The mTOR signaling cascade controls initiation of cap-dependent translation (Hay and Sonenberg, 2004; Narayanan et al., 2008; Hoeffer and Klann, 2010). Its downstream effector ribosomal protein S6 kinase (S6K1) is a regulator of translation initiation and elongation in cap-dependent protein synthesis (Narayanan et al., 2008; Hoeffer and Klann, 2010). S6K1 is a major kinase which phosphorylates and regulates FMRP following group 1 mGluR or dopamine D1 receptor activation (Narayanan et al., 2008; Wang et al., 2010a). The basal levels of mTOR phosphorylation and activity were found to be elevated in the hippocampus of *Fmr1* knockout mice (Sharma et al., 2010). In addition, group 1 mGluR activation of mTOR is absent is those mice (Ronesi and Huber, 2008b). The misregulation of mTOR signaling was also observed in fragile X patients (Hoeffer et al., 2012), suggesting that mTOR could be a target or biomarker for treatment of fragile X syndrome.

Treatment of *Fmr1* knockout mice with temsirolimus, an mTOR inhibitor, prevented object recognition memory deficits and reduced audiogenic seizure susceptibility in those mice (Busquets-Garcia et al., 2013). Elevated phosphorylation of translational control molecules and exaggerated protein synthesis in fragile X mice were corrected through the targeting of S6K1. Genetic deletion of S6K1 also prevented a broad range of fragile X phenotypes, including exaggerated translation, enhanced mGluR-LTD, abnormal dendritic spine morphology, several behavioral characteristics and peripheral features (weight gain and macroorchidism) (Bhattacharya et al., 2012). Notably, administration of the mTORC1 (mTOR complex 1) inhibitor rapamycin improved sociability in the BTBR mouse model of ASDs (Burket et al., 2014); targeting downstream mTOR signaling such as eukaryotic translation initiation factor 4E (eIF4E) also reversed autism (Gkogkas et al., 2013; Wang and Doering, 2013). These studies thus support that mTOR signaling represents a potential therapeutic target for fragile X syndrome and other ASDs.

Glycogen synthase kinase-3

GSK3 is a serine/threonine kinase that exists in two isoforms (GSK3α and GSK3β) and regulates many cellular processes through phosphorylation of their substrates. The activity of GSK3 itself is controlled by inhibitory serine phosphorylation induced by various intracellular pathways including PI3K/Akt and MEK/ERK that converge on GSK3 (Cohen and Goedert, 2004; Jope and Roh, 2006; Sugden et al., 2008). In *Fmr1* knockout mice, GSK3 phosphorylation was reduced in several brain regions resulting in elevated GSK3 signaling (Min et al., 2009; Mines et al., 2010; Yuskaitis et al., 2010). Lithium, a classical drug for psychiatric disorders, is a GSK3 inhibitor that both increases the inhibitory serine-phosphorylation of GSK3 and directly inhibits GSK3 activity (Chiu and Chuang, 2010; Mines and Jope, 2011). Since lithium has many other off-target effects including inhibition of inositol monophosphatase, more selective GSK3 inhibitors have been developed (Chiu and Chuang, 2010; Mines and Jope, 2011). Lithium, as well as the selective GSK3β inhibitor SB216763, was found to be able to correct mutant phenotypes (audiogenic seizure susceptibility and hyperactivity) of *Fmr1* knockout mice. Particularly, lithium remained effective with chronic administration (Min et al., 2009). Acute or chronic lithium treatment could increase inhibitory serine phosphorylation of GSK3 in mouse brain; chronic treatment ameliorated alterations in open-field activity, elevated plus-maze and passive avoidance and impaired cognition in fragile X mice (Yuskaitis et al., 2010; King and Jope, 2013). Chronic treatment with SB216763 corrected hippocampus-dependent learning deficits as well as defects in adult neurogenesis in the hippocampus of fragile x mice (Guo et al., 2012). The specific GSK3 inhibitors TDZD-8 and VP0.7 corrected impairments in hippocampus-related cognitive tasks. Furthermore, the improvements in behaviors correlated to the rescue of deficits in NMDA receptor dependent LTP in the hippocampus of *Fmr1* knockout mice as a result of GSK3 inhibition (Franklin et al., 2014). These studies thus support that targeting GSK3 may provide therapeutic benefits for fragile X syndrome.

In an open-label trial in 15 patients, the two month treatment with lithium was well-tolerated and had positive effects on behavior and adaptive skills in fragile X syndrome (Berry-Kravis et al., 2008). The placebo-controlled trials of lithium or other GSK3 inhibitors in fragile X syndrome will be warranted.

TARGETING PROTEINS REGULATED BY FMRP

Matrix metalloproteinase 9

Matrix metalloproteinases (MMPs) are a family of extracellular proteases that are involved in synaptogenesis, neurotransmission and synaptic plasticity (Ethell and Ethell, 2007; Wright and Harding, 2009; Huntley, 2012). MPP9 mRNA is among the putative mRNA targets of FMRP with increased translation in the absence of FMRP (Janusz et al., 2013). MMP9 is necessary for the development of fragile X phenotypes. Genetic deletion of MMP9 rescued key features of fragile X syndrome, including dendritic spine abnormalities, exaggerated mGluR-LTD, aberrant cognitive and social behaviors as well as macroorchidism in the mouse model (Sidhu et al., 2014). Minocycline, a tetracycline analogue with anti-inflammatory and antiapoptotic activity, has been used to inhibit MMP9 (Bilousova et al., 2009; Siller and Broadie, 2012). Treatment of young mice with minocycline increased phosphorylation and subsequent membrane insertion of AMPA GluR1 receptors (Imbesi et al., 2008). Minocycline rescued maturation of dendritic spines in the hippocampus thereby correcting the spine phenotype in *Fmr1* knockout mice (Bilousova et al., 2009). In addition, chronic minocycline reduced anxiety-related behavior, improved cognitive function in young *Fmr1* knockout mice (Bilousova et al., 2009), and reversed impaired social communication during mating among fragile X mice (Rotschafer et al., 2012). In comparison of the effect of minocycline on young and adult fragile X mice, it was found that minocycline could reduce locomotor activity in both young and adult mice, some behavioral improvements could be long-lasting in young mice, but not in adults. In addition, minocycline reduced audiogenic seizure susceptibility in young mice (Dansie et al., 2013). This study provides further evidence that minocycline can produce long-lasting benefits in the fragile X animal model.

Clinical trials have been conducted to evaluate the safety and efficacy of minocycline. An open-label add-on pilot trial demonstrated that minocycline is well tolerated and can provide significant functional benefits to fragile X patients (Paribello et al., 2010). In a controlled clinical trial, minocycline treatment was observed to lower the elevated plasma activity of MMP9 in individuals with fragile X syndrome. In some cases, changes in MMP9 activity were found to be positively associated with improvement in clinical measures (Dziembowska et al., 2013). In another randomized, double-blind, placebo-controlled and crossover trial, minocycline treatment administered for 3 months was found to be safe and produce greater global improvement than a placebo in children with fragile X syndrome (Leigh et al., 2013). However, longer trials are warranted to further assess the benefits and side effects related to minocycline.

p21-activated kinase

The small GTPase Rac1 and its effector p-21 activated kinase (PAK) are critical for regulation of actin polymerization, dendritic spine morphogenesis and synaptic plasticity (Hayashi et al., 2004; Zhang et al., 2005; Kreis and Barnier, 2009; Murata and Constantine-Paton, 2013). In hippocampal synapses of *Fmr1* knockout mice, physiological activation of the Rac-PAK signaling pathway is impaired (Chen et al., 2010). FMRP directly interacts with PAK1. Inhibition of PAK activity by expression of the dominant negative PAK (dnPAK) transgene results in a dendritic spine phenotype opposite to that of fragile X syndrome (Hayashi et al., 2007). A genetic expression of dnPAK in *Fmr1* knockout mice at least partially corrected abnormalities in spine length and density in the cortex, and fully restored deficits in cortical LTP. Additionally, several behavioral abnormalities including hyperactivity, stereotypy, anxiety, and deficits in trace fear memory were ameliorated (Hayashi et al., 2007). This genetic rescue of fragile X phenotypes in the mouse model suggests that the PAK signaling pathway could be a novel intervention site for fragile X syndrome and autism. Pharmacological treatment with the PAK inhibitor FRAX486 reversed dendritic spine phenotypes, and rescued seizures and behavioral abnormalities such as hyperactivity and repetitive movements in *Fmr1* knockout mice, further supporting PAK as a therapeutic target. Importantly, these effects could be achieved in adult *Fmr1* knockout mice with a single administration of FRAX486, demonstrating the potential for therapy in adults with fragile X syndrome (Dolan et al., 2013).

Amyloid precursor protein

Amyloid precursor protein (APP) is a transmembrane protein that plays roles in synaptogenesis and synaptic plasticity (Gralle and Ferreira, 2007; Randall et al., 2010; Nalivaeva and Turner, 2013). APP is translated upon mGluR5 activation. FMRP binds to APP mRNA and controls its translation (Westmark and Malter, 2007). Absence of FMRP leads to APP overexpression and diminished mGluR-induced synthesis (Westmark and Malter, 2007). Cleavage of APP can produce β-amyloid (Aβ), which is overexpressed in the brain of *Fmr1* knockout mice, suggesting a pathogenic role in fragile X syndrome (Westmark et al., 2010). Genetic reduction of APP/Aβ could partially or completely correct characteristic fragile X phenotypes, including audiogenic seizures, anxiety, dendritic spine morphology and exaggerated mGluR-LTD (Westmark et al., 2011), suggesting drugs directed at reducing Aβ in Alzheimer disease such as the secretase inhibitors or β-site APP cleaving enzyme (BACE-1) inhibitors may be applicable to fragile X syndrome (Malter et al., 2010; Westmark, 2013; Westmark et al., 2013).

Striatal-enriched protein tyrosine phosphatase

STEP, a brain-specific protein tyrosine phosphatase, dephosphorylates key signaling proteins including ERK1/2, p38 MAPK, the tyrosine kinase Fyn, and surface AMPA and NMDA receptors, thereby inactivating the kinases or promoting endocytosis of the receptors and opposing development of synaptic strengthening (Braithwaite et al., 2006; Goebel-Goody et al., 2012b). STEP is translated upon mGluR5 activation and mediates AMPA receptor internalization during mGluR-LTD (Zhang et al., 2008; Goebel-Goody and Lombroso, 2012). FMRP interacts with the transcript encoding STEP. The basal level of STEP is elevated and mGluR-dependent STEP synthesis is absent in *Fmr1* knockout mice (Goebel-Goody et al., 2012a). It is possible that the synaptic deficits and behavioral abnormalities in fragile X syndrome may be linked to the dysregulation of STEP (Goebel-Goody and Lombroso, 2012). Genetic reduction of STEP could attenuate audiogenic seizures, improve characteristic social abnormalities, and reverse anxiety-related behaviors in *Fmr1* knockout mice, suggesting that STEP might be a therapeutic target for treating fragile X patients (Goebel-Goody et al., 2012a).

Potassium channels

Potassium channels control the resting membrane potential and modulate the action potential waveform, mediating homeostasis of neuronal excitability (Misonou, 2010; Lee and Jan, 2012; Kim and Kaczmarek, 2014). In fragile X animal models, defects have been found in several types of potassium channels, such as the sodium-activated potassium Slack (Brown et al., 2010; Zhang et al., 2012), voltage-gated potassium channels Kv3.1b (Strumbos et al., 2010) and Kv4.2 (Gross et al., 2011; Lee et al., 2011), and large-conductance calcium-activated potassium (BK) channels (Deng et al., 2013; Zhang et al., 2014b).

FMRP interacts directly with Slack channels to enhance the channel activity, raising the possibility that Slack-FMRP interaction may link patterns of neuronal firing with changes in protein translation (Brown et al., 2010; Zhang et al., 2012). Disturbance of this link when FMRP is absent may underlie altered neuronal networks in fragile X syndrome. FMRP binds the mRNAs encoding Kv3.1b and is required for rapid experience-dependent regulation of Kv3.1b (Strumbos et al., 2010). FMRP also regulates mRNA translation and protein expression of Kv4.2; absence of FMRP-mediated control of Kv4.2 might contribute to excess neuronal excitability in *Fmr1* KO mice (Gross et al., 2011). Recovery of Kv4.2 after NMDA receptor-mediated degradation also requires FMRP, probably due to NMDA receptor activation-induced FMRP dephosphorylation, which turns off FMRP suppression of Kv4.2 (Lee et al., 2011). Significantly, treating hippocampal slices of *fmr1* KO mice with Kv4 channel blocker HpTx2 restored LTP induced by moderate stimuli, suggesting that potassium channels as an FMRP target could be of potential relevance to fragile X therapy (Lee et al., 2011). FMRP modulates action potential duration via its interaction with beta4 subunits of BK channels, thus regulating neurotransmitter release and synaptic transmission. Loss of these FMRP functions might be responsible for dysregulation of synaptic transmission in fragile X syndrome (Deng et al., 2013). Interestingly, a recent study showed that a selective BK channel opener (BMS-204352) could rescue multiple behavioral impairments (social, emotional and cognitive) in fragile X mice (Hebert et al., 2014), further demonstrating that potassium channels may open up new opportunities for treating fragile X syndrome.

In summary, multiple targeted pharmacological treatments have been found to rescue the phenotypes of fragile X animal models, but few have been beneficial to patients. Acamprosate, lovastatin, lithium and minocycline are the drugs that can be currently prescribed and have shown benefits to patients with fragile X syndrome. However, each single drug may not be effective for all patients. The combination of different drug therapies, together with behavioral interventions, will be necessary for better efficacy in treating fragile X syndrome (Braat and Kooy, 2014; Hagerman et al., 2014; Hagerman and Polussa, 2015).

TARGETED PHARMACOTHERAPY FOR RETT SYNDROME

RTT is a postnatal neurodevelopmental disorder that occurs mainly in females and is the leading cause of intellectual disability in this gender (Hagberg et al., 1983; Laurvick et al., 2006; Neul et al., 2010). Clinical presentation occurs in stages with an initial developmental stagnation that is followed by a rapid regression during which RTT individuals have autistic features, stereotypic hand movements, loss of language, and develop aggressive behaviors (Chahrour and Zoghbi, 2007; Percy et al., 2010). RTT girls also have seizures during childhood, daytime breathing arrythmias, dysautonomia, and develop scoliosis at later stages, which also include Parkinsonian features and loss of mobility (Glaze et al., 2010; Neul et al., 2014).

Loss-of-function mutations in the X-linked gene *MECP2* (methyl-CpG-binding protein-2) are responsible for RTT (Amir et al., 1999). In 95% of classic RTT cases, *MECP2* mutations occur *de novo* in germ cells and are usually on the paternal side (Girard et al., 2001; Trappe et al., 2001; Bienvenu and Chelly, 2006). There is a spectrum of mutations ranging from missense, nonsense, and frameshift mutations (Moretti and Zoghbi, 2006). RTT individuals appear to have a typical development until 6–18 months of age, when they start missing developmental milestones. The *MECP2* gene encodes a predominantly nuclear protein that is expressed ubiquitously but with predominance in the brain (Klose and Bird, 2006). The expression of *MECP2* follows a temporal pattern: it peaks in the early postnatal period when maturation of neurons and activity dependent refinement of synapses occurs (LaSalle et al., 2001; Shahbazian et al., 2002; Cohen et al., 2011). Its expression remains elevated during adulthood, when it is involved in the maintenance of existing neurons and synapses. MeCP2 was initially identified as a transcriptional repressor through its binding to methylated CpG sites in gene promoters (Nan et al., 1998; Jung et al., 2003), although it regulates gene expression through multiple mechanisms (Guy et al., 2011).

From multiple studies using different knockout mouse models, converging data indicates that the pathological deficit in RTT is at the microcircuit level involving the structure and function of synapses that are critical for synaptic transmission and plasticity (Chen et al., 2001; Guy et al., 2001, 2007; **Figure 2**). Therefore, most therapeutic treatments revolve around the restoration of synaptic function and maturation (Gadalla et al., 2011). Current preclinical research on therapeutic strategies and human clinical trials can be divided into drugs that target the primary cause, i.e., loss-of-function mutations in *MECP2*, and drugs that target downstream consequences, including neurotransmitter receptor systems, neurotrophins, and their intracellular signaling pathways (**Tables 3, 4**). Since this review is focused on pharmacological treatments, genetic manipulations will not be discussed here and readers are directed to recent reviews on this topic (Cobb et al., 2010; Gadalla et al., 2011; Guy et al., 2011). Treatment paradigms that have targeted pathways downstream of the *Mecp2* gene in mice, and the current human clinical trials are discussed in detail below.

GROWTH AND NEUROTROPHIC FACTORS

Brain-derived neurotrophic factor

Bdnf, the gene encoding the BDNF protein, is one of the first recognized direct targets of MeCP2 transcriptional regulation (Chen et al., 2003; Martinowich et al., 2003). BDNF binds to the high affinity receptor tropomyosin-related kinase B (TrkB), which activates intracellular signaling cascades critical for neuronal development, synaptic maturation, and learning and memory, like PLCγ-IP3R, PI3K-Akt, and MAPK-CREB (Segal and Greenberg, 1996). *Bdnf* expression is controlled by MeCP2 through complex interactions (Chen et al., 2003; Chang et al., 2006; Li and Pozzo-Miller, 2014), and reduced levels of BDNF mRNA and protein are considered to contribute to the pathophysiological mechanisms of RTT disease progression (Katz, 2014). Over-expression of BDNF in excitatory forebrain

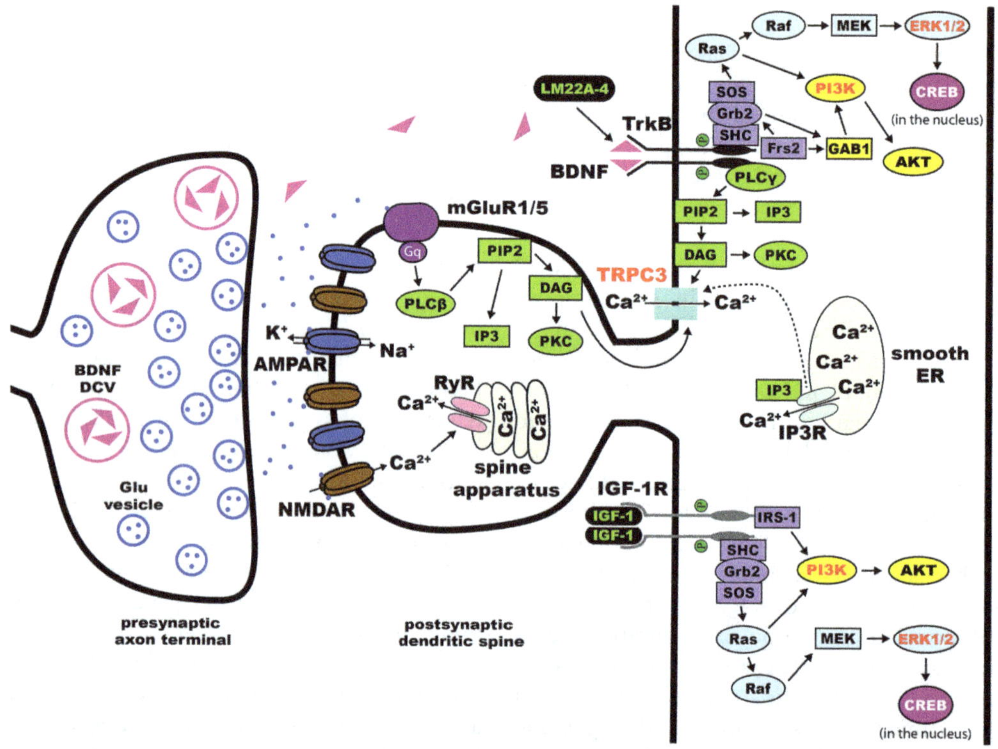

FIGURE 2 | Dendritic spines in Rett syndrome (RTT). Proposed intracellular mechanisms that mediate the effects of BDNF/TrkB on dendritic spine density and morphology. Trk receptors are activated upon binding of neurotophic factors, leading to dimerization and auto-phosphorylation. This process allows for the intracellular binding of adaptor proteins to Trk and activation of major pathways including Ras/ERK, PI3K, and PLCγ. Components of each of these three pathways have been implicated in the effects of BDNF on dendritic spines (highlighted in red text). Potential therapies for the treatment of RTT act on these pathways (highlighted in green text)—LM22A-4 directly phosphorylates TrkB and [1,3]IGF-1 activates the PI3K and Ras/ERK pathways. Abbreviations: AKT(PKB), protein kinase B; AMPAR, α-amino-3-hydroxy-5-methyl-4-isoxazolepropionic acid receptor; BDNF, brain-derived neurotrophic factor; CaMK, Ca2+/calmodulin-dependent protein kinase; cAMP, cyclic adenosine monophosphate; CREB, cAMP response element-binding protein; DAG, diacylglycerol; Frs2, fibroblast growth factor receptor substrate 2; GAB1, GRB2-associated-binding protein 1; Grb2, growth factor receptor-binding protein 2; IGF-1, insulin-like growth factor 1; IGF-1R, IGF-1 receptor; IP3, inositol triphosphate; MAPK, mitogen-activated protein kinase; MEK, MAPK//ERK kinase; NMDAR, *N*-methyl-D-aspartate receptor; PI3K, phosphoinositide 3-kinase; PIP2, phospohatidylinositol 4, 5 bisphosphate; PKC, protein kinase C; PLCγ, phospholipase C-γ; Raf, proto-oncogenic serine/threonine protein kinase; Ras, rat sarcoma proto-oncogenic G-protein; SHC, SH-2-containing protein; SH-2, src homology domain 2; SOS, nucleotide exchange factor son of sevenless; TrkB, tropomyosin related kinase B receptor; TRPC, transient receptor potential channel.

neurons of *Mecp2* deficient mice improved their RTT-like neurological phenotypes (Chang et al., 2006). Over-expression of *BDNF* rescued dendritic atrophy caused by shRNA-mediated *Mecp2* knockdown in cultured hippocampal neurons (Chapleau et al., 2009). The main limitation of recombinant BDNF is its low blood-brain barrier permeability, which prompted the search for BDNF "boosters" or mimetics with sufficient bioavailability in brain.

Currently, there are two clinical trials in RTT individuals testing compounds that boost BDNF levels: a Phase-1 open label trial of Fingolimod, and a Phase-2 open label trial of glatiramer acetate (Copaxone), both FDA-aproved drugs for the treatment of multiple sclerosis. Fingolimod is a modulator of the sphingosine-1 phosphate receptor, which leads to an increase in BDNF expression and activation of TrkB downstream signaling pathways (Deogracias et al., 2012). Glatiramer acetate is an immunomodulatory agent based on the amino acid structure of myelin basic protein (MBP) that is currently used for the treatment of relapsing-remitting multiple sclerosis. One of the proposed mechanisms of action of Copaxone is the increased expression and release of BDNF by autoreactive T-cells (Ziemssen et al., 2002).

Additonal potential leads with preclinical evidence include ampakines, which are known to increase BDNF expression by their action on AMPA-type glutamate receptors (Lauterborn et al., 2003). Peripheral treatment with ampakines significantly improved respiratory dysfunction in male *Mecp2* knockout mice (Ogier et al., 2007) that model the recurrent apneas suffered by RTT girls. Cysteamine and its dimer cystamine increase BDNF levels (Borrell-Pagès et al., 2006), which supports the Phase-2/3 clinical trial of RP103 for Huntington's disease. More recently, a small molecule BDNF loop mimetic (LM22A-4) designed *in silico* to interact with the BDNF binding pocket in the TrkB receptor (Massa et al., 2010), restored respiratory regularity in female *Mecp2* heterozygous mice (Schmid et al., 2012; Kron et al., 2014).

Table 3 | Current preclinical trials in *Mecp2* deficient mice.

Agent or Approach	Sponsor	Action
BDNF boosters		
LM22A-4 (BDNF loop mimetic)	Sigma-Aldrich; RSRT	Partial agonist of TrkB receptors Improves breathing
RP103 (cysteamine)	Raptor Pharmaceuticals	Increases BDNF expression and release Improves breathing
Serotonin agonists		
Sarizotan	Newron Pharmaceuticals	5HT1 agonist Improves breathing
NLX-101	Neurolixis	5HT1 agonist Improves breathing
NMDA receptors		
GluN2A negative allosteric modulator	Mnemosyne Pharmaceuticals	Improved visual cortical functioning
Ketamine	Approved drug	Non-competitive NMDA receptor antagonist Improved respiratory and locomotor function
Antidepressants		
REV-003 (Tianeptine)	Revive Therapeutics	Atypical antidepressant Improves breathing
MECP2 gene		
Read-through compounds	Research labs	Skip premature STOP codon in nonsense mutations

Insulin Growth factor-1

Insulin Growth factor-1 (IGF-1) is a growth factor that, by binding to the IGF-1 receptor, activates similar intracellular signaling cascades to those triggered by BDNF activation of TrkB receptors. Indeed, IGF-1 modulates synaptic plasticity and neuronal maturation through a tyrosine kinase signaling pathway that includes PI3K-Akt and MAPK (Zheng and Quirion, 2004). Unlike BDNF, IGF-1 permeability through the blood brain barrier makes it an attractive compound for therapy. Intraperitoneal injection of the active IGF-1 tripeptide (also known as [1–3]IGF-1, or Glypromate) in male *Mecp2* knockout mice improved survival, locomotor activity, as well as social and anxiety behaviors (Tropea et al., 2009). Full-length IGF-1 (Mecasermin) is already approved by the FDA for the treatment of growth failure in children, and it was shown to have similar effects in male *Mecp2* knockout mice, as well as in female *Mecp2* heterozygous mice (Castro et al., 2014); a cautionary note is that full-length IGF-1 can worsen the metabolic syndrome of *Mecp2* deficient mice (Pitcher et al., 2013). The effects of full-length IGF-1 are due to the direct activation of IGF-1 receptors and its downstream signaling cascades, while the effects of the [1–3]IGF-1 tripeptide may reflect increased expression of IGF-1 (Corvin et al., 2012), although its molecular mechanism-of-action is currently unknown. Based on these promising leads, a Phase-2 double-blinded placebo-controlled clinical trail is underway to treat 3–10 years old RTT patients with full-length IGF-1 (Khwaja et al., 2014). More recently, a Phase-2 double-blinded placebo-controlled clinical trail in 16–45 years old RTT individuals has been initiated to test the efficacy of NNZ-2566, a protease-resistant analogue of the [1–3]IGF-1 tripeptide.

NEUROTRANSMITTER SYSTEMS

Monoamines

Multiple studies have documented low levels of monoamine markers (dopamine, 5-HT, noradrenaline) in autopsy RTT brains and in *Mecp2* deficient mice (Brücke et al., 1987; Lekman et al., 1989; Roux et al., 2008). Desipramine is an antidepressant that blocks the uptake of noradrenaline, and has been shown to reverse the depletion of tyrosine hydroxylase in the brainstem, helping with the regulation of breathing and extending the life-span of male *Mecp2* knockout mice (Roux et al., 2007; Zanella et al., 2008). Desipramine is currently in a Phase-2 double blinded, placebo-controlled clinical trial for RTT. The atypical tricyclic antidepressant tianeptine (REV-003) also improved respiratory activity in *Mecp2* deficient mice, although this effect may reflect modulation of monoamine levels, glutamate receptor function, or BDNF levels (McEwen et al., 2010). Recently, preclinical studies in *Mecp2* deficient mice have demonstrated that the 5-HT1a agonist Sarizotan inhibited expiratory neuron activity, which significantly improved breathing patterns and reduced the frequency of apneas (Abdala et al., 2014).

Glutamate

The NMDA-type of glutamate receptors is altered in *Mecp2* knockout mice (Blue et al., 1999, 2011; Maliszewska-Cyna et al., 2010). Dextromethorphan is a NMDA receptor antagonist that has been tried in an open label clinical trial without any significant benefit. The FDA-approved NMDA receptor antagonist ketamine has been useful in *Mecp2* knockout mice to improve RTT-like phenotypes (Kron et al., 2012); based on these encouraging results, a clinical trial of low dose ketamine is currently planned. A delay in the developmental switch in the expression of GluN2 subunits of the NMDA receptor in the visual cortex contributes to visual acuity deficits in *Mecp2* deficient mice, which were improved by genetic deletion of the GluN2A subunit (Durand et al., 2012); a negative allosteric modulator selective for GluN2A-containing NMDA receptors is currently in preclinical trials in *Mecp2* deficient mice.

GABA

Several studies have shown that GABAergic signaling is impaired in *Mecp2* deficient mice, which alters the excitatory/inhibitory balance. Impaired GABAergic inhibition was described in the brainstem (Medrihan et al., 2008), thalamus (Zhang et al., 2010) and hippocampus (Calfa et al., 2015), and involved impaired evoked and spontaneous inhibitory synaptic transmission and numbers of GABAergic synapses on principal neurons. Furthermore, selective deletion of *Mecp2* in GABAergic neurons led to impaired GABAergic transmission, cortical hyperexcitability and several neurological features of RTT and ASDs (Chao et al., 2010). Also, deletion of *Mecp2* specifically in excitatory neurons caused impaired GABAergic transmission on cortical pyramidal neurons, which led to seizures and cortical hyperexcitation (Zhang et al., 2014a). A preclinical study in female *Mecp2* heterozygous mice demonstrated that

Table 4 | Current clinical trials in RTT individuals.

Agent	Results	Trial outcome	Sponsor	Type
Growth Factors				
Full length IGF-1	Phase 2	Safety confirmed on-going; scheduled through Fall 2015	Approved drug in children with growth failure	Double-blind; placebo controlled; injection
NNZ-2566 [1–3]IGF-1 analogue	Phase 2	Safety confirmed short-term trial positive	Neuren pharmaceuticals	Double-blind; placebo controlled; oral
BDNF Effectors				
Copaxone	Phase 2	Improved ambulation	Approved drug	Open-label; injection
Fingolimod	Phase 1	On-going; scheduled through August 2017	Novartis pharmaceuticals; Approved drug-adults	Open-label; oral
NMDA Antagonist				
Dextromethorphan	Phase 2	On-going; scheduled through June 2015	Approved drug in cough suppressant	Double-blind; placebo controlled
Norepinephrine Effector				
Desipramine	Phase 2	On-going; scheduled through December 2014	Approved drug in Europe	Double-blind; placebo controlled
Mitochondrial Effector				
EPI-743	Phase 2	Safety confirmed Improved head circumference growth	Edison pharmaceuticals	Double-blind; placebo controlled; oral

increasing ambient GABA levels by inhibiting the GABA reuptake transporter improved respiratory patterns (Abdala et al., 2010). Vigabatrin is an antiepileptic drug that irreversibly inhibits GABA transaminase, inhibits GABA catabolism and thereby increases GABA levels (Connelly, 1993). The drug is already FDA approved for use in epilepsy syndromes. Planning for a clinical trial for RTT is underway. However, retinal toxicity may limit the chronic use of this medication.

MITOCHONDRIAL FUNCTION

RTT is associated with high levels of systemic oxidative stress and alteration in mitochondrial morphology, while plasma levels of oxidative stress biomarkers correlate with disease severity and progression (De Felice et al., 2012). Based on these observations, the small molecule EPI-743 was tested in a phase-2 placebo controlled trial of RTT individuals. Results from this exploratory trial revealed improvement in head growth but not in other core features of RTT. The structure of EPI-743 is based on vitamin E and its proposed mechanisms-of-action includes augmenting glutathione synthesis and acting at the mitochondrial level to regulate electron transport.

"READ-THROUGH" COMPOUNDS TO INCREASE MECP2 EXPRESSION

In approximately one-third of RTT individuals, a nonsense mutation in *MECP2* (e.g., R168X, R255X) leads to the premature termination of transcripton due to a premature STOP codon (Schanen et al., 2004; Percy et al., 2007). Clinically, these RTT individuals have a more severe presentation than RTT individuals with missense *MECP2* mutations that result in single amino acid substitutions. Aminoglycoside antibiotics like gentamycin are so-called "read-through" compounds because they allow ribosomal read-through of the premature STOP codon during translation, yielding a full-length functional protein. Aminoglycoside and non-aminoglycoside "read-through" compounds have been tested for therapeutic efficacy in Duchenne muscular dystrophy and cystic fibrosis (Zingman et al., 2007). Preclinical studies relevant to RTT have demonstrated that either gentamycin or geneticin were effective in translating a full-length functional MeCP2 protein in a lymphocyte cell line derived from an individual with a R255X nonsense mutation (Popescu et al., 2010), and in transgenic mice expressing a R168X nonsense mutation (Brendel et al., 2011). Furthermore, gentamycin increased dendritic spine density in neurons derived from induced pluripotent stem cells (iPSC) that were obtained from a RTT individual with a Q244X nonsense mutation (Marchetto et al., 2010). However, the renal and auditory toxicity of gentamycin has limited its progress toward human clinical trials and prompted the development of new "read-through" compounds with better safety profiles.

OPEN QUESTIONS AND CHALLENGES

DESIGN AND QUALITY OF PRECLINICAL STUDIES

Although many targeted treatments have shown efficacy across multiple aspects in ASD animal models, none has thus far demonstrated the same effectiveness in patients (Katz et al., 2012; Hagerman et al., 2014). Hurdles to translational success may include lack of rigorous standards in assessing the effect of treatment, lack of transparency in reporting preclinical data, as well as publication bias caused by disregarding negative results in preclinical studies (Katz et al., 2012). The translational success stories in fragile X and Rett syndromes indicates that the effectiveness of targeted treatments in animal models can turn into clinical efficacy in humans, provided that studies are well designed, the models are reliable and robust, and that preclinical outcome measures are relevant to patients (Anagnostou, 2012; Lipton and Sahin, 2013; Castro et al., 2014; Khwaja et al., 2014). To achieve more translational success in ASDs, efforts are needed to improve the quality of preclinical studies in the future. Strict standards must be implemented for preclinical study designs and result reporting to ensure that clinical trials are grounded on reliable preclinical data (Katz et al., 2012; Landis et al., 2012).

One of the key issues in preclinical studies is that almost every study has applied its own animal behavioral experiment battery to evaluate the effects of genetic or pharmacological manipulations, making comparison of efficacy among different treatments a challenge. This situation will be greatly improved if animal behavioral test batteries for identifying potential therapy could be standardized. Despite the discrepancies in test batteries from different laboratories, many of the targeted treatments achieve predicted effect and rescue at least part of phenotypic features of the disorders in animal models (Braat and Kooy, 2014; Hagerman et al., 2014).

CHALLENGES IN CLINICAL TRIALS

Despite progress made in clinical trials, one of the major concerns for these studies is the lack of appropriate outcome measures for an objective assessment of patients' daily performance (Berry-Kravis et al., 2011; Wijetunge et al., 2013; Berry-Kravis, 2014; Braat and Kooy, 2014; Jacquemont et al., 2014). As a result, some improvements following therapeutic intervention might not be observed without the right measurements. It is helpful that researchers have been trying to formulate suitable outcome measures, which could be adjusted accordingly for patients (Berry-Kravis et al., 2013), such as quantitative event related potential and expressive language outcome measure which have been developed for fragile X patients (Hessl et al., 2009). It is anticipated that these measures will better demonstrate improvements in language and cognition in individual patients. In addition, molecular markers, such as ERK, BDNF and MMP9, can be measured to provide a direct biochemical evidence of improvement with targeted treatments (Hagerman et al., 2014).

Differential responses to one specific treatment have been observed in individuals with ASDs. Some subgroups within the patient cohorts respond to the therapy where others do not, as evident from clinical trials in fragile X syndrome (Jacquemont et al., 2011; Berry-Kravis et al., 2012). It is therefore important and helpful to develop biomarkers for selection of patients that will benefit from a specific therapy depending on their genotypes and/or neurobiological phenotypes. For example, if follow-up studies would confirm that AFQ056 treatment significantly improves behavior in fully methylated patients, detecting the methylation status of *Fmr1* promoter might help identify a subgroup of fragile X patients that will respond well to this treatment (Jacquemont et al., 2011; Braat and Kooy, 2014).

Interference with the molecular pathways disturbed in ASDs has led to the initiation of clinical trials. The fragile X and Rett syndromes are the prototypes of neurodevelopmental disorders for which targeted treatments are becoming realities (Samaco and Neul, 2011; Chapleau et al., 2013a,b; Braat and Kooy, 2014). However, it is unlikely that a single compound will be effective in all individuals with ASDs. Thus, it will be necessary to test combinations of multiple drugs that each rescue part of clinical presentations to find a combination of drugs that works more efficiently than each on its own. Importantly, pharmaceutical interventions need to be paired with appropriate behavioral and cognitive training to maximize the efficacy. This represents a significant step towards more personalized approaches to treating fragile X, RTT and other ASDs in future, with a better chance of success (Castro et al., 2013; Wijetunge et al., 2013; Braat and Kooy, 2014; Hagerman et al., 2014).

THE TIMING OF TREATMENT INITIATION

It is generally believed that earlier interventions in developmental disorders will have better outcomes. Abnormalities occurring during early development have usually been considered irreversible in adulthood. However, studies in mouse models of neurodevelopmental disorders, including fragile X and Rett syndromes, suggest that many pathophysiological aspects associated with the disorders can be reversed by genetic or pharmacological manipulations performed during adulthood (Castrén et al., 2012). Improvements have also been observed in adult patients with fragile X syndrome treated with arbaclofen and AFQ056 (Jacquemont et al., 2011; Henderson et al., 2012). These findings suggest that the pathophysiology associated with the loss of FMRP or MeCP2 may not arise from irreversible developmental brain abnormalities, but result from functional disturbances of neural circuits that could be corrected in adulthood, providing a potential rational basis for treatment of neurodevelopmental disorders in adulthood (Castrén et al., 2012; Wijetunge et al., 2013; Hagerman et al., 2014). Despite these exciting advances, translation from animal experimentation to clinical practice and finding out the right initiation timing for treating individual patients will be challenging issues in future investigation (Castrén et al., 2012; Wijetunge et al., 2013).

CONCLUSIONS

The increasing need for effective treatments of fragile X and Rett syndromes, coupled with the availability of animal models and iPSC-derived neurons from human individuals with these disorders (Marchetto et al., 2010; Wang and Doering, 2012), has promoted translational studies towards identifying potential therapeutics. New opportunities are now emerging that might lead to development of novel pharmacotherapies for patients with fragile X and Rett syndromes. The development of mechanism-based targeted treatments will require more extensive multidisciplinary researches (Chapleau et al., 2013a; Berry-Kravis, 2014; Braat and Kooy, 2014; Hagerman et al., 2014). It is the responsibility of the research community to rigorously validate disease models, outcome measures and study designs that will produce robust and reproducible preclinical findings with clear relevance to human diseases (Katz et al., 2012; Landis et al., 2012).

The rational therapeutics for ASDs requires the knowledge of an entire spectrum of symptoms that relate to each specific disorder. The complicated pathophysiology of fragile X and Rett syndromes should be taken fully into account in designing preclinical and clinical studies. It should be recognized that loss of FMRP or MeCP2 will affect a number of downstream targets which exist not only on neurons, but on glial cells and other tissues (McCauley et al., 2011; Cheng et al., 2012; Derecki et al., 2013; Ausió et al., 2014); that the loss can have direct, as well as indirect and cumulative effects on development and function of the central nervous system or other organs, leading to distinct phenotypic consequences that possibly require different treatment strategies. Understanding these complexities will be essential for selecting relative therapeutics for patients (Chapleau et al., 2013a,b; Delorme et al., 2013; Berry-Kravis, 2014; Hagerman et al., 2014). It is inspiring to see that fragile X and Rett syndromes are becoming role models for how research in animal models could be translated into patients and how management of symptoms of the diseases could extend and improve the quality of life, providing further insights into understanding and treating ASDs and other neurodevelopmental diseases.

ACKNOWLEDGMENTS

HW was supported by the National Natural Science Foundation of China (NSFC, No.30200152) for Rett syndrome studies and the Fragile X Research Foundation of Canada. LP-M was supported by NIH grants NS-065027 and HD-074418, Rettsyndrome.org (former International Rett Syndrome Foundation), and the Rett Syndrome Research Trust (RSRT). LCD was supported by the Natural Sciences and Engineering Research Council of Canada (NSERC) and the Brain Canada/Azrieli Neurodevelopmental Research Program.

REFERENCES

Abdala, A. P., Dutschmann, M., Bissonnette, J. M., and Paton, J. F. (2010). Correction of respiratory disorders in a mouse model of Rett syndrome. *Proc. Natl. Acad. Sci. U S A* 107, 18208–18213. doi: 10.1073/pnas.1012104107

Abdala, A. P., Lioy, D. T., Garg, S. K., Knopp, S. J., Paton, J. F., and Bissonnette, J. M. (2014). Effect of Sarizotan, a 5-HT1a and D2-like receptor agonist, on respiration in three mouse models of Rett syndrome. *Am. J. Respir. Cell Mol. Biol.* 50, 1031–1039. doi: 10.1165/rcmb.2013-0372OC

Abekhoukh, S., and Bardoni, B. (2014). CYFIP family proteins between autism and intellectual disability: links with Fragile X syndrome. *Front. Cell. Neurosci.* 8:81. doi: 10.3389/fncel.2014.00081

Amir, R. E., Van den Veyver, I. B., Wan, M., Tran, C. Q., Francke, U., and Zoghbi, H. Y. (1999). Rett syndrome is caused by mutations in X-linked MECP2, encoding methyl-CpG-binding protein 2. *Nat. Genet.* 23, 185–188. doi: 10.1038/13810

Anagnostou, E. (2012). Translational medicine: mice and men show the way. *Nature* 491, 196–197. doi: 10.1038/491196a

Anagnostou, E., Soorya, L., Brian, J., Dupuis, A., Mankad, D., Smile, S., et al. (2014a). Intranasal oxytocin in the treatment of autism spectrum disorders: a review of literature and early safety and efficacy data in youth. *Brain Res.* 1580, 188–198. doi: 10.1016/j.brainres.2014.01.049.

Anagnostou, E., Zwaigenbaum, L., Szatmari, P., Fombonne, E., Fernandez, B. A., Woodbury-Smith, M., et al. (2014b). Autism spectrum disorder: advances in evidence-based practice. *CMAJ* 186, 509–519. doi: 10.1503/cmaj.121756

Andari, E., Duhamel, J. R., Zalla, T., Herbrecht, E., Leboyer, M., and Sirigu, A. (2010). Promoting social behavior with oxytocin in high-functioning autism spectrum disorders. *Proc. Natl. Acad. Sci. U S A* 107, 4389–4394. doi: 10.1073/pnas.0910249107

Auerbach, B. D., Osterweil, E. K., and Bear, M. F. (2011). Mutations causing syndromic autism define an axis of synaptic pathophysiology. *Nature* 480, 63–68. doi: 10.1038/nature10658

Ausió, J., de Paz, A. M., and Esteller, M. (2014). MeCP2: the long trip from a chromatin protein to neurological disorders. *Trends Mol. Med.* 20, 487–498. doi: 10.1016/j.molmed.2014.03.004

Banerjee, S., Riordan, M., and Bhat, M. A. (2014). Genetic aspects of autism spectrum disorders: insights from animal models. *Front. Cell. Neurosci.* 8:58. doi: 10.3389/fncel.2014.00058

Bassell, G. J., and Warren, S. T. (2008). Fragile X syndrome: loss of local mRNA regulation alters synaptic development and function. *Neuron* 60, 201–214. doi: 10.1016/j.neuron.2008.10.004

Bear, M. F., Huber, K. M., and Warren, S. T. (2004). The mGluR theory of fragile X mental retardation. *Trends Neurosci.* 27, 370–377. doi: 10.1016/j.tins.2004.04.009

Ben-Ari, Y., Khalilov, I., Kahle, K. T., and Cherubini, E. (2012). The GABA excitatory/inhibitory shift in brain maturation and neurological disorders. *Neuroscientist* 18, 467–486. doi: 10.1177/1073858412438697

Berry-Kravis, E. (2014). Mechanism-based treatments in neurodevelopmental disorders: fragile X syndrome. *Pediatr. Neurol.* 50, 297–302. doi: 10.1016/j.pediatrneurol.2013.12.001

Berry-Kravis, E., Hessl, D., Abbeduto, L., Reiss, A. L., Beckel-Mitchener, A., and Urv, T. K. (2013). Outcome measures for clinical trials in fragile X syndrome. *J. Dev. Behav. Pediatr.* 34, 508–522. doi: 10.1097/DBP.0b013e31829d1f20

Berry-Kravis, E., Hessl, D., Coffey, S., Hervey, C., Schneider, A., Yuhas, J., et al. (2009). A pilot open label, single dose trial of fenobam in adults with fragile X syndrome. *J. Med. Genet.* 46, 266–271. doi: 10.1136/jmg.2008.063701

Berry-Kravis, E. M., Hessl, D., Rathmell, B., Zarevics, P., Cherubini, M., Walton-Bowen, K., et al. (2012). Effects of STX209 (arbaclofen) on neurobehavioral function in children and adults with fragile X syndrome: a randomized, controlled, phase 2 trial. *Sci. Transl. Med.* 4:152ra127. doi: 10.1126/scitranslmed.3004214

Berry-Kravis, E., Knox, A., and Hervey, C. (2011). Targeted treatments for fragile X syndrome. *J. Neurodev. Disord.* 3, 193–210. doi: 10.1007/s11689-011-9074-7

Berry-Kravis, E., Krause, S. E., Block, S. S., Guter, S., Wuu, J., Leurgans, S., et al. (2006). Effect of CX516, an AMPA-modulating compound, on cognition and behavior in fragile X syndrome: a controlled trial. *J. Child Adolesc. Psychopharmacol.* 16, 525–540. doi: 10.1089/cap.2006.16.525

Berry-Kravis, E., Sumis, A., Hervey, C., Nelson, M., Porges, S. W., Weng, N., et al. (2008). Open-label treatment trial of lithium to target the underlying defect in fragile X syndrome. *J. Dev. Behav. Pediatr.* 29, 293–302. doi: 10.1097/DBP.0b013e31817dc447

Bhakar, A. L., Dolen, G., and Bear, M. F. (2012). The pathophysiology of fragile, X (and what it teaches us about synapses). *Annu. Rev. Neurosci.* 35, 417–443. doi: 10.1146/annurev-neuro-060909-153138

Bhattacharya, A., Kaphzan, H., Alvarez-Dieppa, A. C., Murphy, J. P., Pierre, P., and Klann, E. (2012). Genetic removal of p70 S6 kinase 1 corrects molecular, synaptic and behavioral phenotypes in fragile X syndrome mice. *Neuron* 76, 325–337. doi: 10.1016/j.neuron.2012.07.022

Bienvenu, T., and Chelly, J. (2006). Molecular genetics of Rett syndrome: when DNA methylation goes unrecognized. *Nat. Rev. Genet.* 7, 415–426. doi: 10.1038/nrg1878

Bilousova, T. V., Dansie, L., Ngo, M., Aye, J., Charles, J. R., Ethell, D. W., et al. (2009). Minocycline promotes dendritic spine maturation and improves behavioural performance in the fragile X mouse model. *J. Med. Genet.* 46, 94–102. doi: 10.1136/jmg.2008.061796

Blue, M. E., Kaufmann, W. E., Bressler, J., Eyring, C., O'driscoll, C., Naidu, S., et al. (2011). Temporal and regional alterations in NMDA receptor expression in Mecp2-null mice. *Anat. Rec. (Hoboken)* 294, 1624–1634. doi: 10.1002/ar.21380

Blue, M. E., Naidu, S., and Johnston, M. V. (1999). Development of amino acid receptors in frontal cortex from girls with Rett syndrome. *Ann. Neurol.* 45, 541–545. doi: 10.1002/1531-8249(199904)45:4<541::aid-ana21>3.0.co;2-2

Boda, B., Mendez, P., Boury-Jamot, B., Magara, F., and Muller, D. (2014). Reversal of activity-mediated spine dynamics and learning impairment in a mouse model of Fragile X syndrome. *Eur. J. Neurosci.* 39, 1130–1137. doi: 10.1111/ejn.12488

Borrell-Pagès, M., Canals, J. M., Cordelières, F. P., Parker, J. A., Pineda, J. R., Grange, G., et al. (2006). Cystamine and cysteamine increase brain levels of BDNF in Huntington disease via HSJ1b and transglutaminase. *J. Clin. Invest.* 116, 1410–1424. doi: 10.1172/jci27607

Bortolotto, Z. A., Fitzjohn, S. M., and Collingridge, G. L. (1999). Roles of metabotropic glutamate receptors in LTP and LTD in the hippocampus. *Curr. Opin. Neurobiol.* 9, 299–304. doi: 10.1016/s0959-4388(99)80044-0

Braat, S., and Kooy, R. F. (2014). Fragile X syndrome neurobiology translates into rational therapy. *Drug Discov. Today* 19, 510–519. doi: 10.1016/j.drudis.2014.01.013

Braithwaite, S. P., Paul, S., Nairn, A. C., and Lombroso, P. J. (2006). Synaptic plasticity: one STEP at a time. *Trends Neurosci.* 29, 452–458. doi: 10.1016/j.tins.2006.06.007

Brendel, C., Belakhov, V., Werner, H., Wegener, E., Gärtner, J., Nudelman, I., et al. (2011). Readthrough of nonsense mutations in Rett syndrome: evaluation of novel aminoglycosides and generation of a new mouse model. *J. Mol. Med. (Berl.)* 89, 389–398. doi: 10.1007/s00109-010-0704-4

Brown, M. R., Kronengold, J., Gazula, V. R., Chen, Y., Strumbos, J. G., Sigworth, F. J., et al. (2010). Fragile X mental retardation protein controls gating of the sodium-activated potassium channel slack. *Nat. Neurosci.* 13, 819–821. doi: 10.1038/nn.2563

Brücke, T., Sofic, E., Killian, W., Rett, A., and Riederer, P. (1987). Reduced concentrations and increased metabolism of biogenic amines in a single case of Rett-syndrome: a postmortem brain study. *J. Neural Transm.* 68, 315–324. doi: 10.1007/bf02098506

Burket, J. A., Benson, A. D., Tang, A. H., and Deutsch, S. I. (2014). Rapamycin improves sociability in the BTBR T(+)Itpr3(tf)/J mouse model of autism spectrum disorders. *Brain Res. Bull.* 100, 70–75. doi: 10.1016/j.brainresbull.2013.11.005

Busquets-Garcia, A., Gomis-González, M., Guegan, T., Agustín-Pavón, C., Pastor, A., Mato, S., et al. (2013). Targeting the endocannabinoid system in the treatment of fragile X syndrome. *Nat. Med.* 19, 603–607. doi: 10.1038/nm.3127

Çaku, A., Pellerin, D., Bouvier, P., Riou, E., and Corbin, F. (2014). Effect of lovastatin on behavior in children and adults with fragile X syndrome: an open-label study. *Am. J. Med. Genet. A* 164A, 2834–2842. doi: 10.1002/ajmg.a.36750

Calfa, G., Li, W., Rutherford, J. M., and Pozzo-Miller, L. (2015). Excitation/inhibition imbalance and impaired synaptic inhibition in hippocampal area CA3 of Mecp2 knockout mice. *Hippocampus* 25, 159–168. doi: 10.1002/hipo.22360

Castrén, E., Elgersma, Y., Maffei, L., and Hagerman, R. (2012). Treatment of neurodevelopmental disorders in adulthood. *J. Neurosci.* 32, 14074–14079. doi: 10.1523/JNEUROSCI.3287-12.2012

Castro, J., Garcia, R. I., Kwok, S., Banerjee, A., Petravicz, J., Woodson, J., et al. (2014). Functional recovery with recombinant human IGF1 treatment in a mouse model of Rett syndrome. *Proc. Natl. Acad. Sci. U S A* 111, 9941–9946. doi: 10.1073/pnas.1311685111

Castro, J., Mellios, N., and Sur, M. (2013). Mechanisms and therapeutic challenges in autism spectrum disorders: insights from Rett syndrome. *Curr. Opin. Neurol.* 26, 154–159. doi: 10.1097/WCO.0b013e32835f19a7

Cerovic, M., d'Isa, R., Tonini, R., and Brambilla, R. (2013). Molecular and cellular mechanisms of dopamine-mediated behavioral plasticity in the striatum. *Neurobiol. Learn. Mem.* 105, 63–80. doi: 10.1016/j.nlm.2013.06.013

Chahrour, M., and Zoghbi, H. Y. (2007). The story of Rett syndrome: from clinic to neurobiology. *Neuron* 56, 422–437. doi: 10.1016/j.neuron.2007.10.001

Chang, S., Bray, S. M., Li, Z., Zarnescu, D. C., He, C., Jin, P., et al. (2008). Identification of small molecules rescuing fragile X syndrome phenotypes in Drosophila. *Nat. Chem. Biol.* 4, 256–263. doi: 10.1038/nchembio.78

Chang, Q., Khare, G., Dani, V., Nelson, S., and Jaenisch, R. (2006). The disease progression of Mecp2 mutant mice is affected by the level of BDNF expression. *Neuron* 49, 341–348. doi: 10.1016/j.neuron.2005.12.027

Chao, H. T., Chen, H., Samaco, R. C., Xue, M., Chahrour, M., Yoo, J., et al. (2010). Dysfunction in GABA signalling mediates autism-like stereotypies and Rett syndrome phenotypes. *Nature* 468, 263–269. doi: 10.1038/nature09582

Chapleau, C. A., Lane, J., Larimore, J., Li, W., Pozzo-Miller, L., and Percy, A. K. (2013b). Recent progress in Rett syndrome and MeCP2 Dysfunction: assessment of potential treatment options. *Future Neurol.* 8, 21–28. doi: 10.2217/fnl.12.79

Chapleau, C. A., Lane, J., Pozzo-Miller, L., and Percy, A. K. (2013a). Evaluation of current pharmacological treatment options in the management of Rett syndrome: from the present to future therapeutic alternatives. *Curr. Clin. Pharmacol.* 8, 358–369. doi: 10.2174/15748847113086660069

Chapleau, C. A., Larimore, J. L., Theibert, A., and Pozzo-Miller, L. (2009). Modulation of dendritic spine development and plasticity by BDNF and vesicular trafficking: fundamental roles in neurodevelopmental disorders associated with mental retardation and autism. *J. Neurodev. Disord.* 1, 185–196. doi: 10.1007/s11689-009-9027-6

Chen, R. Z., Akbarian, S., Tudor, M., and Jaenisch, R. (2001). Deficiency of methyl-CpG binding protein-2 in CNS neurons results in a Rett-like phenotype in mice. *Nat. Genet.* 27, 327–331. doi: 10.1038/85906

Chen, W. G., Chang, Q., Lin, Y., Meissner, A., West, A. E., Griffith, E. C., et al. (2003). Derepression of BDNF transcription involves calcium-dependent phosphorylation of MeCP2. *Science* 302, 885–889. doi: 10.1126/science.1086446

Chen, L. Y., Rex, C. S., Babayan, A. H., Kramár, E. A., Lynch, G., Gall, C. M., et al. (2010). Physiological activation of synaptic Rac>PAK (p-21 activated kinase) signaling is defective in a mouse model of fragile X syndrome. *J. Neurosci.* 30, 10977–10984. doi: 10.1523/JNEUROSCI.1077-10.2010

Cheng, C., Sourial, M., and Doering, L. C. (2012). Astrocytes and developmental plasticity in fragile X. *Neural Plast.* 2012:197491. doi: 10.1155/2012/197491

Chevaleyre, V., Takahashi, K. A., and Castillo, P. E. (2006). Endocannabinoid-mediated synaptic plasticity in the CNS. *Annu. Rev. Neurosci.* 29, 37–76. doi: 10.1146/annurev.neuro.29.051605.112834

Chez, M. G., Burton, Q., Dowling, T., Chang, M., Khanna, P., and Kramer, C. (2007). Memantine as adjunctive therapy in children diagnosed with autistic spectrum disorders: an observation of initial clinical response and maintenance tolerability. *J. Child Neurol.* 22, 574–579. doi: 10.1177/0883073807302611

Chiu, C. T., and Chuang, D. M. (2010). Molecular actions and therapeutic potential of lithium in preclinical and clinical studies of CNS disorders. *Pharmacol. Ther.* 128, 281–304. doi: 10.1016/j.pharmthera.2010.07.006

Chugani, D. C. (2002). Role of altered brain serotonin mechanisms in autism. *Mol. Psychiatry* 7(Suppl. 2), S16–S17. doi: 10.1038/sj.mp.4001167

Cobb, S., Guy, J., and Bird, A. (2010). Reversibility of functional deficits in experimental models of Rett syndrome. *Biochem. Soc. Trans.* 38, 498–506. doi: 10.1042/BST0380498

Cohen, S., Gabel, H. W., Hemberg, M., Hutchinson, A. N., Sadacca, L. A., Ebert, D. H., et al. (2011). Genome-wide activity-dependent MeCP2 phosphorylation regulates nervous system development and function. *Neuron* 72, 72–85. doi: 10.1016/j.neuron.2011.08.022

Cohen, P., and Goedert, M. (2004). GSK3 inhibitors: development and therapeutic potential. *Nat. Rev. Drug Discov.* 3, 479–487. doi: 10.1038/nrd1415

Connelly, J. F. (1993). Vigabatrin. *Ann. Pharmacother.* 27, 197–204.

Corvin, A. P., Molinos, I., Little, G., Donohoe, G., Gill, M., Morris, D. W., et al. (2012). Insulin-like growth factor 1 (IGF1) and its active peptide (1–3)IGF1 enhance the expression of synaptic markers in neuronal circuits through different cellular mechanisms. *Neurosci. Lett.* 520, 51–56. doi: 10.1016/j.neulet.2012.05.029

Costa, L., Spatuzza, M., D'Antoni, S., Bonaccorso, C. M., Trovato, C., Musumeci, S. A., et al. (2012). Activation of 5-HT7 serotonin receptors reverses metabotropic glutamate receptor-mediated synaptic plasticity in wild-type and Fmr1 knockout mice, a model of Fragile X syndrome. *Biol. Psychiatry* 72, 924–933. doi: 10.1016/j.biopsych.2012.06.008

Cuesto, G., Enriquez-Barreto, L., Caramés, C., Cantarero, M., Gasull, X., Sandi, C., et al. (2011). Phosphoinositide-3-kinase activation controls synaptogenesis and spinogenesis in hippocampal neurons. *J. Neurosci.* 31, 2721–2733. doi: 10.1523/JNEUROSCI.4477-10.2011

Curia, G., Gualtieri, F., Bartolomeo, R., Vezzali, R., and Biagini, G. (2013). Resilience to audiogenic seizures is associated with p-ERK1/2 dephosphorylation in the subiculum of Fmr1 knockout mice. *Front. Cell. Neurosci.* 7:46. doi: 10.3389/fncel.2013.00046

Dansie, L. E., Phommahaxay, K., Okusanya, A. G., Uwadia, J., Huang, M., Rotschafer, S. E., et al. (2013). Long-lasting effects of minocycline on behavior in young but not adult Fragile X mice. *Neuroscience* 246, 186–198. doi: 10.1016/j.neuroscience.2013.04.058

Darnell, J. C., and Klann, E. (2013). The translation of translational control by FMRP: therapeutic targets for FXS. *Nat. Neurosci.* 16, 1530–1536. doi: 10.1038/nn.3379

De Felice, C., Signorini, C., Leoncini, S., Pecorelli, A., Durand, T., Valacchi, G., et al. (2012). The role of oxidative stress in Rett syndrome: an overview. *Ann. N Y Acad. Sci.* 1259, 121–135. doi: 10.1111/j.1749-6632.2012.06611.x

Delorme, R., Ey, E., Toro, R., Leboyer, M., Gillberg, C., and Bourgeron, T. (2013). Progress toward treatments for synaptic defects in autism. *Nat. Med.* 19, 685–694. doi: 10.1038/nm.3193

Deng, P. Y., Rotman, Z., Blundon, J. A., Cho, Y., Cui, J., Cavalli, V., et al. (2013). FMRP regulates neurotransmitter release and synaptic information transmission by modulating action potential duration via BK channels. *Neuron* 77, 696–711. doi: 10.1016/j.neuron.2012.12.018

Deogracias, R., Yazdani, M., Dekkers, M. P., Guy, J., Ionescu, M. C., Vogt, K. E., et al. (2012). Fingolimod, a sphingosine-1 phosphate receptor modulator, increases BDNF levels and improves symptoms of a mouse model of Rett syndrome. *Proc. Natl. Acad. Sci. U S A* 109, 14230–14235. doi: 10.1073/pnas.1206093109

Derecki, N. C., Cronk, J. C., and Kipnis, J. (2013). The role of microglia in brain maintenance: implications for Rett syndrome. *Trends Immunol.* 34, 144–150. doi: 10.1016/j.it.2012.10.002

Devlin, B., Cook, E. H. Jr., Coon, H., Dawson, G., Grigorenko, E. L., McMahon, W., et al. (2005). Autism and the serotonin transporter: the long and short of it. *Mol. Psychiatry* 10, 1110–1116. doi: 10.1038/sj.mp.4001724

de Vrij, F. M., Levenga, J., van der Linde, H. C., Koekkoek, S. K., De Zeeuw, C. I., Nelson, D. L., et al. (2008). Rescue of behavioral phenotype and neuronal protrusion morphology in Fmr1 KO mice. *Neurobiol. Dis.* 31, 127–132. doi: 10.1016/j.nbd.2008.04.002

D'Hulst, C., De Geest, N., Reeve, S. P., Van Dam, D., De Deyn, P. P., Hassan, B. A., et al. (2006). Decreased expression of the GABAA receptor in fragile X syndrome. *Brain Res.* 1121, 238–245. doi: 10.1016/j.brainres.2006.08.115

D'Hulst, C., Heulens, I., Brouwer, J. R., Willemsen, R., De Geest, N., Reeve, S. P., et al. (2009). Expression of the GABAergic system in animal models for fragile X syndrome and fragile X associated tremor/ataxia syndrome (FXTAS). *Brain Res.* 1253, 176–183. doi: 10.1016/j.brainres.2008.11.075

Dolan, B. M., Duron, S. G., Campbell, D. A., Vollrath, B., Shankaranarayana Rao, B. S., Ko, H. Y., et al. (2013). Rescue of fragile X syndrome phenotypes in Fmr1 KO mice by the small-molecule PAK inhibitor FRAX486. *Proc. Natl. Acad. Sci. U S A* 110, 5671–5676. doi: 10.1073/pnas.1219383110

Dölen, G., and Bear, M. F. (2008). Role for metabotropic glutamate receptor 5 (mGluR5) in the pathogenesis of fragile X syndrome. *J. Physiol.* 586, 1503–1508. doi: 10.1113/jphysiol.2008.150722

Doll, C. A., and Broadie, K. (2014). Impaired activity-dependent neural circuit assembly and refinement in autism spectrum disorder genetic models. *Front. Cell. Neurosci.* 8:30. doi: 10.3389/fncel.2014.00030

Domes, G., Heinrichs, M., Kumbier, E., Grossmann, A., Hauenstein, K., and Herpertz, S. C. (2013). Effects of intranasal oxytocin on the neural basis of face processing in autism spectrum disorder. *Biol. Psychiatry* 74, 164–171. doi: 10.1016/j.biopsych.2013.02.007

Durand, S., Patrizi, A., Quast, K. B., Hachigian, L., Pavlyuk, R., Saxena, A., et al. (2012). NMDA receptor regulation prevents regression of visual cortical function in the absence of Mecp2. *Neuron* 76, 1078–1090. doi: 10.1016/j.neuron.2012.12.004

Dziembowska, M., Pretto, D. I., Janusz, A., Kaczmarek, L., Leigh, M. J., Gabriel, N., et al. (2013). High MMP-9 activity levels in fragile X syndrome are lowered by minocycline. *Am. J. Med. Genet. A* 161A, 1897–1903. doi: 10.1002/ajmg.a.36023

Eadie, B. D., Cushman, J., Kannangara, T. S., Fanselow, M. S., and Christie, B. R. (2012). NMDA receptor hypofunction in the dentate gyrus and impaired context discrimination in adult Fmr1 knockout mice. *Hippocampus* 22, 241–254. doi: 10.1002/hipo.20890

Ebert, D. H., and Greenberg, M. E. (2013). Activity-dependent neuronal signalling and autism spectrum disorder. *Nature* 493, 327–337. doi: 10.1038/nature11860

Erickson, C. A., and Chambers, J. E. (2006). Memantine for disruptive behavior in autistic disorder. *J. Clin. Psychiatry* 67:1000. doi: 10.4088/jcp.v67n0619h

Erickson, C. A., Mullett, J. E., and McDougle, C. J. (2009). Open-label memantine in fragile X syndrome. *J. Autism Dev. Disord.* 39, 1629–1635. doi: 10.1007/s10803-009-0807-3

Erickson, C. A., Mullett, J. E., and McDougle, C. J. (2010). Brief report: acamprosate in fragile X syndrome. *J. Autism Dev. Disord.* 40, 1412–1416. doi: 10.1007/s10803-010-0988-9

Erickson, C. A., Wink, L. K., Ray, B., Early, M. C., Stiegelmeyer, E., Mathieu-Frasier, L., et al. (2013). Impact of acamprosate on behavior and brain-derived neurotrophic factor: an open-label study in youth with fragile X syndrome. *Psychopharmacology (Berl)* 228, 75–84. doi: 10.1007/s00213-013-3022-z

Ethell, I. M., and Ethell, D. W. (2007). Matrix metalloproteinases in brain development and remodeling: synaptic functions and targets. *J. Neurosci. Res.* 85, 2813–2823. doi: 10.1002/jnr.21273

Franklin, A. V., King, M. K., Palomo, V., Martinez, A., McMahon, L. L., and Jope, R. S. (2014). Glycogen synthase kinase-3 inhibitors reverse deficits in long-term potentiation and cognition in fragile X mice. *Biol. Psychiatry* 75, 198–206. doi: 10.1016/j.biopsych.2013.08.003

Fulks, J. L., O'Bryhim, B. E., Wenzel, S. K., Fowler, S. C., Vorontsova, E., Pinkston, J. W., et al. (2010). Dopamine release and uptake impairments and behavioral alterations observed in mice that model fragile X mental retardation syndrome. *ACS Chem. Neurosci.* 1, 679–690. doi: 10.1021/cn100032f

Gadalla, K. K., Bailey, M. E., and Cobb, S. R. (2011). MeCP2 and Rett syndrome: reversibility and potential avenues for therapy. *Biochem. J.* 439, 1–14. doi: 10.1042/bj20110648

Gandhi, R. M., Kogan, C. S., and Messier, C. (2014). 2-Methyl-6-(phenylethynyl) pyridine (MPEP) reverses maze learning and PSD-95 deficits in Fmr1 knock-out mice. *Front. Cell. Neurosci.* 8:70. doi: 10.3389/fncel.2014.00070

Gantois, I., Pop, A. S., de Esch, C. E., Buijsen, R. A., Pooters, T., Gomez-Mancilla, B., et al. (2013). Chronic administration of AFQ056/Mavoglurant restores social behaviour in Fmr1 knockout mice. *Behav. Brain Res.* 239, 72–79. doi: 10.1016/j.bbr.2012.10.059

Garber, K. B., Visootsak, J., and Warren, S. T. (2008). Fragile X syndrome. *Eur. J. Hum. Genet.* 16, 666–672. doi: 10.1038/ejhg.2008.61

Gassmann, M., and Bettler, B. (2012). Regulation of neuronal GABA(B) receptor functions by subunit composition. *Nat. Rev. Neurosci.* 13, 380–394. doi: 10.1038/nrn3249

Gellynck, E., Heyninck, K., Andressen, K. W., Haegeman, G., Levy, F. O., Vanhoenacker, P., et al. (2013). The serotonin 5-HT7 receptors: two decades of research. *Exp. Brain Res.* 230, 555–568. doi: 10.1007/s00221-013-3694-y

Girard, M., Couvert, P., Carrié, A., Tardieu, M., Chelly, J., Beldjord, C., et al. (2001). Parental origin of de novo MECP2 mutations in Rett syndrome. *Eur. J. Hum. Genet.* 9, 231–236. doi: 10.1038/sj.ejhg.5200618

Gkogkas, C. G., Khoutorsky, A., Ran, I., Rampakakis, E., Nevarko, T., Weatherill, D. B., et al. (2013). Autism-related deficits via dysregulated eIF4E-dependent translational control. *Nature* 493, 371–377. doi: 10.1038/nature11628

Glaze, D. G., Percy, A. K., Skinner, S., Motil, K. J., Neul, J. L., Barrish, J. O., et al. (2010). Epilepsy and the natural history of Rett syndrome. *Neurology* 74, 909–912. doi: 10.1212/wnl.0b013e3181d6b852

Gocel, J., and Larson, J. (2012). Synaptic NMDA receptor-mediated currents in anterior piriform cortex are reduced in the adult fragile X mouse. *Neuroscience* 221, 170–181. doi: 10.1016/j.neuroscience.2012.06.052

Goebel-Goody, S. M., Baum, M., Paspalas, C. D., Fernandez, S. M., Carty, N. C., Kurup, P., et al. (2012b). Therapeutic implications for striatal-enriched protein tyrosine phosphatase (STEP) in neuropsychiatric disorders. *Pharmacol. Rev.* 64, 65–87. doi: 10.1124/pr.110.003053

Goebel-Goody, S. M., and Lombroso, P. J. (2012). Taking STEPs forward to understand fragile X syndrome. *Results Probl. Cell Differ.* 54, 223–241. doi: 10.1007/978-3-642-21649-7_12

Goebel-Goody, S. M., Wilson-Wallis, E. D., Royston, S., Tagliatela, S. M., Naegele, J. R., and Lombroso, P. J. (2012a). Genetic manipulation of STEP reverses behavioral abnormalities in a fragile X syndrome mouse model. *Genes Brain Behav.* 11, 586–600. doi: 10.1111/j.1601-183x.2012.00781.x

Gordon, I., Vander Wyk, B. C., Bennett, R. H., Cordeaux, C., Lucas, M. V., Eilbott, J. A., et al. (2013). Oxytocin enhances brain function in children with autism. *Proc. Natl. Acad. Sci. U S A* 110, 20953–20958. doi: 10.1073/pnas.1312857110

Gralle, M., and Ferreira, S. T. (2007). Structure and functions of the human amyloid precursor protein: the whole is more than the sum of its parts. *Prog. Neurobiol.* 82, 11–32. doi: 10.1016/j.pneurobio.2007.02.001

Gross, C., and Bassell, G. J. (2012). Excess protein synthesis in FXS patient lymphoblastoid cells can be rescued with a p110beta-selective inhibitor. *Mol. Med.* 18, 336–345. doi: 10.2119/molmed.2011.00363

Gross, C., and Bassell, G. J. (2014). Neuron-specific regulation of class I PI3K catalytic subunits and their dysfunction in brain disorders. *Front. Mol. Neurosci.* 7:12. doi: 10.3389/fnmol.2014.00012

Gross, C., Berry-Kravis, E. M., and Bassell, G. J. (2012). Therapeutic strategies in fragile X syndrome: dysregulated mGluR signaling and beyond. *Neuropsychopharmacology* 37, 178–195. doi: 10.1038/npp.2011.137

Gross, C., Nakamoto, M., Yao, X., Chan, C. B., Yim, S. Y., Ye, K., et al. (2010). Excess phosphoinositide 3-kinase subunit synthesis and activity as a novel therapeutic target in fragile X syndrome. *J. Neurosci.* 30, 10624–10638. doi: 10.1523/jneurosci.0402-10.2010

Gross, C., Yao, X., Pong, D. L., Jeromin, A., and Bassell, G. J. (2011). Fragile X mental retardation protein regulates protein expression and mRNA translation of the potassium channel Kv4.2. *J. Neurosci.* 31, 5693–5698. doi: 10.1523/jneurosci.6661-10.2011

Guo, W., Murthy, A. C., Zhang, L., Johnson, E. B., Schaller, E. G., Allan, A. M., et al. (2012). Inhibition of GSK3beta improves hippocampus-dependent learning and rescues neurogenesis in a mouse model of fragile X syndrome. *Hum. Mol. Genet.* 21, 681–691. doi: 10.1093/hmg/ddr501

Guy, J., Cheval, H., Selfridge, J., and Bird, A. (2011). The role of MeCP2 in the brain. *Annu. Rev. Cell Dev. Biol.* 27, 631–652. doi: 10.1146/annurev-cellbio-092910-154121

Guy, J., Gan, J., Selfridge, J., Cobb, S., and Bird, A. (2007). Reversal of neurological defects in a mouse model of Rett syndrome. *Science* 315, 1143–1147. doi: 10.1126/science.1138389

Guy, J., Hendrich, B., Holmes, M., Martin, J. E., and Bird, A. (2001). A mouse Mecp2-null mutation causes neurological symptoms that mimic Rett syndrome. *Nat. Genet.* 27, 322–326. doi: 10.1038/85899

Hagberg, B., Aicardi, J., Dias, K., and Ramos, O. (1983). A progressive syndrome of autism, dementia, ataxia and loss of purposeful hand use in girls: Rett's syndrome: report of 35 cases. *Ann. Neurol.* 14, 471–479. doi: 10.1002/ana.410140412

Hagerman, R. J., Des-Portes, V., Gasparini, F., Jacquemont, S., and Gomez-Mancilla, B. (2014). Translating molecular advances in fragile X syndrome into therapy: a review. *J. Clin. Psychiatry* 75, e294–e307. doi: 10.4088/jcp.13r08714

Hagerman, R. J., Hills, J., Scharfenaker, S., and Lewis, H. (1999). Fragile X syndrome and selective mutism. *Am. J. Med. Genet.* 83, 313–317. doi: 10.1002/(sici)1096-8628(19990402)83:4<313::aid-ajmg15>3.0.co;2-f

Hagerman, R. J., and Polussa, J. (2015). Treatment of the psychiatric problems associated with fragile X syndrome. *Curr. Opin. Psychiatry* 28, 107–112. doi: 10.1097/yco.0000000000000131

Hall, S. S., Lightbody, A. A., McCarthy, B. E., Parker, K. J., and Reiss, A. L. (2012). Effects of intranasal oxytocin on social anxiety in males with fragile X syndrome. *Psychoneuroendocrinology* 37, 509–518. doi: 10.1016/j.psyneuen.2011.07.020

Harrington, R. A., Lee, L. C., Crum, R. M., Zimmerman, A. W., and Hertz-Picciotto, I. (2013). Serotonin hypothesis of autism: implications for selective serotonin reuptake inhibitor use during pregnancy. *Autism Res.* 6, 149–168. doi: 10.1002/aur.1288

Hay, N., and Sonenberg, N. (2004). Upstream and downstream of mTOR. *Genes Dev.* 18, 1926–1945. doi: 10.1101/gad.1212704

Hayashi, M. L., Choi, S. Y., Rao, B. S., Jung, H. Y., Lee, H. K., Zhang, D., et al. (2004). Altered cortical synaptic morphology and impaired memory consolidation in forebrain-specific dominant-negative PAK transgenic mice. *Neuron* 42, 773–787. doi: 10.1016/j.neuron.2004.05.003

Hayashi, M. L., Rao, B. S., Seo, J. S., Choi, H. S., Dolan, B. M., Choi, S. Y., et al. (2007). Inhibition of p21-activated kinase rescues symptoms of fragile X syndrome in mice. *Proc. Natl. Acad. Sci. U S A* 104, 11489–11494. doi: 10.1073/pnas.0705003104

Hays, S. A., Huber, K. M., and Gibson, J. R. (2011). Altered neocortical rhythmic activity states in Fmr1 KO mice are due to enhanced mGluR5 signaling and involve changes in excitatory circuitry. *J. Neurosci.* 31, 14223–14234. doi: 10.1523/jneurosci.3157-11.2011

He, Q., Nomura, T., Xu, J., and Contractor, A. (2014). The developmental switch in GABA polarity is delayed in fragile X mice. *J. Neurosci.* 34, 446–450. doi: 10.1523/jneurosci.4447-13.2014

Hebert, B., Pietropaolo, S., Meme, S., Laudier, B., Laugeray, A., Doisne, N., et al. (2014). Rescue of fragile X syndrome phenotypes in Fmr1 KO mice by a BKCa channel opener molecule. *Orphanet J. Rare Dis.* 9:124. doi: 10.1186/s13023-014-0124-6

Heifets, B. D., and Castillo, P. E. (2009). Endocannabinoid signaling and long-term synaptic plasticity. *Annu. Rev. Physiol.* 71, 283–306. doi: 10.1146/annurev.physiol.010908.163149

Henderson, C., Wijetunge, L., Kinoshita, M. N., Shumway, M., Hammond, R. S., Postma, F. R., et al. (2012). Reversal of disease-related pathologies in the fragile X mouse model by selective activation of GABAB receptors with arbaclofen. *Sci. Transl. Med.* 4:152ra128. doi: 10.1126/scitranslmed.3004218

Hessl, D., Nguyen, D. V., Green, C., Chavez, A., Tassone, F., Hagerman, R. J., et al. (2009). A solution to limitations of cognitive testing in children with intellectual disabilities: the case of fragile X syndrome. *J. Neurodev. Disord.* 1, 33–45. doi: 10.1007/s11689-008-9001-8

Heulens, I., D'Hulst, C., Van Dam, D., De Deyn, P. P., and Kooy, R. F. (2012). Pharmacological treatment of fragile X syndrome with GABAergic drugs in a knockout mouse model. *Behav. Brain Res.* 229, 244–249. doi: 10.1016/j.bbr.2012.01.031

Hoeffer, C. A., and Klann, E. (2010). mTOR signaling: at the crossroads of plasticity, memory and disease. *Trends Neurosci.* 33, 67–75. doi: 10.1016/j.tins.2009.11.003

Hoeffer, C. A., Sanchez, E., Hagerman, R. J., Mu, Y., Nguyen, D. V., Wong, H., et al. (2012). Altered mTOR signaling and enhanced CYFIP2 expression levels in subjects with fragile X syndrome. *Genes Brain Behav.* 11, 332–341. doi: 10.1111/j.1601-183x.2012.00768.x

Hollander, E., Phillips, A., Chaplin, W., Zagursky, K., Novotny, S., Wasserman, S., et al. (2005). A placebo controlled crossover trial of liquid fluoxetine on repetitive behaviors in childhood and adolescent autism. *Neuropsychopharmacology* 30, 582–589. doi: 10.1038/sj.npp.1300627

Hollander, E., Soorya, L., Chaplin, W., Anagnostou, E., Taylor, B. P., Ferretti, C. J., et al. (2012). A double-blind placebo-controlled trial of fluoxetine for repetitive behaviors and global severity in adult autism spectrum disorders. *Am. J. Psychiatry* 169, 292–299. doi: 10.1176/appi.ajp.2011.10050764

Horwood, J. M., Dufour, F., Laroche, S., and Davis, S. (2006). Signalling mechanisms mediated by the phosphoinositide 3-kinase/Akt cascade in synaptic plasticity and memory in the rat. *Eur. J. Neurosci.* 23, 3375–3384. doi: 10.1111/j.1460-9568.2006.04859.x

Hu, H., Qin, Y., Bochorishvili, G., Zhu, Y., van Aelst, L., and Zhu, J. J. (2008). Ras signaling mechanisms underlying impaired GluR1-dependent plasticity associated with fragile X syndrome. *J. Neurosci.* 28, 7847–7862. doi: 10.1523/jneurosci.1496-08.2008

Huguet, G., Ey, E., and Bourgeron, T. (2013). The genetic landscapes of autism spectrum disorders. *Annu. Rev. Genomics Hum. Genet.* 14, 191–213. doi: 10.1146/annurev-genom-091212-153431

Huntley, G. W. (2012). Synaptic circuit remodelling by matrix metalloproteinases in health and disease. *Nat. Rev. Neurosci.* 13, 743–757. doi: 10.1038/nrn3320

Imbesi, M., Uz, T., Manev, R., Sharma, R. P., and Manev, H. (2008). Minocycline increases phosphorylation and membrane insertion of neuronal GluR1 receptors. *Neurosci. Lett.* 447, 134–137. doi: 10.1016/j.neulet.2008.10.006

Jacquemont, S., Berry-Kravis, E., Hagerman, R., von Raison, F., Gasparini, F., Apostol, G., et al. (2014). The challenges of clinical trials in fragile X syndrome. *Psychopharmacology (Berl)* 231, 1237–1250. doi: 10.1007/s00213-013-3289-0

Jacquemont, S., Curie, A., des Portes, V., Torrioli, M. G., Berry-Kravis, E., Hagerman, R. J., et al. (2011). Epigenetic modification of the FMR1 gene in fragile X syndrome is associated with differential response to the mGluR5 antagonist AFQ056. *Sci. Transl. Med.* 3:64ra61. doi: 10.1126/scitranslmed.3001708

Janusz, A., Milek, J., Perycz, M., Pacini, L., Bagni, C., Kaczmarek, L., et al. (2013). The fragile X mental retardation protein regulates matrix metalloproteinase 9 mRNA at synapses. *J. Neurosci.* 33, 18234–18241. doi: 10.1523/JNEUROSCI.2207-13.2013

Jay, T. M. (2003). Dopamine: a potential substrate for synaptic plasticity and memory mechanisms. *Prog. Neurobiol.* 69, 375–390. doi: 10.1016/s0301-0082(03)00085-6

Jope, R. S., and Roh, M. S. (2006). Glycogen synthase kinase-3 (GSK3) in psychiatric diseases and therapeutic interventions. *Curr. Drug Targets* 7, 1421–1434. doi: 10.2174/1389450110607011421

Jung, B. P., Jugloff, D. G., Zhang, G., Logan, R., Brown, S., and Eubanks, J. H. (2003). The expression of methyl CpG binding factor MeCP2 correlates with cellular differentiation in the developing rat brain and in cultured cells. *J. Neurobiol.* 55, 86–96. doi: 10.1002/neu.10201

Jung, K. M., Sepers, M., Henstridge, C. M., Lassalle, O., Neuhofer, D., Martin, H., et al. (2012). Uncoupling of the endocannabinoid signalling complex in a mouse model of fragile X syndrome. *Nat. Commun.* 3:1080. doi: 10.1038/ncomms2045

Katz, D. M. (2014). Brain-derived neurotrophic factor and Rett syndrome. *Handb. Exp. Pharmacol.* 220, 481–495. doi: 10.1007/978-3-642-45106-5_18

Katz, D. M., Berger-Sweeney, J. E., Eubanks, J. H., Justice, M. J., Neul, J. L., Pozzo-Miller, L., et al. (2012). Preclinical research in Rett syndrome: setting the foundation for translational success. *Dis. Model. Mech.* 5, 733–745. doi: 10.1242/dmm.011007

Kelleher, R. J. 3rd, Govindarajan, A., Jung, H. Y., Kang, H., and Tonegawa, S. (2004). Translational control by MAPK signaling in long-term synaptic plasticity and memory. *Cell* 116, 467–479. doi: 10.1016/s0092-8674(04)00115-1

Khwaja, O. S., Ho, E., Barnes, K. V., O'Leary, H. M., Pereira, L. M., Finkelstein, Y., et al. (2014). Safety, pharmacokinetics and preliminary assessment of efficacy of mecasermin (recombinant human IGF-1) for the treatment of Rett syndrome. *Proc. Natl. Acad. Sci. U S A* 111, 4596–4601. doi: 10.1073/pnas.1311141111

Kim, G. E., and Kaczmarek, L. K. (2014). Emerging role of the KCNT1 Slack channel in intellectual disability. *Front. Cell. Neurosci.* 8:209. doi: 10.3389/fncel.2014.00209

Kim, S. H., Markham, J. A., Weiler, I. J., and Greenough, W. T. (2008). Aberrant early-phase ERK inactivation impedes neuronal function in fragile X syndrome. *Proc. Natl. Acad. Sci. U S A* 105, 4429–4434. doi: 10.1073/pnas.0800257105

King, M. K., and Jope, R. S. (2013). Lithium treatment alleviates impaired cognition in a mouse model of fragile X syndrome. *Genes Brain Behav.* 12, 723–731. doi: 10.1111/gbb.12071

Klose, R. J., and Bird, A. P. (2006). Genomic DNA methylation: the mark and its mediators. *Trends Biochem. Sci.* 31, 89–97. doi: 10.1016/j.tibs.2005.12.008

Knobloch, H. S., and Grinevich, V. (2014). Evolution of oxytocin pathways in the brain of vertebrates. *Front. Behav. Neurosci.* 8:31. doi: 10.3389/fnbeh.2014.00031

Kolevzon, A., Mathewson, K. A., and Hollander, E. (2006). Selective serotonin reuptake inhibitors in autism: a review of efficacy and tolerability. *J. Clin. Psychiatry* 67, 407–414. doi: 10.4088/jcp.v67n0311

Kreis, P., and Barnier, J. V. (2009). PAK signalling in neuronal physiology. *Cell. Signal.* 21, 384–393. doi: 10.1016/j.cellsig.2008.11.001

Kron, M., Howell, C. J., Adams, I. T., Ransbottom, M., Christian, D., Ogier, M., et al. (2012). Brain activity mapping in Mecp2 mutant mice reveals functional deficits in forebrain circuits, including key nodes in the default mode network, that are reversed with ketamine treatment. *J. Neurosci.* 32, 13860–13872. doi: 10.1523/JNEUROSCI.2159-12.2012

Kron, M., Lang, M., Adams, I. T., Sceniak, M., Longo, F., and Katz, D. M. (2014). A BDNF loop-domain mimetic acutely reverses spontaneous apneas and respiratory abnormalities during behavioral arousal in a mouse model of Rett syndrome. *Dis. Model. Mech.* 7, 1047–1055. doi: 10.1242/dmm.016030

Krueger, D. D., Osterweil, E. K., Chen, S. P., Tye, L. D., and Bear, M. F. (2011). Cognitive dysfunction and prefrontal synaptic abnormalities in a mouse model of fragile X syndrome. *Proc. Natl. Acad. Sci. U S A* 108, 2587–2592. doi: 10.1073/pnas.1013855108

Krumm, N., O'Roak, B. J., Shendure, J., and Eichler, E. E. (2014). A de novo convergence of autism genetics and molecular neuroscience. *Trends Neurosci.* 37, 95–105. doi: 10.1016/j.tins.2013.11.005

Kumari, R., Castillo, C., and Francesconi, A. (2013). Agonist-dependent signaling by group I metabotropic glutamate receptors is regulated by association with lipid domains. *J. Biol. Chem.* 288, 32004–32019. doi: 10.1074/jbc.M113.475863

Lai, M. C., Lombardo, M. V., and Baron-Cohen, S. (2014). Autism. *Lancet* 383, 896–910. doi: 10.1016/S0140-6736(13)61539-1

Landis, S. C., Amara, S. G., Asadullah, K., Austin, C. P., Blumenstein, R., Bradley, E. W., et al. (2012). A call for transparent reporting to optimize the predictive value of preclinical research. *Nature* 490, 187–191. doi: 10.1038/nature11556

LaSalle, J. M., Goldstine, J., Balmer, D., and Greco, C. M. (2001). Quantitative localization of heterogeneous methyl-CpG-binding protein 2 (MeCP2) expression phenotypes in normal and Rett syndrome brain by laser scanning cytometry. *Hum. Mol. Genet.* 10, 1729–1740. doi: 10.1093/hmg/10.17.1729

Laurvick, C. L., de Klerk, N., Bower, C., Christodoulou, J., Ravine, D., Ellaway, C., et al. (2006). Rett syndrome in Australia: a review of the epidemiology. *J. Pediatr.* 148, 347–352. doi: 10.1016/j.jpeds.2005.10.037

Lauterborn, J. C., Truong, G. S., Baudry, M., Bi, X., Lynch, G., and Gall, C. M. (2003). Chronic elevation of brain-derived neurotrophic factor by ampakines. *J. Pharmacol. Exp. Ther.* 307, 297–305. doi: 10.1124/jpet.103.053694

Lee, H. Y., Ge, W. P., Huang, W., He, Y., Wang, G. X., Rowson-Baldwin, A., et al. (2011). Bidirectional regulation of dendritic voltage-gated potassium channels by the fragile X mental retardation protein. *Neuron* 72, 630–642. doi: 10.1016/j.neuron.2011.09.033.

Lee, H. Y., and Jan, L. Y. (2012). Fragile X syndrome: mechanistic insights and therapeutic avenues regarding the role of potassium channels. *Curr. Opin. Neurobiol.* 22, 887–894. doi: 10.1016/j.conb.2012.03.010

Leigh, M. J., Nguyen, D. V., Mu, Y., Winarni, T. I., Schneider, A., Chechi, T., et al. (2013). A randomized double-blind, placebo-controlled trial of minocycline in children and adolescents with fragile x syndrome. *J. Dev. Behav. Pediatr.* 34, 147–155. doi: 10.1097/DBP.0b013e318287cd17

Lekman, A., Witt-Engerstrom, I., Gottfries, J., Hagberg, B. A., Percy, A. K., and Svennerholm, L. (1989). Rett syndrome: biogenic amines and metabolites in postmortem brain. *Pediatr. Neurol.* 5, 357–362. doi: 10.1016/0887-8994(89)90049-0

Lesch, K. P., and Waider, J. (2012). Serotonin in the modulation of neural plasticity and networks: implications for neurodevelopmental disorders. *Neuron* 76, 175–191. doi: 10.1016/j.neuron.2012.09.013

Levenga, J., Hayashi, S., de Vrij, F. M., Koekkoek, S. K., van der Linde, H. C., Nieuwenhuizen, I., et al. (2011). AFQ056, a new mGluR5 antagonist for treatment of fragile X syndrome. *Neurobiol. Dis.* 42, 311–317. doi: 10.1016/j.nbd.2011.01.022

Li, W., and Pozzo-Miller, L. (2014). BDNF deregulation in Rett syndrome. *Neuropharmacology* 76(Pt. C), 737–746. doi: 10.1016/j.neuropharm.2013.03.024

Lim, C. S., Hoang, E. T., Viar, K. E., Stornetta, R. L., Scott, M. M., and Zhu, J. J. (2014). Pharmacological rescue of Ras signaling, GluA1-dependent synaptic plasticity and learning deficits in a fragile X model. *Genes Dev.* 28, 273–289. doi: 10.1101/gad.232470.113

Lipton, J., and Sahin, M. (2013). Fragile X syndrome therapeutics: translation, meet translational medicine. *Neuron* 77, 212–213. doi: 10.1016/j.neuron.2013.01.009

Maccarrone, M., Rossi, S., Bari, M., De Chiara, V., Rapino, C., Musella, A., et al. (2010). Abnormal mGlu 5 receptor/endocannabinoid coupling in mice lacking FMRP and BC1 RNA. *Neuropsychopharmacology* 35, 1500–1509. doi: 10.1038/npp.2010.19

Maliszewska-Cyna, E., Bawa, D., and Eubanks, J. H. (2010). Diminished prevalence but preserved synaptic distribution of N-methyl-D-aspartate receptor subunits in the methyl CpG binding protein 2(MeCP2)-null mouse brain. *Neuroscience* 168, 624–632. doi: 10.1016/j.neuroscience.2010.03.065

Malter, J. S., Ray, B. C., Westmark, P. R., and Westmark, C. J. (2010). Fragile X syndrome and Alzheimer's disease: another story about APP and beta-amyloid. *Curr. Alzheimer Res.* 7, 200–206. doi: 10.2174/156720510791050957

Marchetto, M. C., Carromeu, C., Acab, A., Yu, D., Yeo, G. W., Mu, Y., et al. (2010). A model for neural development and treatment of Rett syndrome using human induced pluripotent stem cells. *Cell* 143, 527–539. doi: 10.1016/j.cell.2010.10.016

Martinowich, K., Hattori, D., Wu, H., Fouse, S., He, F., Hu, Y., et al. (2003). DNA methylation-related chromatin remodeling in activity-dependent BDNF gene regulation. *Science* 302, 890–893. doi: 10.1126/science.1090842

Massa, S. M., Yang, T., Xie, Y., Shi, J., Bilgen, M., Joyce, J. N., et al. (2010). Small molecule BDNF mimetics activate TrkB signaling and prevent neuronal degeneration in rodents. *J. Clin. Invest.* 120, 1774–1785. doi: 10.1172/JCI41356

Matthys, A., Haegeman, G., Van Craenenbroeck, K., and Vanhoenacker, P. (2011). Role of the 5-HT7 receptor in the central nervous system: from current status to future perspectives. *Mol. Neurobiol.* 43, 228–253. doi: 10.1007/s12035-011-8175-3

McCauley, M. D., Wang, T., Mike, E., Herrera, J., Beavers, D. L., Huang, T. W., et al. (2011). Pathogenesis of lethal cardiac arrhythmias in Mecp2 mutant mice: implication for therapy in Rett syndrome. *Sci. Transl. Med.* 3:113ra125. doi: 10.1126/scitranslmed.3002982

McCoy, P. A., and McMahon, L. L. (2007). Muscarinic receptor dependent long-term depression in rat visual cortex is PKC independent but requires ERK1/2 activation and protein synthesis. *J. Neurophysiol.* 98, 1862–1870. doi: 10.1152/jn.00510.2007

McEwen, B. S., Chattarji, S., Diamond, D. M., Jay, T. M., Reagan, L. P., Svenningsson, P., et al. (2010). The neurobiological properties of tianeptine (Stablon): from monoamine hypothesis to glutamatergic modulation. *Mol. Psychiatry* 15, 237–249. doi: 10.1038/mp.2009.80

Medrihan, L., Tantalaki, E., Aramuni, G., Sargsyan, V., Dudanova, I., Missler, M., et al. (2008). Early defects of GABAergic synapses in the brain stem of a MeCP2 mouse model of Rett syndrome. *J. Neurophysiol.* 99, 112–121. doi: 10.1152/jn.00826.2007

Mefford, H. C., Batshaw, M. L., and Hoffman, E. P. (2012). Genomics, intellectual disability and autism. *N. Engl. J. Med.* 366, 733–743. doi: 10.1056/NEJMra1114194

Meyer-Lindenberg, A., Domes, G., Kirsch, P., and Heinrichs, M. (2011). Oxytocin and vasopressin in the human brain: social neuropeptides for translational medicine. *Nat. Rev. Neurosci.* 12, 524–538. doi: 10.1038/nrn3044

Michalon, A., Bruns, A., Risterucci, C., Honer, M., Ballard, T. M., Ozmen, L., et al. (2014). Chronic metabotropic glutamate receptor 5 inhibition corrects local alterations of brain activity and improves cognitive performance in fragile X mice. *Biol. Psychiatry* 75, 189–197. doi: 10.1016/j.biopsych.2013.05.038

Michalon, A., Sidorov, M., Ballard, T. M., Ozmen, L., Spooren, W., Wettstein, J. G., et al. (2012). Chronic pharmacological mGlu5 inhibition corrects fragile X in adult mice. *Neuron* 74, 49–56. doi: 10.1016/j.neuron.2012.03.009

Min, W. W., Yuskaitis, C. J., Yan, Q., Sikorski, C., Chen, S., Jope, R. S., et al. (2009). Elevated glycogen synthase kinase-3 activity in fragile X mice: key metabolic regulator with evidence for treatment potential. *Neuropharmacology* 56, 463–472. doi: 10.1016/j.neuropharm.2008.09.017

Mines, M. A., and Jope, R. S. (2011). Glycogen synthase kinase-3: a promising therapeutic target for fragile x syndrome. *Front. Mol. Neurosci.* 4:35. doi: 10.3389/fnmol.2011.00035

Mines, M. A., Yuskaitis, C. J., King, M. K., Beurel, E., and Jope, R. S. (2010). GSK3 influences social preference and anxiety-related behaviors during social interaction in a mouse model of fragile X syndrome and autism. *PLoS One* 5:e9706. doi: 10.1371/journal.pone.0009706

Misonou, H. (2010). Homeostatic regulation of neuronal excitability by K(+) channels in normal and diseased brains. *Neuroscientist* 16, 51–64. doi: 10.1177/1073858409341085

Moretti, P., and Zoghbi, H. Y. (2006). MeCP2 dysfunction in Rett syndrome and related disorders. *Curr. Opin. Genet. Dev.* 16, 276–281. doi: 10.1016/j.gde.2006.04.009

Mukherjee, S., and Manahan-Vaughan, D. (2013). Role of metabotropic glutamate receptors in persistent forms of hippocampal plasticity and learning. *Neuropharmacology* 66, 65–81. doi: 10.1016/j.neuropharm.2012.06.005

Murata, Y., and Constantine-Paton, M. (2013). Postsynaptic density scaffold SAP102 regulates cortical synapse development through EphB and PAK signaling pathway. *J. Neurosci.* 33, 5040–5052. doi: 10.1523/jneurosci.2896-12.2013

Murdoch, J. D., and State, M. W. (2013). Recent developments in the genetics of autism spectrum disorders. *Curr. Opin. Genet. Dev.* 23, 310–315. doi: 10.1016/j.gde.2013.02.003

Nakamoto, M., Nalavadi, V., Epstein, M. P., Narayanan, U., Bassell, G. J., and Warren, S. T. (2007). Fragile X mental retardation protein deficiency leads to excessive mGluR5-dependent internalization of AMPA receptors. *Proc. Natl. Acad. Sci. U S A* 104, 15537–15542. doi: 10.1073/pnas.0707484104

Nalivaeva, N. N., and Turner, A. J. (2013). The amyloid precursor protein: a biochemical enigma in brain development, function and disease. *FEBS Lett.* 587, 2046–2054. doi: 10.1016/j.febslet.2013.05.010

Nan, X., Ng, H. H., Johnson, C. A., Laherty, C. D., Turner, B. M., Eisenman, R. N., et al. (1998). Transcriptional repression by the methyl-CpG-binding protein MeCP2 involves a histone deacetylase complex. *Nature* 393, 386–389. doi: 10.3410/f.718020287.793478774

Narayanan, U., Nalavadi, V., Nakamoto, M., Thomas, G., Ceman, S., Bassell, G. J., et al. (2008). S6K1 phosphorylates and regulates fragile X mental retardation protein (FMRP) with the neuronal protein synthesis-dependent mammalian target of rapamycin (mTOR) signaling cascade. *J. Biol. Chem.* 283, 18478–18482. doi: 10.1074/jbc.c800055200

Neul, J. L., Kaufmann, W. E., Glaze, D. G., Christodoulou, J., Clarke, A. J., Bahi-Buisson, N., et al. (2010). Rett syndrome: revised diagnostic criteria and nomenclature. *Ann. Neurol.* 68, 944–950. doi: 10.1002/ana.22124

Neul, J. L., Lane, J. B., Lee, H. S., Geerts, S., Barrish, J. O., Annese, F., et al. (2014). Developmental delay in Rett syndrome: data from the natural history study. *J. Neurodev. Disord.* 6:20. doi: 10.1186/1866-1955-6-20

Neumann, I. D. (2008). Brain oxytocin: a key regulator of emotional and social behaviours in both females and males. *J. Neuroendocrinol.* 20, 858–865. doi: 10.1111/j.1365-2826.2008.01726.x

Neumann, I. D., and Landgraf, R. (2012). Balance of brain oxytocin and vasopressin: implications for anxiety, depression and social behaviors. *Trends Neurosci.* 35, 649–659. doi: 10.1016/j.tins.2012.08.004

Niederhofer, H. (2007). Glutamate antagonists seem to be slightly effective in psychopharmacologic treatment of autism. *J. Clin. Psychopharmacol.* 27, 317–318. doi: 10.1097/01.jcp.0000270082.30500.69

Ogier, M., Wang, H., Hong, E., Wang, Q., Greenberg, M. E., and Katz, D. M. (2007). Brain-derived neurotrophic factor expression and respiratory function improve after ampakine treatment in a mouse model of Rett syndrome. *J. Neurosci.* 27, 10912–10917. doi: 10.1523/jneurosci.1869-07.2007

Olmos-Serrano, J. L., Corbin, J. G., and Burns, M. P. (2011). The GABA(A) receptor agonist THIP ameliorates specific behavioral deficits in the mouse model of fragile X syndrome. *Dev. Neurosci.* 33, 395–403. doi: 10.1159/000332884

Olmos-Serrano, J. L., Paluszkiewicz, S. M., Martin, B. S., Kaufmann, W. E., Corbin, J. G., and Huntsman, M. M. (2010). Defective GABAergic neurotransmission and pharmacological rescue of neuronal hyperexcitability in the amygdala in a mouse model of fragile X syndrome. *J. Neurosci.* 30, 9929–9938. doi: 10.1523/jneurosci.1714-10.2010

O'Neill, M. J., Bleakman, D., Zimmerman, D. M., and Nisenbaum, E. S. (2004). AMPA receptor potentiators for the treatment of CNS disorders. *Curr. Drug Targets CNS Neurol. Disord.* 3, 181–194. doi: 10.2174/1568007043337508

O'Neill, M. J., and Witkin, J. M. (2007). AMPA receptor potentiators: application for depression and Parkinson's disease. *Curr. Drug Targets* 8, 603–620. doi: 10.2174/138945007780618517

Osterweil, E. K., Chuang, S. C., Chubykin, A. A., Sidorov, M., Bianchi, R., Wong, R. K., et al. (2013). Lovastatin corrects excess protein synthesis and prevents epileptogenesis in a mouse model of fragile X syndrome. *Neuron* 77, 243–250. doi: 10.1016/j.neuron.2012.01.034

Osterweil, E. K., Krueger, D. D., Reinhold, K., and Bear, M. F. (2010). Hypersensitivity to mGluR5 and ERK1/2 leads to excessive protein synthesis in the hippocampus of a mouse model of fragile X syndrome. *J. Neurosci.* 30, 15616–15627. doi: 10.1523/jneurosci.3888-10.2010

Oudin, M. J., Hobbs, C., and Doherty, P. (2011). DAGL-dependent endocannabinoid signalling: roles in axonal pathfinding, synaptic plasticity and adult neurogenesis. *Eur. J. Neurosci.* 34, 1634–1646. doi: 10.1111/j.1460-9568.2011.07831.x

Pacey, L. K., and Doering, L. C. (2007). Developmental expression of FMRP in the astrocyte lineage: implications for fragile X syndrome. *Glia* 55, 1601–1609. doi: 10.1002/glia.20573

Pacey, L. K., Heximer, S. P., and Hampson, D. R. (2009). Increased GABA(B) receptor-mediated signaling reduces the susceptibility of fragile X knockout mice to audiogenic seizures. *Mol. Pharmacol.* 76, 18–24. doi: 10.1124/mol.109.056127

Pacey, L. K., Tharmalingam, S., and Hampson, D. R. (2011). Subchronic administration and combination metabotropic glutamate and GABAB receptor drug therapy in fragile X syndrome. *J. Pharmacol. Exp. Ther.* 338, 897–905. doi: 10.1124/jpet.111.183327

Paluszkiewicz, S. M., Martin, B. S., and Huntsman, M. M. (2011). Fragile X syndrome: the GABAergic system and circuit dysfunction. *Dev. Neurosci.* 33, 349–364. doi: 10.1159/000329420

Paribello, C., Tao, L., Folino, A., Berry-Kravis, E., Tranfaglia, M., Ethell, I. M., et al. (2010). Open-label add-on treatment trial of minocycline in fragile X syndrome. *BMC Neurol.* 10:91. doi: 10.1186/1471-2377-10-91

Paul, K., Venkitaramani, D. V., and Cox, C. L. (2013). Dampened dopamine-mediated neuromodulation in prefrontal cortex of fragile X mice. *J. Physiol.* 591, 1133–1143. doi: 10.1113/jphysiol.2012.241067

Penagarikano, O., Mulle, J. G., and Warren, S. T. (2007). The pathophysiology of fragile x syndrome. *Annu. Rev. Genomics Hum. Genet.* 8, 109–129. doi: 10.1146/annurev.genom.8.080706.092249

Percy, A. K., Lane, J. B., Childers, J., Skinner, S., Annese, F., Barrish, J., et al. (2007). Rett syndrome: North American database. *J. Child Neurol.* 22, 1338–1341. doi: 10.1177/0883073807308715

Percy, A. K., Neul, J. L., Glaze, D. G., Motil, K. J., Skinner, S. A., Khwaja, O., et al. (2010). Rett syndrome diagnostic criteria: lessons from the natural history study. *Ann. Neurol.* 68, 951–955. doi: 10.1002/ana.22154

Picciotto, M. R., Higley, M. J., and Mineur, Y. S. (2012). Acetylcholine as a neuromodulator: cholinergic signaling shapes nervous system function and behavior. *Neuron* 76, 116–129. doi: 10.1016/j.neuron.2012.08.036

Pilpel, Y., Kolleker, A., Berberich, S., Ginger, M., Frick, A., Mientjes, E., et al. (2009). Synaptic ionotropic glutamate receptors and plasticity are developmentally altered in the CA1 field of Fmr1 knockout mice. *J. Physiol.* 587, 787–804. doi: 10.1113/jphysiol.2008.160929

Pitcher, M. R., Ward, C. S., Arvide, E. M., Chapleau, C. A., Pozzo-Miller, L., Hoeflich, A., et al. (2013). Insulinotropic treatments exacerbate metabolic syndrome in mice lacking MeCP2 function. *Hum. Mol. Genet.* 22, 2626–2633. doi: 10.1093/hmg/ddt111

Pop, A. S., Levenga, J., de Esch, C. E., Buijsen, R. A., Nieuwenhuizen, I. M., Li, T., et al. (2014). Rescue of dendritic spine phenotype in Fmr1 KO mice with the mGluR5 antagonist AFQ056/Mavoglurant. *Psychopharmacology (Berl)* 231, 1227–1235. doi: 10.1007/s00213-012-2947-y

Popescu, A. C., Sidorova, E., Zhang, G., and Eubanks, J. H. (2010). Aminoglycoside-mediated partial suppression of MECP2 nonsense mutations responsible for Rett syndrome in vitro. *J. Neurosci. Res.* 88, 2316–2324. doi: 10.1002/jnr.22409

Prasad, H. C., Steiner, J. A., Sutcliffe, J. S., and Blakely, R. D. (2009). Enhanced activity of human serotonin transporter variants associated with autism. *Philos. Trans. R. Soc. Lond. B Biol. Sci.* 364, 163–173. doi: 10.1098/rstb.2008.0143

Preti, A., Melis, M., Siddi, S., Vellante, M., Doneddu, G., and Fadda, R. (2014). Oxytocin and autism: a systematic review of randomized controlled trials. *J. Child Adolesc. Psychopharmacol.* 24, 54–68. doi: 10.1089/cap.2013.0040

Randall, A. D., Witton, J., Booth, C., Hynes-Allen, A., and Brown, J. T. (2010). The functional neurophysiology of the amyloid precursor protein (APP) processing pathway. *Neuropharmacology* 59, 243–267. doi: 10.1016/j.neuropharm.2010.02.011

Raymond, C. R., Thompson, V. L., Tate, W. P., and Abraham, W. C. (2000). Metabotropic glutamate receptors trigger homosynaptic protein synthesis to prolong long-term potentiation. *J. Neurosci.* 20, 969–976.

Roberts, J. E., Symons, F. J., Johnson, A. M., Hatton, D. D., and Boccia, M. L. (2005). Blink rate in boys with fragile X syndrome: preliminary evidence for altered dopamine function. *J. Intellect. Disabil. Res.* 49, 647–656. doi: 10.1111/j.1365-2788.2005.00713.x

Rogers, T. D., Dickson, P. E., McKimm, E., Heck, D. H., Goldowitz, D., Blaha, C. D., et al. (2013). Reorganization of circuits underlying cerebellar modulation of prefrontal cortical dopamine in mouse models of autism spectrum disorder. *Cerebellum* 12, 547–556. doi: 10.1007/s12311-013-0462-2

Ronemus, M., Iossifov, I., Levy, D., and Wigler, M. (2014). The role of de novo mutations in the genetics of autism spectrum disorders. *Nat. Rev. Genet.* 15, 133–141. doi: 10.1038/nrg3585

Ronesi, J. A., and Huber, K. M. (2008a). Metabotropic glutamate receptors and fragile x mental retardation protein: partners in translational regulation at the synapse. *Sci. Signal.* 1:pe6. doi: 10.1126/stke.15pe6

Ronesi, J. A., and Huber, K. M. (2008b). Homer interactions are necessary for metabotropic glutamate receptor-induced long-term depression and translational activation. *J. Neurosci.* 28, 543–547. doi: 10.1523/jneurosci.5019-07.2008

Rotschafer, S. E., Trujillo, M. S., Dansie, L. E., Ethell, I. M., and Razak, K. A. (2012). Minocycline treatment reverses ultrasonic vocalization production deficit in a mouse model of Fragile X syndrome. *Brain Res.* 1439, 7–14. doi: 10.1016/j.brainres.2011.12.041

Roux, J. C., Dura, E., Moncla, A., Mancini, J., and Villard, L. (2007). Treatment with desipramine improves breathing and survival in a mouse model for Rett syndrome. *Eur. J. Neurosci.* 25, 1915–1922. doi: 10.1111/j.1460-9568.2007.05466.x

Roux, J. C., Dura, E., and Villard, L. (2008). Tyrosine hydroxylase deficit in the chemoafferent and the sympathoadrenergic pathways of the Mecp2 deficient mouse. *Neurosci. Lett.* 447, 82–86. doi: 10.1016/j.neulet.2008.09.045

Samaco, R. C., and Neul, J. L. (2011). Complexities of Rett syndrome and MeCP2. *J. Neurosci.* 31, 7951–7959. doi: 10.1523/jneurosci.0169-11.2011

Santoro, M. R., Bray, S. M., and Warren, S. T. (2012). Molecular mechanisms of fragile X syndrome: a twenty-year perspective. *Annu. Rev. Pathol.* 7, 219–245. doi: 10.1146/annurev-pathol-011811-132457

Schanen, C., Houwink, E. J., Dorrani, N., Lane, J., Everett, R., Feng, A., et al. (2004). Phenotypic manifestations of MECP2 mutations in classical and atypical Rett syndrome. *Am. J. Med. Genet. A* 126A, 129–140. doi: 10.1002/ajmg.a.20571

Scheele, D., Kendrick, K. M., Khouri, C., Kretzer, E., Schläpfer, T. E., Stoffel-Wagner, B., et al. (2014). An oxytocin-induced facilitation of neural and emotional responses to social touch correlates inversely with autism traits. *Neuropsychopharmacology* 39, 2078–2085. doi: 10.1038/npp.2014.78

Schmid, D. A., Yang, T., Ogier, M., Adams, I., Mirakhur, Y., Wang, Q., et al. (2012). A TrkB small molecule partial agonist rescues TrkB phosphorylation deficits and improves respiratory function in a mouse model of Rett syndrome. *J. Neurosci.* 32, 1803–1810. doi: 10.1523/JNEUROSCI.0865-11.2012

Schmit, T. L., Dowell, J. A., Maes, M. E., and Wilhelm, M. (2013). c-Jun N-terminal kinase regulates mGluR-dependent expression of post-synaptic FMRP target proteins. *J. Neurochem.* 127, 772–781. doi: 10.1111/jnc.12453

Seamans, J. K., and Yang, C. R. (2004). The principal features and mechanisms of dopamine modulation in the prefrontal cortex. *Prog. Neurobiol.* 74, 1–58. doi: 10.1016/j.pneurobio.2004.05.006

Segal, R. A., and Greenberg, M. E. (1996). Intracellular signaling pathways activated by neurotrophic factors. *Annu. Rev. Neurosci.* 19, 463–489. doi: 10.1146/annurev.neuro.19.1.463

Shahbazian, M. D., Antalffy, B., Armstrong, D. L., and Zoghbi, H. Y. (2002). Insight into Rett syndrome: MeCP2 levels display tissue- and cell-specific differences and correlate with neuronal maturation. *Hum. Mol. Genet.* 11, 115–124. doi: 10.1093/hmg/11.2.115

Sharma, A., Hoeffer, C. A., Takayasu, Y., Miyawaki, T., McBride, S. M., Klann, E., et al. (2010). Dysregulation of mTOR signaling in fragile X syndrome. *J. Neurosci.* 30, 694–702. doi: 10.1523/jneurosci.3696-09.2010

Sidhu, H., Dansie, L. E., Hickmott, P. W., Ethell, D. W., and Ethell, I. M. (2014). Genetic removal of matrix metalloproteinase 9 rescues the symptoms of fragile x syndrome in a mouse model. *J. Neurosci.* 34, 9867–9879. doi: 10.1523/jneurosci.1162-14.2014

Sidorov, M. S., Auerbach, B. D., and Bear, M. F. (2013). Fragile X mental retardation protein and synaptic plasticity. *Mol. Brain* 6:15. doi: 10.1186/1756-6606-6-15

Sigel, E., and Steinmann, M. E. (2012). Structure, function and modulation of GABA(A) receptors. *J. Biol. Chem.* 287, 40224–40231. doi: 10.1074/jbc.R112.386664

Siller, S. S., and Broadie, K. (2012). Matrix metalloproteinases and minocycline: therapeutic avenues for fragile X syndrome. *Neural Plast.* 2012:124548. doi: 10.1155/2012/124548

Straiker, A., Min, K. T., and Mackie, K. (2013). Fmr1 deletion enhances and ultimately desensitizes CB(1) signaling in autaptic hippocampal neurons. *Neurobiol. Dis.* 56, 1–5. doi: 10.1016/j.nbd.2013.04.002

Strumbos, J. G., Brown, M. R., Kronengold, J., Polley, D. B., and Kaczmarek, L. K. (2010). Fragile X mental retardation protein is required for rapid experience-dependent regulation of the potassium channel Kv3.1b. *J. Neurosci.* 30, 10263–10271. doi: 10.1523/jneurosci.1125-10.2010

Sugden, P. H., Fuller, S. J., Weiss, S. C., and Clerk, A. (2008). Glycogen synthase kinase 3 (GSK3) in the heart: a point of integration in hypertrophic signalling and a therapeutic target? A critical analysis. *Br. J. Pharmacol.* 153(Suppl 1), S137–S153. doi: 10.1038/sj.bjp.0707659

Surmeier, D. J., Plotkin, J., and Shen, W. (2009). Dopamine and synaptic plasticity in dorsal striatal circuits controlling action selection. *Curr. Opin. Neurobiol.* 19, 621–628. doi: 10.1016/j.conb.2009.10.003

Suvrathan, A., Hoeffer, C. A., Wong, H., Klann, E., and Chattarji, S. (2010). Characterization and reversal of synaptic defects in the amygdala in a mouse model of fragile X syndrome. *Proc. Natl. Acad. Sci. U S A* 107, 11591–11596. doi: 10.1073/pnas.1002262107

Tavoulari, S., Forrest, L. R., and Rudnick, G. (2009). Fluoxetine (Prozac) binding to serotonin transporter is modulated by chloride and conformational changes. *J. Neurosci.* 29, 9635–9643. doi: 10.1523/jneurosci.0440-09.2009

Thomas, A. M., Bui, N., Graham, D., Perkins, J. R., Yuva-Paylor, L. A., and Paylor, R. (2011). Genetic reduction of group 1 metabotropic glutamate receptors alters select behaviors in a mouse model for fragile X syndrome. *Behav. Brain Res.* 223, 310–321. doi: 10.1016/j.bbr.2011.04.049

Thomas, A. M., Bui, N., Perkins, J. R., Yuva-Paylor, L. A., and Paylor, R. (2012). Group I metabotropic glutamate receptor antagonists alter select behaviors in a mouse model for fragile X syndrome. *Psychopharmacology (Berl)* 219, 47–58. doi: 10.1007/s00213-011-2375-4

Thomas, G. M., and Huganir, R. L. (2004). MAPK cascade signalling and synaptic plasticity. *Nat. Rev. Neurosci.* 5, 173–183. doi: 10.1038/nrn1346

Trappe, R., Laccone, F., Cobilanschi, J., Meins, M., Huppke, P., Hanefeld, F., et al. (2001). MECP2 mutations in sporadic cases of Rett syndrome are almost exclusively of paternal origin. *Am. J. Hum. Genet.* 68, 1093–1101. doi: 10.1086/320109

Tropea, D., Giacometti, E., Wilson, N. R., Beard, C., McCurry, C., Fu, D. D., et al. (2009). Partial reversal of Rett syndrome-like symptoms in MeCP2 mutant mice. *Proc. Natl. Acad. Sci. U S A* 106, 2029–2034. doi: 10.1073/pnas.0812394106

Tyzio, R., Nardou, R., Ferrari, D. C., Tsintsadze, T., Shahrokhi, A., Eftekhari, S., et al. (2014). Oxytocin-mediated GABA inhibition during delivery attenuates autism pathogenesis in rodent offspring. *Science* 343, 675–679. doi: 10.1126/science.1247190

Upreti, C., Zhang, X. L., Alford, S., and Stanton, P. K. (2013). Role of presynaptic metabotropic glutamate receptors in the induction of long-term synaptic plasticity of vesicular release. *Neuropharmacology* 66, 31–39. doi: 10.1016/j.neuropharm.2012.05.004

Uutela, M., Lindholm, J., Rantamäki, T., Umemori, J., Hunter, K., Võikar, V., et al. (2014). Distinctive behavioral and cellular responses to fluoxetine in the mouse model for fragile X syndrome. *Front. Cell. Neurosci.* 8:150. doi: 10.3389/fncel.2014.00150

Veenstra-VanderWeele, J., Muller, C. L., Iwamoto, H., Sauer, J. E., Owens, W. A., Shah, C. R., et al. (2012). Autism gene variant causes hyperserotonemia, serotonin receptor hypersensitivity, social impairment and repetitive behavior. *Proc. Natl. Acad. Sci. U S A* 109, 5469–5474. doi: 10.1073/pnas.1112345109

Veeraragavan, S., Bui, N., Perkins, J. R., Yuva-Paylor, L. A., Carpenter, R. L., and Paylor, R. (2011b). Modulation of behavioral phenotypes by a muscarinic M1 antagonist in a mouse model of fragile X syndrome. *Psychopharmacology (Berl)* 217, 143–151. doi: 10.1007/s00213-011-2276-6

Veeraragavan, S., Bui, N., Perkins, J. R., Yuva-Paylor, L. A., and Paylor, R. (2011a). The modulation of fragile X behaviors by the muscarinic M4 antagonist, tropicamide. *Behav. Neurosci.* 125, 783–790. doi: 10.1037/a0025202

Veeraragavan, S., Graham, D., Bui, N., Yuva-Paylor, L. A., Wess, J., and Paylor, R. (2012). Genetic reduction of muscarinic M4 receptor modulates analgesic response and acoustic startle response in a mouse model of fragile X syndrome (FXS). *Behav. Brain Res.* 228, 1–8. doi: 10.1016/j.bbr.2011.11.018

Vinueza Veloz, M. F., Buijsen, R. A., Willemsen, R., Cupido, A., Bosman, L. W., Koekkoek, S. K., et al. (2012). The effect of an mGluR5 inhibitor on procedural memory and avoidance discrimination impairments in Fmr1 KO mice. *Genes Brain Behav.* 11, 325–331. doi: 10.1111/j.1601-183x.2011.00763.x

Volk, L. J., Pfeiffer, B. E., Gibson, J. R., and Huber, K. M. (2007). Multiple Gq-coupled receptors converge on a common protein synthesis-dependent long-term depression that is affected in fragile X syndrome mental retardation. *J. Neurosci.* 27, 11624–11634. doi: 10.1523/jneurosci.2266-07.2007

Volpicelli, L. A., and Levey, A. I. (2004). Muscarinic acetylcholine receptor subtypes in cerebral cortex and hippocampus. *Prog. Brain Res.* 145, 59–66. doi: 10.1016/s0079-6123(03)45003-6

Wang, H. (2014). Lipid rafts: a signaling platform linking cholesterol metabolism to synaptic deficits in autism spectrum disorders. *Front. Behav. Neurosci.* 8:104. doi: 10.3389/fnbeh.2014.00104

Wang, L. W., Berry-Kravis, E., and Hagerman, R. J. (2010b). Fragile X: leading the way for targeted treatments in autism. *Neurotherapeutics* 7, 264–274. doi: 10.1016/j.nurt.2010.05.005

Wang, T., Bray, S. M., and Warren, S. T. (2012a). New perspectives on the biology of fragile X syndrome. *Curr. Opin. Genet. Dev.* 22, 256–263. doi: 10.1016/j.gde.2012.02.002

Wang, H., and Doering, L. C. (2012). Induced pluripotent stem cells to model and treat neurogenetic disorders. *Neural Plast.* 2012:346053. doi: 10.1155/2012/346053

Wang, H., and Doering, L. C. (2013). Reversing autism by targeting downstream mTOR signaling. *Front. Cell. Neurosci.* 7:28. doi: 10.3389/fncel.2013.00028

Wang, H., Kim, S. S., and Zhuo, M. (2010a). Roles of fragile X mental retardation protein in dopaminergic stimulation-induced synapse-associated protein synthesis and subsequent alpha-amino-3-hydroxyl-5-methyl-4-isoxazole-4-propionate (AMPA) receptor internalization. *J. Biol. Chem.* 285, 21888–21901. doi: 10.1074/jbc.M110.116293

Wang, H., Ku, L., Osterhout, D. J., Li, W., Ahmadian, A., Liang, Z., et al. (2004). Developmentally-programmed FMRP expression in oligodendrocytes: a potential role of FMRP in regulating translation in oligodendroglia progenitors. *Hum. Mol. Genet.* 13, 79–89. doi: 10.1093/hmg/ddh009

Wang, G. X., Smith, S. J., and Mourrain, P. (2014). Fmr1 KO and fenobam treatment differentially impact distinct synapse populations of mouse neocortex. *Neuron* 84, 1273–1286. doi: 10.1016/j.neuron.2014.11.016

Wang, X., Snape, M., Klann, E., Stone, J. G., Singh, A., Petersen, R. B., et al. (2012b). Activation of the extracellular signal-regulated kinase pathway contributes to the behavioral deficit of fragile x-syndrome. *J. Neurochem.* 121, 672–679. doi: 10.1111/j.1471-4159.2012.07722.x

Wang, H., Wu, L. J., Kim, S. S., Lee, F. J., Gong, B., Toyoda, H., et al. (2008b). FMRP acts as a key messenger for dopamine modulation in the forebrain. *Neuron* 59, 634–647. doi: 10.1016/j.neuron.2008.06.027

Wang, H., Wu, L. J., Zhang, F., and Zhuo, M. (2008a). Roles of calcium-stimulated adenylyl cyclase and calmodulin-dependent protein kinase IV in the regulation of FMRP by group I metabotropic glutamate receptors. *J. Neurosci.* 28, 4385–4397. doi: 10.1523/JNEUROSCI.0646-08.2008

Wang, H., and Zhuo, M. (2012). Group I metabotropic glutamate receptor-mediated gene transcription and implications for synaptic plasticity and diseases. *Front. Pharmacol.* 3:189. doi: 10.3389/fphar.2012.00189

Watanabe, T., Abe, O., Kuwabara, H., Yahata, N., Takano, Y., Iwashiro, N., et al. (2014). Mitigation of sociocommunicational deficits of autism through oxytocin-induced recovery of medial prefrontal activity: a randomized trial. *JAMA Psychiatry* 71, 166–175. doi: 10.1001/jamapsychiatry.2013.3181

Wei, H., Dobkin, C., Sheikh, A. M., Malik, M., Brown, W. T., and Li, X. (2012). The therapeutic effect of memantine through the stimulation of synapse formation and dendritic spine maturation in autism and fragile X syndrome. *PLoS One* 7:e36981. doi: 10.1371/journal.pone.0036981

Weiler, I. J., and Greenough, W. T. (1993). Metabotropic glutamate receptors trigger postsynaptic protein synthesis. *Proc. Natl. Acad. Sci. U S A* 90, 7168–7171. doi: 10.1073/pnas.90.15.7168

Weinshenker, D., and Warren, S. T. (2008). Neuroscience: fragile dopamine. *Nature* 455, 607–608. doi: 10.1038/455607a

Weng, N., Weiler, I. J., Sumis, A., Berry-Kravis, E., and Greenough, W. T. (2008). Early-phase ERK activation as a biomarker for metabolic status in fragile X syndrome. *Am. J. Med. Genet. B Neuropsychiatr. Genet.* 147B, 1253–1257. doi: 10.1002/ajmg.b.30765

Wernicke, J. F. (2004). Safety and side effect profile of fluoxetine. *Expert Opin. Drug Saf.* 3, 495–504. doi: 10.1517/14740338.3.5.495

Westmark, C. J. (2013). What's hAPPening at synapses? The role of amyloid beta-protein precursor and β-amyloid in neurological disorders. *Mol. Psychiatry* 18, 425–434. doi: 10.1038/mp.2012.122

Westmark, C. J., Berry-Kravis, E. M., Ikonomidou, C., Yin, J. C., and Puglielli, L. (2013). Developing BACE-1 inhibitors for FXS. *Front. Cell. Neurosci.* 7:77. doi: 10.3389/fncel.2013.00077

Westmark, C. J., and Malter, J. S. (2007). FMRP mediates mGluR5-dependent translation of amyloid precursor protein. *PLoS Biol.* 5:e52. doi: 10.1371/journal.pbio.0050052

Westmark, C. J., Westmark, P. R., and Malter, J. S. (2010). MPEP reduces seizure severity in Fmr-1 KO mice over expressing human Abeta. *Int. J. Clin. Exp. Pathol.* 3, 56–68.

Westmark, C. J., Westmark, P. R., O'Riordan, K. J., Ray, B. C., Hervey, C. M., Salamat, M. S., et al. (2011). Reversal of fragile X phenotypes by manipulation of AβPP/Aβ levels in Fmr1KO mice. *PLoS One* 6:e26549. doi: 10.1371/journal.pone.0026549

Wiegert, J. S., and Bading, H. (2011). Activity-dependent calcium signaling and ERK-MAP kinases in neurons: a link to structural plasticity of the nucleus and gene transcription regulation. *Cell Calcium* 49, 296–305. doi: 10.1016/j.ceca.2010.11.009

Wijetunge, L. S., Chattarji, S., Wyllie, D. J., and Kind, P. C. (2013). Fragile X syndrome: from targets to treatments. *Neuropharmacology* 68, 83–96. doi: 10.1016/j.neuropharm.2012.11.028

Wong, D. T., Perry, K. W., and Bymaster, F. P. (2005). Case history: the discovery of fluoxetine hydrochloride (Prozac). *Nat. Rev. Drug Discov.* 4, 764–774. doi: 10.1038/nrd1821

Wright, J. W., and Harding, J. W. (2009). Contributions of matrix metalloproteinases to neural plasticity, habituation, associative learning and drug addiction. *Neural Plast.* 2009:579382. doi: 10.1155/2009/579382

Yan, Q. J., Rammal, M., Tranfaglia, M., and Bauchwitz, R. P. (2005). Suppression of two major fragile X syndrome mouse model phenotypes by the mGluR5 antagonist MPEP. *Neuropharmacology* 49, 1053–1066. doi: 10.1016/j.neuropharm.2005.06.004

Yun, S. H., and Trommer, B. L. (2011). Fragile X mice: reduced long-term potentiation and N-Methyl-D-Aspartate receptor-mediated neurotransmission in dentate gyrus. *J. Neurosci. Res.* 89, 176–182. doi: 10.1002/jnr.22546

Yuskaitis, C. J., Mines, M. A., King, M. K., Sweatt, J. D., Miller, C. A., and Jope, R. S. (2010). Lithium ameliorates altered glycogen synthase kinase-3 and behavior in a mouse model of fragile X syndrome. *Biochem. Pharmacol.* 79, 632–646. doi: 10.1016/j.bcp.2009.09.023

Zanella, S., Mebarek, S., Lajard, A. M., Picard, N., Dutschmann, M., and Hilaire, G. (2008). Oral treatment with desipramine improves breathing and life span in Rett syndrome mouse model. *Respir. Physiol. Neurobiol.* 160, 116–121. doi: 10.1016/j.resp.2007.08.009

Zhang, L., and Alger, B. E. (2010). Enhanced endocannabinoid signaling elevates neuronal excitability in fragile X syndrome. *J. Neurosci.* 30, 5724–5729. doi: 10.1523/JNEUROSCI.0795-10.2010

Zhang, Y., Bonnan, A., Bony, G., Ferezou, I., Pietropaolo, S., Ginger, M., et al. (2014b). Dendritic channelopathies contribute to neocortical and sensory hyperexcitability in Fmr1(-/y) mice. *Nat. Neurosci.* 17, 1701–1709. doi: 10.1038/nn.3864

Zhang, Y., Brown, M. R., Hyland, C., Chen, Y., Kronengold, J., Fleming, M. R., et al. (2012). Regulation of neuronal excitability by interaction of fragile X mental retardation protein with slack potassium channels. *J. Neurosci.* 32, 15318–15327. doi: 10.1523/JNEUROSCI.2162-12.2012

Zhang, W., Peterson, M., Beyer, B., Frankel, W. N., and Zhang, Z. W. (2014a). Loss of MeCP2 from forebrain excitatory neurons leads to cortical hyperexcitation and seizures. *J. Neurosci.* 34, 2754–2763. doi: 10.1523/JNEUROSCI.4900-12.2014

Zhang, Y., Venkitaramani, D. V., Gladding, C. M., Kurup, P., Molnar, E., Collingridge, G. L., et al. (2008). The tyrosine phosphatase STEP mediates AMPA receptor endocytosis after metabotropic glutamate receptor stimulation. *J. Neurosci.* 28, 10561–10566. doi: 10.1523/JNEUROSCI.2666-08.2008

Zhang, H., Webb, D. J., Asmussen, H., Niu, S., and Horwitz, A. F. (2005). A GIT1/PIX/Rac/PAK signaling module regulates spine morphogenesis and synapse formation through MLC. *J. Neurosci.* 25, 3379–3388. doi: 10. 1523/jneurosci.3553-04.2005

Zhang, Z. W., Zak, J. D., and Liu, H. (2010). MeCP2 is required for normal development of GABAergic circuits in the thalamus. *J. Neurophysiol.* 103, 2470–2481. doi: 10.1152/jn.00601.2009

Zheng, W. H., and Quirion, R. (2004). Comparative signaling pathways of insulin-like growth factor-1 and brain-derived neurotrophic factor in hippocampal neurons and the role of the PI3 kinase pathway in cell survival. *J. Neurochem.* 89, 844–852. doi: 10.1111/j.1471-4159.2004.02350.x

Ziemssen, T., Kümpfel, T., Klinkert, W. E., Neuhaus, O., and Hohlfeld, R. (2002). Glatiramer acetate-specific T-helper 1- and 2-type cell lines produce BDNF: implications for multiple sclerosis therapy. Brain-derived neurotrophic factor. *Brain* 125, 2381–2391. doi: 10.1093/brain/awf252

Zingman, L. V., Park, S., Olson, T. M., Alekseev, A. E., and Terzic, A. (2007). Aminoglycoside-induced translational read-through in disease: overcoming nonsense mutations by pharmacogenetic therapy. *Clin. Pharmacol. Ther.* 81, 99–103. doi: 10.1038/sj.clpt.6100012

Zoghbi, H. Y., and Bear, M. F. (2012). Synaptic dysfunction in neurodevelopmental disorders associated with autism and intellectual disabilities. *Cold Spring Harb. Perspect. Biol.* 4, pii:a009886. doi: 10.1101/cshperspect.a009886

Zupan, B., and Toth, M. (2008). Inactivation of the maternal fragile X gene results in sensitization of GABAB receptor function in the offspring. *J. Pharmacol. Exp. Ther.* 327, 820–826. doi: 10.1124/jpet.108.143990

15

A selective histone deacetylase-6 inhibitor improves BDNF trafficking in hippocampal neurons from *Mecp2* knockout mice: Implications for Rett syndrome

Xin Xu*[1], *Alan P. Kozikowski*[2] and *Lucas Pozzo-Miller*[1]

[1] *Department of Neurobiology, Civitan International Research Center, The University of Alabama at Birmingham, Birmingham, AL, USA*
[2] *Drug Discovery Program, Department of Medicinal Chemistry and Pharmacognosy, University of Illinois at Chicago, Chicago, IL, USA*

***Correspondence:**
Lucas Pozzo-Miller, Department of Neurobiology, The University of Alabama at Birmingham, SHEL-1002, 1825 University Blvd., Birmingham, AL 35294-2182, USA
e-mail: lucaspm@uab.edu

Rett syndrome (RTT) is a neurodevelopmental disorder caused by loss-of-function mutations in the transcriptional modulator methyl-CpG-binding protein 2 (*MECP2*). One of the most prominent gene targets of MeCP2 is brain-derived neurotrophic factor (*Bdnf*), a potent modulator of activity-dependent synaptic development, function and plasticity. Dysfunctional BDNF signaling has been demonstrated in several pathophysiological mechanisms of RTT disease progression. To evaluate whether the dynamics of BDNF trafficking is affected by *Mecp2* deletion, we analyzed movements of BDNF tagged with yellow fluorescent protein (YFP) in cultured hippocampal neurons by time-lapse fluorescence imaging. We found that both anterograde and retrograde vesicular trafficking of BDNF-YFP are significantly impaired in *Mecp2* knockout hippocampal neurons. Selective inhibitors of histone deacetylase 6 (HDAC6) show neuroprotective effects in neurodegenerative diseases and stimulate microtubule-dependent vesicular trafficking of BDNF-containing dense core vesicles. Here, we show that the selective HDAC6 inhibitor Tubastatin-A increased the velocity of BDNF-YFP vesicles in *Mecp2* knockout neurons in both directions by increasing α–tubulin acetylation. Tubastatin-A also restored activity-dependent BDNF release from *Mecp2* knockout neurons to levels comparable to those shown by wildtype neurons. These findings demonstrate that a selective HDAC6 inhibitor is a potential pharmacological strategy to reverse cellular and synaptic impairments in RTT resulting from impaired BDNF signaling.

Keywords: Rett syndrome, dense core vesicle, activity-dependent BDNF release, Tubastatin-A, tubulin acetylation

INTRODUCTION

Rett syndrome (RTT), an X-linked postnatal neurodevelopmental disorder associated with intellectual disabilities, is primarily caused by mutations in methyl-CpG-binding protein 2 (*MECP2*), the gene encoding MeCP2, a transcriptional modulator that binds to methylated CpG sites in promoter regions of DNA (Nan et al., 1997; Amir et al., 1999; Percy and Lane, 2005). A number of genes including brain-derived neurotrophic factor (*Bdnf*) were identified to be regulated by MeCP2 and relevant to the pathogenesis of RTT (Bievenu and Chelly, 2006; Chahrour and Zoghbi, 2007). MeCP2 binds to the *Bdnf* promoter and directly modulates *Bdnf* expression in an activity-dependent manner (Chen et al., 2003; Martinowich et al., 2003; Zhou et al., 2006). Several studies have reported lower BDNF mRNA and protein levels in various brain regions of *Mecp2* deficient mice and RTT individuals (Chang et al., 2006; Wang et al., 2006; Ogier et al., 2007; Li et al., 2012). Reduced overall neuronal activity caused by MeCP2 deficiency is thought to contribute to BDNF downregulation. Conditional *Bdnf* mutant mice showed similar RTT phenotypes as *Mecp2* knockout mice, while *Bdnf* overexpression rescued some of the functional deficits observed in *Mecp2* mutants and extended their lifespan (Chang et al., 2006; Chahrour and Zoghbi, 2007). These findings strongly indicate BDNF plays a critical role in neurological dysfunctions in RTT.

Prior to RTT, BDNF had been implicated in other neurological disorders due to its widespread function in neuronal development, plasticity, differentiation, and survival (Poo, 2001; Fahnestock et al., 2002; Gines et al., 2010; Hartmann et al., 2012). Common among these BDNF-related disorders, such as Alzheimer's disease (AD), Huntington disease (HD), is the irregular trafficking of dense-core vesicles containing BDNF, as well as activity-dependent BDNF release from those vesicles (Gauthier et al., 2004; Chapleau et al., 2009; Poon et al., 2011). Intriguingly, the single nucleotide polymorphism Val66Met observed in the human *BDNF* gene resulted in more severe RTT symptoms and an increased risk of seizure onset, suggesting that in addition to BDNF expression levels, BDNF trafficking and release are altered in RTT (Zeev et al., 2009; Hartmann et al., 2012). Live BDNF-YFP imaging in cultured neurons offers the ability to investigate dynamic trafficking of BDNF, which was reported to be identical to that of endogenous BDNF in terms of its cellular localization, processing and secretion (Haubensak et al., 1998; Kohara et al., 2001; Lessmann and Brigadski, 2009; Hartmann et al., 2012). Here, we report that vesicular trafficking of BDNF, as well as its activity-dependent release are significantly impaired in hippocampal neurons of *Mecp2* knockout mice, providing further support for the role of BDNF signaling in RTT pathophysiology.

Histone deacetylase-6 (HDAC6), a member of the class II histone deacetylases, is a unique cytosolic enzyme that regulates cell motility (Hubbert et al., 2002; Matsuyama et al., 2002; Zhang et al., 2003; Tran et al., 2007), endocytosis (Gao et al., 2007), vesicle transport (Dompierre et al., 2007), cell migration and degradation of misfolded proteins (Iwata et al., 2005; Valenzuela-Fernandez et al., 2008) and other cellular process by deacetylating α-tubulin, Hsp90 and cortactin (Fukada et al., 2012). HDAC6 has emerged as an attractive target for pharmacological intervention in several CNS diseases. Selective inhibition of HDAC6 is thought to promote neuronal survival and regrowth after injury, offering a potential therapy for various neurodegenerative diseases (Kazantsev and Thompson, 2008; Rivieccio et al., 2009; Butler et al., 2010). For example, the non-selective HDAC inhibitor trichostatin A (TSA) improves microtubule (MT)-dependent transport of BDNF-GFP in cultured neurons expressing mutant Huntingtin; this effect was ascribed to increased α–tubulin acetylation through the inhibition of cytoplasmic HDAC6 (Dompierre et al., 2007). Indeed, Tubastatin-A (TBA), a more selective HDAC6 inhibitor, showed neuroprotective effects in a model of oxidative stress, and exhibited no toxicity compared to TSA (Butler et al., 2010). Furthermore, TBA rescued the impairment of mitochondrial transport in axons and mitochondrial elongation caused by Aβ exposure (Kim et al., 2012). We report that TBA improves BDNF-YFP trafficking and activity-dependent release in *Mecp2* knockout hippocampal neurons to reach wildtype levels, suggesting that HDAC6 is a potential therapeutic target to restore BDNF-dependent neurological function in the absence of functional MeCP2, which provides a novel approach for therapeutic intervention in RTT.

MATERIALS AND METHODS

ANIMALS

Breeding pairs of mice lacking exon 3 of the X chromosome-linked *Mecp2* gene (B6.Cg-$Mecp2^{tm1.1Jae}$, "Jaenisch" strain in a pure C57BL/6 background) (Chen et al., 2001) were purchased from the Mutant Mouse Regional Resource Center at the University of California, Davis. A colony was established at The University of Alabama at Birmingham (UAB) by mating wildtype males with heterozygous $Mecp2^{tm1.1Jae}$ mutant females, as recommended by the supplier. Genotyping was performed by PCR of DNA sample from tail clips. Hemizygous $Mecp2^{tm1.1Jae}$ mutant males are healthy until 5–6 weeks of age, when they exhibit RTT-like motor symptoms, such as hypoactivity, hind limb clasping, and reflex impairments (Chen et al., 2001). Animals were handled and housed according to the Committee on Laboratory Animal Resources of the National Institutes of Health. All experimental protocols were annually reviewed and approved by the Institutional Animals Care and Use Committee of UAB.

PRIMARY CULTURES OF HIPPOCAMPAL NEURONS AND TRANSFECTION

Both hippocampi were dissected from anesthetized postnatal day 0 or 1 (P0-1) male *Mecp2* knockout mice and wildtype littermates, and dissociated in papain (20 U/ml) plus DNAse I (Worthington, Lakewood, NJ) for 20-30 min at 37°C, as described (Amaral and Pozzo-Miller, 2007). The tissue was then triturated to obtain a single-cell suspension, and the cells were plated at a density of 50,000 cells/cm^2 on 12 mm poly-L-lysine/laminin coated glass coverslips, and immersed in Neurobasal medium supplemented with 2% B27 and 0.5 mM glutamine (Life Technologies, Carlsbad, CA). Neurons were grown in 37°C, 5% CO_2, 90% relative humidity incubators (Thermo-Forma), with half of the fresh medium changed every 3-4 days. After 11 days *in vitro* (DIV), neurons were transfected with cDNA encoding BDNF-YFP (a gift from M. Kojima) using Lipofectamine 2000 (Life Technologies) (0.8 μg DNA) according to the manufacturer's protocol.

IMMUNOCYTOCHEMISTRY

All experiments were performed at 12-14 DIV. For localization of endogenous native BDNF, neurons were fixed with 4% (wt/vol) paraformaldehyde/sucrose in phosphate buffer (PB; 23 mM NaH_2PO4, 2 mM Na_2HPO4 pH 7.4) for 10 min, and incubated in 0.25% (vol/vol) Triton X-100 for 10 min, then washed with PB saline (PBS). After blocking with 10% (vol/vol) goat serum in PBS, cells were incubated with anti-BDNF antibody (2μg/ml, Santa Cruz Biotechnology #SC-546) overnight at 4°C, rinsed in PBS, and incubated with Alexa Fluor-488 secondary antibody (Life Technologies) for 1 h; coverslips were then mounted with Vectashield (Vector Laboratories). Images were acquired in a laser-scanning confocal microscope using a solid-state 488 nm laser for excitation, and a 60 X 1.4 NA oil immersion lens, and standard FITC dichroic and emission filters (FluoView-300, Olympus; Center Valley, PA). For dual immunocytochemistry, BDNF-YFP-expressing neurons were fixed with 3% formaldehyde in PB at 0°C for 20 min, permeabilized for 10 min at room temperature with 3% formaldehyde containing 0.25% Triton X-100, and blocked with 10% bovine serum albumin (BSA) for 1 h at 37°C. Primary goat anti-chromogranin B (1:100; Santa Cruz) and rabbit anti-BDNF (1:100, Santa Cruz) antibodies, as well as fluorescently-conjugated anti-goat and anti-rabbit secondary antibodies (Molecular Probes) were diluted in 1X PBS and 3% horse serum. Coverslips were mounted with Vectashield (Vector Laboratories), and fluorescence images were acquired with a cooled CCD camera (CoolSnap HQ2, Photometics) on a wide-field fluorescence microscope (Eclipse TE2000-U, Nikon Instruments); BDNF-YFP was imaged with a standard FITC filter, and fluorescently-conjugated secondary antibodies with standard FITC and TRITC filters. Images were deconvolved using Metamorph (Molecular Devices).

TIME-LAPSE FLUORESCENCE IMAGING

Time-lapse imaging was performed 24–48 h after BDNF-YFP transfection. For mitochondria trafficking, neurons were incubated for 15 min with MitoTracker Red (200 nM; Life Technologies) prior to live imaging. Individual coverslips with cultured neurons were transferred to a recording chamber mounted on a fixed-stage upright microscope (Leica DM-LFS with either a 63 × 0.9 NA or a Zeiss 63 × 1.0 NA water-immersion objective), and continuously perfused (1 ml/min) with HEPES buffered artificial CSF (aCSF) at 32–34°C, containing (mM): 119 NaCl, 5 KCl, 2 $CaCl_2$, 1.3 $MgCl_2$, 10 glucose, 10 HEPES (pH 7.4). YFP was excited with 490 ± 12 nm light using a galvanometric monochromator (Polychrome-II, TILL Photonics; Germany), and its emission (>510 nm, FITC-LP cube) was filtered and detected with an electron-multiplying cooled CCD camera operating in frame-transfer mode (QuantEM: 512SC, Photometrics, Tucson AZ). MitoTracker Red was excited with 560 ± 12 nm and imaged through a standard TRITC cube. Digital images were acquired every 5 s (50–100 ms exposures for ~100 × 200 pixel sub-arrays, 1 × 1 binning) for a total time of 10 min. The position of fluorescent puncta was tracked as a function of time using the Particle Tracking module of Imaris (Bitplane).

DRUG TREATMENTS AND CELL VIABILITY ASSAYS

BDNF-YFP-transfected neurons were treated with the HDAC6 inhibitor Tubastatin A (1 μM, prepared in 0.01% DMSO vehicle) for 48 h; 0.01% DMSO was used as control. Cell viability was assessed by trypan blue exclusion. Cells were rinsed with HBSS, and incubated with 0.4% trypan blue solution (Gibco) for 2 min at room temperature. After washing with HBSS, dead and live cells were counted in ten random fields per coverslip.

SURFACE STAINING OF BDNF-YFP IMMUNOFLUORESCENCE

The procedure for BDNF-YFP immunostaining on the surface of cultured neurons was as described (Sadakata et al., 2012). Twenty-four hours after BDNF-YFP transfection, cultured neurons were stimulated with 50 mM KCl for 10 min in the absence or presence of the voltage-gated Ca^{2+} channel blocker nifedipine (50 μM), the ionotropic glutamate receptor antagonists CNQX (10 μM) and D-APV (50 μM), the $GABA_AR$ antagonist bicuculline (10 μM), or the voltage-gated Na^+ channel blocker TTX (0.5 μM), fixed with 4% (wt/vol) paraformaldehyde/sucrose for 5 min, and then washed with PBS. After blocking with 10% (vol/vol) goat serum in PBS, cells were incubated with anti-GFP antibody (which also recognized YFP; Abcam) overnight at 4°C, rinsed in PBS, and incubated with anti-rabbit secondary antibody conjugated to Cy3 (Millipore) for 1 h; coverslips were then mounted with Vectashield medium (Vector Laboratories). Images were acquired in a laser-scanning confocal microscope using a solid-state 488 nm laser for YFP excitation, a 543 nm HeNe green laser for Cy3 excitation, a 60 × 1.4 NA oil immersion lens, and standard FITC and TRITC dichroic and emission filters (FluoView-300, Olympus). Quantification of co-localized pixels was performed using Colocalization module in Imaris. The ratio of surface-bound BDNF-YFP to total BDNF-YFP was estimated as volumetric percentage of co-localized signals over the threshold.

WESTERN IMMUNOBLOTTING

For biochemical measurements of the levels of acetylated and total α-tubulin, total cell lysates were obtained by rinsing 4 × 10^5 treated hippocampal neurons with cold PBS followed by lysis in NP-40 lysis buffer (20 mM Tris at pH 8.0, 137 mM NaCl, 10% glycerol, 1% Nonidet P-40, 2 mM EDTA) containing protease inhibitor. The cell lysates were maintained with constant agitation for 30 min at 4°C and centrifuged at 12,000 g for 20 min. The supernatants were aspirated and protein concentrations were quantified by the Lowry method. Fifteen micrograms of total lysate were subjected to SDS-PAGE (Bio-Rad) and Western blot analysis with primary antibodies against acetylated α-tubulin (1:1000; Sigma) and total α-tubulin (1:2000; Life Technologies). Immunodetection was performed using Odyssey infrared imaging system (Li-Cor Bioscience).

STATISTICAL ANALYSES

All the experiments were performed at least 3 different times, from at least 3 different neuronal culture preparations. Data are presented as mean ± standard error of the mean (SEM), and were compared using unpaired Student's t-test for two groups or One Way ANOVA with Tukey post test for more than three groups; percentages were compared using Chi-square test. All analyses were performed using Prism software (GraphPad Software, San Diego, CA). $P < 0.05$ was considered significant.

RESULTS

BDNF-YFP TRAFFICKING IS IMPAIRED IN *MECP2* KNOCKOUT NEURONS

The cellular localization, processing and secretion of exogenously expressed BDNF-xFP have been reported to be identical to those of endogenous native BDNF, including its co-localization to secretory granule cargoes like chromogranin-B and SGA2 (Haubensak et al., 1998; Kohara et al., 2001; Lessmann and Brigadski, 2009; Hartmann et al., 2012) (**Supplemental Figure 1**). To evaluate whether the dynamics of dendritic BDNF trafficking is altered by *Mecp2* deletion, time-lapse fluorescence imaging of BDNF-YFP was performed in primary cultures of hippocampal neurons (12–14 days *in vitro*, DIV) from male *Mecp2* knockouts and wildtype littermates. BDNF-YFP puncta are widely distributed and move bi-directionally in live neurons (**Figures 1A,B**), as previously described (Park et al., 2008; Matsuda et al., 2009). The average velocity of BDNF-YFP puncta was significantly slower in *Mecp2* knockout neurons (0.10 ± 0.01 μm/s, $n = 261$ puncta from 8 cells) compared to wildtype cells (WT 0.25 ± 0.01 μm/s, $n = 225$ puncta from 8 cells; $p < 0.001$). Analyses of the distributions of the velocity of BDNF-YFP puncta revealed that the number of fast moving puncta (velocity >0.4 μm/s) is significantly smaller in *Mecp2* knockout neurons (*Mecp2* 1.30 % vs. WT 16.77 %; $p < 0.001$; **Figures 1C,D**). To quantify BDNF transport efficiency, we compared the persistence of each BDNF-YFP puncta, estimated as the ratio of total distance traveled during an image sequence over the minimum displacement between image frames (Gauthier et al., 2004). Consistent with impaired and slower BDNF trafficking, the persistence of BDNF-YFP puncta was higher in *Mecp2* knockout neurons (*Mecp2* 7.14 ± 0.98 vs. WT 3.91 ± 0.43; $p < 0.05$; **Figure 1E**). Then, we tested whether the transport of other organelles such as mitochondria is also affected by *Mecp2* deletion. Intriguingly, time-lapse imaging of MitoTracker-Red puncta revealed a lower percentage of fast moving mitochondria in *Mecp2* knockout neurons (*Mecp2* 6.08 % vs. WT 12.39 %; $p < 0.01$; **Figure 1F**), but no significant differences in their average velocity or persistence between *Mecp2* knockout ($n = 410$ puncta from 13 cells) and wildtype neurons ($n = 359$ puncta from 14 cells; $p > 0.05$; **Figures 1G,H**).

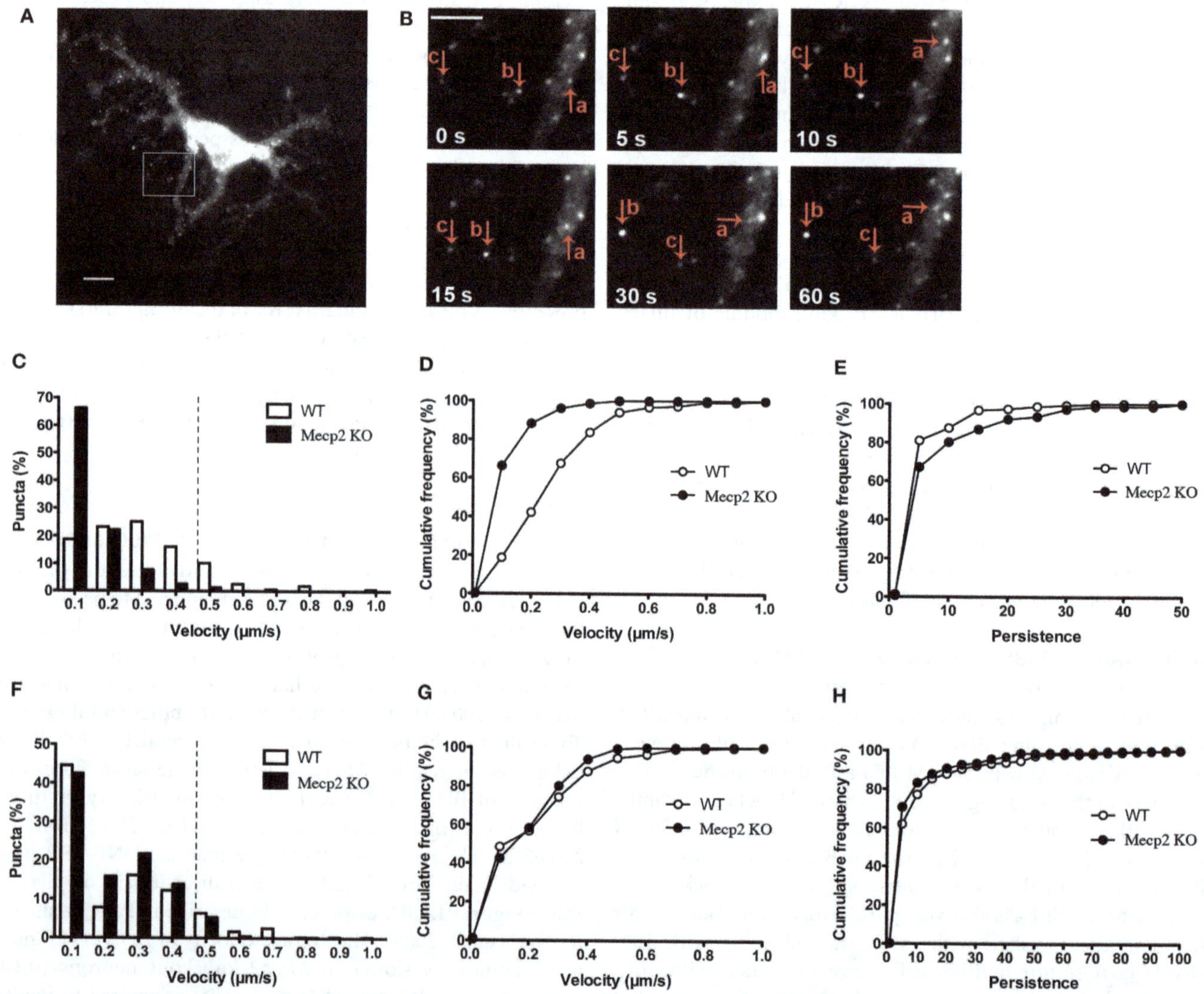

FIGURE 1 | BDNF-YFP trafficking is impaired in *Mecp2* knockout neurons. (A) Representative example of a cultured pyramidal neuron expressing BDNF-YFP; scale bar = 10 µm. The white square is enlarged in **(B)**. **(B)** Movement of BDNF-YFP punta (a, b, and c); scale bar = 5 µm. Each image was taken at the time point indicated at bottom left. **(C)** Distributions of velocities of BDNF-YFP puncta in wildtype and *Mecp2* knockout neurons. **(D)** Cumulative frequency of velocities of BDNF-YFP puncta from the histograms shown in **(C)**. **(E)** Cumulative frequency of persistence of BDNF-YFP puncta. **(F)** Distributions of velocities of MitoTracker-Red puncta in wildtype and *Mecp2* knockout neurons. **(G)** Cumulative frequency of velocities of MitoTracker-Red puncta from the histograms shown in **(F)**. **(H)** Cumulative frequency of persistence of MitoTracker-Red puncta.

THE IMPAIRMENT OF BDNF-YFP TRAFFICKING IN *MECP2* KNOCKOUT NEURONS IS BI-DIRECTIONAL

Anterograde BDNF transport from somata to dendrites and axon terminals is important for activity-dependent BDNF release to participate in synaptic plasticity, while retrograde BDNF transport back to the soma is critical for neurotrophin recycling and nuclear signaling (Egan et al., 2003; Park et al., 2008). When BDNF-YFP puncta were separated by their trafficking direction, *Mecp2* knockout neurons showed significantly fewer BDNF puncta moving in both anterograde and retrograde directions than wildtype neurons, with a significantly shorter total distance traveled in either direction in *Mecp2* knockout cells ($p < 0.001$; **Figures 2A,B**). Consistently, the average velocity of BDNF-YFP puncta moving in both anterograde and retrograde directions was significantly slower ($p < 0.001$; **Figure 2C**), and their persistence higher ($p < 0.05$ in retrograde direction; **Figure 2D**), in *Mecp2* knockout neurons.

THE HDAC6-SELECTIVE INHIBITOR TBA IMPROVES BI-DIRECTIONAL BDNF-YFP TRAFFICKING IN *MECP2* KNOCKOUT NEURONS

HDAC6 removes acetyl groups from α-tubulin (Hubbert et al., 2002; Matsuyama et al., 2002; Zhang et al., 2003), which makes microtubules less stable. Since BDNF is transported along microtubules (Gauthier et al., 2004), inhibiting HDAC6 is expected to improve BDNF trafficking by stabilizing microtubules (Dompierre et al., 2007). We tested whether treatment with the selective HDAC6 inhibitor enhances BDNF-YFP trafficking in cultured hippocampal neurons. Treatment with Tubastatin A for 48 h (TBA, 1 µM, prepared in 0.01% DMSO) was not neurotoxic, as determined by trypan blue exclusion ($p > 0.05$;

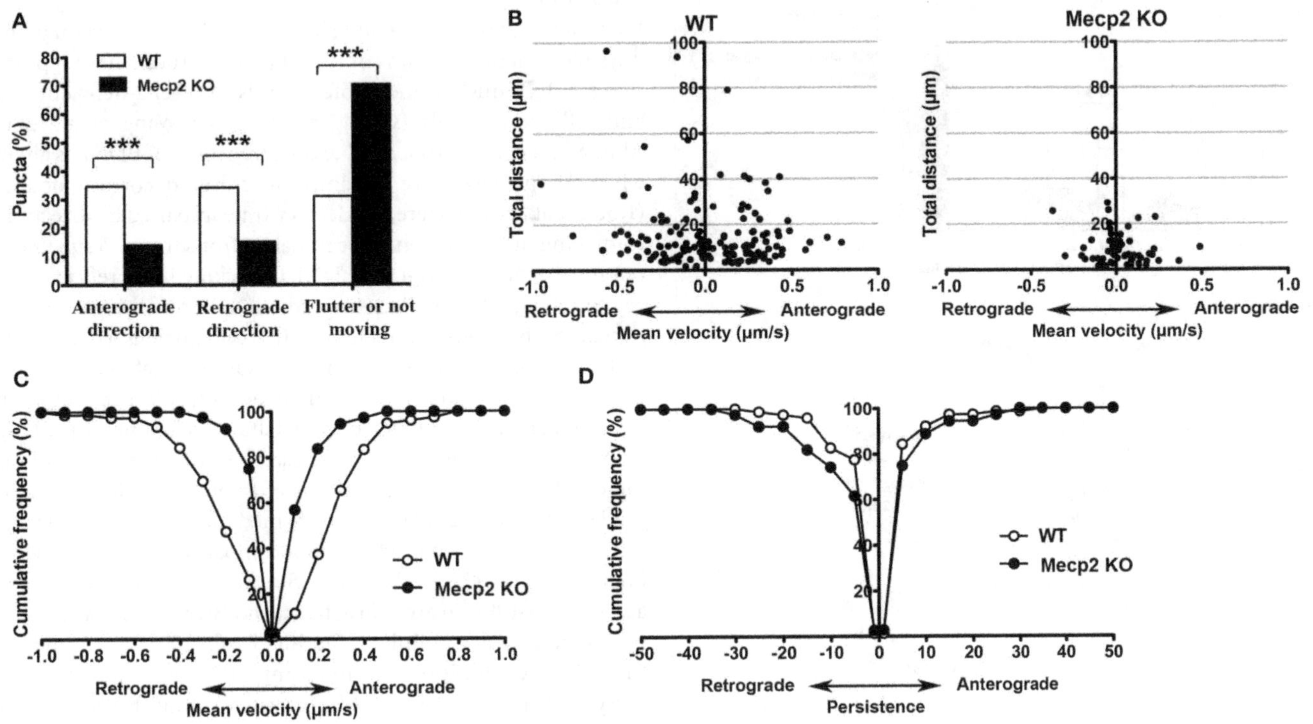

FIGURE 2 | Bi-directional BDNF-YFP trafficking is impaired in *Mecp2* knockout neurons. (A) Proportion of BDNF-YFP puncta that moves in the anterograde or retrograde directions, flutter within a small distance (10 μm) or not moving at all in wildtype and *Mecp2* knockout neurons. **(B)** Scatter plots showing analyses of movement of BDNF-YFP puncta in anterograde and retrograde directions. **(C)** Average velocity of BDNF-YFP puncta was significantly slower in *Mecp2* knockout neurons for both directions. **(D)** Persistence of BDNF-YFP puncta was also higher in *Mecp2* knockout neurons for both directions. $^{***}p < 0.001$ wildtype vs. *Mecp2* knockout.

Supplemental Figure 2A). Then, we confirmed that TBA affected the acetylation state of α-tubulin under our experimental conditions. Western immunoblots of cultured hippocampal neurons (DIV12) treated with TBA showed that the levels of acetylated tubulin were significantly increased in wildtype neurons ($p < 0.01$; **Supplemental Figure 2B**), and elevated by two times in *Mecp2* knockout neurons ($p < 0.001$; **Supplemental Figure 2B**).

Next, we tested the effect of HDAC6 inhibition on BDNF-YFP trafficking. Compared to vehicle-treated neurons (162 puncta from 7 cells), TBA increased the proportion of retrogradely moving BDNF puncta (159 puncta from 7 cells; $p < 0.01$; **Figure 3A**), as well as the average velocity of puncta moving anterogradely and retrogradely in *Mecp2* knockout neurons ($p < 0.001$; **Figure 3B**). However, TBA did not affect the persistence of BDNF puncta in *Mecp2* knockout neurons ($p > 0.05$; **Figure 3C**). On the other hand, TBA had no effect in any of these BDNF-YFP trafficking parameters in wildtype neurons (DMSO 106 puncta from 5 cells; TBA 149 puncta from 7 cells; $p > 0.05$; **Figures 3A–C**).

ACTIVITY-DEPENDENT BDNF RELEASE WAS IMPAIRED IN *MECP2* KNOCKOUT NEURONS, AND IMPROVED BY INHIBITING HDAC6

Improving BDNF transport to release sites could in principle also enhance its activity-dependent release. To estimate activity-dependent BDNF secretion, BDNF-YFP-expressing neurons were depolarized with 50 mM KCl, followed by immunostaining with anti-YFP antibody before cell permeabilization. The degree of co-colocalization between immunopositive puncta (labeled with red-conjugated anti-YFP secondary antibody), and native YFP fluorescent puncta after fixation is directly proportional to BDNF-YFP secreted during neuronal depolarization (**Figure 4A**), as described (Sadakata et al., 2012). KCl-induced postsynaptic secretion of BDNF depends on Ca^{2+} influx (Hartmann et al., 2001; Kolarow et al., 2007), mainly through L-type voltage-gated Ca^{2+} channels (Wang et al., 2002). Here, we confirmed that elevated KCl-induced BDNF secretion was absent in a Ca^{2+} free solution ($n = 18$ cells), or in the presence of the L-type Ca^{2+}channel blocker nifedipine (50 μM; $n = 16$; $p < 0.05$; **Figure 4B**). Ca^{2+} channels can also be activated by depolarization from $GABA_A$ receptor activity in immature neurons with high intracellular Cl^- concentration (Fiorentino et al., 2009; Porcher et al., 2011). Indeed, the $GABA_A$ receptor antagonist bicuculline also prevented KCl-induced BDNF secretion (10 μM; $n = 15$; $p < 0.05$; **Figure 4B**). In addition, KCl-induced BDNF secretion required functional ionotropic glutamate receptor activity (10 μM CNQX, 50 μM D-APV; $n = 17$; $p < 0.01$), and voltage-sensitive Na^+ channels (0.5 μM TTX; $n = 19$; $p < 0.05$; **Figure 4B**), as previously described (Lessmann et al., 2003). **Figure 5** illustrates the different mechanisms leading to Ca^{2+}-dependent BDNF release during KCl-induced depolarization.

Consistent with reports of impaired activity-dependent BDNF release using different assays (Li et al., 2012), the

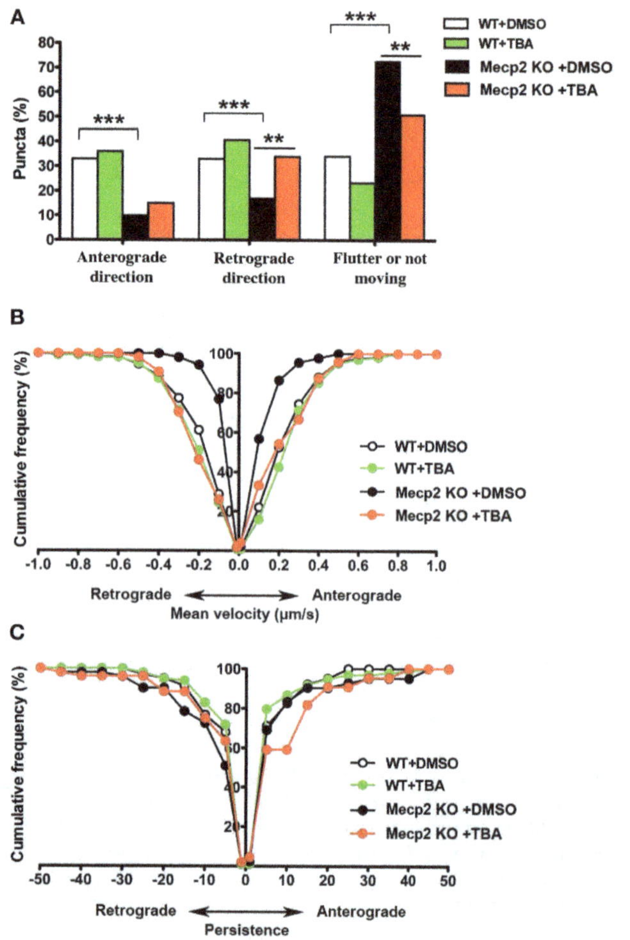

FIGURE 3 | TBA improves BDNF-YFP trafficking in *Mecp2* knockout neurons. (A) Proportion of BDNF-YFP puncta that moves in anterograde or retrograde directions, flutter or not move in wildtype and *Mecp2* knockout neurons, with or without TBA. **(B)** TBA increased the average velocity of both anterograde and retrograde BDNF-YFP puncta only in *Mecp2* knockout neurons. **(C)** TBA did not affect BDNF puncta persistence in neither wildtype nor *Mecp2* knockout neurons. $^{**}p < 0.01$; $^{***}p < 0.001$ wildtype vs. *Mecp2* knockout.

proportion of BDNF secreted during KCl-induced depolarization was significantly smaller in *Mecp2* knockout neurons ($n = 21$) than in wildtype neurons ($n = 25$; $p < 0.01$; **Figure 4B**). In addition, there was no evidence of BDNF secretion in *Mecp2* knockout neurons under any of the conditions of activity blockade described above (Ca^{2+} free $n = 15$; nifedipine $n = 13$; CNQX/D-APV $n = 16$; bicuculline $n = 15$; TTX $n = 13$; $p > 0.05$; **Figure 4B**). Intriguingly, TBA significantly improved the proportion of BDNF secreted during KCl-induced depolarization in *Mecp2* knockout neurons ($n = 14$; $p < 0.001$; **Figure 4B**), but not in wildtype neurons ($n = 22$; $p > 0.05$; **Figure 4B**). These results suggest that improved microtubule-dependent trafficking allowed a larger pool of BDNF to be transported to release sites and be available for activity-dependent release, underscoring the potential therapeutic benefit of this approach to restore BDNF signaling in RTT.

DISCUSSION

Dysfunctional BDNF signaling likely contributes to several pathophysiological mechanisms of RTT. Previous studies have reported lower BDNF mRNA and protein levels in *Mecp2*-deficient mice and RTT individuals (Chang et al., 2006; Wang et al., 2006; Abuhatzira et al., 2007). Also, axonal transport of BDNF is altered when *Mecp2* levels are modified in cultured cortical neurons (Roux et al., 2012). Here, we demonstrate impaired bi-directional trafficking of BDNF in hippocampal neurons from *Mecp2* knockout mice. Since anterograde BDNF trafficking likely reflects delivery to release sites, while retrograde BDNF trafficking represents signaling endosomes directed to the cell nucleus (Egan et al., 2003; Park et al., 2008), our results suggest that both activity-dependent BDNF release, as well as neurotrophin recycling and nuclear signaling are affected in MeCP2-deficient neurons. Using a novel assay of BDNF secretion based on surface immunostaining of BDNF-YFP in live neurons after neuronal depolarization (Sadakata et al., 2012), we confirmed that activity-dependent BDNF release is impaired in hippocampal neurons from *Mecp2* knockout mice (Li et al., 2012). Since microtubules containing acetylated α-tubulin are more stable, and BDNF vesicles are transported along microtubules (Gauthier et al., 2004), we confirmed that selective inhibition of cytoplasmic HDAC6—which increases acetylated α-tubulin levels—improves not only BDNF trafficking, but also its activity-dependent secretion. Taken together, our findings suggest that, in addition to BDNF mRNA and protein levels, dysfunctional BDNF trafficking and release contribute to RTT neuropathology. Thus, targeting the molecular machinery responsible for BDNF trafficking and release represents a novel strategy to reverse BDNF-dependent neurological deficits in RTT.

Is this impairment in trafficking specific for BDNF-containing vesicles, or does it affect other cellular elements transported along microtubules? *Mecp2* deficiency impairs axonal transport of amyloid precursor protein (App) without affecting its mRNA and protein levels (Roux et al., 2012). Also, we showed here that *Mecp2* knockout neurons have fewer fast-moving mitochondria than wildtype neurons, suggesting that MeCP2 deficiency affects microtubule-dependent transport in general. Whether and how the molecular motors responsible for anterograde (kinesin-1), and retrograde transport (dynein/dynactin) are affected in RTT needs to be further explored.

We showed that the selective HDAC6 inhibitor TBA improves BDNF trafficking in *Mecp2* knockout neurons by increasing the proportion of moving BDNF puncta and their average velocity in both anterograde and retrograde directions. TBA also restored activity-dependent BDNF release in *Mecp2* knockout neurons to levels comparable to those of wildtype neurons. How did HDAC6 inhibition produce these effects? It is known that acetylation of α-tubulin at Lys-40 promotes axonal transport of cargo proteins by increasing microtubule stability (Reed et al., 2006; Bulinski, 2007), and that inhibition of HDAC6 is responsible for such increased α-tubulin acetylation that leads to enhanced axonal transport of lysosomes and other secretory vesicles (Dompierre et al., 2007). Consistently, *in vivo* treatment with TBA improves axonal trafficking in a mouse model of Charcot-MarieTooth disease by increasing α-tubulin acetylation and enhancing microtubule rigidity (d'Ydewalle et al., 2011).

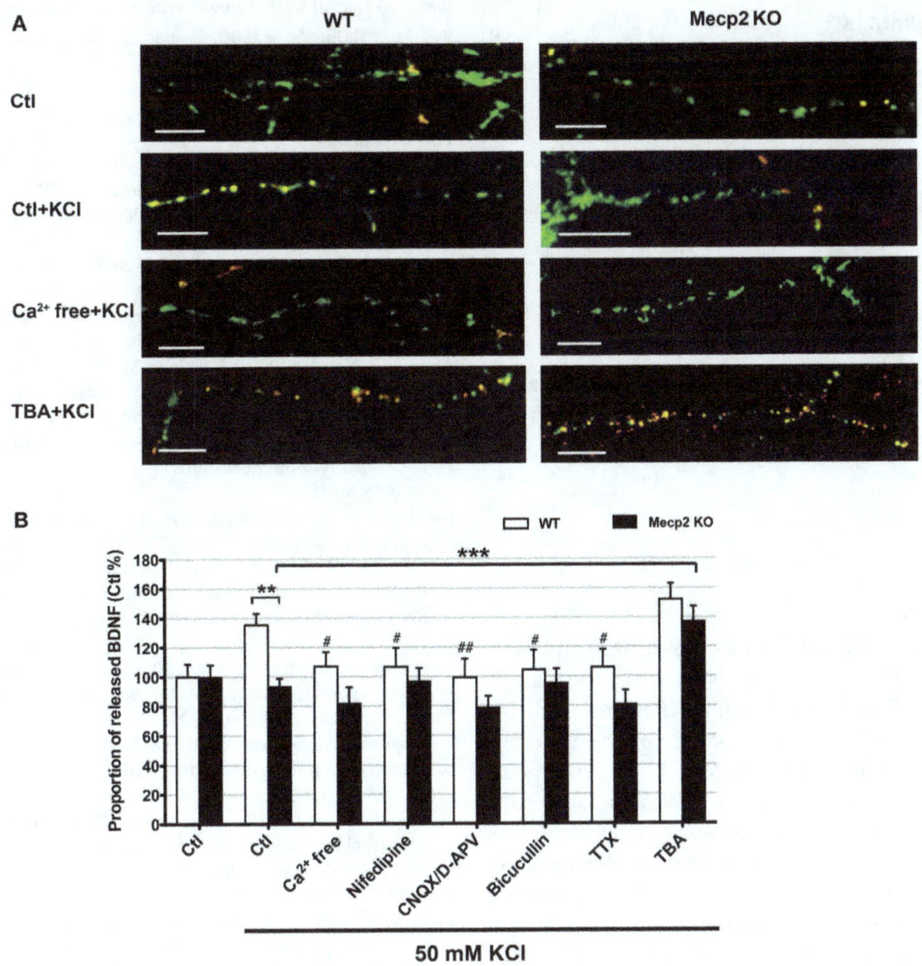

FIGURE 4 | Activity-dependent release of BDNF-YFP is impaired in *Mecp2* knockout neurons. (A) Representative examples of BDNF release in wildtype and *Mecp2* knockout neurons: no treatment, stimulated with KCl, stimulated with KCl in the absence of extracellular Ca^{2+} and stimulated with KCl upon TBA treatment; scale bar = 10 μm. BDNF-YFP is shown in green, while YFP immunoreactivity is shown in red. Yellow pixels represent colocalization of green and red pixels, i.e., secreted BDNF. **(B)** Proportion of released BDNF per total BDNF upon KCl stimulation in wildtype neurons and *Mecp2* knockout neurons in the absence or presence of extracellular Ca^{2+}, nifedipine (50 μM), CNQX (10 μM) /D-APV (50 μM), Bicuculline (10 μM), TTX (0.5 μM) or TBA (1 μM). The proportion of released BDNF per total BDNF was normalized to that in non-stimulated neurons (Ctl), and expressed as % of Ctl. $^{**}p < 0.01$; wildtype vs. *Mecp2* knockout; $^{***}p < 0.001$ compared to *Mecp2* knockout Ctl group stimulated with KCl; $^{\#}p < 0.05$; $^{\#\#}p < 0.01$ compared to wildtype Ctl group stimulated with KCl.

Therefore, HDAC6 inhibitors represent a potential therapeutic strategy for neurodegenerative disorders in which microtubule-dependent intracellular transport is impaired (Dompierre et al., 2007; Kim et al., 2012). Our results also showed that TBA increased α-tubulin acetylation in wildtype neurons, but not as much as in *Mecp2* knockout neurons. However, we didn't find any effect of TBA in wildtype neurons. This might be because BDNF trafficking is in the optimal state in wildtype neurons. TBA restored impaired BDNF trafficking in *Mecp2* knockout neurons to wildtype levels.

In the present study with BDNF-YFP transfected in hippocampal neurons, we cannot exclude an artifact of BDNF overexpression to endogenous levels. However, the intracellular localization of BDNF-YFP is similar to that of endogenous BDNF, including its co-localization to secretory granule cargoes like chromogranin-B and SGA2 (Haubensak et al., 1998; Kohara et al., 2001; Lessmann and Brigadski, 2009; Hartmann et al., 2012) (**Supplemental Figure 1**), suggesting that the trafficking properties of BDNF-YFP can be comparable to those of endogenous BDNF. Even though BDNF expression is higher, we cannot ignore the differences of BDNF trafficking and release between wildtype and *Mecp2* knockout neurons.

In conclusion, our findings revealed that bi-directional trafficking of BDNF and its activity-dependent release are significantly impaired in hippocampal neurons of *Mecp2* knockout mice, and that this deficit can be improved by enhancing tubulin acetylation with a selective HDAC6 inhibitor, which should improve microtubule-based transport. Targeting molecular components responsible for microtubule-based trafficking of BDNF-containing dense core vesicles is a potential strategy to reverse cellular and synaptic impairments in RTT.

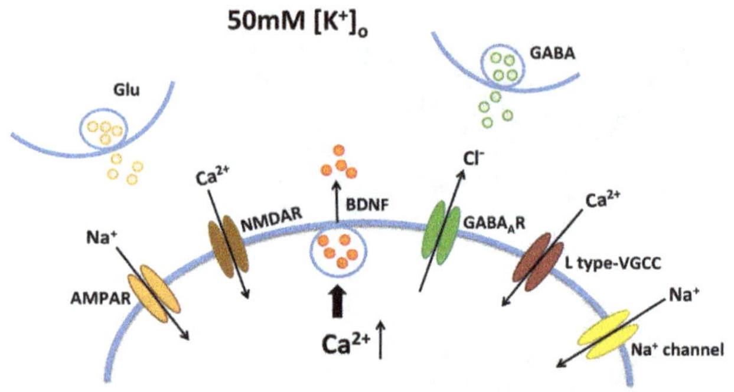

FIGURE 5 | Mechanisms of Ca^{2+}-dependent BDNF release during KCl-induced depolarization. KCl-induced BDNF secretion depends on Ca^{2+} influx, which can be mediated by L type-VGCC, AMPA receptors, NMDA receptors, $GABA_A$ receptors and voltage-sensitive Na^+ channels.

ACKNOWLEDGMENTS

This work was supported by NIH grants NS-065027 and HD-074418 (to Lucas Pozzo-Miller), and NS-79183 (to Alan P. Kozikowski). We thank Drs. Masami Kojima (Research Institute for Cell Engineering, NIAIST, Osaka, Japan) for the generous gift of BDNF-YFP encoding plasmids, Wei Li for comments on the manuscript, and Takafumi Inoue (Waseda University, Tokyo, Japan) for data acquisition and analysis software. We are indebted to Ms. Lili Mao for mouse colony management. Drs. Shardey Ewell and Anne Theibert (UAB) contributed examples of BDNF-YFP-expressing cultured neurons immunostained for chromogranin-B (**Supplemental Figures 1A,B**). The UAB Intellectual and Developmental Disabilities Research Center (HD-38985), and the UAB Neuroscience Core (NS-47466) provided instrumentation.

SUPPLEMENTARY MATERIAL

Supplemental Figure 1| Distribution of exogenously expressed BDNF-YFP is comparable to that of endogenous native BDNF. (A) Representative example of a cultured hippocampal pyramidal neuron after dual immunostaining for endogenously expressed native BDNF (red) with chromogranin-B (green), a marker of secretory granules. The inset shows colocalization in a dendritic segment. **(B)** Immunostaining for chromogranin-B (red) on a BDNF-YFP-expressing neuron (green) reveals essentially the same patter of colocalization. **(C,D)** The same pattern of co-localization between exogenous BDNF-YFP and endogenous BDNF is observed in cultured hippocampal pyramidal neurons from either WT **(C)** mice or *Mecp2* knockout mice **(D)**. Scale bar = 10 μm.

Supplemental Figure 2| TBA increases tubulin acetylation. (A) Cell viability assessed by trypan blue exclusion. **(B)** Extracts from DIV12 wildtype cells and *Mecp2* knockout neurons treated with or without TBA (1 μM) for 48 h were processed by Western blot and analyzed for acetylated tubulin and total tubulin. GAPDH was performed as loading control (top). Quantification of protein levels for acetylated tubulin in each group ($n = 4$) was normalized to that in wildtype neurons (WT) and expressed as % of WT. $^*p < 0.05$; $^{**}p < 0.01$ compared to WT group; $^{***}p < 0.001$ compared to *Mecp2* knockout group (bottom).

REFERENCES

Abuhatzira, L., Makedonski, K., Kaufman, Y., Razin, A., and Shemer, R. (2007). MeCP2 deficiency in the brain decreases BDNF levels by REST/CoREST-mediated repression and increases TRKB production. *Epigenetics* 2, 214–222. doi: 10.4161/epi.2.4.5212

Amaral, M. D., and Pozzo-Miller, L. (2007). TRPC3 channels are necessary for brain-derived neurotrophic factor to activate a non-selective cationic current and to induce dendritic spine formation. *J. Neurosci.* 27, 5179–5189. doi: 10.1523/JNEUROSCI.5499-06.2007

Amir, R. E., Van den Veyver, I. B., Wan, M., Tran, C. Q., Francke, U., and Zoghbi, H. Y. (1999). Rett syndrome is caused by mutations in X-linked MECP2, encoding methyl-CpG-binding protein 2. *Nat. Genet.* 23, 185–188. doi: 10.1038/13810

Bievenu, T., and Chelly, J. (2006). Molecular genetics of Rett syndrome: when DNA methylation goes unrecognized. *Nat. Rev. Genet.* 7, 415–426. doi: 10.1038/nrg1878

Bulinski, J. C. (2007). Microtubule modification: acetylation speeds anterograde traffic flow. *Curr. Biol.* 17, R18–R20. doi: 10.1016/j.cub.2006.11.036

Butler, K. V., Kalin, J., Brochier, C., Vistoli, G., Langley, B., and Kozikowski, A. P. (2010). Rational design and simple chemistry yield a superior, neuroprotective HDAC6 inhibitor, tubastatin A. *J. Am. Chem. Soc.* 132, 10842–10846. doi: 10.1021/ja102758v

Chahrour, M., and Zoghbi, H. Y. (2007). The story of Rett syndrome: from clinic to neurobiology. *Neuron* 56, 422–437. doi: 10.1016/j.neuron.2007.10.001

Chang, Q., Khare, G., Dani, V., Nelson, S., and Jaenisch, R. (2006). The disease progression of Mecp2 mutant mice is affected by the level of BDNF expression. *Neuron* 49, 341–348. doi: 10.1016/j.neuron.2005.12.027

Chapleau, C. A., Larimore, J. L., Theibert, A., and Pozzo-Miller, L. (2009). Modulation of dendritic spine development and plasticity by BDNF and vesicular trafficking: fundamental roles in neurodevelopmental disorders associated with mental retardation and autism. *J. Neurodev. Disord.* 1, 185–196. doi: 10.1007/s11689-009-9027-6

Chen, R. Z., Akbarian, S., Tudor, M., and Jaenisch, R. (2001). Deficiency of methyl-CpG binding protein-2 in CNS neurons results in a Rett-like phenotype in mice. *Nat. Genet.* 27, 327–331. doi: 10.1038/85906

Chen, W. G., Chang, Q., Lin, Y., Meissner, A., West, A. E., Griffith, E. C., et al. (2003). Derepression of BDNF transcription involves calcium-dependent phosphorylation of MeCP2. *Science* 302, 885–889. doi: 10.1126/science.1086446

Dompierre, J. P., Godin, J. D., Charrin, B. C., Cordelières, F. P., King, S. J., Humbert, S., et al. (2007). Histone deacetylase 6 inhibition compensates for the transport deficit in Huntington's disease by increasing tubulin acetylation. *J. Neurosci.* 27, 3571–3583. doi: 10.1523/JNEUROSCI.0037-07.2007

d'Ydewalle, C., Krishnan, J., Chiheb, D. M., Van Damme, P., Irobi, J., Kozikowski, A. P., et al. (2011). HDAC6 inhibitors reverse axonal loss in a mouse model of mutant HSPB1-induced Charcot-Marie-Tooth disease. *Nat. Med.* 17, 968–974. doi: 10.1038/nm.2396

Egan, M. F., Kojima, M., Callicott, J. H., Goldberg, T. E., Kolachana, B. S., Bertolino, A., et al. (2003). The BDNF val66met polymorphism affects activity-dependent secretion of BDNF and human memory and hippocampal function. *Cell* 112, 257–269. doi: 10.1016/S0092-8674(03)00035-7

Fahnestock, M., Garzon, D., Holsinger, R. M., and Michalski, B. (2002). Neurotrophic factors and Alzheimer's disease: are we focusing on the wrong molecule? *J. Neural Transm. Suppl.* 62, 241–252. doi: 10.1007/978-3-7091-6139-5_22

Fiorentino, H., Kuczewski, N., Diabira, D., Ferrand, N., Pangalos, M. N., Porcher, C., et al. (2009). GABA(B) receptor activation triggers BDNF release and promotes the maturation of GABAergic synapses. *J. Neurosci.* 29, 11650–11661. doi: 10.1523/JNEUROSCI.3587-09.2009

Fukada, M., Hanai, A., Nakayama, A., Suzuki, T., Miyata, N., Rodriguiz, R. M., et al. (2012). Loss of Deacetylation activity of Hdac6 affects emotional behavior in mice. *PLoS ONE* 7:e30924. doi: 10.1371/journal.pone.0030924

Gao, Y. S., Hubbert, C., Lu, J., Lee, Y. S., and Yao, T. P. (2007). Histone deacetylase 6 regulates growth factor-induced actin remodeling and endocytosis. *Mol. Cell Biol.* 27, 8637–8647. doi: 10.1128/MCB.00393-07

Gauthier, L. R., Charrin, B. C., Borrell-Pages, M., Dornpierre, J. P., Rangone, H., Cordelieres, F. P., et al. (2004). Huntingtin controls neurotrophic support and survival of neurons by enhancing BDNF vesicular transport along microtubules. *Cell* 118, 127–138. doi: 10.1016/j.cell.2004.06.018

Gines, S., Paoletti, P., and Alberch, J. (2010). Impaired, TrkB-mediated ERK1/2 activation in Huntington disease knock-in striatal cells involves reduced p52/p46 Shc expression. *J. Biol. Chem.* 285, 21537–21548. doi: 10.1074/jbc.M109.084202

Hartmann, D., Drummond, J., Handberg, E., Ewell, S., and Pozzo-Miller, L. (2012). Multiple approaches to investigate the transport and activity-dependent release of BDNF and their application in neurogenetic disorders. *Neural Plast.* 2012:203734. doi: 10.1155/2012/203734

Hartmann, M., Heumann, R., and Lessmann, V. (2001). Synaptic secretion of BDNF after high-frequency stimulation of glutamatergic synapses. *EMBO J.* 20, 5887–5897. doi: 10.1093/emboj/20.21.5887

Haubensak, W., Narz, F., Heumann, R., and Lessmann, V. (1998). BDNF-GFP containing secretory granules are localized in synaptic junctions of cultured cortical neurons. *J. Cell Sci.* 111, 1483–1493.

Hubbert, C., Guardiola, A., Shao, R., Kawaguchi, Y., Ito, A., Nixon, A., et al. (2002). HDAC6 is a microtubule-associated deacetylase. *Nature* 417, 455–458. doi: 10.1038/417455a

Iwata, A., Riley, B. E., Johnston, J. A., and Kopito, R. (2005). HDAC6 and microtubules are required for autophagic degradation of aggregated huntingtin. *J. Biol. Chem.* 280, 40282–40292. doi: 10.1074/jbc.M508786200

Kazantsev, A. G., and Thompson, L. M. (2008). Therapeutic application of histone deacetylase inhibitors for central nervous system disorders. *Nat. Rev. Drug Discov.* 7, 854–868. doi: 10.1038/nrd2681

Kim, C., Choi, H., Jung, E. S., Lee, W., Oh, S., Jeon, N. L., et al. (2012). HDAC6 inhibitor blocks amyloid beta-induced impairment of mitochondrial transport in hippocampal neurons. *PLoS ONE* 7:e42983. doi: 10.1371/journal.pone.0042983

Kohara, K., Kitamura, A., Morishima, M., and Tsumoto, T. (2001). Activity-dependent transfer of brain-derived neurotrophic factor to postsynaptic neurons. *Science* 291, 2419–2423. doi: 10.1126/science.1057415

Kolarow, R., Brigadski, T., and Lessmann, V. (2007). Postsynaptic secretion of BDNF and NT-3 from hippocampal neurons depends on calcium calmodulin kinase II signaling and proceeds via delayed fusion pore opening. *J. Neurosci.* 27, 10350–10364. doi: 10.1523/JNEUROSCI.0692-07.2007

Lessmann, V., and Brigadski, T. (2009). Mechanisms, locations, and kinetics of synaptic BDNF secretion: an update. *Neurosci. Res.* 65, 11–22. doi: 10.1016/j.neures.2009.06.004

Lessmann, V., Gottmann, K., and Malcangio, M. (2003). Neurotrophin secretion: current facts and future prospects. *Prog. Neurobiol.* 69, 341–374. doi: 10.1016/S0301-0082(03)00019-4

Li, W., Calfa, G., Larimore, J., and Pozzo-Miller, L. (2012). Activity-dependent BDNF release and TRPC signaling is impaired in hippocampal neurons of Mecp2 mutant mice. *Proc. Natl. Acad. Sci. U.S.A.* 109, 17087–17092. doi: 10.1073/pnas.1205271109

Martinowich, K., Hattori, D., Wu, H., Fouse, S., He, F., Hu, Y., et al. (2003). DNA methylation-related chromatin remodeling in activity-dependent BDNF gene regulation. *Science* 302, 890–893. doi: 10.1126/science.1090842

Matsuda, N., Lu, H., Fukata, Y., Noritake, J., Gao, H., Mukherjee, S., et al. (2009). Differential activity-dependent secretion of brain-derived neurotrophic factor from axon and dendrite. *J. Neurosci.* 29, 14185–14198. doi: 10.1523/JNEUROSCI.1863-09.2009

Matsuyama, A., Shimazu, T., Sumida, Y., Saito, A., Yoshimatsu, Y., Seigneurin-Berny, D., et al. (2002). *In vivo* destabilization of dynamic microtubules by HDAC6-mediated deacetylation. *EMBO J.* 21, 6820–6831. doi: 10.1093/emboj/cdf682

Nan, X., CamPoy, F. J., and Bird, A. (1997). MeCP2 is a transcriptional repressor with abundant binding sites in genomic chromatin. *Cell* 88, 471–481. doi: 10.1016/S0092-8674(00)81887-5

Ogier, M., Wang, H., Hong, E., Wang, Q., Greenberg, M. E., and Katz, D. M. (2007). Brain-derived neurotrophic factor expression and respiratory function improve after ampakine treatment in a mouse model of Rett syndrome. *J. Neurosci.* 27, 10912–10917. doi: 10.1523/JNEUROSCI.1869-07.2007

Park, J., Cawley, N. X., and, Loh, Y. P. (2008). A bi-directional carboxypeptidase E-driven transport mechanism controls BDNF vesicle homeostasis in hippocampal neurons. *Mol. Cell Neurosci.* 39, 63–73. doi: 10.1016/j.mcn.2008.05.016

Percy, A. K., and Lane, J. B. (2005). Rett syndrome: model of neurodevelopmental disorders. *J. Child Neurol.* 20, 718–721. doi: 10.1177/08830738050200090301

Poo, M. (2001). Neurotrophins as synaptic modulators. *Nat. Rev. Neurosci.* 2, 24–32. doi: 10.1038/35049004

Poon, W., Blurton-Jones, M., Tu, C. H., Feinberg, L. M., Chabrier, M. A., Harris, J. W., et al. (2011). β-Amyloid impairs axonal BDNF retrograde trafficking. *Neurobiol. Aging.* 32, 821–833. doi: 10.1016/j.neurobiolaging.2009.05.012

Porcher, C., Hatchett, C., Longbottom, R. E., McAinch, K., Sihra, T. S., Moss, S. J., et al. (2011). Positive feedback regulation between gamma-aminobutyric acid type A (GABA(A)) receptor signaling and brain-derived neurotrophic factor (BDNF) release in developing neurons. *J. Biol. Chem.* 286, 21667–21677. doi: 10.1074/jbc.M110.201582

Reed, N. A., Cai, D., Blasius, T. L., Jih, G. T., Meyhofer, E., Gaertig, J., et al. (2006). Microtubule acetylation promotes kinesin-1 binding and transport. *Curr. Biol.* 16, 2166–2172. doi: 10.1016/j.cub.2006.09.014

Rivieccio, M. A., Brochier, C., Willis, D. E., Walker, B. A., D'Annibale, M. A., McLaughlin, K., et al. (2009). HDAC6 is a target for protection and regeneration following injury in the nervous system. *Proc. Natl. Acad. Sci. U.S.A.* 106, 19599–19604. doi: 10.1073/pnas.0907935106

Roux, J. C., Zala, D., Panayotis, N., Borges-Correia, A., Saudou, F., and Villard, L. (2012). Modification of Mecp2 dosage alters axonal transport through the Huntingtin/Hap1 pathway. *Neurobiol. Dis.* 45, 786–795. doi: 10.1016/j.nbd.2011.11.002

Sadakata, T., Shinoda, Y., Oka, M., Sekine, Y., Sato, Y., Saruta, C., et al. (2012). Reduced axonal localization of a Caps2 splice variant impairs axonal release of BDNF and causes autistic-like behavior in mice. *Proc. Natl. Acad. Sci. U.S.A.* 109, 21104–21109. doi: 10.1073/pnas.1210055109

Tran, A. D. A., Marmo, T. P., Salam, A., Che, S., Finkelstein, E., Kabarriti, R., et al. (2007). HDAC6 deacetylation of tubulin modulates dynamics of cellular adhesions. *J. Cell Sci.* 120, 1469–1479. doi: 10.1242/jcs.03431

Valenzuela-Fernandez, A., Cabrero, J. R., Serrador, J. M., and Sanchez-Madrid, F. (2008). HDAC6: a key regulator of cytoskeleton, cell migration and cell-cell interactions. *Trends Cell Biol.* 18, 291–297. doi: 10.1016/j.tcb.2008.04.003

Wang, X., Butowt, R., Vasko, M. R., and von Bartheld, C. S. (2002). Mechanisms of the release of anterogradely transported neurotrophin-3 from axon terminals. *J. Neurosci.* 22, 931–945.

Wang, H., Chan, S. A., Ogier, M., Hellard, D., Wang, Q., Smith, C., et al. (2006). Dysregulation of brain-derived neurotrophic factor expression and neurosecretory function in Mecp2 null mice. *J. Neurosci.* 26, 10911–10915. doi: 10.1523/JNEUROSCI.1810-06.2006

Zeev, B., Bebbington, A., Ho, G., Leonard, H., de Klerk, N., Gak, E., et al. (2009). The common BDNF polymorphism may be a modifier of disease severity in Rett syndrome. *Neurology* 72, 1242–1247. doi: 10.1212/01.wnl.0000345664.72220.6a

Zhang, Y., Li, N., Caron, C., Matthias, G., Hess, D., Khochbin, S., et al. (2003). HDAC-6 interacts with and deacetylates tubulin and microtubules *in vivo*. *EMBO J.* 22, 1168–1179. doi: 10.1093/emboj/cdg115

Zhou, Z., Hong, E. J., Cohen, S., Zhao, W. N., Ho, H. Y., Schmidt, L., et al. (2006). Brain-specific phosphorylation of MeCP2 regulates activity-dependent Bdnf transcription, dendritic growth, and spine maturation. *Neuron* 52, 255–269. doi: 10.1016/j.neuron.2006.09.037

16

Optimizing neuronal differentiation from induced pluripotent stem cells to model ASD

Dae-Sung Kim*[1], *P. Joel Ross*[1], *Kirill Zaslavsky*[1,2] *and James Ellis*[1,2]

[1] Program in Developmental and Stem Cell Biology, The Hospital for Sick Children, Toronto, ON, Canada
[2] Department of Molecular Genetics, University of Toronto, Toronto, ON, Canada

***Correspondence:**
James Ellis, Program in Developmental and Stem Cell Biology, The Hospital for Sick Children, Peter Gilgan Centre for Research and Learning, Room 16-9-715, 686 Bay Street, Toronto, ON M5G 0A4, Canada
e-mail: jellis@sickkids.ca

Autism spectrum disorder (ASD) is an early-onset neurodevelopmental disorder characterized by deficits in social communication, and restricted and repetitive patterns of behavior. Despite its high prevalence, discovery of pathophysiological mechanisms underlying ASD has lagged due to a lack of appropriate model systems. Recent advances in induced pluripotent stem cell (iPSC) technology and neural differentiation techniques allow for detailed functional analyses of neurons generated from living individuals with ASD. Refinement of cortical neuron differentiation methods from iPSCs will enable mechanistic studies of specific neuronal subpopulations that may be preferentially impaired in ASD. In this review, we summarize recent accomplishments in differentiation of cortical neurons from human pluripotent stems cells and efforts to establish *in vitro* model systems to study ASD using personalized neurons.

Keywords: human pluripotent stem cells, neural differentiation, neocortical neurons, disease modeling, autism spectrum disorders (ASD), cellular phenotype

INTRODUCTION

Autism spectrum disorder (ASD) is a debilitating neurodevelopmental disorder characterized by impaired communication and social interactions, as well as restricted interests and repetitive behaviors (Devlin and Scherer, 2012). Approximately 1/50 children in North America are diagnosed with ASD, typically by the age of 3 years (Blumberg et al., 2013). The severity of symptoms varies greatly and the prevalence of intellectual disability, epilepsy, attention deficit/hyperactivity disorder, and obsessive-compulsive disorder is markedly higher in people with ASD than in unaffected individuals (Huguet et al., 2013). Despite the complexity and heterogeneity of ASD, genetic studies, post-mortem brain analyses, and functional imaging studies have resulted in the widely accepted hypothesis the ASD arises from dysfunctional neuronal communication in the neocortex (Zikopoulos and Barbas, 2013).

ASD is primarily viewed as a genetic disorder, although the genetic underpinnings of ASD are complex. Family and twin studies have revealed that the heritability of ASD is as high as 90%, but causal genomic variations have only been identified in ~25% of cases. These have mostly consisted of relatively rare genetic variations, none of which account for more than ~1% of ASD cases (Devlin and Scherer, 2012). To date, several dozen high priority ASD candidate genes have been identified, many of which encode proteins that localize to synapses [e.g., SH3 and multiple ankyrin repeat domains (SHANK) 2, SHANK3, Neuroligin (NLGN)-1, NLGN-3, NLGN-4X, Neurexin (NRXN)-1, and NRXN-3] and regulate their development, maturation, and function (Zoghbi and Bear, 2012). ASD-associated genomic variations can occur *de novo* in affected individuals. In familial cases, these variants are often inherited from unaffected parents, suggesting either incomplete penetrance or modifier genes. For example, four autistic individuals with *de novo SHANK2* mutations have additional genetic variations at ASD candidate loci, suggesting a "mutliple hit" model of ASD (Leblond et al., 2012; Chilian et al., 2013).

Mice engineered to encode human ASD-associated mutations often recapitulate behavioral hallmarks of the disorder and are readily amenable to experimental analyses (Silverman et al., 2010; Jiang and Ehlers, 2013). Many synapse-associated ASD candidate genes have been knocked-out in mice, revealing a wide range of synaptic phenotypes that may contribute to ASD. *Nlgn-1* knockout mice exhibited altered excitatory synaptic transmission (Blundell et al., 2010) and knockdown results in decreased cortical synapse numbers (Kwon et al., 2012). *Nrxn-1α* knockouts exhibit reduced spontaneous excitatory synaptic activity, with no change in inhibitory synapse function (Etherton et al., 2009). Mice with the ASD-associated *Nlgn-3* R451C mutation exhibit increased inhibitory neurotransmission in the cortex (Tabuchi et al., 2007; Etherton et al., 2011), but increased excitatory neurotransmission in the hippocampus (Etherton et al., 2011). Finally, knockouts of *Shank2* and *Shank3* support a role for SHANKs in excitatory synapse function, although distinct phenotypes were observed in different models (Durand et al., 2007; reviewed in Jiang and Ehlers, 2013). Unfortunately, mice with ASD-associated mutations rarely exhibit phenotypes unless these mutations are homozygous, which are exceptionally rare in people with ASD (Ey et al., 2011; Won et al., 2012). These findings suggest that heterozygous disruption of individual candidate genes may be necessary, but not sufficient for development of the disorder, and that other genetic variables may play a role (Huguet et al., 2013). An alternative explanation is that ASD candidate genes have slightly different functions in human neurons. Both of these limitations of mouse models can be overcome with the use of induced pluripotent stem (iPSC) technology, which allows the generation of personalized human neurons from people with ASD.

iPSCs represent an incredible new avenue for the modeling of ASD (Ross and Ellis, 2010). Donor-derived cells (e.g., dermal fibroblasts from a skin biopsy or peripheral blood mononuclear cells) are reprogrammed into iPSCs by forced expression of four pluripotency-associated transcription factors: OCT4, SOX2, KLF4, and c-MYC (Takahashi et al., 2007). Resultant iPSC lines exhibit functional properties of human embryonic stem cells (hESCs), including the ability to differentiate into any cell type in the human body. For experimental analyses, iPSCs provide an unlimited supply of ASD-specific neurons. To date, iPSC-derived neurons have been used to generate personalized neurons from individuals with neurodevelopmental disorders that include autistic features—RTT (Marchetto et al., 2010; Cheung et al., 2011), Timothy syndrome (TS) (Paşca et al., 2011), and Phelan McDermid syndrome (PMDS) (Shcheglovitov et al., 2013)—and have revealed disorder-specific neuronal phenotypes, including dysfunctional synaptic connectivity. However, this approach has yet to be applied to ASD as the fifth edition of the Diagnostic and Statistical Manual of Mental Disorders excludes individuals with syndromic neurodevelopmental disorders from an ASD diagnosis (American Psychiatric Association, 2013). Although iPSC-derived neurons have been generated from people with ASD, no functional experiments were described (DeRosa et al., 2012). As such, the potential of iPSC technology has yet to be fully applied to modeling ASD, although many groups are actively pursuing this approach.

The generation of iPSCs has become commonplace. However, efficient differentiation of these cells into specific neuronal subtypes remains challenging. As discussed above, one of the prevailing hypotheses suggest that ASD arises due to dysfunctional synaptic communication in the neocortex. Successful generation of ASD-specific cortical neurons will improve our understanding of how ASD develops and may allow for identification of novel therapeutics. In this review, we discuss (1) recent advances in technology of cortical differentiation from human pluripotent stem cells (hPSCs) based on the knowledge of *in vivo* cortical development, (2) recent findings from human iPSC (hiPSC)-based models of RTT, TS, and PMDS, and (3) future directions for optimization of cortical differentiation and modeling of ASD, as well as potential applications of this exciting technology.

DEVELOPMENT OF THE NEOCORTEX

A thorough understanding of neocortical development can inform methodology for cortical neuron differentiation from hPSCs and define neuronal characteristics that should be considered in validating the identity and functionality of resultant neurons. This is especially important for hPSC-based ASD modeling, as abnormal neocortical development has been directly associated with the etiology of some ASDs (Kwan, 2013). Thus, we first give an overview of neuronal composition in the neocortex and its origins, based on the studies of animal models.

The mammalian neocortex has a well-organized six-layered structure. Each cortical layer contains a characteristic distribution of neuronal cells with distinctive shape, size, and neurochemical and electrophysiological properties, which make local or long distance connections with other cortical region or subcortical compartments (Douglas and Martin, 2004; Migliore and Shepherd, 2005). Neurons in the neocortex can be broadly categorized into two types: excitatory projection neurons and inhibitory interneurons. Excitatory projection neurons, which comprise around 80% of the neocortical neuronal population, mainly originate from neuroepithelial cells of the germinal zone in the dorsal telencephalon (pallium) (Molyneaux et al., 2007). They have a characteristic pyramidal shape with a long apical dendrite, multiple basal dendritic branches with spines receiving signals from other neurons, and a long axon making synaptic connections via the excitatory neurotransmitter glutamate (Spruston, 2008). On the other hand, inhibitory interneurons develop and migrate from distinct progenitors of the germinal zone of the ventral telencephalon (subpallium), mostly from the medial ganglionic eminence (MGE) and caudal ganglionic eminence (CGE) (Wonders and Anderson, 2006). They make up the remaining 20% of cortical neurons and make local connections using the inhibitory neurotransmitter GABA. Inhibitory interneurons in the neocortex display an astonishing diversity with over 20 subtypes based on morphology, electrophysiological properties, and expression of calcium binding proteins and neuropeptides (Petilla Interneuron Nomenclature Group, 2008).

DEVELOPMENT OF NEOCORTICAL EXCITATORY NEURONS

In the widely accepted model of vertebrate neural induction, the first emerging neuroectodermal cells in the neural plate develop an anterior fate characterized by expression of transcription factors such as forkhead box G1 (*Foxg1*, also known as brain factor 1, *Bf1*) or orthodenticle homoebox 1/2 (*Otx1/2*) (Stern, 2001; Hébert and Fishell, 2008) (**Figure 1A**). As neural induction proceeds, the cells that position in relatively posterior regions are influenced by patterning factors, such as Wnts and retinoic acid (RA), and are subsequently reprogrammed to a caudal fate. In contrast, the cells in the anterior part of neural plate are less influenced by caudalizing factors due to the endogenous expression of their antagonists [e.g., Dickkopf-related protein 1 (DKK1, a Wnt signal antagonist)], and maintain the acquired anterior character (Glinka et al., 1998; Wilson and Houart, 2004). Once the neural tube forms, the most anterior region rapidly expands to form the telencephalon, which is divided into two distinctive regions, the dorsal telencephalon and the ventral telencephalon by gradients of dorso-ventral patterning factors (Wilson and Rubenstein, 2000).

The pallial neural progenitors, the main source of neocortical projection neurons, are developed under the influence of Wnt and BMP signaling. They can be defined by the expression of a set of transcription factors, which includes Foxg1, paired box 6 (*Pax6*), empty spiracles homolog 1/2 (*Emx1/2*) in mice (**Figures 1A,B**) (Molyneaux et al., 2007). Mouse genetic studies have provided evidence that these transcription factors are responsible for the establishment and maintenance of neocortical progenitors and suppress alternative fates. For example, removal of *Foxg1* in the mouse embryo causes the absolute absence of neocortical progenitors, which eventually results in

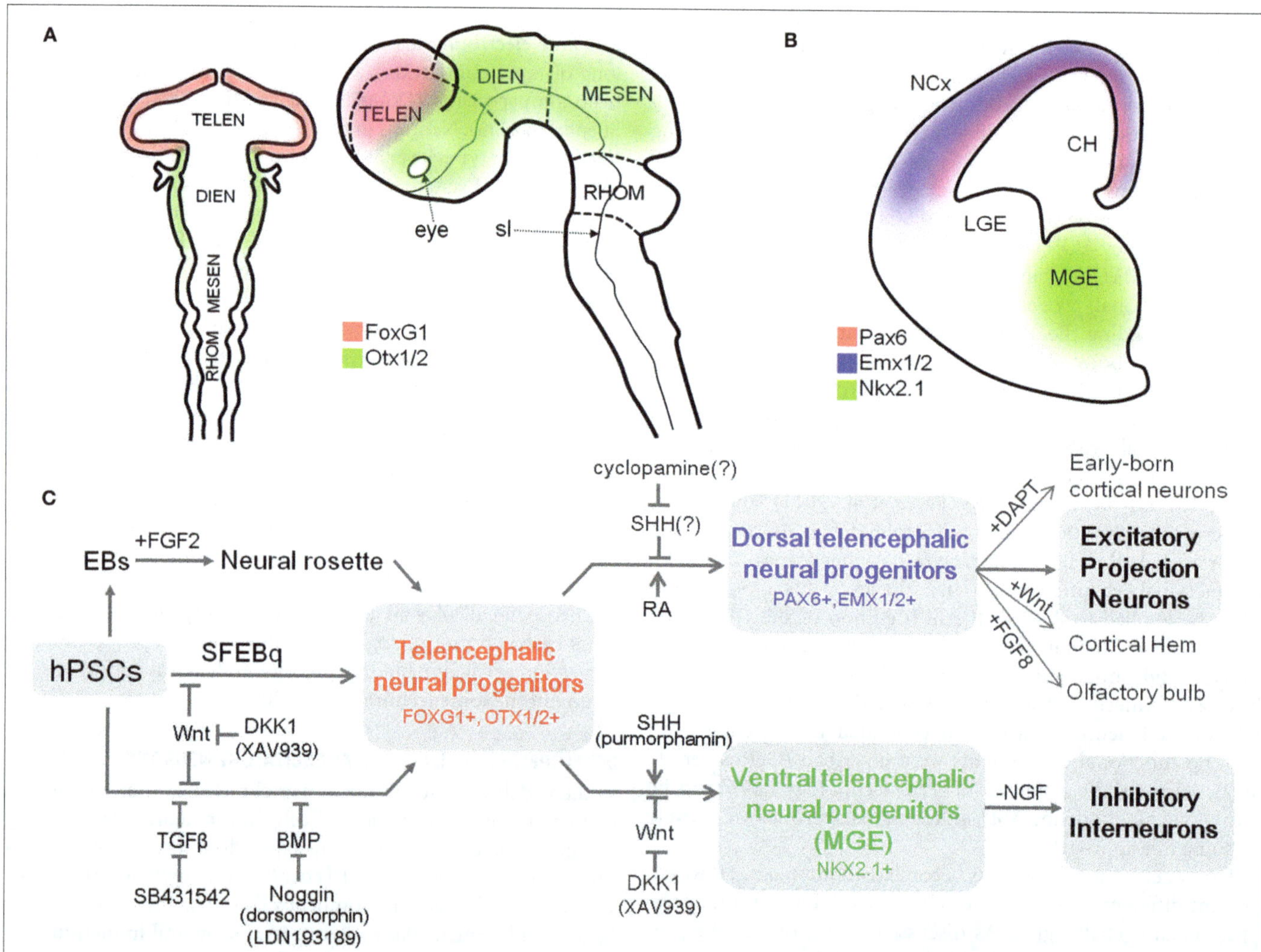

FIGURE 1 | A summary of differentiation from hPSCs into neocortical excitatory projection neurons and inhibitory interneurons. (A) Schematic mouse brain at E8 (left) and at E10.5 (right) depicting the expression domain of Foxg1 and Otx1/2. **(B)** Coronal hemi-section view of mouse brain at E13 showing the distinctive expression domains of Emx1/2, Pax6, and Nkx2.1, abbreviation: TELEN, telencephalon; DIEN, diencephalon; MESEN, mesencephalon; RHOM, rhombencephalon; sl, sulcus limitans; NCx, neocortex; LGE, lateral ganglionic eminence; MGE, medial ganglionic eminence; CH, cortical hem. **(C)** Human PSCs are induced into telencephalic neural progenitors in three main ways: (1) culturing EBs in suspension and isolation of neural rosette cell from the subsequent adherent culture of EBs (Zhang et al., 2001), (2) SFEBq method (Eiraku et al., 2008), and (3) dual-SMAD inhibition method (Chambers et al., 2009). Telencephalic fate can be facilitated by inhibition of the Wnt pathway during neural induction (Eiraku et al., 2008; Maroof et al., 2013; Nicholas et al., 2013). Telencephalic neural progenitors can be specified either to dorsal fate by blockade of endogenous SHH signal (Vazin et al., 2013) or exogenous RA treatment (Shi et al., 2012), or to ventral fate by additional activation of SHH signal (Liu et al., 2013a; Maroof et al., 2013; Nicholas et al., 2013) combined with Wnt inhibition (Li et al., 2009). Dorsal telencephalic progenitors can generate a variety of excitatory projection neurons (Eiraku et al., 2008; Shi et al., 2012; Lancaster et al., 2013), and also be further specified into (1) early-born cortical neurons such as Reelin-positive Cajal-Retzius cells or CTIP2-positive deep layer neurons depending on timing of DAPT treatment; (2) cortical hem by exogenous Wnt; and (3) olfactory bulb by FGF8 treatment (Eiraku et al., 2008). In contrast, ventral telencephalic progenitors can differentiate into functional GABAergic inhibitory neurons by either withdrawal of NGF in the culture medium (Liu et al., 2013b) or by adjusting the temporal window for SHH treatment during the ventralization step (Maroof et al., 2013).

severe malformation of the neocortex (Xuan et al., 1995; Muzio and Mallamaci, 2005). In turn, *Pax6* is essential for proliferation of progenitors in the pallium (Estivill-Torrus et al., 2002), and its absence in the murine embryonic brain results in the expansion of a domain expressing ventral progenitor makers, suggesting that it is essential for the establishment and maintenance of pallial progenitors (Stoykova et al., 2000). Accordingly, the appropriate expression of these transcription factors in cortical progenitors is a prerequisite for their progressive specification to projection neurons. Their expression can be used as a reliable marker for dorsal telencephalic identity of the progenitor stage during neural differentiation of hPSCs.

Once neurogenesis begins, neuroepithelial cells in the dorsal telencephalon acquire features of neural stem cells known as radial glial cells (RGCs). Through asymmetric cell division, RGCs give rise to (1) self-renewed RGCs that remain in the ventricular zone (VZ) throughout corticogenesis, and (2) committed daughter cells that can migrate out (Kriegstein and Alvarez-Buylla, 2009). The committed daughter cells either become early-born cortical neurons or remain in a defined domain next to the VZ called the subventricular zone (SVZ), where they undergo cell division as intermediate progenitors to generate diverse cortical projection neurons across multiple neocortical layers (Götz and Huttner, 2005). Recent clonal analysis of progenitors in the SVZ of human cortex revealed the appearance of distinctive progenitors called outer radial glial cells (oRGCs) immediately outside the SVZ (Hansen et al., 2010). The diversity of the progenitor population in the human brains contributes to their structural complexity, and results in a vast increase in the number of projection neurons and overall volume of the neocortex relative to those of rodents and other carnivores (Lui et al., 2011).

In general, early-born projection neurons migrate out from the proliferative area settling in the deep layer first, and later-born projection neurons migrate beyond those in deeper layers to reach the upper layers. Such "inside-out" patterning of post-mitotic neurons in a spatio-temporally controlled manner accounts for the well-organized layered structure of neocortex (Rash and Grove, 2006). Recent studies in the mouse show that each subtype and laminar specification in the neocortex is programmed by expression of particular transcription factors in cortical progenitors and neurons (reviewed by Molyneaux et al., 2007; Kwan et al., 2012). These genes play essential roles in refining the specific molecular identity of each layer (neuronal migration and the proper positioning) (Alcamo et al., 2008; Chen et al., 2008), layer-dependent axonal connectivity (Han et al., 2011), and even dendritic arborization and spine morphology (Cubelos et al., 2010). In addition, many studies have suggested that alteration in the proper expression of cortical layer-specific genes is associated with human neurodevelopmental disorders, including ASD (reviewed by Kwan, 2013).

DEVELOPMENT OF NEOCORTICAL GABAergic INTERNEURON

Unlike excitatory projection neurons, neocortical inhibitory neurons arise from progenitors in the subpallial region, where cells are under the influence of SHH. Progenitors in the MGE are characterized by expression of Nkx2 homeobox 1 (Nkx2.1, also known as thyroid transcription factor 1, TTF-1) (**Figure 1B**) and Foxg1, which are both regulated by SHH (Sussel et al., 1999; Gulacsi and Anderson, 2006). In particular, Nkx2.1 plays a pivotal role in the induction of neocortical GABAergic neurons. Mutation of Nkx2.1 in mice results in significant loss of parvalbumin (PV)- and somatostatin (STT)-positive GABAergic neurons in the cortex (Sussel et al., 1999). On the other hand, GS homeobox 2 (Gsx2) specifies progenitors in CGE, where SHH-independent calreticulin (CR)-expressing GABAergic neurons are derived (Xu et al., 2010).

A remarkable feature in the development of neocortical interneurons is that they—unlike projection neurons—undergo tangential migration from their place of origin to their cortical destination. Several genetic studies in humans and mice have implicated dysfunctional development or migration of GABAergic interneurons with many psychiatric and neurodevelopmental disorders (Powell et al., 2003; Gant et al., 2009; Poitras et al., 2010). Together, these data emphasize the critical role of GABAergic neurons in proper function of the neocortex.

CURRENT PROGRESS IN CORTICAL NEURON DERIVATION FROM hPSCs

Impairment of proper development and migration of both excitatory projection neurons and inhibitory interneurons in the neocortex contributes to neurodevelopmental disorders. Therefore, the ability to generate those neurons from hPSCs is a powerful approach for assessing their molecular and cellular phenotypes and essential mechanisms underlying disease onset. Currently, most protocols for cortical differentiation from hPSCs are based on a few core methods that were developed using hESCs (**Table 1**). Understanding how these methods work and the basic characteristics of neural progenitors they generate is critical for developing novel protocols for differentiation of specific subtypes of cortical neurons. Thus, we first introduce several methods that are most frequently used to generate neural progenitors from hPSCs. After that, we discuss recent accomplishments in differentiation of cortical excitatory projection and inhibitory neurons from hPSCs (summarized in **Figure 1C**).

NEURAL DIFFERENTIATION FROM hPSCs

Zhang and colleagues published the first report on neural differentiation from human ESCs (Zhang et al., 2001). In their study, embryoid bodies (EBs) are generated by lifting hESC colonies and cultured in suspension devoid of mitogens for a short period of time. Next the EBs are grown in adherent culture in defined media containing N2 supplement and basic fibroblast growth factor (bFGF) and allowed to form "neural rosettes." This unique cellular arrangement of epithelial cells is reminiscent of cross sections of the developing neural tube and is now considered a hallmark of successful neural induction. These cells extensively express many neural stem cell markers such as Nestin, Musashi-1, and polysialylated-neuronal cell adhesion molecule, vigorously proliferating in the presence of bFGF after enzymatic isolation, and generate neurons, astrocytes, and oligodendrocytes both *in vitro* and *in vivo* (Zhang et al., 2001). In a subsequent study, Zhang's group found that neural progenitors generated in this manner mainly exhibit the anterior identity even though no regional cues were used throughout the differentiation (Pankratz et al., 2007). The regional identity of hESC-derived neural progenitors appears to be convertible by patterning cues. Timely treatment with particular morphogens such as SHH and Wnts, or their agonists/antagonists redirects the regional identity of hESC-derived neural progenitors to either ventral or caudal fate. The fate plasticity of hESC-derived neural progenitors has led to the development of many methods for generating different neuronal subtypes, such as midbrain dopaminergic neurons (Yan et al., 2005), spinal motor neurons (Li et al., 2005), as well as cortical neurons (Li et al., 2009).

Another EB-like structure-based neural differentiation method was published by Sasai's group. Their first study described a serum-free EB-like protocol (which they called SFEB) to generate neurons from mouse ESCs (mESCs). Quantitative analysis revealed that around 80% of total cells were Sox1-positive neural lineage in 5 days. Substantial numbers of cells derived

Table 1 | Comparison among common methods for neural differentiation of hPSCs.

	Culture method	Strategy for neural differentiation	Regional identity of neural progenitors	Advantage	References
EB formation-neural rosette isolation method	EB formation by lifting hPSC colonies and following adherent culture of EBs	Induction and isolation of neural rosettes without morphogens	Dorsal telen-diencephalon (PAX6+, OTX2+, FOXG1+)	Highly reproducible across many hPSC lines	Zhang et al., 2001; Pankratz et al., 2007
Dual-SMAD inhibition method	Adherent monolayer culture of dissociated hPSCs	Inhibition of BMP/ Nodal signals	Dorsal telen-diencephalon (PAX6+, OTX2+, FOXG1+)	Highly rapid and efficient	Chambers et al., 2009
SFEBq method	EB formation by re-aggregation of dissociated hPSCs	Inhibition of WNT/BMP/Nodal signals	Dorsal telencephalon (FOXG1+, EMX1+)	Suitable for cortical differentiation	Watanabe et al., 2005; Eiraku et al., 2008

by SFEB culture express forebrain markers such as *Foxg1* and *Otx2*, although this number was still low (~20% of total cells) compared to the number in hESC differentiation (Watanabe et al., 2005; Pankratz et al., 2007). A key step in this protocol was the dissociation of mESCs to single cells to form EB-like structures of a defined size, and cultured in serum-free media. However, this protocol was difficult to adapt to hESCs, which are remarkably vulnerable to apoptosis upon dissociation (Ohgushi et al., 2010). To circumvent this problem, Sasai's group employed Rho-dependent protein kinase (ROCK) inhibitor, which promotes the survival of dissociated hESCs. With it, they successfully reproduced the SFEB method with hESCs (Watanabe et al., 2007). As was observed with mESCs, human neural cells differentiated by SFEB culture were frequently positive for FOXG1 (~32% of total cells), and could be patterned toward either ventral or dorsal fate. More recently, the same research group further optimized this method in terms of speed, efficiency, and reproducibility of neural conversion by quick re-aggregation of ESCs in round-bottom well-plates (Eiraku et al., 2008). In this manner, over 95% of total cells exhibited features of neuroepithelial cells at day 5 of differentiation. Most interestingly, the majority expressed dorsal telencephalic markers. Since this method exhibited a striking resemblance with *in vivo* corticogenesis and mainly generated cortical excitatory neurons, we will return to it in the next section.

Another approach that has been used to induce neural progenitors from ESCs was co-culturing with mouse stromal feeder cells that are known to have neural inducing activity (Kawasaki et al., 2000; Elkabetz et al., 2008). Despite the method's robustness, the involvement of non-human cells and the requirement of relatively long period of time for neural induction (>3 weeks) made this method less attractive for biomedical applications.

Recently, Studer's group reported a remarkably simple and robust method for neural induction of hESCs (Chambers et al., 2009). In adherent single cell-culture of hESCs under serum-free conditions, simultaneous modulation of endogenous BMP and Activin/Nodal signaling by treatment with Noggin (BMP inhibitor) and SB431542 (Activin/Nodal inhibitor) converted hESCs to largely PAX6-positive neuroectodermal cells competent to form neural rosettes in 11 days of differentiation. Since each signaling pathway recruits SMAD proteins as intracellular signal transducers, this was often referred to as the dual-SMAD inhibition approach. Interestingly, most neural cells generated by this method express FOXG1 and OTX2, along with robust expression of PAX6, suggesting dorsal telencephalic identity (Chambers et al., 2009). The feasibility and robustness of this method has resulted in its relative popularity in the field, as it provides highly enriched neural precursors for disease modeling (Lee et al., 2009).

Given that hESC-derived neural progenitors from different research groups exhibit regional identity of the dorsal telencephalon, hPSCs are likely to have an innate program for differentiation into neural cells found in this brain region regardless of method (Pankratz et al., 2007; Elkabetz et al., 2008; Chambers et al., 2009). This seems consistent with the theory that the first neural precursors generated during vertebrate neural induction acquire dorsal telencephalic identity by default (Muñoz-Sanjuán and Brivanlou, 2002). However, current protocols for neural differentiation were developed and tested with only a few widely-used cell lines (e.g., H9). Moreover, a recent report argued that neural progenitors generated from different hESC lines differ in regional identity when derived by the same protocol, potentially due to differences in epigenetic programming (Wu et al., 2007). The assumption hPSC lines all follow a default pathway to a dorsal telencephalic identity may be a hasty generalization. Thus, we recommend determination of the regional identity of neural progenitors from new hPSC lines before further neuronal specification.

GENERATION OF EXCITATORY PROJECTION NEURONS FROM hPSCs

Sasai's group pioneered directed cortical differentiation from both mouse and human ESC by SFEB method and regional patterning. They optimized the previous SFEB method by allowing a defined number of cells to re-aggregate quickly in round-bottom 96-well plates under the influence of several regionalizing factors (referred to as the SFEBq method). This remarkably improved the differentiation efficiency of mESCs to dorsal telencephalic neural precursors, evidenced by expression of *Foxg1* (~65–75% of total cells) and *Emx1* (~89% of *Foxg1*-positive cells) (Eiraku et al., 2008). Interestingly, this system generated self-organized cellular aggregates of cortical progenitors and cortical neurons from mESC in the spatio-temporal manner reminiscent of *in vivo* corticogenesis. SFEBq-induced cortical progenitors even respond to cues directing regional pallial induction, such as FGF, which refines the pallial fate along the rostro-caudal axis, and BMP/Wnt, which induces expression of choroid flexus or cortical hem markers (Eiraku et al., 2008). However, well-organized laminar formation of cortical neurons did not appear within SFEBq-induced mouse cortical tissues, and hESCs failed to generate neurons of upper cortical layers in this system.

Upon further refinement, SFEBq approaches have been successfully applied to hPSCs. Vaccarino and colleagues reproduced this approach by generating hiPSC-derived multilayered cortical structures, which predominantly exhibited the gene expression profile of dorsal telencephalon (Mariani et al., 2012). More recently, Knoblich and colleagues developed an advanced *in vitro* differentiation method adapting the SFEBq system by culturing matrigel-embedded EBs in a spinning bioreactor (Lancaster et al., 2013). This system succeeded in establishing a cerebral organoid culture system, which reproduces many features of human cortical development in a more precise manner. In particular, they found characteristic progenitor zone organization, including abundant RGC and oRGC populations, with ventral telencephalic progenitors migrating into a cortical layer-like structure. Moreover, the ability to produce mature cortical neuron subtypes in an "inside-out laminar pattern" was unique in recapitulating *in vivo* corticogenesis not observed with the original SFEBq method. Most interestingly, cerebral organoids from hiPSCs with a CDK5RAP2 mutation, which causes microcephaly in humans, resulted in smaller neural tissues with impaired progenitor regions, which has never before been recapitulated in animal models (Lancaster et al., 2013). Most recently, Sasai's group optimized their SFEBq method by culturing cell aggregates in enriched medium and high oxygen (40%), thereby generating a three-dimensional neuronal mass with features resembling human fetal cortex in the early second trimester. Their new method surpassed the limitations of their previous method and achieved axial polarity, human specific oRGC populations, and "inside-out" laminar structure of cortical neurons (Kadoshima et al., 2013). By providing a robust methodology for efficient generation of cortical neurons from hPSCs, these three-dimensional differentiation approaches represent a powerful tool for investigation of human brain development and neurodevelopmental disorders. The potential to characterize electrophysiological properties, function, and connectivity of targeted neuronal populations organized in a multi-layered cortical pattern is of great utility for the study of ASD.

In contrast to the three-dimensional differentiation system, the adherent monolayer-differentiation system may provide a more feasible tool to examine morphology and synaptic connectivity, which are of interest as the main cellular phenotype of ASD neurons. It can also be scaled-up for drug screening platforms. Livesey and colleagues described a defined cortical differentiation condition by employing the monolayer culture and dual-SMAD inhibition (Shi et al., 2012). Interestingly, they found that RA was an essential factor for robust differentiation of cortical progenitors with PAX6 and OTX1/2-immunoreactivity. Cortical progenitors generated by their method displayed neural rosette structures with the apico-basal polarity and characteristic interkinetic nuclear migration during cell division. More importantly, this method recapitulated complex human progenitor populations including intermediate progenitors and oRGCs with unipolar basal processes, as seen in the developing human brain. In addition, birth-dating analysis using BrdU labeling revealed the appearance of both deep-layer and upper-layer cortical neurons in a temporal manner, paralleling *in vivo* corticogenesis over 90 days of neuronal maturation (Shi et al., 2012). With this protocol, the same group generated cortical neurons derived from Down syndrome (DS)-specific iPSCs. These neurons exhibited pathological features of early-onset Alzheimer's disease seen in DS patients, demonstrating the applicability of this protocol for modeling cortical disease (Shi et al., 2013). Although the role of RA as a modulator for cortical differentiation needs further mechanistic characterization, this study was the first to recapitulate the diversity of cortical progenitors and generation of cortical subtypes from hPSCs in a temporally-controlled manner.

There have also been attempts to obtain cortical projection neurons by inhibiting cellular signal(s) that drive alternative fates. Since the cerebral cortex develops in the dorsal telencephalic region of the embryonic brain, blockade of intrinsic ventralizing and/or caudalizing signals during neural induction of ESCs may lead to neural precursors with dorsal telencephalic fate. Vanderhaeghen's group was the first to test this hypothesis in mESCs (Gaspard et al., 2008). They found that a low density culture of mESCs in chemically defined media devoid of any regional cues generated Otx1/2-positive neural progenitors, many of which were co-labeled with Nkx2.1. Therefore, at least in the mESC system, the default differentiation condition may favorably generate ventralized telencephalic progenitors, possibly because of high endogenous Shh levels. As support for this hypothesis, the same group showed that the inhibition of intrinsic Shh signaling by treatment with cyclopamine, a small molecule inhibitor of Shh signal, abolished ventral marker expression in neural progenitors, whereas it largely elevated dorsal marker expression. Cortical progenitors differentiated in this manner could mainly differentiate into functional excitatory neurons with pyramidal shape that expressed a series of transcription factors corresponding to each cortical layer in a temporal manner reminiscent of *in vivo* corticogenesis (Gaspard et al., 2008).

Unlike those in the mESC system, neural progenitors derived from hESCs tend to retain dorsal telencephalic fate in many cases, as discussed above. The difference in dorso-ventral patterning between these systems may be explained by distinctive intracellular programming. While endogenous Shh signal dominates during early neural induction of mESCs (Gaspard et al., 2008), Zhang and colleagues found that Wnt signaling prevails during neural induction of hESCs. In addition, they showed that Wnt inhibition facilitated the ventralization of neural progenitors by exogenous SHH, supporting the idea that the endogenous Wnt signaling underlies the differentiation inclination of hPSC toward dorsal fate (Li et al., 2009). Consistent with this, a recent study from Vanderhaeghen's group showed that cyclopamine treatment was not required for induction of the dorsal telencephalic fate in the hPSC system (Espuny-Camacho et al., 2013). However, Schaffer and colleagues recently showed that SHH inhibition by cyclopamine was necessary to generate excitatory neurons expressing cortical markers from hPSCs (Vazin et al., 2013). Thus far, the involvement of SHH signaling in the induction of dorsal telencephalic fate of hPSC-derived neurons is controversial and needs further study.

Ghosh and colleagues suggested a procedure for efficient differentiation of forebrain-type neurons via aggregate formation in multi-well plates in the presence of Noggin (Kim et al., 2011a). After adherent culture of aggregates on matrigel for a few days, most colonies developed neural rosettes that highly expressed transcripts of several dorsal telencephalic markers, such as *SOX1*, *PAX6*, *SIX3*, and *EMX2*. Continuous treatment with Noggin seemed critical for maintaining rosette structure and inducing telencephalic fate, and SHH-inhibition by cyclopamine did not facilitate the acquisition of dorsal fate. Further differentiation by dissociating neural rosette cells and coculturing them with rat astrocytes generated functional excitatory neurons. This study also assessed synaptic dysfunction by employing an artificial synapse formation assay, in which hPSC-derived neurons were co-cultured with HEK293T cells that expressed either normal or mutant types of *NLGN-3* and *NLGN-4*. In this system, hPSC-derived neurons were able to form presynaptic specializations on the HEK293T cells that expressed wild-type NLGNs more efficiently than on those that expressed ASD-associated mutant NLGNs (Kim et al., 2011a). This study was a practical example of an efficient cortical differentiation method combined with an assay of synapse formation to assess the functional impact of ASD-associated mutations.

In recent years, several studies have provided multiple methods for generating cortical excitatory neurons from hPSCs that recapitulate *in vivo* corticogenesis and even human-specific features not seen in animal models. Although *in vitro* modeling ASD using cortical differentiation technology is still in its infancy, it is becoming clear that the current accomplishments already provide robust models for investigating cellular phenotypes that are directly relevant to ASD pathophysiology.

DIFFERENTIATION OF NEOCORTICAL INHIBITORY NEURONS FROM hPSCs

In recent years, many studies of autistic people and ASD animal models have strongly implicated dysfunction of the GABAergic system in the pathophysiology of ASD (reviewed by Chattopadhyaya and Cristo, 2012). Perturbation of subtle excitatory-inhibitory balance due to loss or dysfunction of GABAergic interneurons can lead to hyperexcitability and/or impaired cortical oscillations, thereby resulting in various psychiatric and neurodevelopmental disorders. Given that epilepsy is more prevalent in children with ASD (Viscidi et al., 2013) and epileptiform activity in the prefrontal cortex is associated with deficits in social interaction (Hernan et al., 2013), dysfunction of the GABAergic system may be an especially important mechanism of ASD pathophysiology. Therefore, the ability to efficiently generate human cortical interneurons from people with ASD could serve as a valuable tool for investigating GABAergic system dysfunction in ASD pathophysiology, as well as facilitating drug discovery. Here, we summarize recent results in obtaining GABAergic interneurons from hPSCs.

Zhang and colleagues obtained human neuroepithelial cells predominantly expressing PAX6 around 8–15 days of neural induction. This was achieved using the EB formation-neural rosette isolation method without exogenous morphogens, which exploits the default telencephalic specification of hESCs (Liu et al., 2013a). By exposing those cells to high doses of SHH (over 500 ng/ml) or purmorphamine (1.5 μM), a small molecule agonist of SHH signaling, they succeeded in generating MGE-like neural progenitors, mainly characterized by expression of NKX2.1, and abolished PAX6 and EMX1-positive dorsal telencephalon and MEIS1/2-positive lateral ganglionic eminence population. Neuronal maturation of NKX2.1-positve cells on hESC-derived astrocytes in the presence of nerve growth factor (NGF) gave rise to both functional choline acetyl-transferase-positive basal forebrain cholinergic neurons and GABAergic neurons in similar proportions, faithfully recapitulating *in vivo* differentiation from MGE precursors (Liu et al., 2013a). Interestingly, they also found that depletion of NGF, a simple modification, favored GABAergic differentiation with a purity of over 90% in the same conditions (Liu et al., 2013b).

Two different groups sought a direct way to pattern hPSC-derived neural precursors into cortical GABAergic interneurons. Specifically, they directed telencephalic fate prior to subsequent ventralization for differentiation, instead of depending on spontaneous telencephalic specification. Studer and colleagues described a robust pharmacological method that allows efficient modulation of signals implicated in neural patterning. In particular, they inhibited endogenous Wnt signaling to facilitate telencephalic differentiation (Maroof et al., 2013), inspired by previous findings that Wnt can suppress forebrain induction in several vertebrates (Yamaguchi, 2001; Nordström et al., 2002). Treatment with XAV939, a small molecule inhibitor of the canonical Wnt pathway, during neural induction through dual-SMAD inhibition significantly increased the proportion of neural progenitors expressing FOXG1. In subsequent dorso-ventral patterning, activation of SHH signaling by the treatment of purmorphamine in a specific temporal window (day 6–18) was efficient for robust co-induction of NKX2.1 with FOXG1. Interestingly, fine temporal tuning of SHH signal activation (day 10–18) even discriminated between different subtypes of ventral progenitors, those co-expressing OLIG2 with NKX2.1 and FOXG1, and telencephalic GABAergic neurons expressing SST or PV after further differentiation. Such robustness makes this method more attractive for future investigations of specific roles for interneuron subtypes in the pathophysiology of neuropsychiatric disorders (Maroof et al., 2013).

Kriegstein and colleagues took a similar approach to enrich for neural progenitors with a telencephalic ventral fate from hPSCs (Nicholas et al., 2013). In this study, they exposed *NKX2.1::GFP* knockin reporter hESCs to DKK1 and purmorphamine under the combination of the SFEBq method (Eiraku et al., 2008), and the EB formation-neural rosette isolation method (Zhang et al., 2001). As a result, about 90% of differentiated cells were positive for GFP, 81.5% of which co-expressed FOXG1 at particular temporal conditions of DKK1 (for initial 15 days) and purmorphamine treatment (for initial 35 days). Co-expression of OLIG2 and MASH1 at the neural progenitor stage, and doublecortin or GABA immunoreactivity after further differentiation supported their MGE-like identity. Further differentiation after cell sorting GFP-positive cells efficiently generated multiple subtypes of functional forebrain GABAergic neurons both *in vitro* and *in vivo* (Nicholas et al., 2013).

Recently, another approach was developed for generation of cortical interneurons from the CGE. In contrast to STT and PV-expressing GABAergic neurons, which mostly originate from the MGE, the developmental mechanism of calreticulin (CR)-type interneurons that arise mostly in the CGE was not well-known. Rodríguez and colleagues illustrated that activation of Activin signaling facilitated the induction of CGE identity during neural differentiation of mouse and human ESCs, and enriched for CR-expressing GABAergic neurons (Cambray et al., 2012). Given the implication of CR-expressing interneurons in cases of epilepsy (Tóth et al., 2010), this approach may also be used for investigating impairment of the inhibitory system in people with ASD.

Despite differences in the details of differentiation methods, the studies described above showed that strong SHH signaling promotes the ventralization of telencephalic progenitors and generates MGE-like neocortical GABAergic interneurons (Sousa and Fishell, 2010). More importantly, each approach presented not only efficient methodologies for generating neocortical GABAergic interneurons, but also provided new insights into developmental mechanisms of these cells, which not been observed in previous mouse studies. Thus, current advances in the development of neocortical interneurons from hPSCs are promising for elucidating the role of inhibitory interneurons in the etiology of ASD.

DERIVING NEURONS FROM hPSCs TO MODEL NEURODEVELOPMENTAL DISORDERS

Several research groups have recently used hPSCs to model neurodevelopmental disorders that include autistic features, such as Rett syndrome (RTT) (Marchetto et al., 2010; Ananiev et al., 2011; Cheung et al., 2011; Kim et al., 2011b; Li et al., 2013), Fragile X-syndrome (Urbach et al., 2010; Sheridan et al., 2011; Bar-Nur et al., 2012; Liu et al., 2012), Prader-Willi/Angelman syndrome (Chamberlain et al., 2010; Yang et al., 2010), Timothy syndrome (Paşca et al., 2011; Krey et al., 2013), and Phelan-McDermid syndrome (Shcheglovitov et al., 2013). Most of the studies obtained mature neurons by employing existing neural differentiation protocols and showed that neurons differentiated from affected individuals or from genetically modified hPSCs exhibited disease-related phenotypes (summarized in **Table 2**). Here, we discuss a few accomplishments in *in vitro* modeling for these disorder using iPSCs, and discuss the efforts to make effective and meaningful iPSC-based models of ASD.

RTT is a severe neurodevelopmental disorder caused primarily by mutations in the X-linked gene *MECP2* (Methyl CpG-binding protein 2) (Chahrour and Zoghbi, 2007). Muotri and colleagues provided the first example of *in vitro* modeling of RTT by establishing iPSCs from individuals with various mutations in *MECP2*. They found that neural precursors derived from RTT-iPSCs did not show a distinct impairment in differentiation, proliferation, or survival. In contrast, RTT-neurons had fewer synapses, smaller soma size, and showed deficits in both calcium signaling and spontaneous excitatory synaptic communication compared to unaffected control neurons. Furthermore, they showed that some disease-related phenotypes (e.g., synaptic density) could be partially reversed by insulin-like growth factor 1 (IGF1) or gentamycin treatment, providing proof-of-principle evidence for the application of RTT-patient derived neurons for drug discovery (Marchetto et al., 2010). Importantly, smaller soma and nuclei have been repeatedly observed in RTT-iPSC derived neurons established by other research groups, regardless of the mutation or differentiation methods (Marchetto et al., 2010; Cheung et al., 2011; Li et al., 2013), suggesting that this phenotype might be a possible biomarker for future biomedical applications.

More recently, Jaenisch and colleagues established hESC lines with *MECP2* mutations using TALEN-mediated gene editing. By comparing mutant neurons to isogenic neurons from the parental hESCs, they investigated key molecular and cellular features of RTT (Li et al., 2013). MAP2-positive neuronal cells differentiated by the dual SMAD-inhibition method were mainly comprised of VGluT1-positive excitatory neurons, and displayed many typical deficits of RTT neurons previously shown in mouse models and neurons from RTT-specific iPSCs, such as smaller soma and nuclei, reduced neurite complexity, and electrophysiological deficits. Beyond this, they also detected a global translational impairment due to reduced AKT/mTOR activity, mitochondrial defects, an absence in activity-dependent gene transcription in hESC-derived neurons that lacked MECP2, which had not been observed previously in *in vivo* and *in vitro* models (Li et al., 2013).

Individuals with mutation of the cyclin-dependent kinase-like 5 (*CDKL5*) gene present with clinical features similar to RTT (Tao et al., 2004; Weaving et al., 2004). However, the mechanism underlying RTT-like symptoms caused by *CDKL5* mutations is largely unknown. Broccoli and colleagues addressed the function of *Cdkl5* in mouse hippocampal neurons by short-hairpin RNA-mediated knock-down of *Cdkl5*. These experiments showed that this *Cdkl5* is essential for proper dendritic spine structure and for activity of excitatory synapses by stimulating the phosphorylation-dependent interaction between NGL-1 (netrin-G1 ligand) and PSD95 (Ricciardi et al., 2012). They validated their finding in human neurons by generating iPSC lines from two individuals with *CDKL5* mutations and differentiating them into cortical neurons. Indeed, human neurons with a defective *CDKL5* gene had reduced numbers of synapses and long dendritic protrusions, as seen in mouse hippocampal neurons with knock-down of *Cdkl5*. Although the proposed mechanism was not fully addressed in human neurons, evidence from iPSC-modeling supports that the functional defect due to loss of *CDKL5* in affected individual results in disease-related phenotypes similar to RTT.

Many individuals with TS, caused by mutations in the L-type calcium channel *CACNA1C* gene, display features of ASDs (Splawski et al., 2004). Recently, Dolmetsch and colleagues established iPSC lines from individuals with TS and explored potential abnormalities in neuronal development or function (Paşca et al., 2011). iPSC-derived neurons with TS mutations had altered electrophysiological properties and activity-dependent

Table 2 | A summary of neural differentiation methods and cellular phenotypes in current iPSC models for ASD-related syndromes.

Disorder (Genetic defects)	Differentiation method	Regional induction	Neuronal subtype	Neural phenotypes	Cellular phenotypes of mutant neurons	References
RTT (*MeCP2*)	NPCs: EB formation-neural rosette isolation method Neurons*: Culturing EBs (without RA for 1 week and with RA for following 3 weeks) and plating them after dissociation	N/A	Excitatory neuron	TUJ1, MAP2, VGLUT1,	Fewer synapses, Reduced spine density, Smaller soma size, Altered calcium signal, Electrophysiological defect Reduced synaptic density was restored by treatment of IGF1 or gentamycin	Marchetto et al., 2010
RTT (*MeCP2*)	EB formation-neural rosette isolation method	N/A	N/D	MAP2	Smaller soma size	Cheung et al., 2011
RTT (*MeCP2*)	EB formation-neural rosette isolation method	N/A	N/D	Nestin, TUJ1	Defect in neuronal maturation	Kim et al., 2011b
RTT (*MeCP2*)	EB formation-neural rosette isolation method	N/A	N/D	TUJ1	Smaller nuclear size	Ananiev et al., 2011
Atypical RTT (*CDKL5*)	EB formation-neural rosette isolation method	N/A	Cortical excitatory neurons	TUJ1, MAP2, VGLUT1, CTIP2	Reduced number of synaptic puncta Lengthy spine protrusion	Ricciardi et al., 2012
RTT (*MeCP2*[†])	Dual-SMAD inhibition in adherent culture	N/A	Excitatory neurons	MAP2, TUJ1, VGLUT1	Smaller soma/nuclear size Reduced dendritic complexity, Electrophysiological deficits Global reduction in transcription Impaired AKT/mTOR activity Mitochondria deficit	Li et al., 2013
TS (*CACNA1C*)	EB formation-neural rosette isolation method	N/A	Cortical neurons	46 neural/neuronal markers were assessed by Fluidigm array	Defects in calcium-channel function Altered activity-dependent gene-expression/dendritic retraction Abnormality of lower cortical layer and callosal projection differentiation Abnormal catecholaminergic differentiation	Paşca et al., 2011; Krey et al., 2013
FXS (*FMR1*)	Manual isolation of neural rosette cells or isolation of PSA-NCAM-positive cells by MACS from the spontaneously differentiating iPSCs	N/A	N/D	TUJ1, GFAP	Fewer and shorter processes	Sheridan et al., 2011

(Continued)

Table 2 | Continued

Disorder (Genetic defects)	Differentiation method	Regional induction	Neuronal subtype	Neural phenotypes	Cellular phenotypes of mutant neurons	References
FXTAS (*FMR1*)	EB formation-neural rosette isolation method accompanied by dual-SMAD inhibition	N/A	Excitatory neurons	MAP2, VGLUT1,	Shorter neurite length Fewer PSD95-positive synaptic puncta Sustained calcium response after glutamate application	Liu et al., 2012
AS (deletion in maternal chromosome 15q11-q13) PWS (deletion in paternal chromosome 15q11-q13)	EB formation-neural rosette isolation method	N/A	N/D	TUJ1	Phenotypic impairment was not specified	Chamberlain et al., 2010
PWS (translocation in maternal 15q11 and 4q27)	EB formation-neural rosette isolation method	N/A	N/D	MAP2, TUJ1	Phenotypic impairment was not specified	Yang et al., 2010
ASD (*NRXN1*)‡	EB formation-neural rosette isolation method	N/A	N/D	TUJ1, GFAP, and Global transcript-tome alteration was monitored by RNA-seq and Q-PCR	Reduced glial differentiation Altered gene expression related to cell adhesion and neuron differentiation	Zeng et al., 2013
PMDS (deletion in chromosome 22q13)	Dual-SMAD inhibition in adherent culture	Dorsal forebrain	Cortical neurons (both excitatory and inhibitory neurons)	MAP2, CaMKIIa, TBR1, CTIP2, SATB2, GAD67, and 66 sets of neural/neuronal marker expression were assessed by Fluidigm array	Impaired excitatory (both AMPA and NMDA-mediated) but not inhibitory synaptic transmission mainly due to loss of function of SHANK3 Reintroduction of SHANK3 and IGF1 application restore excitatory synaptic transmission	Shcheglovitov et al., 2013

**In this study, the authors used different methods to derive NPCs and neurons, respectively.*

†This study used genetically modified hESCs by deletion of exon 3 in the MECP2 locus by TALEN-mediated targeting.

Abbreviations: NPC, neural progenitor cells; EBs, embryoid bodies; N/A, not applicable; N/D, not defined; VGLUT1, vesicular glutamate transporter1; MAP2, microtubule-associated protein2; IGF1, insulin-like growth factor1, TUJ1, neuron-specific class III β-tubulin; mTOR, mammalian target of rapamycin; MACS, magnetic-activated cell sorting; GFAP, glial fibrillary acidic protein, CaMKIIa, calcium/calmodulin-dependent protein kinase IIa; GAD67, glutamic acid decarboxylase 67; TBR1; T-box brain 1; CTIP2, COUP-TF interacting protein2; SATB2, special AT-rich sequence-binding protein2; AMPA, α-amino-3-hydroxy-5-methyl-4-isoxazolepropionic acid; NMDA, N-methyl-D-aspartic acid.

‡Small-hairpin RNA was used for knocking-down NRXN1 in hiPSC-derived neural stem cells.

gene expression, mainly resulting from aberrant calcium signaling. Interestingly, comparison of single-cell gene expression array profiles revealed reduced numbers of deep layer neurons expressing SATB2 in TS neurons compared to control neurons. This finding was confirmed in the brains of transgenic mice carrying mutation associated with type-1 TS. Since SATB2 is a critical transcription factor for development of callosal projection neurons (Alcamo et al., 2008), this finding strongly supported the idea that autistic symptoms seen in TS patients result from defects in cortical connectivity through the corpus callosum. In addition, the authors observed an abnormal increase in tyrosine hydroxylase-expression, consistent with the idea that altered synthesis of catecholamine may underlie ASD pathophysiology (D'Souza et al., 2009). In a follow-up study, both rodent cortical neurons with TS mutations and human neurons derived from TS-iPSCs exhibited activity-dependent dendritic retraction, which was caused by erroneous regulation of RhoA signaling by the mutated calcium channel (Krey et al., 2013).

Fragile X syndrome (FXS) is the most commonly inherited mental impairment, and is caused by expansion of CGG-repeats in the 5′ untranslated region of the fragile X mental retardation 1 (*FMR1*) gene, which leads to silencing of FMR1 expression. While Benvenisty and colleagues were the first to report the establishment of iPSC lines from FXS patients (Urbach et al., 2010), the first phenotypes of neurons derived from FXS-iPSCs were reported by Haggarty and colleagues, who showed that FXS-iPSCs preferentially generated Tuj1-positive neurons with shorter and fewer processes and more compact astrocytes (Sheridan et al., 2011). More recently, Hagerman and colleagues established isogenic pairs of iPSC lines from individuals with the related disorder fragile X-associated tremor ataxia syndrome (FXTAS) (Liu et al., 2012). iPSC-derived FXTAS neurons exhibited altered synapse formation, possibly caused by aberrant calcium currents. Interestingly, the mutant neurons exhibited a sustained calcium elevation after glutamate application, implying that enhanced type-I metabotropic glutamate activity may result in the imbalance of excitatory-inhibitory neuronal transmission (Liu et al., 2012).

AS and PWS are neurogenetic disorders caused by disruption of genes in imprinted regions of chromosome 15q11-13 (Ramocki and Zoghbi, 2008). AS results from loss of the maternal copy of the gene UBE3A, while the imprinted paternal gene is silenced; conversely, PWS results from loss of paternal genes (including the HBII-85 small nucleolar RNA cluster) and imprinting of maternal allele. Individuals with AS or PWS frequently exhibit intellectual disability, autism, severe seizures, and unusual or problematic behavior (Cassidy et al., 2012; Dagli et al., 2012). Chamberlain and colleagues provided the first example of disease modeling of AS and PWS and found that AS- and PWS-iPSCs retained the appropriate DNA methylation patterns. During neuronal differentiation, AS-iPSCs specifically repressed the paternal copy of *UBE3A*, concomitant with upregulation of UBE3A antisense transcripts, which is only expressed in neurons (Chamberlain et al., 2010). Similarly, Esteban and colleagues observed that iPSCs derived from individuals with PWS mutations bear an intact imprinting signature on the maternal allele, as seen in fibroblasts from which they originated (Yang et al., 2010). Although functional differences between affected neurons and normal neurons were not clearly addressed, these studies proved that iPSC-disease modeling of neurodevelopmental disorders of genomic imprinting is applicable.

Studies of hPSCs have also examined the function of ASD candidate genes. Wang and colleagues recently addressed the functional role of NRXN-1, a presynaptic protein of which mutation is highly associated with ASD pathogenesis, during the neurodevelopment of hPSC by functional knockdown. This study showed that reduction of NRXN-1 expression in hPSC-derived neural stem cells alters expression of many genes for the cell adhesion pathway (20 genes) and neuronal differentiation pathway (13 genes) with impairment of astrocyte differentiation, suggesting its functional impact on human neurodevelopment (Zeng et al., 2013). Dolmetsch and colleagues recently reported *in vitro* modeling of a rare neurodevelopmental disorder, Phelan-McDermid syndrome (PMDS), by generating iPSC lines from individual with heterozygous deletion of chromosomal locus 22q13.3 (Shcheglovitov et al., 2013). This locus includes the *SHANK3* gene, which is also mutated in ASD (Durand et al., 2007; Phelan and McDermid, 2012). In this study, the authors illustrated that *SHANK3* mutation causes important physiological defects in PMDS neurons, such as an imbalance of excitatory and inhibitory transmission due to impaired excitatory synapses. Importantly, they also found that PMDS neuronal phenotypes could be reversed by SHANK3 overexpression or treatment with IGF1.

These early studies highlight the remarkable promise of using personalized stem cell-derived neurons to investigate mechanisms underlying ASD pathophysiology. Even without aiming to generate specific neuronal subtypes, these experiments demonstrated deficits in neuronal specification (Paşca et al., 2011), synapse formation (Marchetto et al., 2010; Shcheglovitov et al., 2013), and excitatory neurotransmission (Shcheglovitov et al., 2013) in distinct ASD-related syndromes. However, an important consideration for most studies is the maturation status of iPSC-derived neurons. Neuronal age typically varies from 2 weeks to 3 months, with considerable variation in differentiation protocols and culture conditions. Furthermore, few markers are used to assess neuronal regional specificity, expression of ion channels, and neurotransmitter receptors. While single-cell expression profiling (using a platform like Fluidigm) can provide a snapshot of these characteristics (Paşca et al., 2011), it is currently limited to a fraction of the transcriptome and is relatively costly. Transcriptome profiling can overcome this drawback at the expense of single-cell resolution. For example, Vaccarino and colleagues (Mariani et al., 2012) used genome-wide expression microarrays to compare hPSC-derived cortical neurons to the developing human brain; these experiments revealed remarkable similarity between these neurons and the human frontal cortex at 8–10 weeks post-conception. Comparative expression analyses between cortical neurons derived from ASD-iPSCs and control-iPSCs could generate hypotheses regarding differences in the maturity, the functionality (for example, by expression changes of neurotransmitter receptors), and even regional identity of differentiated cortical neurons.

To date, most iPSC-based studies of neurodevelopmental disorders have been restricted to recapitulating the cellular phenotypes that were previously observed in animal models and postmortem examinations. To inform iPSC-based disease modeling, studies should aim to complement and extend this knowledge. A recent transcriptome analysis of postmortem brain tissues between individuals with ASD and control individuals identified 444 differentially expressed genes, and revealed the alteration of two distinct gene-expression modules related to synaptic communication and immune induction (Voineagu et al., 2011). Given that these features were observed in the postmortem brain, comparative transcriptomic analyses between neurons derived from ASD-iPSCs and control-iPSCs could highlight difference in gene expression during the development and progression of disease. To complement transcriptome-wide studies, comparative analyses of protein-protein interactions (the protein interactome) between ASD and control neurons may reveal alterations in normal cellular mechanisms. Considering the heterogeneity in ASD presentation and the underlying genetic lesions, multifaceted approaches with customized neurons will greatly improve our understanding of molecular mechanisms of ASD. By identifying the mechanistic pathways involved in ASD pathophysiology, with time, the data may converge on a unified mechanistic model for ASD, facilitating development of therapeutic interventions (Casci, 2011).

FUTURE DIRECTIONS

Over the last decade great progress has been made in establishing methods for generation of cortical projection neurons or inhibitory interneurons from hPSCs, but many challenges remain. Methods for the generation of layer- or subregion-specific cortical neurons from hPSCs would be beneficial for studies of ASD pathophysiology. Impairment of specific cortico-striatal (CStr) connectivity has been implicated in ASD, and many ASD-associated genes are involved in CStr synapses (reviewed by Shepherd, 2013). A recent study also showed that differences in gene expression between the frontal and temporal cortices in the normal brain are significantly attenuated in the autistic brain, which implies altered cortical patterning (Voineagu et al., 2011). This finding supports the notion that layer- or subregion-specific neuronal subtypes would be tremendously valuable for *in vitro* modeling of ASD. Although a direct method for layer- or sub-regional specific cortical neurons from hPSCs has not been developed yet, accumulating evidence from studies on mESC differentiation and mouse development suggest possible approaches for achieving this goal (Eiraku et al., 2008).

Differentiation of functionally mature neurons from hPSCs is a long process with multiple steps requiring a few months. This may increase heterogeneity of the final neuronal population, even if the protocol was intended to enrich for a specific neuronal subtype. One way to overcome these difficulties is to convert patient-derived somatic cells directly into neurons, skipping cellular reprogramming and differentiation. A recently introduced method for direct conversion of fibroblasts to functional cortical neurons relies on forced expression of neural-lineage specific transcription factors (Vierbuchen et al., 2010; Pang et al., 2011). The low conversion efficiency (2–4% of cells) of the method is a major obstacle for disease modeling, although small molecule-based modulation reportedly improved differentiation efficiencies to ~80% (Ladewig et al., 2012). Regardless of differentiation efficiencies, the disease modeling potential for direct conversion from fibroblasts to terminally differentiated neurons is limited by the number of patient-derived somatic cells that are available. Südhof and colleagues recently developed a robust and simple method for conversion of hPSCs to functional cortical neurons with 100% efficiency in 3 weeks by expressing a single transcription factor (Zhang et al., 2013). This approach is not limited by available cell numbers, but it does require pre-existing patient-specific iPSC lines for disease modeling. Despite the method's robustness and feasibility, one should be cautious in utilizing direct conversion for disease modeling for ASD because it skips the normal developmental process, which may be critical for manifestation of ASD-associated phenotypes (Sandoe and Eggan, 2013). Furthermore, forced expression of key transcription factors may override pathological mechanisms underlying ASD (Brennand and Gage, 2012). Therefore, it is more desirable to use direct conversion approaches as a complement for screening disease phenotypes or to reinforce results obtained by neurons differentiated from hiPSCs.

Significant line-to-line variability has been observed in the neuronal differentiation of hPSCs (Wu et al., 2007; Hu et al., 2010; Kim et al., 2010) and efforts have been made to overcome this issue. One suggestion for bypassing such variation among iPSC lines is to pre-screen iPSC lines to select those with good responsiveness to lineage specification procedures (Bock et al., 2011; Boulting et al., 2011). However, reduced neural differentiation/specification may be a biologically relevant phenotype in studies of ASD, which would be unintentionally excluded by using this screening approach (Sandoe and Eggan, 2013). Melton et al. recently showed that priming human iPSCs with 1–2% demethylsulfoxide (DMSO) prompted exit from the cell cycle and improved differentiation efficiency of hiPSCs (Chetty et al., 2013). Given the recent evidence that the cell cycle is highly implicated in maintenance of pluripotency and fate decision, and elaborate modulation of cell cycle leads to lineage specification from hPSCs, this strategy may provide a solution for taming the variation in differentiation resulting from cell line-specific characteristics (Pauklin and Vallier, 2013). However, it is important to determine whether specific ASD-associated genetic variations influence cell cycle progression prior to applying these methods.

Finally, neuronal differentiation *in vitro* may not fully recapitulate neuronal development as it happens *in vivo*. Proliferation and differentiation of cortical progenitors occurs within specific niche environments characterized by signaling from the VZ, differentiated daughter cells, as well as signaling from non-neural sources, such as astrocytes, blood vessels, meninges (reviewed by Johansson et al., 2010), and microglia (Antony et al., 2011). The contribution of vascular endothelial cells to cortical development has been appreciated for a decade (Shen et al., 2004). Furthermore, increasing evidence suggests that microglial dysregulation may underlie several neuropsychiatric conditions including ASD (reviewed by Frick et al., 2013). Therefore, the absence of non-neuronal components during *in vitro* differentiation culture may obscure disease-relevant phenotypes using neurons generated from hPSCs. In line with this idea, it would be quite informative to determine whether co-culturing healthy cortical neurons with endothelial cells or microglia derived from individuals with ASD impairs neuronal function. Astrocytes are often supplied during the maturation of hPSC-derived neurons, as they promote synaptogenesis (Johnson et al., 2007). However, astrocytes contribute to the pathophysiology of neurodevelopmental disorders. Indeed, hiPSC-derived RTT astrocytes adversely affect the function of control neurons (Williams et al., 2014). The availability of protocols for generating hiPSC-derived astrocytes will allow co-culture experiments to examine the role of astrocytes in neuronal dysfunction associated with ASD. Finally, investigation of niche effects may help determine optimal *in vitro* conditions for cortical differentiation, and provide clues for therapeutic approaches.

CONCLUSION

With rapid progress in our ability to precisely manipulate hiPSCs, the tremendous knowledge gap between ASD genetics and our understanding of its pathophysiology is beginning to close. Using iPSC technology, it is possible to generate limitless supplies of human ASD-specific cortical neurons, which can revolutionize experimental analyses of ASD. Already, studies of the neurodevelopmental disorders RTT, TS, AS, and PMDS have shown that neuronal phenotypes can be identified using iPSC-derived neurons, and that these phenotypes can be corrected. Given the genetic heterogeneity of idiopathic ASD and the diversity in its clinical presentation, robust and highly reproducible methods for hiPSC manipulation is essential for linking genotype to phenotype. With the advent of facile mammalian genome engineering methods (reviewed in Hsu and Zhang, 2012; Mali et al., 2013) allowing for generation of gene-corrected cells from patient hiPSCs, precise neuronal differentiation methods will greatly facilitate the determination of causal mechanisms underlying ASD pathophysiology. However, there is still a great need for optimized and standardized cortical differentiation protocols that are efficient, swift, scalable, and produce desired neuronal subpopulations. Upon identification of ASD-associated neuronal phenotypes, iPSC-derived cortical neurons may be used for screens of chemical libraries, which will greatly facilitate drug discovery. With continued progress in neuronal differentiation from hiPSCs, the stage is set for understanding how ASD develops and how it may be treated.

ACKNOWLEDGMENTS

The authors thank Wesley Lai and Ugljesa Djuric for comments on the manuscript. This work was supported by grants from the Canadian Institutes of Health Research (EPS-129129), the Ontario Brain Institute, Canadian Institute for Military and Veteran Health Research (W7714-125624/001/SV), and the National Institutes of Health (R33MH087908). Dae-Sung Kim was supported by Basic Science Research Program through the National Research Foundation of Korea (NRF) funded by the Ministry of Education, Science and Technology (#2012039296). P. Joel Ross was supported by postdoctoral fellowships from the Ontario Stem Cell Initiative and Kirill Zaslavsky was funded by the Canada Vanier Graduate Scholarship.

REFERENCES

Alcamo, E. A., Chirivella, L., Dautzenberg, M., Dobreva, G., Fariñas, I., Grosschedl, R., et al. (2008). Satb2 regulates callosal projection neuron identity in the developing cerebral cortex. *Neuron* 57, 364–377. doi: 10.1016/j.neuron.2007.12.012

American Psychiatric Association. (2013). *Diagnostic and Statistical Manual of Mental Disorders, 5th Edn.* Arlington, VA: American Psychiatric Publishing.

Ananiev, G., Williams, E. C., Li, H., and Chang, Q. (2011). Isogenic pairs of wild type and mutant induced pluripotent stem cell (iPSC) lines from Rett syndrome patients as *in vitro* disease model. *PLoS ONE* 6:e25255. doi: 10.1371/journal.pone.0025255

Antony, J. M., Paquin, A., Nutt, S. L., Kaplan, D. R., and Miller, F. D. (2011). Endogenous microglia regulate development of embryonic cortical precursor cells. *J. Neurosci. Res.* 89, 286–298. doi: 10.1002/jnr.22533

Bar-Nur, O., Caspi, I., and Benvenisty, N. (2012). Molecular analysis of FMR1 reactivation in fragile-X induced pluripotent stem cells and their neuronal derivatives. *J. Mol. Cell Biol.* 4, 180–183. doi: 10.1093/jmcb/mjs007

Blumberg, S. J., Bramlett, M. D., Kogan, M. D., Schieve, L. A., Jones, J. R., and Lu, M. C. (2013). Changes in prevalence of parent-reported autism spectrum disorder in school-aged U.S. children: 2007 to 2011–2012. *Natl. Health Stat. Rep.* 65, 1–11.

Blundell, J., Blaiss, C. A., Etherton, M. R., Espinosa, F., Tabuchi, K., Walz, C., et al. (2010). Neuroligin-1 deletion results in impaired spatial memory and increased repetitive behavior. *J. Neurosci.* 30, 2115–2129. doi: 10.1523/JNEUROSCI.4517-09.2010

Bock, C., Kiskinis, E., Verstappen, G., Gu, H., Boulting, G., Smith, Z. D., et al. (2011). Reference Maps of human ES and iPS cell variation enable high-throughput characterization of pluripotent cell lines. *Cell* 14, 439–452. doi: 10.1016/j.cell.2010.12.032

Boulting, G. L., Kiskinis, E., Croft, G. F., Amoroso, M. W., Oakley, D. H., Wainger, B. J., et al. (2011). A functionally characterized test set of human induced pluripotent stem cells. *Nat. Biotechnol.* 29, 279–286. doi: 10.1038/nbt.1783

Brennand, K. J., and Gage, F. H. (2012). Modeling psychiatric disorders through reprogramming. *Dis. Model. Mech.* 5, 26–32. doi: 10.1242/dmm.008268

Cambray, S., Arber, C., Little, G., Dougalis, A. G., de Paola, V., Ungless, M. A., et al. (2012). Activin induces cortical interneuron identity and differentiation in embryonic stem cell-derived telencephalic neural precursors. *Nat. Commun.* 3, 841. doi: 10.1038/ncomms1817

Casci, T. (2011). Disease genetics: converging models for autism. *Nat. Rev. Genet.* 12, 456–457. doi: 10.1038/nrg3022

Cassidy, S. B., Schwartz, S., Miller, J. L., and Driscoll, D. J. (2012). Prader-Willi syndrome. *Genet. Med.* 14, 10–26. doi: 10.1038/gim.0b013e31822bead0

Chahrour, M., and Zoghbi, H. Y. (2007). The story of Rett syndrome: from clinic to neurobiology. *Neuron* 56, 422–437. doi: 10.1016/j.neuron.2007.10.001

Chamberlain, S. J., Chen, P. F., Ng, K. Y., Bourgois-Rocha, F., Lemtiri-Chlieh, F., Levine, E. S., et al. (2010). Induced pluripotent stem cell models of the genomic imprinting disorders angelman and prader-willi syndromes. *Proc. Natl. Acad. Sci. U.S.A.* 107, 17668–17673. doi: 10.1073/pnas.1004487107

Chambers, S. M., Fasano, C. A., Papapetrou, E. P., Tomishima, M., Sadelain, M., and Studer, L. (2009). Highly efficient neural conversion of human ES and iPS cells by dual inhibition of SMAD signaling. *Nat. Biotechnol.* 27, 275–280. doi: 10.1038/nbt.1529

Chattopadhyaya, B., and Cristo, G. D. (2012). GABAergic circuit dysfunctions in neurodevelopmental disorders. *Front. Psychiatry* 3:51. doi: 10.3389/fpsyt.2012.00051

Chen, B., Wang, S. S., Hattox, A. M., Rayburn, H., Nelson, S. B., and McConnell, S. K. (2008). The Fezf2-Ctip2 genetic pathway regulates the fate choice of subcortical projection neurons in the developing cerebral cortex. *Proc. Natl. Acad. Sci. U.S.A.* 105, 11382–11387. doi: 10.1073/pnas.0804918105

Chetty, S., Pagliuca, F. W., Honore, C., Kweudjeu, A., Rezania, A., and Melton, D. A. (2013). A simple tool to improve pluripotent stem cell differentiation. *Nat. Methods* 10, 553–556. doi: 10.1038/nmeth.2442

Cheung, A. Y., Horvath, L. M., Grafodatskaya, D., Pasceri, P., Weksberg, R., Hotta, A., et al. (2011). Isolation of MECP2-null Rett Syndrome patient hiPS cells and isogenic controls through X-chromosome inactivation. *Hum. Mol. Genet.* 20, 2103–2015. doi: 10.1093/hmg/ddr093

Chilian, B., Abdollahpour, H., Bierhals, T., Haltrich, I., Fekete, G., Nagel, I., et al. (2013). Dysfunction of SHANK2and CHRNA7in a patient with intellectual disability and language impairment supports genetic epistasis of the two loci. *Clin. Genet.* 84, 560–565. doi: 10.1111/cge.12105

Cubelos, B., Sebastián-Serrano, A., Beccari, L., Calcagnotto, M. E., Cisneros, E., Kim, S., et al. (2010). Cux1 and Cux2 regulate dendritic branching, spine morphology, and synapses of the upper layer neurons of the cortex. *Neuron* 66, 523–535. doi: 10.1016/j.neuron.2010.04.038

Dagli, A., Buiting, K., and Williams, C. A. (2012). Molecular and clinical aspects of angelman syndrome. *Mol. Syndromol.* 2, 100–112. doi:10.1159/000328837

DeRosa, B. A., Van Baaren, J. M., Dubey, G. K., Lee, J. M., Cuccaro, M. L., Vance, J. M., et al. (2012). Derivation of autism spectrum disorder-specific induced pluripotent stem cells from peripheral blood mononuclear cells. *Neurosci. Lett.* 516, 9–14. doi: 10.1016/j.neulet.2012.02.086

Devlin, B., and Scherer, S. W. (2012). Genetic architecture in autism spectrum disorder. *Curr. Opin. Genet. Dev.* 22, 229–237. doi: 10.1016/j.gde.2012.03.002

Douglas, R. J., and Martin, K. A. (2004). Neuronal circuits of the neocortex. *Annu. Rev. Neurosci.* 27, 419–451 doi: 10.1146/annurev.neuro.27.070203.144152

D'Souza, A., Onem, E., Patel, P., La Gamma, E. F., and Nankova, B. B. (2009). Valproic acid regulates catecholaminergic pathways by concentration-dependent threshold effects on TH mRNA synthesis and degradation. *Brain Res.* 1247, 1–10. doi: 10.1016/j.brainres.2008.09.088

Durand, C. M., Betancur, C., Boeckers, T. M., Bockmann, J., Chaste, P., Fauchereau, F., et al. (2007). Mutations in the gene encoding the synaptic scaffolding protein SHANK3 are associated with autism spectrum disorders. *Nat. Genet.* 39, 25–27. doi: 10.1038/ng1933

Eiraku, M., Watanabe, K., Matsuo-Takasaki, M., Kawada, M., Yonemura, S., Matsumura, M., et al. (2008). Self-organized formation of polarized cortical tissues from ESCs and its active manipulation by extrinsic signals. *Cell Stem Cell* 3, 519–532. doi: 10.1016/j.stem.2008.09.002

Elkabetz, Y., Panagiotakos, G., Al Shamy, G., Socci, N. D., Tabar, V., and Studer, L. (2008). Human ES cell-derived neural rosettes reveal a functionally distinct early neural stem cell stage. *Genes Dev.* 22, 152–165. doi: 10.1101/gad.1616208

Espuny-Camacho, I., Michelsen, K. A., Gall, D., Linaro, D., Hasche, A., Bonnefont, J., et al. (2013). Pyramidal neurons derived from human pluripotent stem cells integrate efficiently into mouse brain circuits *in vivo*. *Neuron* 77, 440–456. doi: 10.1016/j.neuron.2012.12.011

Estivill-Torrus, G., Pearson, H., van Heyningen, V., Price, D. J., and Rashbass, P. (2002). Pax6 is required to regulate the cell cycle and the rate of progression from symmetrical to asymmetrical division in mammalian cortical progenitors. *Development* 129, 455–466.

Etherton, M., Foldy, C., Sharma, M., Tabuchi, K., Liu, X., Shamloo, M., et al. (2011). Autism-linked neuroligin-3 R451C mutation differentially alters hippocampal and cortical synaptic function. *Proc. Natl. Acad. Sci. U.S.A.* 108, 13764–13769. doi: 10.1073/pnas.1111093108

Etherton, M. R., Blaiss, C. A., Powell, C. M., and Südhof, T. C. (2009). Mouse neurexin-1alpha deletion causes correlated electrophysiological and behavioral changes consistent with cognitive impairments. *Proc. Natl. Acad. Sci. U.S.A.* 106, 17998–18003. doi: 10.1073/pnas.0910297106

Ey, E., Leblond, C. S., and Bourgeron, T. (2011). Behavioral profiles of mouse models for autism spectrum disorders. *Autism Res.* 4, 5–16. doi: 10.1002/aur.175

Frick, L. R., Williams, K., and Pittenger, C. (2013). Microglial dysregulation in psychiatric disease. *Clin. Dev. Immunol.* 2013:608654. doi: 10.1155/2013/608654

Gant, J. C., Thibault, O., Blalock, E. M., Yang, J., Bachstetter, A., Kotick, J., et al. (2009). Decreased number of interneurons and increased seizures in neuropilin 2 deficient mice: implications for autism and epilepsy. *Epilepsia* 50, 629–645. doi: 10.1111/j.1528-1167.2008.01725.x

Gaspard, N., Bouschet, T., Hourez, R., Dimidschstein, J., Naeije, G., van den Ameele, J., et al. (2008). An intrinsic mechanism of corticogenesis from embryonic stem cells. *Nature* 455, 351–357. doi: 10.1038/nature07287

Glinka, A., Wu, W., Delius, H., Monaghan, A. P., Blumenstock, C., and Niehrs, C. (1998). Dickkopf-1 is a member of a new family of secreted proteins and functions in head induction. *Nature* 391, 357–362. doi: 10.1038/34848

Götz, M., and Huttner, W. B. (2005). The cell biology of neurogenesis. *Nat. Rev. Mol. Cell Biol.* 6, 777–788. doi: 10.1038/nrm1739

Gulacsi, A., and Anderson, S. A. (2006). Shh maintains Nkx2.1 in the MGE by a Gli3-independent mechanism. *Cereb. Cortex* 16, i89–i95. doi: 10.1093/cercor/bhk018

Han, W., Kwan, K. Y., Shim, S., Lam, M. M., Shin, Y., Xu, X., et al. (2011). TBR1 directly represses Fezf2 to control the laminar origin and development of the corticospinal tract. *Proc. Natl. Acad. Sci. U.S.A.* 108, 3041–3046. doi: 10.1073/pnas.1016723108

Hansen, D. V., Lui, J. H., Parker, P. R., and Kriegstein, A. R. (2010). Neurogenic radial glia in the outer subventricular zone of human neocortex. *Nature* 464, 554–561. doi: 10.1038/nature08845

Hébert, J. M., and Fishell, G. (2008). The genetics of early telencephalon patterning: some assembly required. *Nat. Rev. Neurosci.* 9, 678–685. doi: 10.1038/nrn2463

Hernan, A. E., Alexander, A., Jenks, K. R., Barry, J., Lenck-Santini, P. P., Isaeva, E., et al. (2013). Focal epileptiform activity in the prefrontal cortex is associated with long-term attention and sociability deficits. *Neurobiol. Dis.* 63, 25–34. doi: 10.1016/j.nbd.2013.11.012

Hsu, P. D., and Zhang, F. (2012). Dissecting neural function using targeted genome engineering technologies. *ACS Chem. Neurosci.* 3, 603–610. doi: 10.1021/cn300089k

Hu, B. Y., Weick, J. P., Yu, J., Ma, L. X., Zhang, X. Q., Thomson, J. A., et al. (2010). Neural differentiation of human induced pluripotent stem cells follows developmental principles but with variable potency. *Proc. Natl. Acad. Sci. U.S.A.* 107, 4335–4340. doi: 10.1073/pnas.0910012107

Huguet, G., Ey, E., and Bourgeron, T. (2013). The genetic landscapes of autism spectrum disorders. *Annu. Rev. Genomics Hum. Genet.* 14, 191–213. doi: 10.1146/annurev-genom-091212-153431

Jiang, Y. H., and Ehlers, M. D. (2013). Modeling autism by SHANK gene mutations in mice. *Neuron.* 78, 8–27. doi: 10.1016/j.neuron.2013.03.016

Johansson, P. A., Cappello, S., and Götz, M. (2010). Stem cells niches during development-lessons from the cerebral cortex. *Curr. Opin. Neurobiol.* 20, 400–407. doi: 10.1016/j.conb.2010.04.003

Johnson, M. A., Weick, J. P., Pearce, R. A., and Zhang, S. C. (2007). Functional neural development from human embryonic stem cells: accelerated synaptic activity via astrocyte coculture. *J. Neurosci.* 27, 3069–3077. doi: 10.1523/JNEUROSCI.4562-06.2007

Kadoshima, T., Sakaguchi, H., Nakano, T., Soen, M., Ando, S., Eiraku, M., et al. (2013). Self-organization of axial polarity, inside-out layer pattern, and species-specific progenitor dynamics in human ES cell-derived neocortex. *Proc. Natl. Acad. Sci. U.S.A.* 110, 20284–20289. doi: 10.1073/pnas.1315710110

Kawasaki, H., Mizuseki, K., Nishikawa, S., Kaneko, S., Kuwana, Y., Nakanishi, S., et al. (2000). Induction of midbrain dopaminergic neurons from ES cells by stromal cell-derived inducing activity. *Neuron* 28, 31–40. doi: 10.1016/S0896-6273(00)00083-0

Kim, D. S., Lee, J. S., Leem, J. W., Huh, Y. J., Kim, J. Y., Kim, H. S., et al. (2010). Robust enhancement of neural differentiation from human ES and iPS cells regardless of their innate difference in differentiation propensity. *Stem Cell Rev.* 6, 270–281. doi: 10.1007/s12015-010-9138-1

Kim, J. E., O'Sullivan, M. L., Sanchez, C. A., Hwang, M., Israel, M. A., Brennand, K., et al. (2011a). Investigating synapse formation and function using human pluripotent stem cell-derived neurons. *Proc. Natl. Acad. Sci. U.S.A.* 108, 3005–3010. doi: 10.1073/pnas.1007753108

Kim, K. Y., Hysolli, E., and Park, I. H. (2011b). Neuronal maturation defect in induced pluripotent stem cells from patients with Rett syndrome. *Proc. Natl. Acad. Sci. U.S.A.* 108, 14169–14174. doi: 10.1073/pnas.1018979108

Krey, J. F., Paşca, S. P., Shcheglovitov, A., Yazawa, M., Schwemberger, R., Rasmusson, R., et al. (2013). Timothy syndrome is associated with activity-dependent dendritic retraction in rodent and human neurons. *Nat. Neurosci.* 16, 201–209. doi: 10.1038/nn.3307

Kriegstein, A., and Alvarez-Buylla, A. (2009). The glial nature of embryonic and adult neural stem cells. *Annu. Rev. Neurosci.* 32, 149–184. doi: 10.1146/annurev.neuro.051508.135600

Kwan, K. Y. (2013). Transcriptional dysregulation of neocortical circuit assembly in ASD. *Int. Rev. Neurobiol.* 113, 167–205. doi: 10.1016/B978-0-12-418700-9.00006-X

Kwan, K. Y., Sestan, N., and Anton, E. S. (2012). Transcriptional co-regulation of neuronal migration and laminar identity in the neocortex. *Development* 139, 1535–1546. doi: 10.1242/dev.069963

Kwon, H. B., Kozorovitskiy, Y., Oh, W. J., Peixoto, R. T., Akhtar, N., Saulnier, J. L., et al. (2012). Neuroligin-1-dependent competition regulates cortical synaptogenesis and synapse number. *Nat. Neurosci.* 15, 1667–1674. doi: 10.1038/nn.3256

Ladewig, J., Mertens, J., Kesavan, J., Doerr, J., Poppe, D., Glaue, F., et al. (2012). Small molecules enable highly efficient neuronal conversion of human fibroblasts. *Nat. Methods* 9, 575–578. doi: 10.1038/ncomms3183

Lancaster, M. A., Renner, M., Martin, C. A., Wenzel, D., Bicknell, L. S., Hurles, M. E., et al. (2013). Cerebral organoids model human brain development and microcephaly. *Nature.* 501, 373–379. doi: 10.1038/nature12517

Leblond, C. S., Heinrich, J., Delorme, R., Proepper, C., Betancur, C., Huguet, G., et al. (2012). Genetic and functional analyses of SHANK2 mutations suggest a multiple hit model of autism spectrum disorders. *PLoS Genet.* 8:e1002521. doi: 10.1371/journal.pgen.1002521

Lee, G., Papapetrou, E. P., Kim, H., Chambers, S. M., Tomishima, M. J., Fasano, C. A., et al. (2009). Modelling pathogenesis and treatment of familial dysautonomia using patient-specific iPSCs. *Nature* 461, 402–406. doi: 10.1038/nature08320

Li, X. J., Du, Z. W., Zarnowska, E. D., Pankratz, M., Hansen, L. O., Pearce, R. A., et al. (2005). Specification of motoneurons from human embryonic stem cells. *Nat. Biotechnol.* 23, 215–221. doi: 10.1038/nbt1063

Li, X. J., Zhang, X., Johnson, M. A., Wang, Z. B., Lavaute, T., and Zhang, S. C. (2009). Coordination of sonic hedgehog and Wnt signaling determines ventral and dorsal telencephalic neuron types from human embryonic stem cells. *Development* 136, 4055–4063. doi: 10.1242/dev.036624

Li, Y., Wang, H., Muffat, J., Cheng, A. W., Orlando, D. A., Lovén, J., et al. (2013). Global transcriptional and translational repression in human-embryonic-stem-cell-derived Rett syndrome neurons. *Cell Stem Cell* 13, 446–458. doi: 10.1016/j.stem.2013.09.001

Liu, J., Koscielska, K. A., Cao, Z., Hulsizer, S., Grace, N., Mitchell, G., et al. (2012). Signaling defects in iPSC-derived fragile X premutation neurons. *Hum. Mol. Genet.* 21, 3795–3805. doi: 10.1093/hmg/dds207

Liu, Y., Liu, H., Sauvey, C., Yao, L., Zarnowska, E. D., and Zhang, S. C. (2013a). Directed differentiation of forebrain GABA interneurons from human pluripotent stem cells. *Nat. Protoc.* 8, 1670–1679. doi: 10.1038/nprot.2013.106

Liu, Y., Weick, J. P., Liu, H., Krencik, R., Zhang, X., Ma, L., et al. (2013b). Medial ganglionic eminence-like cells derived from human embryonic stem cells correct learning and memory deficits. *Nat. Biotechnol.* 31, 440–447. doi: 10.1038/nbt.2565

Lui, J. H., Hansen, D. V., and Kriegstein, A. R. (2011). Development and evolution of the human neocortex. *Cell* 146, 18–36. doi: 10.1016/j.cell.2011.06.030

Mali, P., Esvelt, K. M., and Church, G. M. (2013). Cas9 as a versatile tool for engineering biology. *Nat. Methods* 10, 957–963 doi: 10.1038/nmeth.2649

Marchetto, M. C., Carromeu, C., Acab, A., Yu, D., Yeo, G. W., Mu, Y., et al. (2010). A model for neural development and treatment of Rett syndrome using human induced pluripotent stem cells. *Cell* 143, 527–539. doi: 10.1016/j.cell.2010.10.016

Mariani, J., Simonini, M. V., Palejev, D., Tomasini, L., Coppola, G., Szekely, A. M., et al. (2012). Modeling human cortical development *in vitro* using induced pluripotent stem cells. *Proc. Natl. Acad. Sci. U.S.A.* 109, 12770–12775. doi: 10.1073/pnas.1202944109

Maroof, A. M., Keros, S., Tyson, J. A., Ying, S. W., Ganat, Y. M., Merkle, F. T., et al. (2013). Directed differentiation and functional maturation of cortical interneurons from human embryonic stem cells. *Cell Stem Cell* 12, 559–572. doi: 10.1016/j.stem.2013.04.008

Migliore, M., and Shepherd, G. M. (2005). Opinion: an integrated approach to classifying neuronal phenotypes. *Nat. Rev. Neurosci.* 6, 810–818. doi: 10.1038/nrn1769

Molyneaux, B. J., Arlotta, P., Menezes, J. R., and Macklis, J. D. (2007). Neuronal subtype specification in the cerebral cortex. *Nat. Rev. Neurosci.* 8, 427–437. doi: 10.1038/nrn2151

Muñoz-Sanjuán, I., and Brivanlou, A. H. (2002). Neural induction, the default model and embryonic stem cells. *Nat. Rev. Neurosci.* 3, 271–280. doi: 10.1038/nrn786

Muzio, L., and Mallamaci, A. (2005). Foxg1 confines Cajal-Retzius neuronogenesis and hippocampal morphogenesis to the dorsomedial pallium. *J. Neurosci.* 25, 4435–4441. doi: 10.1523/JNEUROSCI.4804-04.2005

Nicholas, C. R., Chen, J., Tang, Y., Southwell, D. G., Chalmers, N., Vogt, D., et al. (2013). Functional maturation of hPSC-derived forebrain interneurons requires an extended timeline and mimics human neural development. *Cell Stem Cell* 12, 573–586. doi: 10.1016/j.stem.2013.04.005

Nordström, U., Jessell, T. M., and Edlund, T. (2002). Progressive induction of caudal neural character by graded Wnt signaling. *Nat. Neurosci.* 5, 525–532. doi: 10.1038/nn854

Ohgushi, M., Matsumura, M., Eiraku, M., Murakami, K., Aramaki, T., Nishiyama, A., et al. (2010). Molecular pathway and cell state responsible for dissociation-induced apoptosis in human pluripotent stem cells. *Cell Stem Cell* 7, 225–239. doi: 10.1016/j.stem.2010.06.018

Pang, Z. P., Yang, N., Vierbuchen, T., Ostermeier, A., Fuentes, D. R., Yang, T. Q., et al. (2011). Induction of human neuronal cells by defined transcription factors. *Nature* 476, 220–223. doi: 10.1038/nature10202

Pankratz, M. T., Li, X. J., Lavaute, T. M., Lyons, E. A., Chen, X., and Zhang, S. C. (2007). Directed neural differentiation of human embryonic stem cells via an obligated primitive anterior stage. *Stem Cells* 25, 1511–1520. doi: 10.1634/stemcells.2006-0707

Paşca, S. P., Portmann, T., Voineagu, I., Yazawa, M., Shcheglovitov, A., Paşca, A. M., et al. (2011). Using iPSC-derived neurons to uncover cellular phenotypes associated with Timothy syndrome. *Nat. Med.* 17, 1657–1662. doi: 10.1038/nm.2576

Pauklin, S., and Vallier, L. (2013). The cell-cycle state of stem cells determines cell fate propensity. *Cell* 155, 135–147. doi: 10.1016/j.cell.2013.08.031

Petilla Interneuron Nomenclature Group. (2008). Petilla terminology: nomenclature of features of GABAergic interneurons of the cerebral cortex. *Nat. Rev. Neurosci.* 9, 557–568. doi: 10.1038/nrn2402

Phelan, K., and McDermid, H. E. (2012). The 22q13.3 Deletion Syndrome (Phelan-McDermid Syndrome). *Mol. Syndromol.* 2, 186–201. doi: 10.1159/000334260

Poitras, L., Yu, M., Lesage-Pelletier, C., Macdonald, R. B., Gagné, J. P., Hatch, G., et al. (2010). An SNP in an ultraconserved regulatory element affects Dlx5/Dlx6 regulation in the forebrain. *Development* 137, 3089–3097. doi: 10.1242/dev.051052

Powell, E. M., Campbell, D. B., Stanwood, G. D., Davis, C., Noebels, J. L., and Levitt, P. (2003). Genetic disruption of cortical interneuron development causes region- and GABA cell type-specific deficits, epilepsy, and behavioral dysfunction. *J. Neurosci.* 23, 622–631.

Ramocki, M. B., and Zoghbi, H. Y. (2008). Failure of neuronal homeostasis results in common neuropsychiatric phenotypes. *Nature* 455, 912–918. doi: 10.1038/nature07457

Rash, B. G., and Grove, E. A. (2006). Area and layer patterning in the developing cerebral cortex. *Curr. Opin. Neurobiol.* 16, 25–34. doi: 10.1016/j.conb.2006.01.004

Ricciardi, S., Ungaro, F., Hambrock, M., Rademacher, N., Stefanelli, G., Brambilla, D., et al. (2012). CDKL5 ensures excitatory synapse stability by reinforcing NGL-1-PSD95 interaction in the postsynaptic compartment and is impaired in patient iPSC-derived neurons. *Nat. Cell Biol.* 14, 911–923. doi: 10.1038/ncb2566

Ross, P. J., and Ellis, J. (2010). Modeling complex neuropsychiatric disease with induced pluripotent stem cells. *F1000 Biol. Rep.* 2:84. doi: 10.3410/B2-84

Sandoe, J., and Eggan, K. (2013). Opportunities and challenges of pluripotent stem cell neurodegenerative disease models. *Nat. Neurosci.* 16, 780–789. doi: 10.1038/nn.3425

Shcheglovitov, A., Shcheglovitova, O., Yazawa, M., Portmann, T., Shu, R., Sebastiano, V., et al. (2013). SHANK3 and IGF1 restore synaptic deficits in neurons from 22q13 deletion syndrome patients. *Nature* 503, 267–271. doi: 10.1038/nature12618

Shen, Q., Goderie, S. K., Jin, L., Karanth, N., Sun, Y., Abramova, N., et al. (2004). Endothelial cells stimulate self-renewal and expand neurogenesis of neural stem cells. *Science* 304, 1338–1340. doi: 10.1126/science.1095505

Shepherd, G. M. (2013). Corticostriatal connectivity and its role in disease. *Nat. Rev. Neurosci.* 14, 278–291. doi: 10.1038/nrn3469

Sheridan, S. D., Theriault, K. M., Reis, S. A., Zhou, F., Madison, J. M., Daheron, L., et al. (2011). Epigenetic characterization of the FMR1 gene and aberrant neurodevelopment in human inducedpluripotent stem cell models of fragile X syndrome. *PLoS ONE* 6:e26203. doi: 10.1371/journal.pone.0026203

Shi, Y., Kirwan, P., Smith, J., MacLean, G., Orkin, S. H., and Livesey, F. J. (2013). A human stem cell model of early Alzheimer's disease pathology in down syndrome. *Sci. Transl. Med.* 4:124ra29. doi: 10.1126/scitranslmed.3003771

Shi, Y., Kirwan, P., Smith, J., Robinson, H. P., and Livesey, F. J. (2012). Human cerebral cortex development from pluripotent stem cells to functional excitatory synapses. *Nat. Neurosci.* 15, 477–486. doi: 10.1038/nn.3041

Silverman, J. L., Yang, M., Lord, C., and Crawley, J. N. (2010). Behavioural phenotyping assays for mouse models of autism. *Nat. Rev. Neurosci.* 11, 490–502. doi: 10.1038/nrn2851

Sousa, V. H., and Fishell, G. (2010). Sonic hedgehog functions through dynamic changes in temporal competence in the developing forebrain. *Curr. Opin. Genet. Dev.* 20, 391–399. doi: 10.1016/j.gde.2010.04.008

Splawski, I., Timothy, K. W., Sharpe, L. M., Decher, N., Kumar, P., Bloise, R., et al. (2004). Ca(V) 1.2 calcium channel dysfunction causes a multisystem disorder including arrhythmia and autism. *Cell* 119, 19–31. doi: 10.1016/j.cell.2004.09.011

Spruston, N. (2008). Pyramidal neurons: dendritic structure and synaptic integration. *Nat. Rev. Neurosci.* 9, 206–221. doi: 10.1038/nrn2286

Stern, C. D. (2001). Initial patterning of the central nervous system: how many organizers? *Nat. Rev. Neurosci.* 2, 92–98. doi: 10.1038/35053563

Stoykova, A., Treichel, D., Hallonet, M., and Gruss, P. (2000). Pax6 modulates the dorsoventral patterning of the mammalian telencephalon. *J. Neurosci.* 20, 8042–8050.

Sussel, L., Marin, O., Kimura, S., and Rubenstein, J. L. (1999). Loss of Nkx2.1 homeobox gene function results in a ventral to dorsal molecular respecification within the basal telencephalon: evidence for a transformation of the pallidum into the striatum. *Development* 126, 3359–3370.

Tabuchi, K., Blundell, J., Etherton, M. R., Hammer, R. E., Liu, X., Powell, C. M., et al. (2007). A neuroligin-3 mutation implicated in autism increases inhibitory synaptic transmission in mice. *Science* 318, 71–76. doi: 10.1126/science.1146221

Takahashi, K., Tanabe, K., Ohnuki, M., Narita, M., Ichisaka, T., Tomoda, K., et al. (2007). Induction of pluripotent stem cells from adult human fibroblasts by defined factors. *Cell* 131, 861–872. doi: 10.1016/j.cell.2007.11.019

Tao, J., Van Esch, H., Hagedorn-Greiwe, M., Hoffmann, K., Moser, B., Raynaud, M., et al. (2004). Mutations in the X-linked cyclin-dependent kinase-like 5 (CDKL5/STK9) gene are associated with severe neurodevelopmental retardation. *Am. J. Hum. Genet.* 75, 1149–1154. doi: 10.1086/426460

Tóth, K., Eross, L., Vajda, J., Halász, P., Freund, T. F., and Maglóczky, Z. (2010). Loss and reorganization of calretinin-containing interneurons in the epileptic human hippocampus. *Brain* 133, 2763–2777. doi: 10.1093/brain/awq149

Urbach, A., Bar-Nur, O., Daley, G. Q., and Benvenisty, N. (2010). Differential modeling of fragile X syndrome by human embryonic stem cells and inducedpluripotent stem cells. *Cell Stem Cell* 6, 407–411. doi: 10.1016/j.stem.2010.04.005

Vazin, T., Ball, K. A., Lu, H., Park, H., Ataeijannati, Y., Head-Gordon, T., et al. (2013). Efficient derivation of cortical glutamatergic neurons from human pluripotent stem cells: a model system to study neurotoxicity in Alzheimer's disease. *Neurobiol. Dis.* 62C, 62–72. doi: 10.1016/j.nbd.2013.09.005

Vierbuchen, T., Ostermeier, A., Pang, Z. P., Kokubu, Y., Südhof, T. C., and Wernig, M. (2010). Direct conversion of fibroblasts to functional neurons by defined factors. *Nature.* 463, 1035–1041. doi: 10.1038/nature08797

Viscidi, E. W., Johnson, A. L., Spence, S. J., Buka, S. L., Morrow, E. M., and Triche, E. W. (2013). The association between epilepsy and autism symptoms and maladaptive behaviors in children with autism spectrum disorder. *Autism* doi: 10.1177/1362361313508027. [Epub ahead of print].

Voineagu, I., Wang, X., Johnston, P., Lowe, J. K., Tian, Y., Horvath, S., et al. (2011). Transcriptomic analysis of autistic brain reveals convergent molecular pathology. *Nature* 474, 380–384. doi: 10.1038/nature10110

Watanabe, K., Kamiya, D., Nishiyama, A., Katayama, T., Nozaki, S., Kawasaki, H., et al. (2005). Directed differentiation of telencephalic precursors from embryonic stem cells. *Nat. Neurosci.* 8, 288–296. doi: 10.1038/nn1402

Watanabe, K., Ueno, M., Kamiya, D., Nishiyama, A., Matsumura, M., Wataya, T., et al. (2007). A ROCK inhibitor permits survival of dissociated human embryonic stem cells. *Nat. Biotechnol.* 25, 681–686. doi: 10.1038/nbt1310

Weaving, L. S., Christodoulou, J., Williamson, S. L., Friend, K. L., McKenzie, O. L., Archer, H., et al. (2004). Mutations of CDKL5 cause a severe neurodevelopmental disorder with infantile spasms and mental retardation. *Am. J. Hum. Genet.* 75, 1079–1093. doi: 10.1086/426462

Williams, E. C., Zhong, X., Mohamed, A., Li, R., Liu, Y., Dong, Q., et al. (2014). Mutant astrocytes differentiated from Rett syndrome patients-specific iPSCs have adverse effects on wild-type neurons. *Hum. Mol. Genet.* doi: 10.1093/hmg/ddu008. [Epub ahead of print].

Wilson, S. W., and Houart, C. (2004). Early steps in the development of the forebrain. *Dev. Cell* 6, 167–181. doi: 10.1016/S1534-5807(04)00027-9

Wilson, S. W., and Rubenstein, J. L. (2000). Induction and dorsoventral patterning of the telencephalon. *Neuron* 28, 641–651. doi: 10.1016/S0896-6273(00)00171-9

Won, H., Lee, H. R., Gee, H. Y., Mah, W., Kim, J. I., Lee, J., et al. (2012). Autistic-like social behaviour in Shank2-mutant mice improved by restoring NMDA receptor function. *Nature* 486, 261–265. doi: 10.1038/nature11208

Wonders, C. P., and Anderson, S. A. (2006). The origin and specification of cortical interneurons. *Nat. Rev. Neurosci.* 7, 687–696. doi: 10.1038/nrn1954

Wu, H., Xu, J., Pang, Z. P., Ge, W., Kim, K. J., Blanchi, B., et al. (2007). Integrative genomic and functional analyses reveal neuronal subtype differentiation bias in human embryonic stem cell lines. *Proc. Natl. Acad. Sci. U.S.A.* 104, 13821–13826. doi: 10.1073/pnas.0706199104

Xu, Q., Guo, L., Moore, H., Waclaw, R. R., Campbell, K., and Anderson, S. A. (2010). Sonic hedgehog signaling confers ventral telencephalic progenitors with distinct cortical interneuron fates. *Neuron* 65, 328–340. doi: 10.1016/j.neuron.2010.01.004

Xuan, S., Baptista, C. A., Balas, G., Tao, W., Soares, V. C., and Lai, E. (1995). Winged helix transcription factor BF-1 is essential for the development of the cerebral hemispheres. *Neuron* 14, 1141–1152. doi: 10.1016/0896-6273(95)90262-7

Yamaguchi, T. P. (2001). Heads or tails: Wnts and anterior-posterior patterning. *Curr. Biol.* 11, R713–R724. doi: 10.1016/S0960-9822(01)00417-1

Yan, Y., Yang, D., Zarnowska, E. D., Du, Z., Werbel, B., Valliere, C., et al. (2005). Directed differentiation of dopaminergic neuronal subtypes from human embryonic stem cells. *Stem Cells* 23, 781–790. doi: 10.1634/stemcells.2004-0365

Yang, J., Cai, J., Zhang, Y., Wang, X., Li, W., Xu, J., et al. (2010). Induced pluripotent stem cells can be used to model the genomic imprinting disorder Prader-Willi syndrome. *J. Biol. Chem.* 285, 40303–40311. doi: 10.1074/jbc.M110.183392

Zeng, L., Zhang, P., Shi, L., Yamamoto, V., Lu, W., and Wang, K. (2013). Functional impacts of NRXN1 knockdown on neurodevelopment in stem cell models. *PLoS ONE* 8:e59685. doi: 10.1371/journal.pone.0059685

Zhang, S. C., Wernig, M., Duncan, I. D., Brüstle, O., and Thomson, J. A. (2001). *In vitro* differentiation of transplantable neural precursors from human embryonic stem cells. *Nat. Biotechnol.* 19, 1129–1133. doi: 10.1038/nbt1201-1129

Zhang, Y., Pak, C., Han, Y., Ahlenius, H., Zhang, Z., Chanda, S., et al. (2013). Rapid single-step induction of functional neurons from human pluripotent stem cells. *Neuron* 78, 785–798. doi: 10.1016/j.neuron.2013.05.029

Zikopoulos, B., and Barbas, H. (2013). Altered neural connectivity in excitatory and inhibitory cortical circuits in autism. *Front. Hum. Neurosci.* 7:609. doi: 10.3389/fnhum.2013.00609

Zoghbi, H. Y., and Bear, M. F. (2012). Synaptic dysfunction in neurodevelopmental disorders associated with autism and intellectual disabilities. *Cold Spring Harb. Perspect. Biol.* 4:a009886. doi: 10.1101/cshperspect.a009886

Permissions

All chapters in this book were first published by Frontiers; hereby published with permission under the Creative Commons Attribution License or equivalent. Every chapter published in this book has been scrutinized by our experts. Their significance has been extensively debated. The topics covered herein carry significant findings which will fuel the growth of the discipline. They may even be implemented as practical applications or may be referred to as a beginning point for another development.

The contributors of this book come from diverse backgrounds, making this book a truly international effort. This book will bring forth new frontiers with its revolutionizing research information and detailed analysis of the nascent developments around the world.

We would like to thank all the contributing authors for lending their expertise to make the book truly unique. They have played a crucial role in the development of this book. Without their invaluable contributions this book wouldn't have been possible. They have made vital efforts to compile up to date information on the varied aspects of this subject to make this book a valuable addition to the collection of many professionals and students.

This book was conceptualized with the vision of imparting up-to-date information and advanced data in this field. To ensure the same, a matchless editorial board was set up. Every individual on the board went through rigorous rounds of assessment to prove their worth. After which they invested a large part of their time researching and compiling the most relevant data for our readers.

The editorial board has been involved in producing this book since its inception. They have spent rigorous hours researching and exploring the diverse topics which have resulted in the successful publishing of this book. They have passed on their knowledge of decades through this book. To expedite this challenging task, the publisher supported the team at every step. A small team of assistant editors was also appointed to further simplify the editing procedure and attain best results for the readers.

Apart from the editorial board, the designing team has also invested a significant amount of their time in understanding the subject and creating the most relevant covers. They scrutinized every image to scout for the most suitable representation of the subject and create an appropriate cover for the book.

The publishing team has been an ardent support to the editorial, designing and production team. Their endless efforts to recruit the best for this project, has resulted in the accomplishment of this book. They are a veteran in the field of academics and their pool of knowledge is as vast as their experience in printing. Their expertise and guidance has proved useful at every step. Their uncompromising quality standards have made this book an exceptional effort. Their encouragement from time to time has been an inspiration for everyone.

The publisher and the editorial board hope that this book will prove to be a valuable piece of knowledge for researchers, students, practitioners and scholars across the globe.

List of Contributors

Grace E. Kim and Leonard K. Kaczmarek
Departments of Pharmacology and Cellular & Molecular Physiology, Yale University School of Medicine, New Haven, CT, USA

Caleb A. Doll
Department of Biological Sciences, Vanderbilt University, Nashville, TN, USA

Kendal Broadie
Department of Biological Sciences, Vanderbilt University, Nashville, TN, USA
Kennedy Center for Research on Human Development, Vanderbilt University, Nashville, TN, USA

Oliwia A. Janc and Michael Müller
Center for Nanoscale Microscopy and Molecular Physiology of the Brain, Georg-August-Universität Göttingen, Göttingen, Germany
Zentrum für Physiologie und Pathophysiologie, Institut für Neuro-und Sinnesphysiologie, Universitätsmedizin, Georg-August-Universität Göttingen, Göttingen, Germany

Elisa Bellini and Maria M. Valente
Division of Neuroscience, San Raffaele Rett Research Center, San Raffaele Scientific Institute, Milan, Italy

Giulio Pavesi
Department of Biosciences, University of Milan, Milan, Italy

Nicoletta Landsberger
Division of Neuroscience, San Raffaele Rett Research Center, San Raffaele Scientific Institute, Milan, Italy
Section of Biomedical Research, Laboratory of Genetic and Epigenetic Control of Gene Expression, Department of Theoretic and Applied Sciences, University of Insubria, Busto Arsizio, Italy

Isabella Barbiero, Anna Bergo, Chetan Chandola, Mohammad S. Nawaz, Laura Rusconi, Gilda Stefanelli, Marta Strollo and Charlotte Kilstrup-Nielsen
Section of Biomedical Research, Laboratory of Genetic and Epigenetic Control of Gene Expression, Department of Theoretic and Applied Sciences, University of Insubria, Busto Arsizio, Italy

Russell G. Port, Steven J. Siegel and Gregory C. Carlson
Department of Psychiatry, Perelman School of Medicine, University of Pennsylvania, Philadelphia, PA, USA

Michael J. Gandal
Semel Institute for Neuroscience and Human Behavior, University of California at Los Angeles, Los Angeles, CA, USA

Timothy P. L. Roberts
Bioengineering Graduate Group, University of Pennsylvania, Philadelphia, PA, USA

Sabiha Abekhoukh and Barbara Bardoni
CNRS, Institute of Molecular and Cellular Pharmacology, UMR 7275, Valbonne, France
University of Nice Sophia-Antipolis, Nice, France
CNRS, International Associated Laboratories–NEOGENEX, Valbonne, France

M. Mar Gámez-Del-Estal, Israel Contreras, Rocío Prieto-Pérez and Manuel Ruiz-Rubio
Departamento de Genética, Universidad de Córdoba, Hospital Universitario Reina Sofía, Instituto Maimónides de Investigación Biomédica de Córdoba, Córdoba, Spain

Jianling Chen, Shunying Yu and Yingmei Fu
Shanghai Key Laboratory of Psychotic Disorders, Shanghai Mental Health Center, Shanghai Jiao Tong University School of Medicine, Shanghai, China

Xiaohong Li
Department of Neurochemistry, New York State Institute for Basic Research in Developmental Disabilities, Staten Island, NY, USA

Sarah E. Rotschafer and Khaleel A. Razak
Graduate Neuroscience Program, Department of Psychology, University of California, Riverside, CA, USA

Christian A. Cea-Del Rio
Department of Pharmaceutical Sciences, Skaggs School of Pharmacy and Pharmaceutical Sciences, University of Colorado, Anschutz Medical Campus, Aurora, CO, USA

Molly M. Huntsman
Department of Pharmaceutical Sciences, Skaggs School of Pharmacy and Pharmaceutical Sciences, University of Colorado, Anschutz Medical Campus, Aurora, CO, USA
Department of Pediatrics, School of Medicine, University of Colorado, Anschutz Medical Campus, Aurora, CO, USA

Henry G. S. Martin and Olivier J. Manzoni
INSERM U901 Pathophysiology of Synaptic Plasticity Group, Marseille, France
Institut de Neurobiologie de la Méditerranée (INMED),Marseille, France
Université de Aix-Marseille, Marseille, France

Lucia Ciranna
Department of Biomedical Sciences, University of Catania, Catania, Italy

Maria Vincenza Catania
Institute of Neurological Sciences, the National Research Council of Italy (CNR) Catania, Italy
Laboratory of Neurobiology, IRCCS Oasi Maria SS, Troina, Italy

Swati Banerjee, Maeveen Riordan and Manzoor A. Bhat
Department of Physiology, Center for Biomedical Neuroscience, School of Medicine, University of Texas Health Science Center, San Antonio, TX, USA

Hansen Wang
Faculty of Medicine, University of Toronto, 1 King's College Circle, Toronto, ON, Canada

Sandipan Pati
Department of Neurology, Epilepsy Division, The University of Alabama at Birmingham, Birmingham, AL, USA

Lucas Pozzo-Miller
Department of Neurobiology, Civitan International Research Center, The University of Alabama at Birmingham, Birmingham, AL, USA

Laurie C. Doering
Faculty of Health Sciences, Department of Pathology and Molecular Medicine, McMaster University, Hamilton, ON, Canada

Xin Xu and Lucas Pozzo-Miller
Department of Neurobiology, Civitan International Research Center, The University of Alabama at Birmingham, Birmingham, AL, USA

Alan P. Kozikowski
Drug Discovery Program, Department of Medicinal Chemistry and Pharmacognosy, University of Illinois at Chicago, Chicago, IL, USA

Dae-Sung Kim and P. Joel Ross
Program in Developmental and Stem Cell Biology, The Hospital for Sick Children, Toronto, ON, Canada

Kirill Zaslavsky and James Ellis
Program in Developmental and Stem Cell Biology, The Hospital for Sick Children, Toronto, ON, Canada
Department of Molecular Genetics, University of Toronto, Toronto, ON, Canad

Index

www.ingramcontent.com/pod-product-compliance
Lightning Source LLC
LaVergne TN
LVHW060558210926
848485LV00005B/1335